MEDICAL CARE CHARTBOOK

Seventh Edition

Avedis Donabedian, M.D.
Solomon J. Axelrod, M.D.
Leon Wyszewianski, Ph.D.

Department of Medical Care Organization
School of Public Health
The University of Michigan

AUPHA Press
1980

Copyright © 1980 by the Regents of the
University of Michigan. All rights reserved.
Printed in the United States of America.

This book or parts thereof may not be reproduced in any form
without written permission of the publisher.

Library of Congress Card No.: 80-69098
ISBN 0-914904-61-2
ISBN 0-914904-62-0 pbk.

AUPHA Press is an imprint of Health Administration Press.

Health Administration Press
School of Public Health
University of Michigan
Ann Arbor, Michigan 48109

313-764-1380

AUPHA Press
One DuPont Circle
Washington, D.C. 20036

202-659-4354

Preface

This Seventh Edition of the *Chartbook* marks an important turning point in its history, one which will assure its continued success. This and subsequent editions will be published by the Health Administration Press.

From its first edition in 1962, the *Chartbook* has been published by the Department of Medical Care Organization. With Drs. Axelrod and Donabedian as its originators and senior editors throughout that period, the *Chartbook* represents a Departmental commitment to contribute to improved teaching and increased information in the field of health services organization. The Department will continue that commitment. A sign of that continuation is the appearance, for the first time, of the name of Leon Wyszewianski, the Department's newest Assistant Professor, along with those of Professor Donabedian and Professor Emeritus Axelrod.

Under its excellent editorship and with the contribution of the technical excellence of the Health Administration Press, we are pleased to present this *Chartbook* in a new and improved format.

S.E. Berki, Chairman
Department of Medical Care Organization

Ann Arbor, Michigan
July, 1980

Introduction

Almost two decades ago the immediate predecessor of this *Chartbook* appeared as a thin sheaf of dittoed charts that were passed out to students for use as a visual aid during our lectures, and as material for more thorough study out of class. Since then, it has grown in size and readership, being used by many people for a variety of purposes. But, we have always seen it primarily as a device for learning and teaching. Accordingly, we have chosen each chart because it carries part of a message that we believe to be important to our field, and we have arranged the charts in sequences which allow a coherent story to unfold. Admittedly, we do not always find the most appropriate material to illustrate the points that we wish to make; there are gaps in our plot, and our story line sometimes falters. But, in general, the *Chartbook* has a meaning that any teacher of health services administration can easily see, and which every student can be encouraged to discover.

The *Chartbook* has a number of additional objectives which, fortunately, can be served jointly, often with an appreciable amount of mutual reinforcement. The most obvious and important of these is its usefulness as a handy compendium of facts and figures that are valuable to the student, the scholar, the administrator and the planner. In the pursuit of this objective we have tried very hard to update all our charts using the latest information we could find. To do so we have sometimes used unpublished material; but we have generally avoided seeking such sources (except to clarify already published information) partly because of the immense labor involved, and partly because we believe that the reader ought to be able to verify, and expand upon, the information in the charts by going to a reasonably accessible source.

No doubt, we have not always succeeded in tracing the most recent published information pertaining to each chart. But often, when we may seem to have failed, the reason is that the information is no longer available in the form we need, or that it appears only at intervals, perhaps every three or four years, and our publication date is out of step with that cycle. In such cases, the sources of the charts, which we have taken great care to specify, can be a handy key to information that may become available subsequently. It may also be that a newer edition of the Chartbook, which we hope to put out every four years, will, by then, have become available!

Recency of information is, of course, only one objective among several. At times, old material has been kept because we consider it to be of historical importance in the development of our field, because it provides a background against which more recent data can be better understood, or because it carries a message that we want to convey at least as well as anything more recent that we know of. By retaining such material, the *Chartbook* gains in scope and usefulness as an introduction to the literature of our field, while it pays homage to its notable pioneers. At the other end of the time scale, we have made an effort in the selection of charts to also represent important current trends in research, though our ability to do so comprehensively or fairly is limited both by the nature of the *Chartbook* and its size.

A brief note on the organization of the Chartbook will make it easier to use for any purpose. Its most notable feature is its division into nine sections. The first, on Population Characteristics, attempts, rather sketchily, to characterize the general context for the organization and delivery of health services in the U.S. The following two sections, on Mortality and Morbidity and on Use of Service, correspond roughly to need and demand for health services. These sections deal with the magnitude of the two sets of phenomena, the ways in which they are measured, the factors that influence them, and the degree to which need and demand correspond. In this way we introduce an evaluative perspective that dominates the *Chartbook* in all its parts.

The fourth section, on Costs and Expenditures, may be seen as a bridge between the first two sections and those that follow. Costs and expenditures are, of course, the consequences of action taken to satisfy the need for care. The monetary resources which costs and expenditures represent can also take their place with the topics for the next two sections, Health Personnel, and Facilities, as the instrumentalities required to meet that need. Similarly, the last two sections of the *Chartbook*, one on Tax-Supported Programs and the other on Medical Care Insurance, can be seen to be concerned with a higher order of the organization of these instrumentalities, as society is called upon to finance and deliver personal health care.

In all these sections, the emphasis is on providing information that has important evaluative connotations. But in one section, that on the Quality of Care, the subject matter is evaluation itself, though the focus is rather narrowly on the assessment of clinical practice. The material that is more important to program evaluation, inclusively defined, is distributed throughout the *Chartbook*.

Of course, there is no one right way either to group the charts into sections or to sequence them within any section. Many charts could fit almost as well in one place as in another. For that reason, we have taken pains to provide a rather extensive index which allows the reader to find the charts that fit any particular subject. An alternative, or additional, means of searching for the needed information would be to go through the Table of Contents, where every chart is listed and briefly described.

All the features that we have described so far have characterized the *Chartbook* for some time, so that they are familiar to many of our readers. With this edition, we make some changes. Although the charts have been designed to be as self-explanatory as possible, we have added an Appendix which defines the geographic terms used in many of the charts. In addition, a glossary of terms which involve rather fine distinctions that may not always be apparent introduces two of the sections: the one on Costs and Expenditures, and the one on Medical Care Insurance.

The most obvious change, of course, is that the Chartbook now has a new, smaller format, even though we have considerably increased the number of charts included. Moreover, all the charts have been redrawn, with attention to legibility, uniformity and appearance. These changes are the result of our new association with the Health Administration Press, which will publish and distribute this and future editions. Editorial responsibility for the content of the *Chartbook* will remain, as before, with the senior editors and with the Department of Medical Care Organization.

And now it is time to thank all those who have helped us in this work. Because the *Chartbook* has grown by accretion it is important not to forget those who have contributed to its previous editions. We list their names, as well as those of the research staff for this edition, following this preface. We have always had the support of a competent and dedicated research staff, and in this respect the current edition was particularly well served. We have also called upon, and received, many kinds of help from other friends and colleagues in the Department and elsewhere. We are indebted to Jean Thorby for making available to us her outstanding skills in the construction of the index. Richard Lichtenstein, as an experienced teacher of courses on health services administration, has reviewed in detail a large number of the charts in this edition to see how they would hold up in the classroom. Several other colleagues have given us help on charts in their particular areas of expertise. Among these, John R.C. Wheeler has been particularly helpful as our consultant on health economics.

We believe that our ability to prepare any of the editions of the *Chartbook* has depended most critically on the availability of our School's Reference Collection of materials on health services organization. Jack Tobias and Lillian Fagin have served as our constant guides to that collection, giving us a great deal of their valuable time. We have also called on Barbara Black, the Department's Administrative Associate, for much additional work in connection with the financing and staffing of the production of this edition, and of previous ones.

Our work on the *Chartbook*, whether now or in the past, has depended heavily on formal endorsement and support by the School of Public Health, in general, and by the Department of Medical Care Organization, in particular. Therefore, we are happy to acknowledge our indebtedness to Richard Remington, Dean of the School, and to S.E. Berki, the Department's current Chairman, and to Rashid Bashshur, its immediate past Chairman.

Many friends and colleagues outside the University have also been very helpful to us. We want to thank, in particular, the many friends in many governmental and other agencies who were willing to take on the additional work of responding to our repeated requests for information and verification. The contributions of some of them are acknowledged in the sources to the charts. There are many more who remain anonymous, but whose kindness we deeply appreciate.

The expansion and updating of the section on the Quality of Care reflects the support that one of the editors, Avedis Donabedian, has received to review the literature on quality assessment, first from the National Center for Health Services Research, and more recently from the Commonwealth Fund. More particularly, the new charts included in that section have been selected from a larger set that will be used in an *Annotated Chartbook on Quality Assessment and Monitoring* that is being sponsored by the Carnegie Corporation of New York.

Finally, the extent of our indebtedness to the Director and staff of the Health Administration Press will be clear to those of our readers who can compare this edition with its predecessors. But only we can testify to the spirit of cooperation and dedication of all those with whom we worked at the Press. In particular, we are indebted to Susan Sweeney, who supervised the critical process that transformed our rough sketches into the finished illustrations of the *Chartbook*.

In collaboration with the Health Administration Press we have tried to make this edition as accurate, as useful, and as pleasant to use as we could. Nevertheless, we expect that there are errors that we have not detected, as well as improvements that we have failed to make. We encourage our readers to call these things to our attention, and, in general, to let us know how we may serve them better in the future. They can write to any of us at the Department of Medical Care Organization, School of Public Health, The University of Michigan, Ann Arbor, MI 48109.

And while we wait to hear from them, we thank all our former readers for their continued support, and welcome all new ones to our circle of friends. We hope that the *Chartbook* will be as profitable to them to use, as it has been rewarding to us to produce.

The Editors
Ann Arbor, Michigan
June 1980

RESEARCH AND TECHNICAL STAFF FOR THE SEVENTH EDITION

Chris A. Thomas Elizabeth H. Bikoff
Laurie R. Silver Colleen O'Neal
Evelyn R. Neuhaus Barbara A. Bahlke
Amy B. Bernstein Sara B. Benton

ART STAFF

Susan L. Sweeney — Designer
Richard M. Fritzler — Medical Illustrator
Jeffrey A. Gretzinger — Technical Artist
David A. Boyer — Technical Artist

CO-EDITORS AND STAFF FOR EARLIER EDITIONS

First Edition (1963) Staff: Marshall Becker.
Second Edition (1964) Staff: Thea Zelman, David Chandler.
Third Edition (1967) and *Fourth Edition (1968)* Co-Editor: Judith Agard.
Fifth Edition (1972) Co-Editors: Judy Jameson, Christine Swearingen.
Sixth Edition (1976) Co-Editor: Douglas W. Gentry;
Staff: Jacob Bomberg, Mary Farrell, Jean E. Maier,
Shelly Malin, Ann P. Munro, Steven J. Speil.

Table of Contents

PREFACE iii
INTRODUCTION v
RESEARCH AND TECHNICAL STAFF viii

A. POPULATION CHARACTERISTICS

   1. Number and Percent of Aged 3
   2. Percent of Females Employed 4
   3. Residence: Urban and Rural 5
   4. Residence: Metropolitan Areas 6
   5. Population Mobility 7
   6. Median Income: Trends by Color 8
   7. Income Distribution: Color: 9
   8. Share of Income 10
   9. Percent Below Poverty Level: Trends 11

B. MORTALITY AND MORBIDITY

   1. Life Expectancy: Trends 15
   2. Life Expectancy: Sex and Race 16
   3. Life Expectancy: With and Without Disability 17
   4. Life Expectancy at Birth: International Comparison ... 18
   5. Life Expectancy of Males at Age 45: International Comparison 19
   6. Mortality: Leading Causes 20
   7. Infant Mortality: International Comparison 21
   8. Infant Mortality: Trends by Color 22
   9. Infant Mortality: Trends by Social Class 23
  10. Infant Mortality: Risk and Care 24
  11. Infant Mortality: Income and Education 25
  12. Acute Conditions: Activity Restriction 26
  13. Acute Conditions: Activity Restriction and Bed Disability, by Age 27
  14. Chronic Conditions: Limitation of Activity 28
  15. Chronic Conditions: Age and Sex 29
  16. Disability Days: Age and Sex 30
  17. Disability and Activity Restriction: Income 31
  18. Chronic Conditions: Age and Income 32

C. USE OF SERVICE

   1. Physician Visits: Trends by Place of Visit 35
   2. Physician Visits: Place of Visit by Color 36

3. Physician Visits: Physician Specialty and Patient Color 37
  4. Physician Visits: Age and Sex 38
  5. Physician Visits: Age, Education and Residence 39
  6. Physician Visits: Age and Income 40
  7. Physician Visits and Income: Trends 41
  8. Preventive and Curative Visits: Income 42
  9. Prenatal Care Trends: Education 43
 10. Prenatal Care: Education and Income 44
 11. Maternity Care: Color, Source of Care and Occupation of Father . . . 45
 12. Prenatal Care: Judgment of Need by Income 46
 13. Recognition of Symptoms: Social Class 47
 14. Physician Visits and Disability: Income 48
 15. Family Physician and Family Dentist: Social Class 49
 16. Type of Psychological Care: Social Class 50
 17. Physician Visits and Income: Effect of National Health
      Service 51
 18. Ambulatory Care Visits: Effect of Universal Health Insurance 52
 19. Physician Visits and Income: Effect of Universal Health
      Insurance 53
 20. Maternity Care and Income: Effect of Health Insurance 54
 21. Consultation of Pharmacists: Family Income 55
 22. Prenatal Care and Ethnicity: Prepaid Group Practice 56
 23. Physician Services: Fashions in Surgery 57
 24. Surgical Operations: Trends 58
 25. Amount of Surgery and Supply of Surgeons 59
 26. Hysterectomies: Risk for Different Groups of Women 60
 27. Physician Services and Caseload 61
 28. Physician Services and Supply of Physicians in Prepaid Group
      Practice 62
 29. Surgical Rates: Variation Attributable to Availability of
      Beds, General Practitioners, and Specialists 63
 30. Utilization of Services: Type and Distance 64
 31. Utilization of General Medical Care Services: Distance 65
 32. Maternity Care: Effect of Distance on Referral and Outcome 66
 33. Abortions: Color and Effect of Liberalized Law 67
 34. Services: Effect of Presence of Clinic Facilities 68
 35. Physician Services: Having a Family Doctor 69
 36. Physician Services: Perception of Medical Care Need 70
 37. Amount of Surgery and Additional Charges: Geographic Variation . 71
 38. Physician Services: Method of Payment 72
 39. Physician Services: Differential Use in Prepaid Group
      Practice, H.I.P. 73
 40. Physician Services: Differential Use in Prepaid Group
      Practice, C.H.A. 74
 41. Physician Services: Differential Use in Insured Population 75
 42. Dental and Physician Visits: Age and Sex 76
 43. Dental Visits: Time Since Last Visit 77
 44. Dental and Physician Visits: Income, Residence and Color 78

45. Dental Visits: Extractions by Education, Color and Geographic Area 79
46. Hospital Supply and Utilization: International Comparison 80
47. Hospital Utilization: Trends 81
48. Hospital Utilization: Age and Sex 82
49. Hospital Utilization: Age 83
50. Hospital Utilization: Psychiatric by Color 84
51. Hospital Utilization: Geographic Area and Residence 85
52. Hospital Utilization: Effect of Insurance, U.S., Canada and Saskatchewan 86
53. Hospital Utilization: Effect of Insurance, by Age 87
54. Hospital Utilization: Effect of Insurance, by Income 88
55. Hospital Utilization: Effect of Insurance, Amount of Care 89
56. Hospital Utilization: Effect of Multiple Insurance 90
57. Hospital Utilization: Source of Payment and Length of Stay 91
58. Hospital Utilization: Appropriateness of Use 92
59. Hospital Utilization: Influence of Physician 93
60. Hospital Utilization: Effect of Bed Supply 94
61. Hospital Utilization: Multiple Admissions 95
62. Hospital Utilization: Effect of Outpatient Psychiatric Intervention 96
63. Corrective Lenses: Type of Prescriber and Education 97
64. Visits to Selected Practitioners and Income 98
65. Prescribed Drugs: Demographic Factors in Acquisition 99

D. COSTS AND EXPENDITURES

    Glossary of Selected Terms 103
1. Medical Care Costs and Wages Lost Due to Illness 105
2. Direct and Indirect Costs: Selected Illnesses 106
3. Present Value of Lifetime Earnings 107
4. National Expenditures: Health, Defense and Education 108
5. National Expenditures: Health and Education, Public and Private 109
6. National Health Expenditures: Percent of Gross National Product, U.S.A. and Selected Countries 110
7. National Health Expenditures: Rate of Increase, Percent of Gross National Product, Selected Countries 111
8. National Health Expenditures: Public and Private, Trends 112
9. National Health Expenditures: Public and Private by Category ... 113
10. National Health Expenditures: Public Relative to Private 114
11. Health Services Expenditures: Type of Expenditure 115
12. Public Expenditures for Health Services: Programs 116
13. Personal Health Care Expenditures: Direct and Third Party Payment 117
14. Personal Health Care Expenditures: Components of Increase 118
15. Consumer Price Index: Relative Increases in Components 119
16. Medical Care Price Index: Trends in Components 120
17. Hospital Costs: Trends 121

18. Effect of Economic Stabilization Program on the Consumer Price Index ... 122
19. Hospital Charges: Size of Hospital and Length of Stay ... 123
20. Out-of-Pocket Health Expenses and Disposable Personal Income ... 124
21. Consumer Dollar ... 125
22. Medical Care Dollar: Trends ... 126
23. Distribution of Families by Level of Out-of-Pocket Health Expense ... 127
24. Family Out-of-Pocket Health Expenses by Income: Amount and Percent of Income ... 128
25. Out-of-Pocket Health Expenses: Type and Income ... 129
26. Out-of-Pocket Health Expenses by Age: Trends ... 130
27. Personal Health Care Expenditures by Age: Type of Service ... 131
28. Drug Costs: Population Characteristics ... 132
29. New Pharmaceuticals: Trends ... 133
30. Drug Prices: Generic and Brand Name ... 134
31. Drug Costs: Generic Equivalents and Savings ... 135
32. Drug Industry: Profit ... 136

E. HEALTH PERSONNEL

1. Physician-Population Ratio: Continents and Selected Countries ... 139
2. Physician-Population Ratio: Selected Countries ... 140
3. Physicians and All Other Health Personnel: Trends ... 141
4. Physicians, Dentists, Nurses: Ratio to Population, Trends ... 142
5. Physician-Population Ratio: Geographic Area ... 143
6. Physician-Population Ratio: Type of Practice and Area ... 144
7. Relative Supply of Selected Health Personnel: Type of Location ... 145
8. Physician-Population Ratio: Per Capita Income of States ... 146
9. Physician-Population Ratio: Poverty Areas ... 147
10. Physician-Population Ratio: Socioeconomic Status of Population ... 148
11. Physician-Population Ratio: Disability and Income, 1965–1967 ... 149
12. Physician-Population Ratio: Disability and Income, 1976–1977 ... 150
13. Medical Schools and Applicants and Acceptances by Sex: Trends ... 151
14. Medical School Enrollment: Percent Black ... 152
15. Medical School Applicants Accepted: Trends ... 153
16. Medical School Applicants and Accepted Applicants: Family Income ... 154
17. Residencies and Internships: Trends ... 155
18. Male and Female Specialists: Distribution by Specialty ... 156
19. Residencies, Filled and Unfilled: Trends ... 157
20. Foreign Graduates: Internships, Residencies and Licensure ... 158
21. Physicians in Private Practice: Trends in Specialization ... 159
22. Primary Care Physicians: Trends in Number and Type ... 160
23. Selected Nonphysician Health Care Providers: Education, Certification, and Licensure Requirements ... 161

24. Selected Nonphysician Health Care Providers: Distribution by Type of Practice, Sex, and Color 162
25. Choice of Practice by Medical Students: Rating by Faculty 163
26. Specialty Board Certificates: Trends 164
27. Obstetrical Care: Volume and Outcome by Type of Physician 165
28. Physicians in Group Practice: Trends 166
29. Physicians in Group Practice: Geographic Distribution........... 167
30. Group Practice: Distribution of Groups and Percent of Physicians in General Practice by Size of Group 168
31. Group Practice: Groups and Physicians by Type of Group 169
32. Group Practice: Form of Organization 170
33. Group Practice: Attitudes of Physicians 171
34. Group Practice: Attrition Rate of Physicians................... 172
35. Physician Hours Worked: Age and Specialty................... 173
36. Physician Workload: Specialty and Place of Visit................ 174
37. Physician Income: Age..................................... 175
38. Physician Income and Workload: Type of Practice 176
39. Physician Income: Specialty 177
40. Physician Fees: Specialty and Type of Visit 178
41. Methods of Payment: Pathologists and Radiologists, Trends...... 179
42. Dentists and Dental Personnel: Trends 180
43. Dentist-Population Ratio: Geographic Distribution 181
44. Dentist-Population Ratio: Per Capita Income of States 182
45. Dentists and Physicians: Type of Practice..................... 183
46. Dentists: Organization of Practice and Employment 184
47. Dentist Income: Type of Practice 185
48. Dentist Workload: Age 186
49. Dentist Productivity: Use of Auxiliary Personnel 187
50. Nursing Personnel: Types and Trends 188
51. Nurse-Population Ratio: Geographic Distribution 189
52. Nurses: Educational Programs 190
53. Nurse Training: Trends.................................... 191
54. Nurses: Type of Practice 192
55. Selected Health Personnel: Ratio to Population, Trends 193
56. Selected Health Professionals: Percent Black 194

F. FACILITIES
1. Hospitals and Hospital Beds: Trends 197
2. Selected Hospital Statistics: Type of Control 198
3. Hospital Bed-Population Ratios: Geographic Area 199
4. Hospitals and Hospital Beds: Type of Control 200
5. Hospitals and Hospital Beds: Type of Ownership 201
6. Hospital Beds: Type of Hospital and Ownership 202
7. Change in Admissions to Long-term and Short-term Hospitals by Ownership 203
8. Hospitals and Hospital Beds: Type of Hospital 204
9. Hospital Mean Size and Hospital Bed-Population Ratios: Type of Hospital 205

10. Hospitals and Hospital Beds: Size of Hospital 206
11. Hospitals and Hospital Beds: Percent Distribution by Size 207
12. Occupancy Rate and Length of Stay: Size of Hospital 208
13. Length of Stay: Size of Hospital and Age of Patient 209
14. Accreditation and Medicare Certification: Size of Hospital 210
15. Accreditation: Size and Ownership of Hospital 211
16. Hospital Maternity Services and Capabilities: Size of Service 212
17. Hospital Discharges: Percent by Length of Stay and Age of Patient 213
18. Hospital Discharges: Cumulative Distribution by Length of Stay and Age of Patient 214
19. Discharges and Patient Days: Length of Stay 215
20. Length of Stay, Discharges and Patient Days: Region 216
21. Length of Stay: Selected Diagnoses by Region................... 217
22. Hospitals with Specified Characteristics: Trends 218
23. Hospitals with Specified Facilities and Services: Trends 1950-1978 219
24. Hospitals with Specified Facilities and Services: Trends by Size... 220
25. Hospitals with Specified Facilities and Services: Trends 1960-1978 221
26. Change in Use: Selected Hospital Services..................... 222
27. Hospital Care, Myocardial Infarction: Trends in Amount and Type of Services 223
28. Effect of Length of Stay on Hospital Charges, Medicare Patients 224
29. Hospital Personnel and Payroll Expenses: Trends 225
30. Judgments on Level of Care Required by Hospital Patients 226
31. Appropriateness of Hospitalization and Suggested Alternative Levels of Care 227
32. Emergency Visits, Outpatient Visits, and Hospital Admissions: Trends 228
33. Emergency Service Use: Reason for Visit 229
34. Emergency Visits: Type of Visits and Source of Payment 230
35. Emergency Service Patients: Triage and Disposition............. 231
36. Emergency Department Patients Not Needing Emergency Treatment: Color, Age, and Shift............................. 232
37. Hospital Emergency Facilities Meeting Specified Criteria: Hospital Size 232
38. Emergency Department Patients: Match Between Need and Facility..234
39. Emergency Department Patients: Match Between Need and Facility, by Insurance Coverage 235
40. Emergency Department Physician Staffing Patterns: Trends 236
41. Nursing Care Homes and Beds: Trends 237
42. Nursing Care and Related Homes and Beds: Type of Care 238
43. Nursing Care Home Beds: Supply by Geographic Region 239

44. Nursing Care Homes and Hospitals: Facilities and Beds by Ownership 240
45. Nursing Care Homes and Beds: Size of Nursing Home 241
46. Nursing Home Residents and Discharges: Primary Source of Payment 242
47. Skilled Nursing Home Employees: Type of Employee 243
48. Appropriateness of Skilled Nursing Care for Patients in Long-term Care Facilities 244
49. Appropriateness of Skilled Nursing Care for Patients in Long-term Care Facilities: Facility Characteristics 245
50. Home Health Agencies and Skilled Nursing Facilities Participating in Medicare: Trends 246
51. Home Health Agencies by Type: Trends 247
52. Home Health Care: Visits and Reimbursement Under Medicare, Trends 248
53. Home Health Agencies Providing Selected Services 249
54. Use of Services With and Without Organized Home Care 250
55. Percent Change in Hospital Use With and Without Organized Home Care 251
56. Home Health Visits Reimbursed by Medicare: Type of Agency and Type of Services 252
57. Total Medicare Payments per Person With and Without Day Care and Homemaker Services 253
58. Aged Population: Type of Care Received and Needed 254

G. QUALITY OF CARE
1. Hospital Care: Opinion of Patient and Experts 257
2. Changes in Cancer Survival: Types of Hospital 258
3. Perinatal Mortality: Preventable Deaths 259
4. Perinatal Mortality: Contributing Factors 260
5. Maternal Mortality: Size of Service 261
6. Maternal Mortality: Preventable Deaths........................ 262
7. Fatality Rates: Type of Condition and Hospital 263
8. Crude and Adjusted Death Rates: Type of Hospital 264
9. Post-Operative Mortality Ratios: Patient Characteristics 265
10. Hospital Mortality Ratio: Diagnostic Categories 266
11. Appendectomy Rates and Mortality: Service Area 267
12. Tonsillectomy Rates: Trends................................... 268
13. Tonsillectomies: Percent Recommended at Successive Examinations 269
14. Appendectomies: Physician Variability by Hospital............. 270
15. Hysterectomies: Justification 271
16. Unjustified Appendectomies: Type of Hospital and Patient Pay Status 272
17. Suspected Appendicitis, Operated and Not Operated: Consequences 273
18. Appendicitis: Propensity to Operate and Consequences 274
19. Appendectomies: Risk of True Appendicitis and Expected Deaths, Costs, and Convalescent Days 275
20. Appendicitis: Surgical and Nonsurgical Treatment 276
21. Elective Surgery: Second Opinion Program 277

22. Abdominal Hysterectomies: Unjustified Operations Before and After Institution of External Review 278
23. Clinic Care: Comparative Assessments......................... 279
24. Deficiencies in Hospital Care: Comparison of Two Measures 280
25. Hospital Care: Necessity for Admission and Quality by Specialty 281
26. Hospital Care: Unnecessary Admissions by Hospital and Physician Characteristics 282
27. Hospital Care: Accreditation and Type of Hospital 283
28. Hospital Care: Type of Hospital and Physician Qualifications 284
29. Hospital Care: Surgical and Non-surgical Admissions, by Type of Hospital and Physician Qualifications 285
30. Physician Performance and Appropriateness of Use: Physician and Hospital Characteristics 286
31. Physician Performance and Appropriateness of Use: Type of Practice 287
32. Physician Performance: Specialty Status 288
33. Physician Performance: Type of Practice 289
34. Physician Performance: Size and Type of Hospital 290
35. Physician Performance: Type of Hospital and Physician Qualifications 291
36. General Practice: Overall Performance 292
37. General Practice: Performance of Specific Procedures 293
38. General Practice: Overall Performance, Canadian Physicians 294
39. Ambulatory Care: Diagnosis, Specialty of Physician and Site of Care 295
40. Ambulatory Care: Institutional Source and Category of Care 296
41. Ambulatory Care: Physician Performance and Type of Delivery Site 297
42. Injections: Approval for Payment and Type of Physician 298
43. Emergency Room Care: Deficiencies in Successive Stages of Management 299
44. Ambulatory Care: Deficiencies in Outcome of Care 300
45. Ambulatory Care: Correspondence Between Implicit and Explicit Assessment Criteria 301
46. Laboratory Tests: Costs of Tests Ordered and Clinical Capability of Physician 302
47. Diagnostic X-rays: Frequency and Type of Examination by Type of Physician 303
48. Antibiotics: Appropriate Use Before and After Medical Audit and Education Program 304
49. Performance of Pharmacists: Activity Categories and Location of Pharmacy 305
50. Pharmacists' Performance and Charges 306
51. Nursing Care: Performance by Component of Care 307
52. Eyeglasses: Need for and Appropriateness..................... 308
53. Deficiencies in Optometric Care: Frequency and Type 309
54. Hebdomadal Deaths: Effect of Health Department Supervision 310

55. Operations: Effect of Medical Audit 311
56. Appendectomy: Effect of Tissue Committee 312
57. Laboratory Findings: Physician Response 313
58. Performance of Studies Using Health Accounting Method for Improving Outcomes 314
59. Hospital Care: Length of Stay Before and After Certification Program 315
60. Hospital Care: Length of Stay Before and After Predischarge Utilization Review Program 316
61. Likelihood of Being Discharged by Time Since Admission 317
62. Hospital Care: Approved Length of Stay at Admission 318
63. Hospital Care: Appropriateness of Stay by Type of Service 319
64. Hospital Care: Appropriateness of Continued Stay 320
65. Professional Standards Review Organizations: Structure and Activities 321
66. Professional Standards Review Organizations: Admissions and Stay Certification Process 322
67. Professional Standards Review Organizations: Planning, Conditional, and Not Funded Areas 323
68. Professional Standards Review Organizations: Review of Care and Delegation of Review 324
69. Professional Standards Review Organizations: Medicare Utilization Rates in Active and Inactive PSRO Areas 325
70. Rheumatic Fever: Incidence and Access to Care 326
71. Ambulatory Care: Course of Treatment and Outcome 327

H. TAX-SUPPORTED PROGRAMS
1. Social Welfare Expenditures: Trends 331
2. Federal Health Expenditures: Percent of Total Federal Expenditures, Trends 332
3. Federal Health Expenditures: Percent of National Health Expenditures, Trends 333
4. Federal Health Expenditures by Type: Trends.................. 334
5. Federal Health Expenditures by Agency 335
6. Programs Dealing With Dependency 336
7. Public Income Maintenance Programs: Trends 337
8. Public Income Maintenance Programs for Aged: Trends 338
9. Medicare and Medicaid: Total Expenditures, State and Federal Share, Trends 339
10. Medicare: Percent of Total Income Derived from General Revenues 340
11. Medicare: Expenditures by Type of Service 341
12. Medicare: Enrollment, Payments, Utilization, Trends 342
13. Medicare: Physicians' Services Covered by Place of Service 343
14. Medicare: Hospital Use by Aged and Others, Trends 344
15. Medicare: Change in Hospital Use by Patient Characteristics 345
16. Medicare: Change in Number and Site of Physicians' Visits 346
17. Medicare: Change in Out-of-Pocket Expenditures by Type 347

xvii

18. Medicare: Personal Health Expenditures for Aged, Trends 348
19. Personal Health Care Expenditures for the Aged: Sources of Funds 349
20. Medicare: Premiums and Deductibles, Trends 350
21. Medicare: Reimbursable and Out-of-Pocket Charges 351
22. Medicare: Change in Physicians' Opinions 352
23. Medicaid: Distribution of Expenditures by Type of Service, Compared with Medicare 353
24. Medicaid: Distribution of Recipients and Expenditures, by Category 354
25. Medicaid: Distribution of Expenditures by Eligibility Categories and Receipt of Public Assistance 355
26. Medicaid: Recipients and Payments by State 356
27. Medicaid: Benefits by per Capita Income of States 357
28. Medicaid: Change in Source of Care 358
29. Medicaid: Effect of Cutbacks 359

I. MEDICAL CARE INSURANCE

Glossary of Selected Terms 363
1. Types of Protection 365
2. Workers' Compensation: Coverage, Benefits, Trends 366
3. Workers' Compensation: Cases and Losses, by Type of Disability 367
4. Insurance Coverage for Income Loss from Short-term Sickness: Trends 368
5. Enrollment: Trends by Type of Insurance 369
6. Enrollment: Trends in Benefits by Age 370
7. Enrollment: Growth in Hospital Insurance 371
8. Enrollment: Population Characteristics 372
9. Enrollment: Hospital Insurance, Type of Insurer, Trends 373
10. Enrollment: Surgical and Physician's Expense Insurance, Type of Insurer 374
11. Enrollment: Type of Insurer by Type of Insurance 375
12. Enrollment: Type of Benefits 376
13. Enrollment: Employee Benefit Plans, Type of Benefit 377
14. Choice of Insurer and Coverage: Federal Employees Program ... 378
15. Expenditures Covered: Trends 379
16. Loss Ratio: Type of Insurer 380
17. Hospital Utilization: Blue Cross Subscribers and U.S. Population, Trends 381
18. Type of Enrollment: Use of Hospital 382
19. Duration of Enrollment: Use of Services 383
20. Prepaid Health Plans: Number of Visits by Duration of Membership 384
21. Prepaid Health Plans: Trends 385
22. Prepaid Health Plans and Enrollment: Federal Qualification .. 386
23. Prepaid Health Plans and Enrollment: Size of Plan 387
24. Prepaid Health Plans and Enrollment: Type of Practice 388
25. Prepaid Health Plans: Hospital Utilization by Type of Practice and Federal Qualification 389
26. Utilization: Insurance Coverage 390

27. Utilization: Group Practice and Other Plans, California 391
28. Utilization: Group Practice and Other Plans, New York City 392
29. Medicare: Effect of Prepaid Group Practice on Program Costs 393
30. Hospital Utilization: Type of Insurer, Trends 394
31. Hospital Utilization: Group Health Association and Blue
    Cross-Blue Shield, Federal Employees 395
32. Utilization: Group Practice and Blue Shield, Federal
    Employees 396
33. Utilization, Expenses and Satisfaction: Group Practice and
    Other Plans 397
34. Satisfaction With Coverage and Medical Care: Group Practice
    and Other Plans 398
35. Consumer Preference: Group Practice Compared With
    Solo Practice 399
36. Consumer Approval: Multispecialty Group Practice 400
37. Disenrollments from Medicaid Program: Voluntary and
    Involuntary by Time Since Enrollment 401
38. Choice of Health Insurance Plan: Having a Private Physician 402

APPENDIX: Geographic Terms 403
INDEX 409

SECTION A
Population Characteristics

Chart A-1

Aged Persons by Age Groups: Number and Percent of Total Population (U.S.A., Selected Years, 1900–1980).

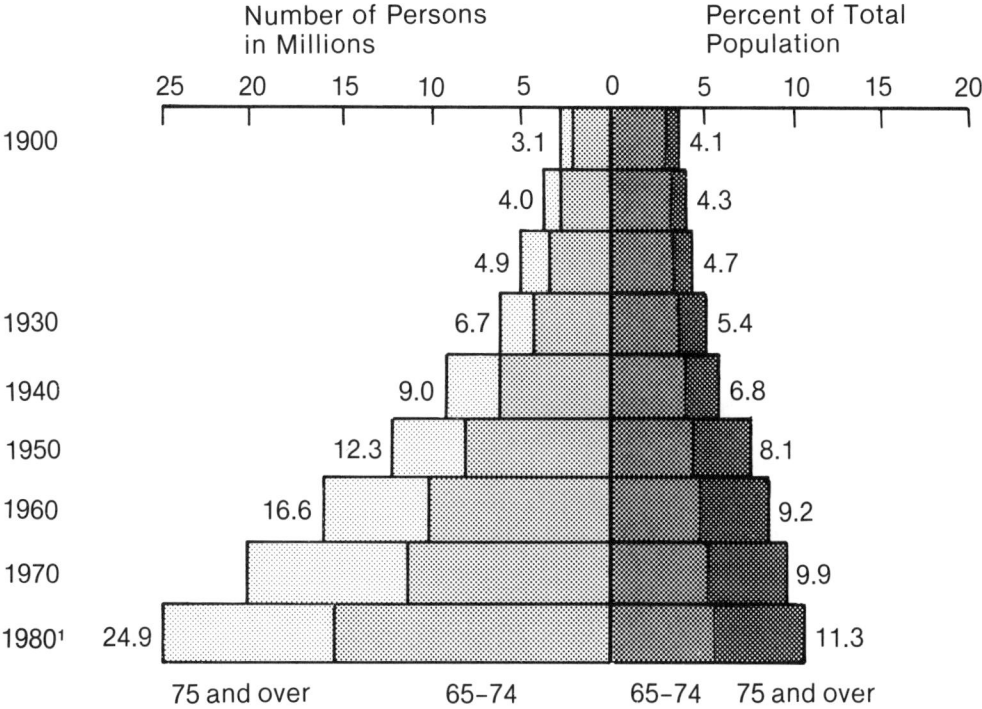

[1]Estimated

SOURCES: For population: U.S. Department of Commerce, Bureau of the Census, *Statistical Abstract of the U.S., 1978*, Washington, D.C., 1978, Table 2, p. 6; for age breakdown: U.S. Department of Commerce, Bureau of the Census, *Current Population Reports: Special Studies—Some Demographic Aspects of Aging in the United States*, Series p. 23, No. 43, February 1973, Washington, D.C., Table 1, p. 2.

Chart A-2

Percent of Females 16 Years and Older Who are Employed (U.S.A., Selected Years, 1950-1978).

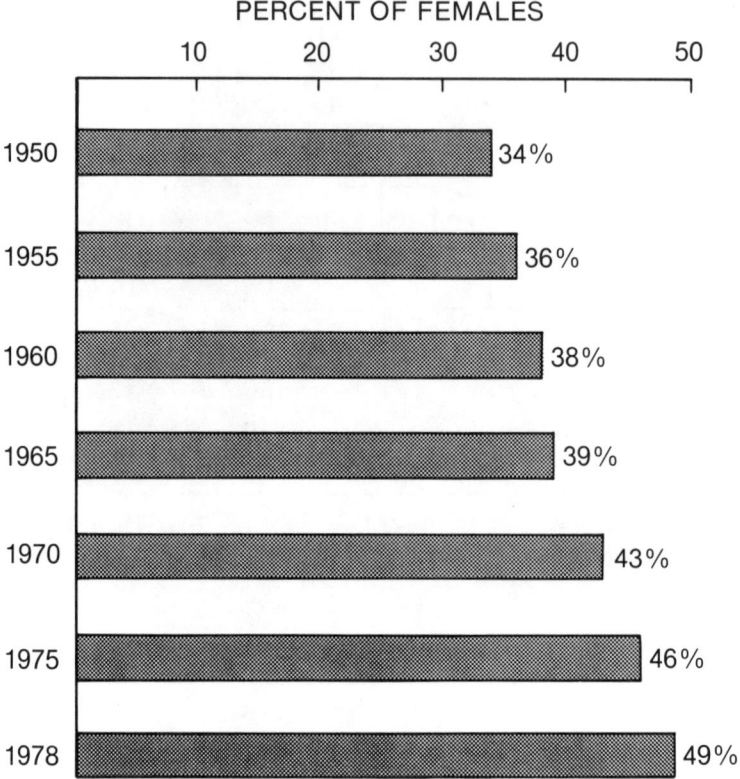

SOURCES: For 1950 and 1955: U.S. Department of Commerce, Bureau of the Census, *Historical Statistics of the U.S., Colonial Times to 1970*, Bicentennial Edition, Part I, Washington, D.C., 1975, p. 128; for 1960-1978: U.S. Department of Commerce, Bureau of the Census, *Statistical Abstract of the United States, 1978*, Washington, D.C., 1978, Table 645, p. 399.

Chart A-3

Percent Distribution of Population Residing in Urban and Rural Areas (U.S.A., Selected Years, 1900-1970).

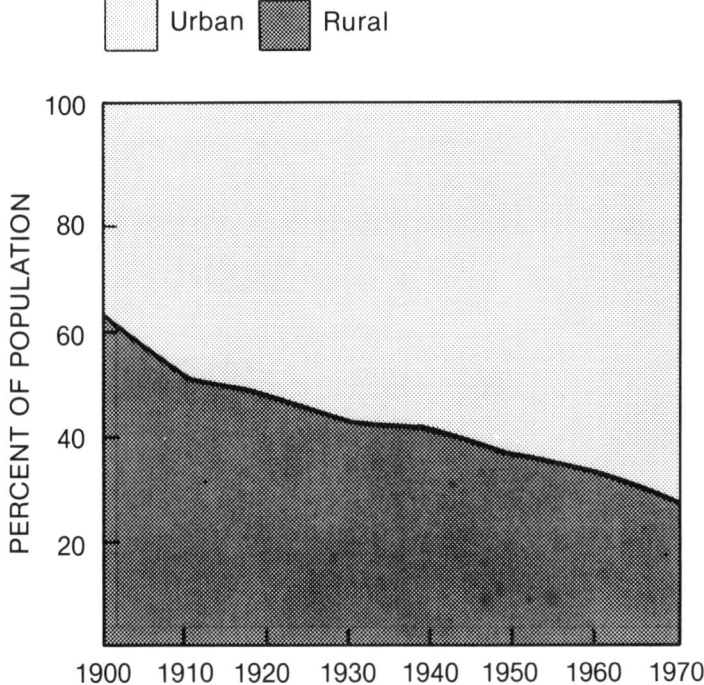

SOURCE: U.S. Department of Commerce, Bureau of the Census, *Historical Statistics of the U.S., Colonial Times to 1970*, Bicentennial Edition, Part 1, Washington, D.C., 1975, p. 12.

Chart A-4

Percent Distribution of Population in Relation to Standard Metropolitan Statistical Areas (U.S.A., Selected Years, 1950–1977).

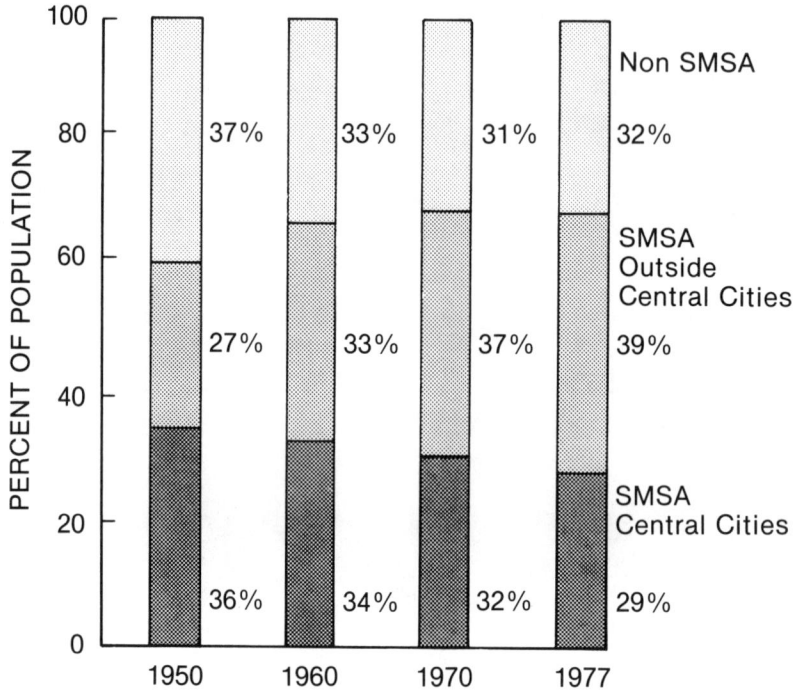

SOURCE: U.S. Department of Commerce, Bureau of the Census, *Statistical Abstract of the United States, 1978,* Washington, D.C., 1978, Table 16, p. 17.

Population Characteristics

Chart A-5

Percent of 1975 Population Having Changed Residence in the Five-Year Period from 1970–1975 (U.S.A.).

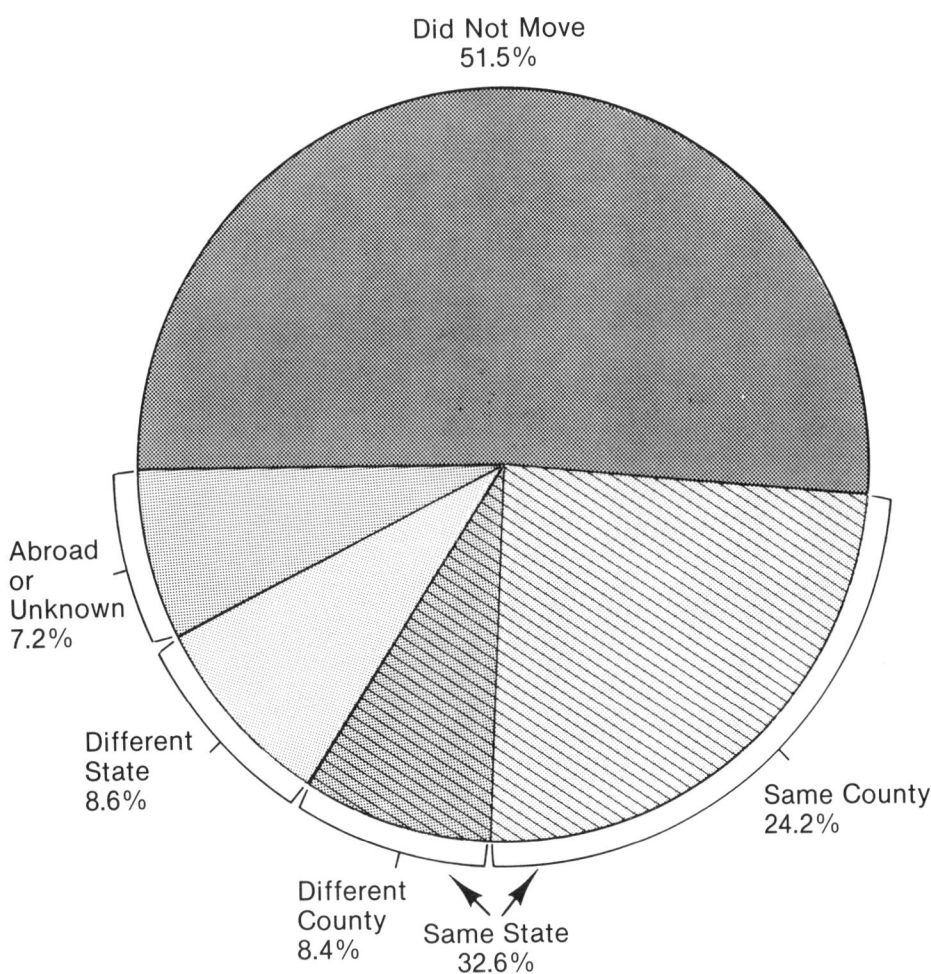

SOURCE: U.S. Department of Commerce, Bureau of the Census, *Statistical Abstract of the United States, 1978,* Washington, D.C., 1978, Table 46, p. 39.

Population Characteristics

Chart A-6

Median Income of Families, by Color of Family Head, in Constant 1977 Dollars (U.S.A., Selected Years 1950-1977).

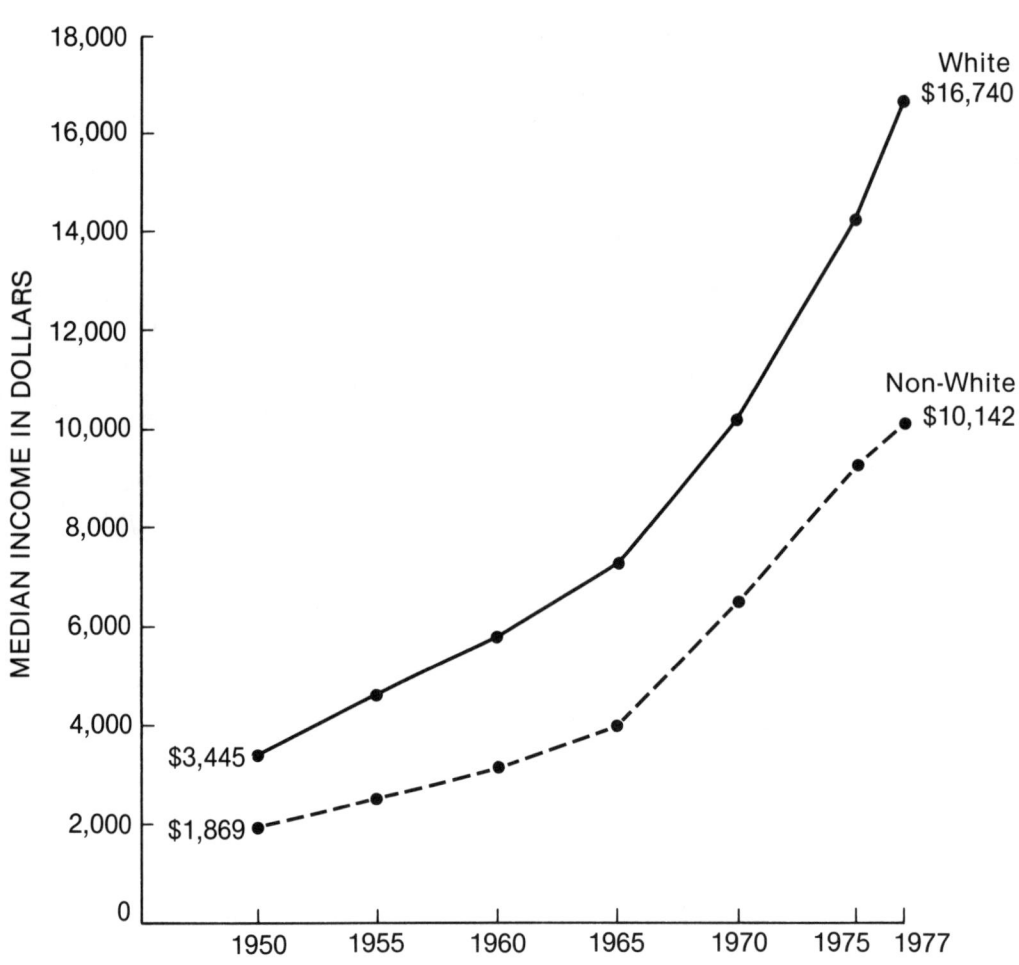

SOURCE: U.S. Department of Commerce, Bureau of the Census, *Current Population Reports,* U.S. Government Printing Office, Washington, D.C., Series p-60, No. 118, 1978, Table 10, pp. 32-33.

Chart A-7

Percent Distribution of Families, by Income Level and Color (U.S.A., 1977).

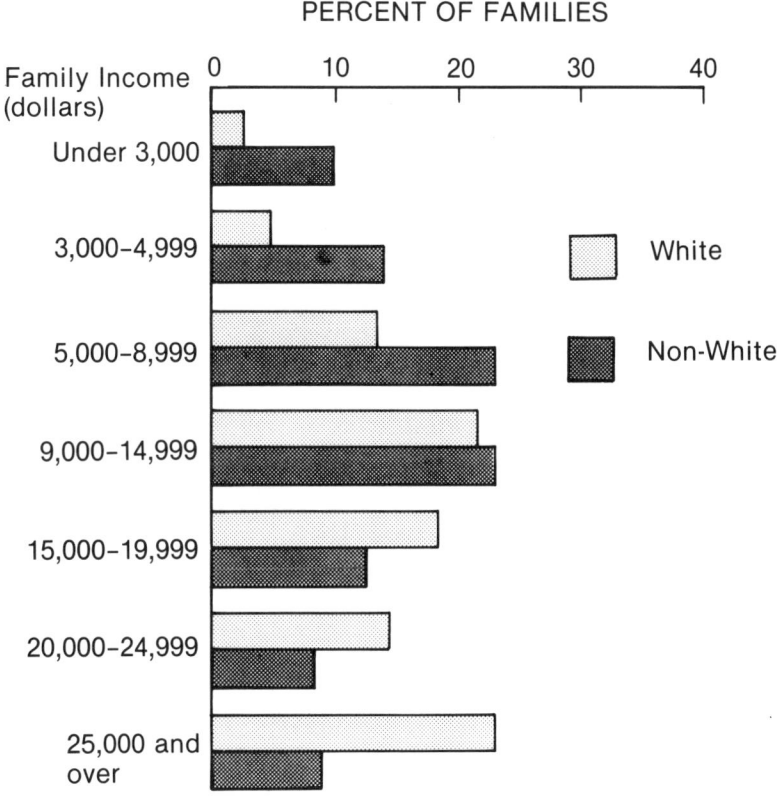

SOURCE: U.S. Department of Commerce, Bureau of the Census, *Statistical Abstract of the United States, 1978,* Washington, D.C., 1978, Table 731, p. 453.

Population Characteristics

Chart A-8

Percent of Aggregate Income Received by Each Fifth of Families
(U.S.A., 1950 and 1977).

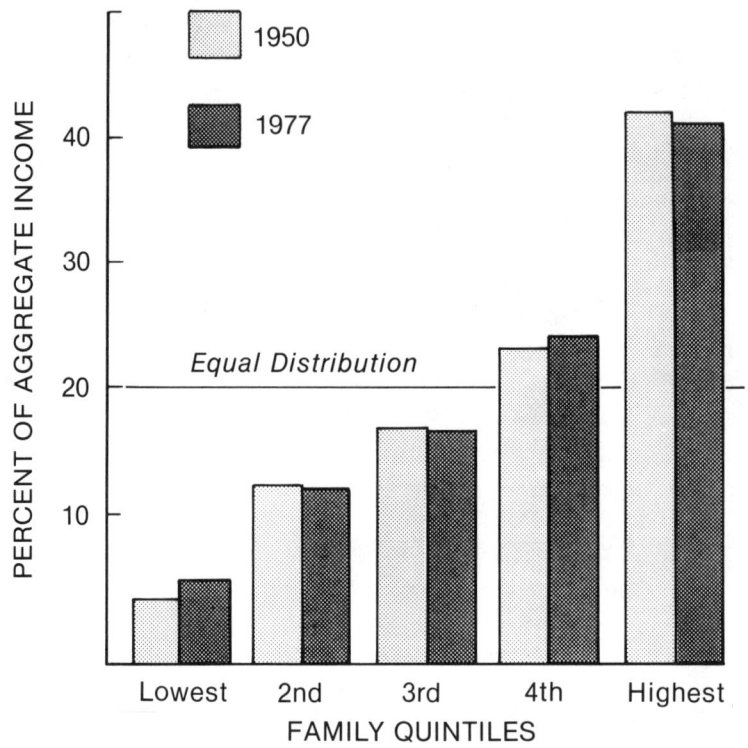

SOURCE: U.S. Department of Commerce, Bureau of the Census, *Statistical Abstract of the United States, 1978,* Washington, D.C., 1978, Table 734, p. 455.

Chart A-9

Percent of Persons Below the Poverty Level as Defined by the Social Security Administration (U.S.A., Selected Years, 1960–1977).

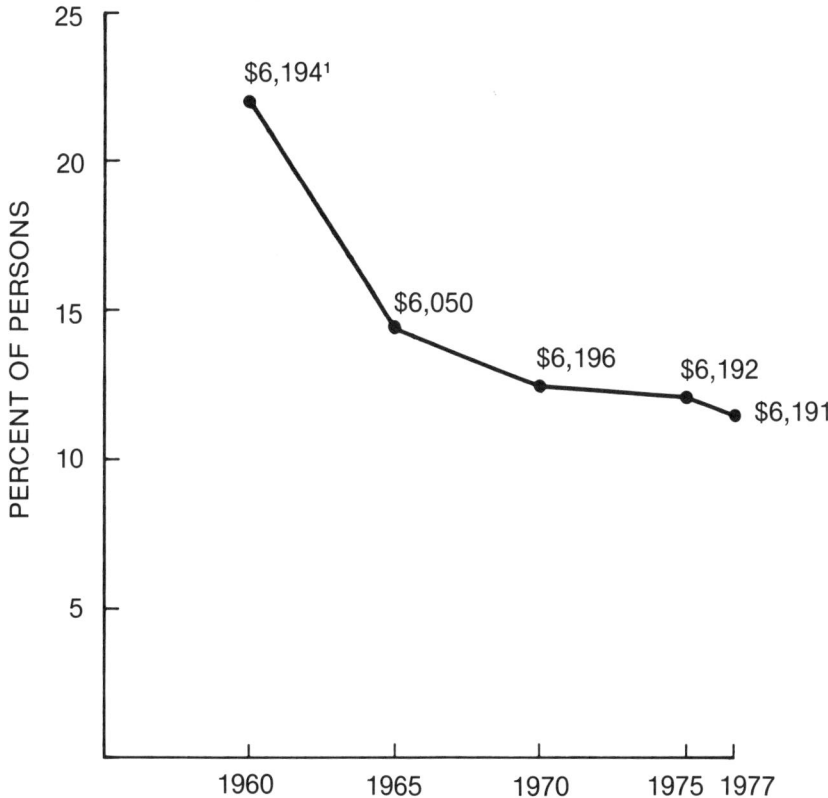

[1]The dollar figures shown indicate the Social Security Administration's definition of poverty for a non-farm family of four, in constant 1977 dollars.

SOURCE: U.S. Department of Commerce, Bureau of the Census, *Statistical Abstract of the United States: 1978,* Washington, D.C., 1978, Table 754, p. 465.

SECTION B
Mortality and Morbidity

Chart B-1

Average Remaining Years of Life at Birth and at Age 65, by Sex and Color (U.S.A., 1900–1902 and 1976).

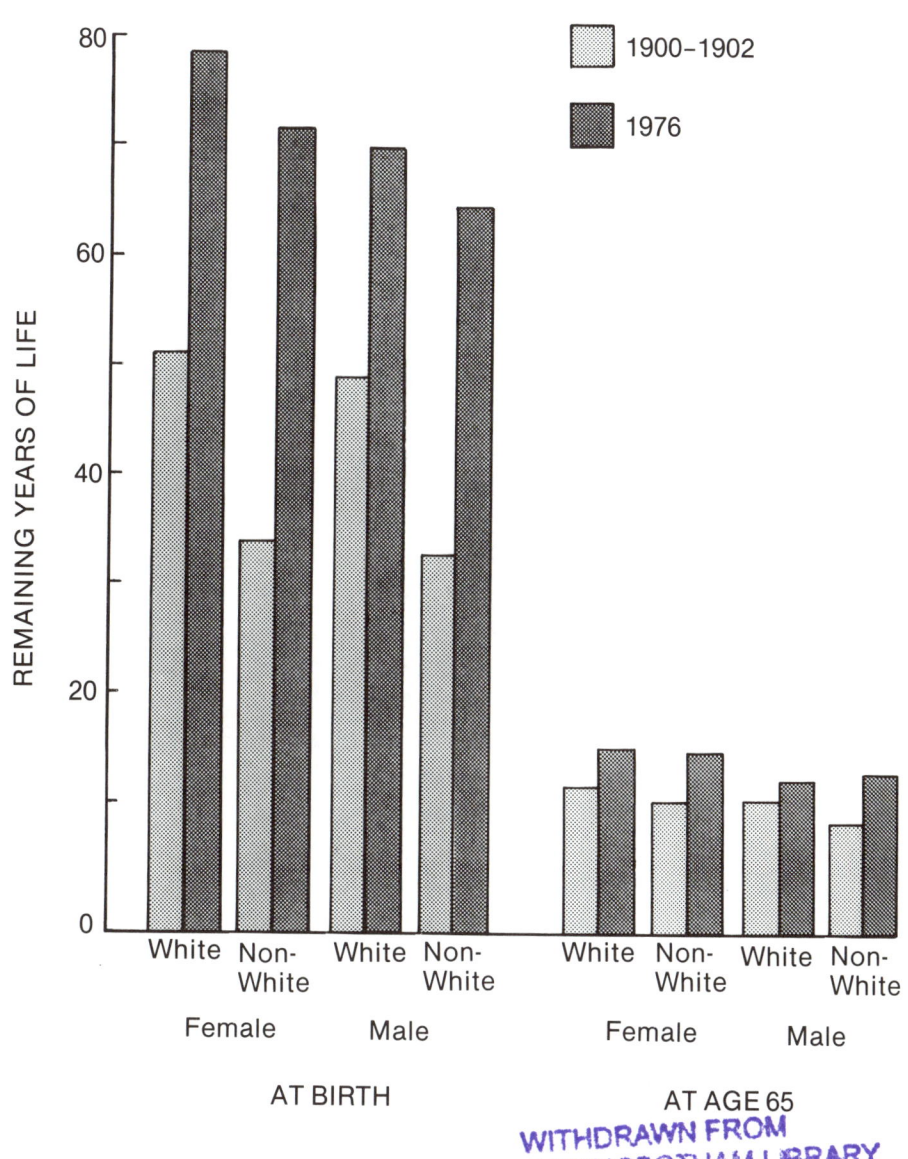

SOURCES: For 1900–1902: U.S. Department of Congress, Bureau of the Census, *Statistical Abstract of the United States, 1966,* Washington, D.C., July 1966, Table 63, p.54; for 1976: U.S. Department of Commerce, Bureau of the Census, *Statistical Abstract of the United States, 1978,* Washington, D.C., 1978, Table 100, p. 70.

Mortality and Morbidity

Chart B-2

Expected Years of Life Remaining, by Age, Sex, and Color (U.S.A., 1976).

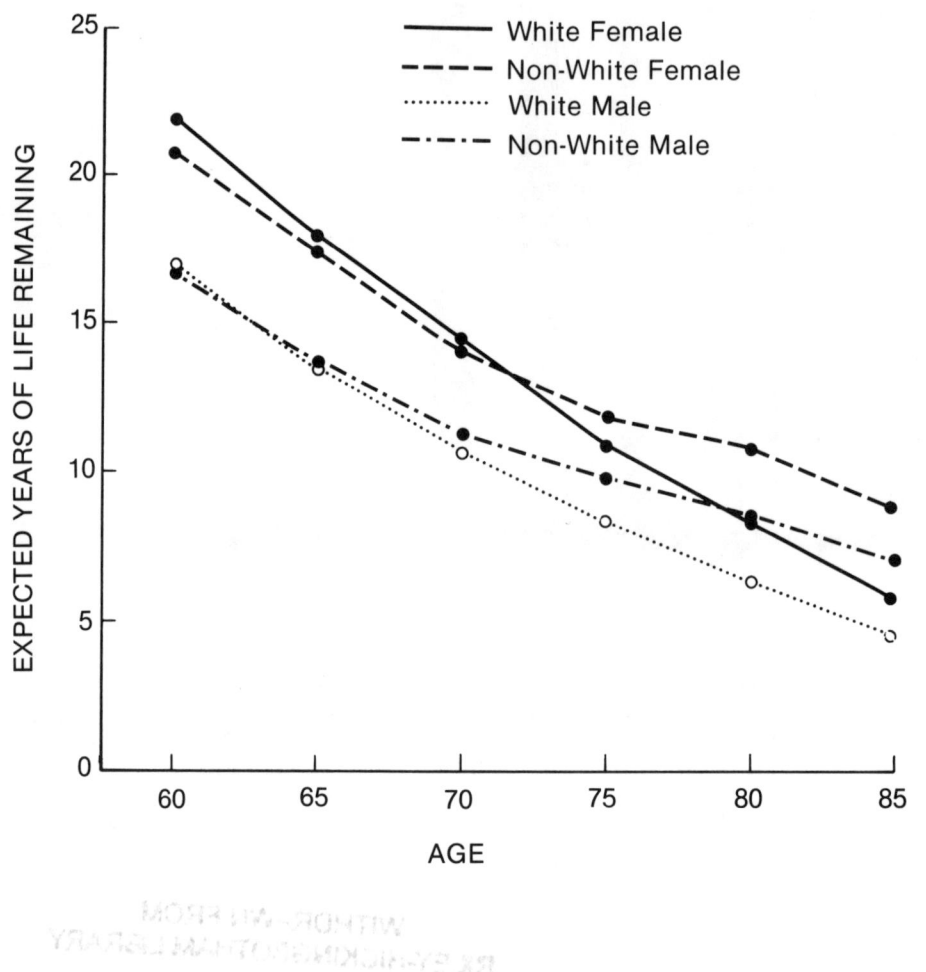

SOURCE: U.S. Department of Commerce, Bureau of the Census, *Statistical Abstract of the United States, 1978,* Washington, D.C., 1978, Table 100, p. 70.

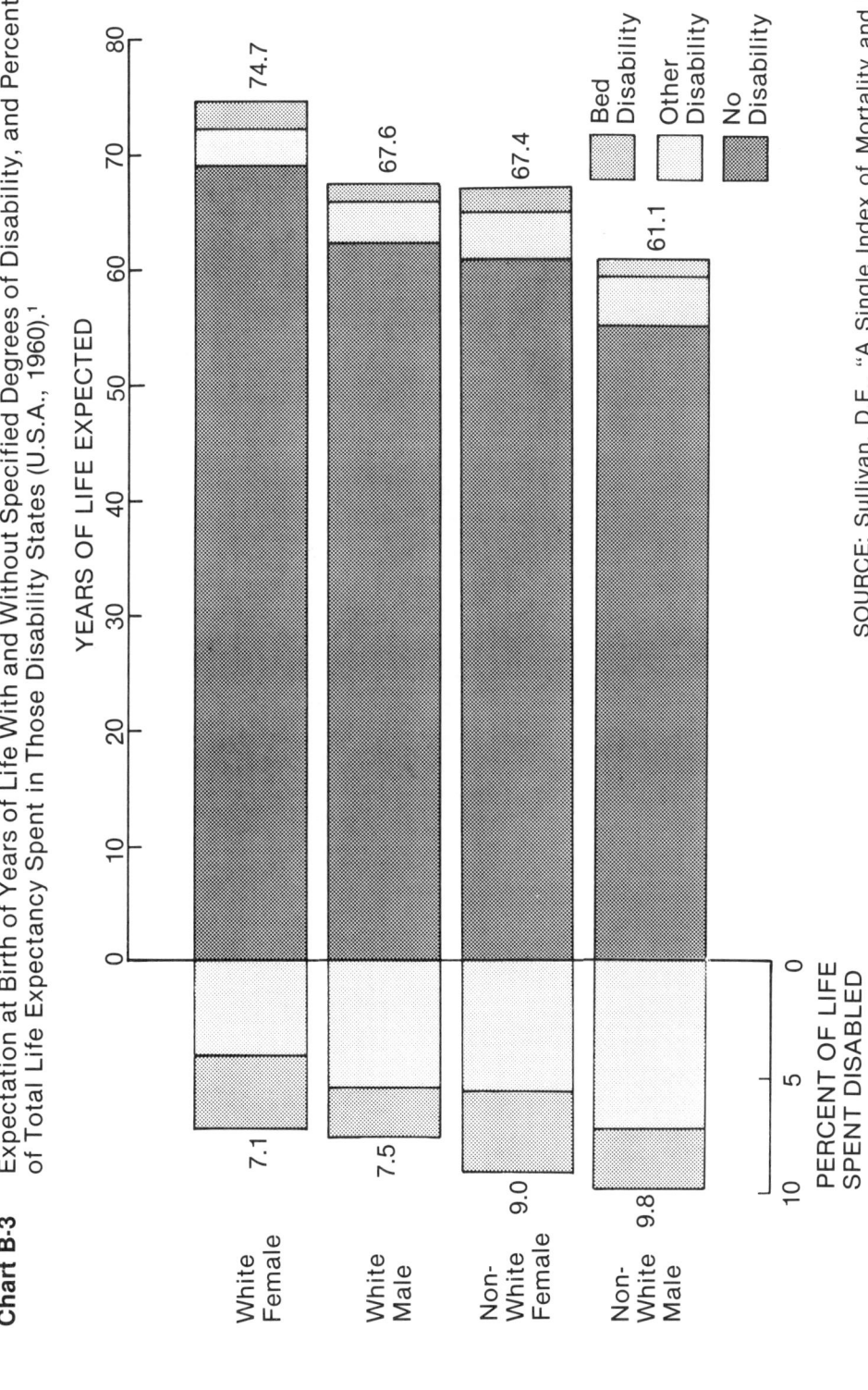

Chart B-3 Expectation at Birth of Years of Life With and Without Specified Degrees of Disability, and Percent of Total Life Expectancy Spent in Those Disability States (U.S.A., 1960).[1]

[1]Applying to a cohort of births the age-specific death and disability rates observed in the United States in the mid 1960's.

SOURCE: Sullivan, D.E., "A Single Index of Mortality and Morbidity," *HSMHA Health Reports*, Vol. 86, April 1971, Tables 1 and 2, pp. 347–354.

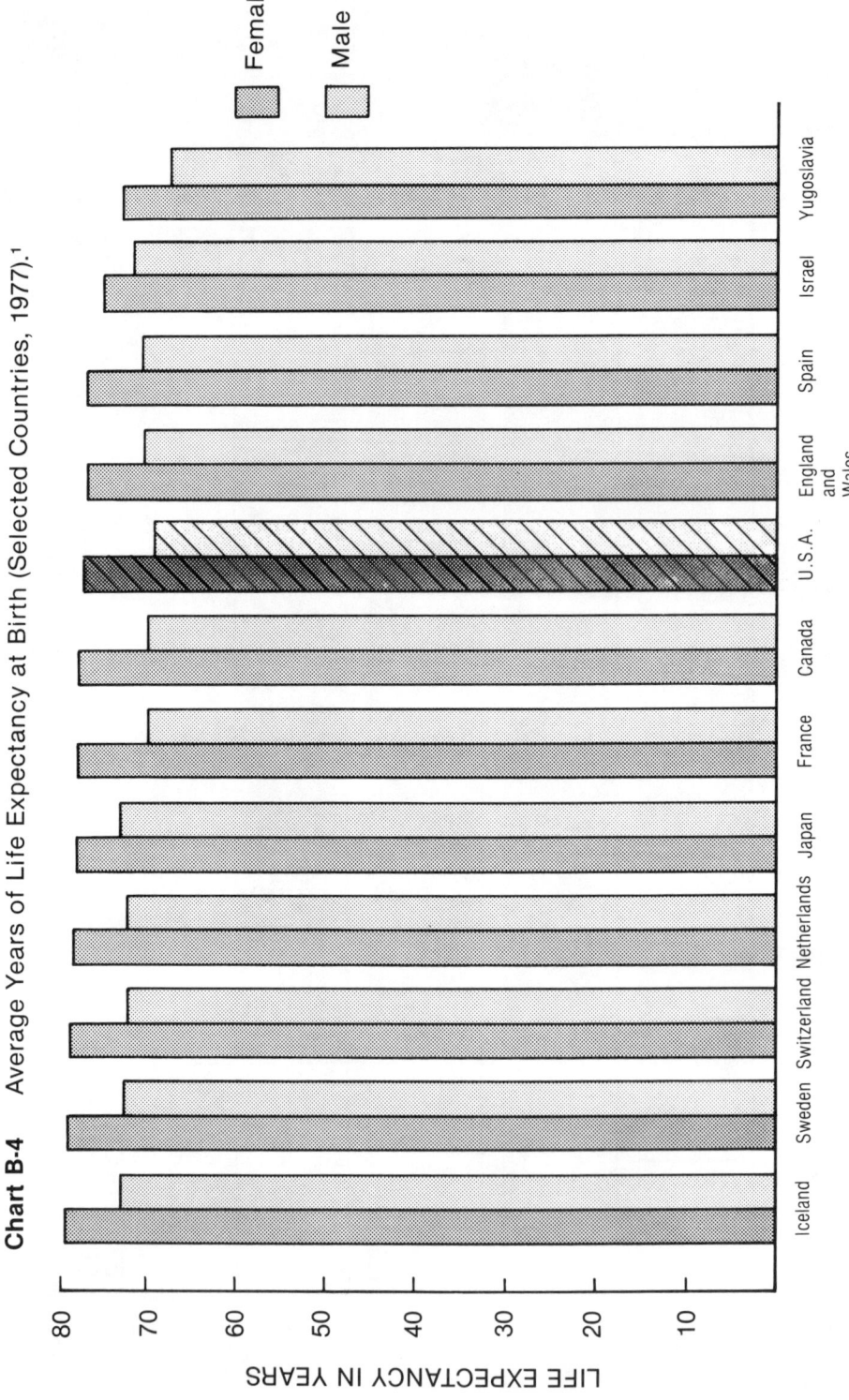

Chart B-4 Average Years of Life Expectancy at Birth (Selected Countries, 1977).[1]

[1] Data for Canada and Spain are for 1975; for France, U.S.A., and Yugoslavia data are for 1976.

SOURCE: World Health Organization, *World Health Statistics Annual, 1979, Vital Statistics and Causes of Death*, Geneva, Switzerland, 1979, Table 10, pp. 510–511.

Chart B-5

Ranking of Selected Countries by Expected Remaining Years of Life for Males at Age 45 (1975-1976).

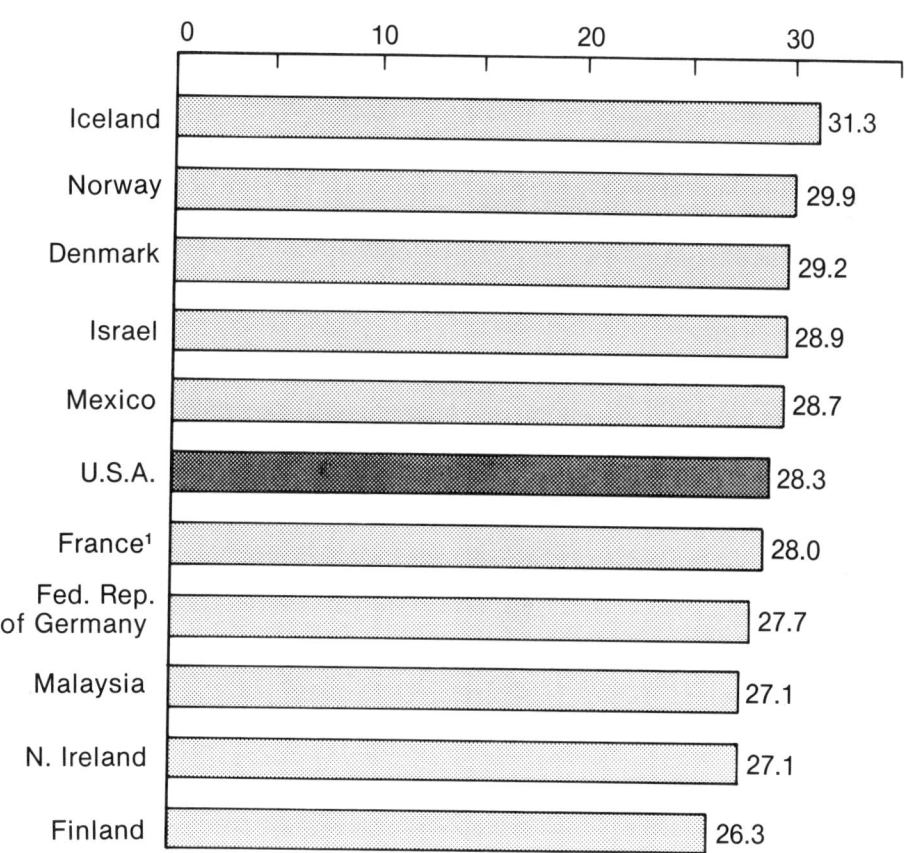

[1] 1974 data

SOURCE: Statistical Office of the United Nations, *Demographic Yearbook 1977*, Department of International Economic and Social Affairs, United Nations, New York, 1978, Table 22, pp. 442-463.

Chart B-6

Percent of All Deaths, by Specified Causes of Death[1] (U.S.A., 1900 and 1976).

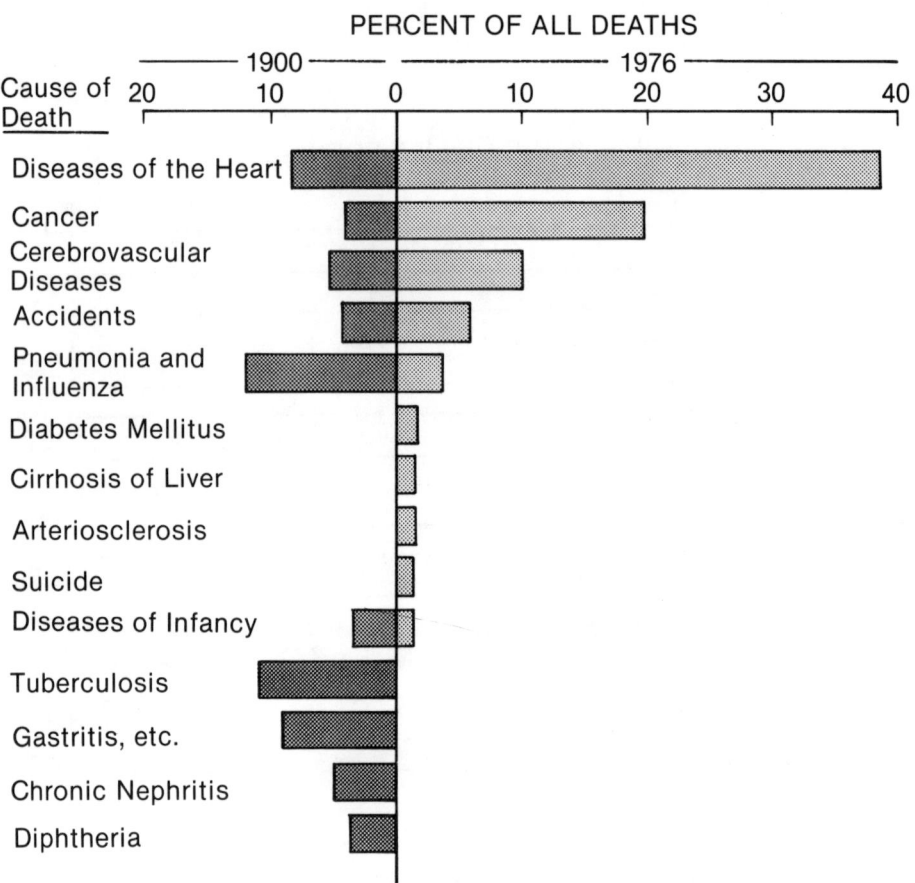

[1] Shows the 10 leading causes of death in 1900 (based on data from states that had death registration) and in 1976, with the latter arranged in descending order of importance.

SOURCES: For 1900: U.S. Department of Commerce and Labor, Bureau of the Census, *Mortality Statistics, 1900–1904*, U.S. Census Office, Washington, 1906, p. xx; for 1976: American Cancer Society, *Ca-A Cancer Journal for Clinicians*, Vol. 29, No. 1, 1979, p. 7.

Chart B-7

Infant Mortality Rates (Selected Countries, 1951 and 1976).

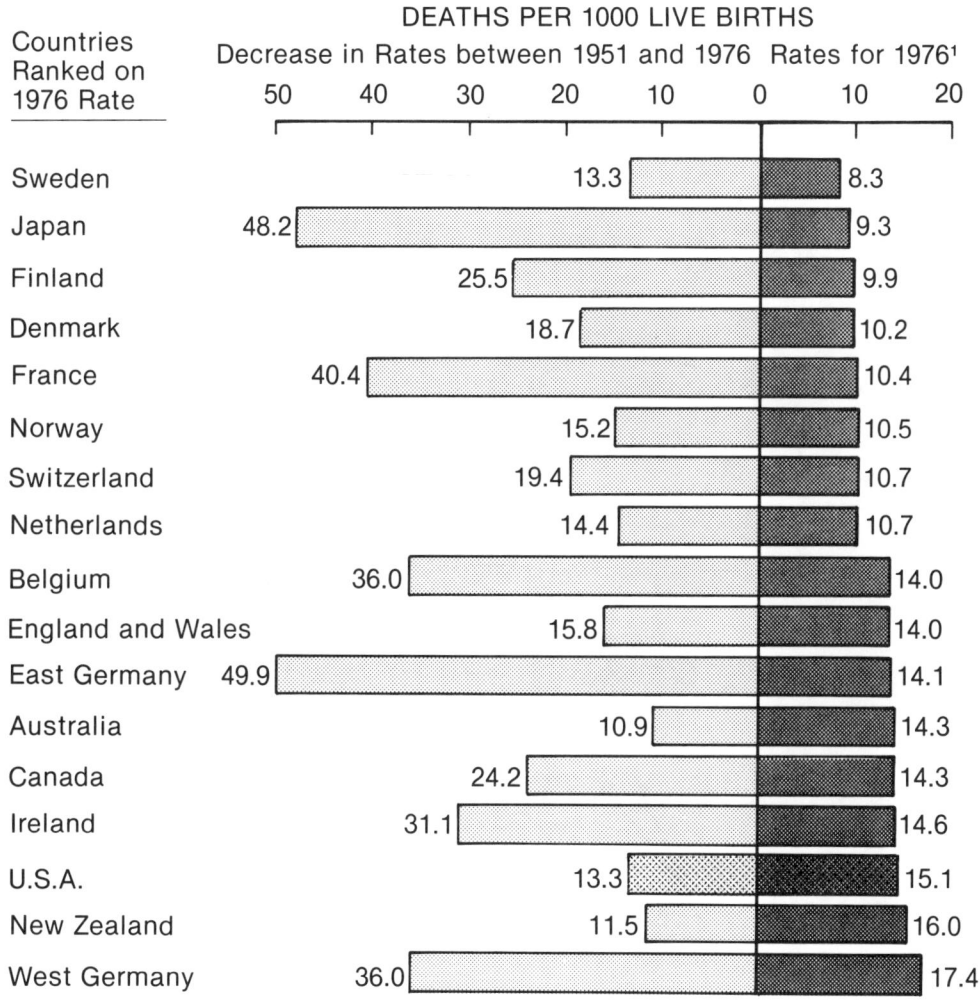

[1] Data for Canada, New Zealand, and Australia are for 1975.

SOURCES: For 1950: United Nations, *Demographic Yearbook, Ninth Issue*, New York, 1957, Table 9, pp. 200-209; for 1976: United Nations, *Demographic Yearbook, 29th Issue*, New York, 1978, Table 15, pp. 332-335.

Chart B-8 Neonatal and Post-neonatal Mortality Rates, by Color, in Logarithmic and Non-logarithmic Scales (U.S.A., Selected Years, 1915–1976).

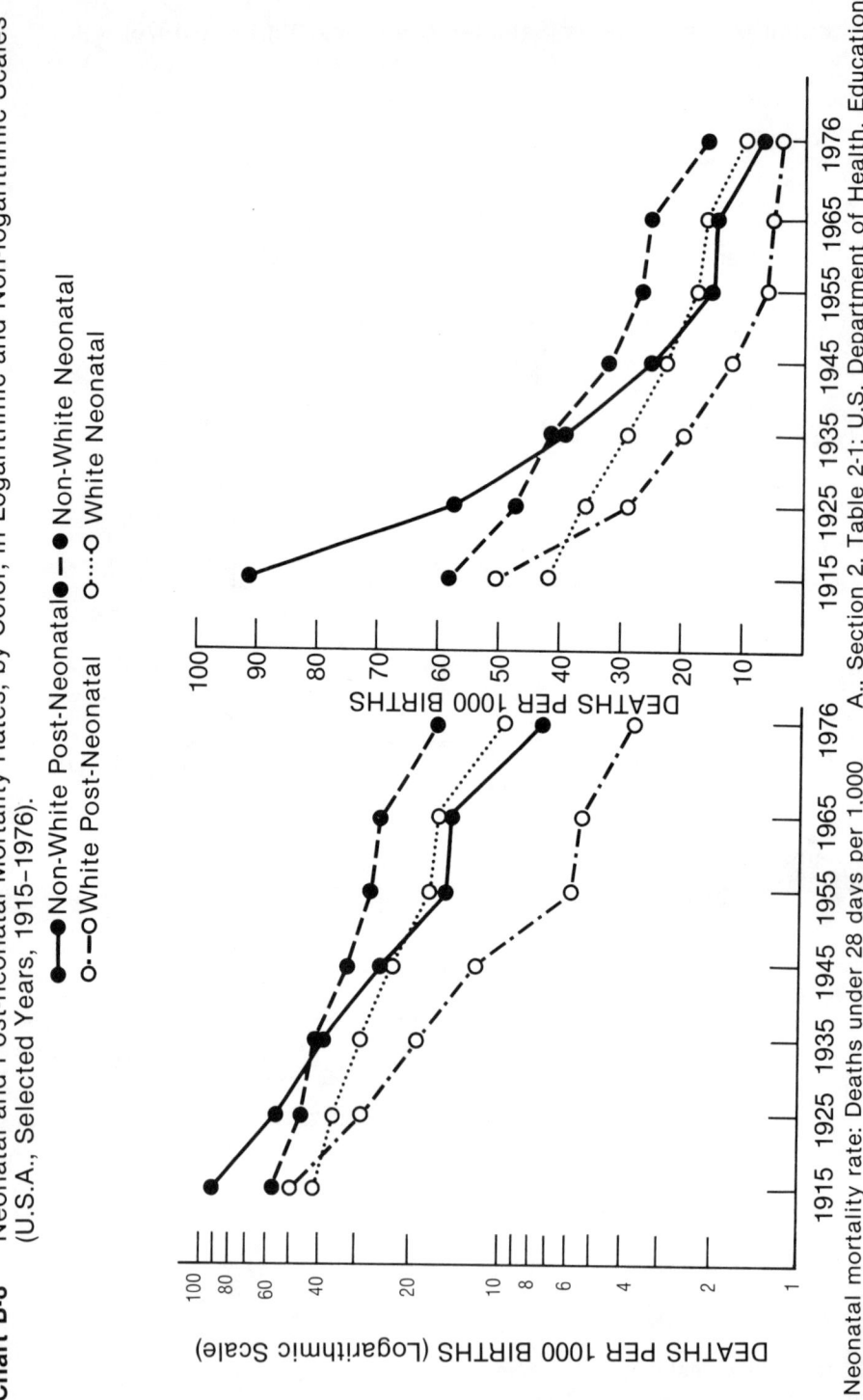

NOTE: Neonatal mortality rate: Deaths under 28 days per 1,000 live births; post-neonatal mortality rate: Deaths from 28 days to 11 months per 1,000 live births.

SOURCES: U.S. Department of Health, Education, and Welfare, *Vital Statistics of the United States, 1967*, Vol. II, Mortality, Part A., Section 2, Table 2-1; U.S. Department of Health, Education, and Welfare, *Vital Statistics of the United States, Provisional Statistics, Annual Summary for U.S., 1977*, "Births, Marriages, and Divorces," Vol. 26, No. 13, December 7, 1978, Table H, p. 10.

Chart B-9

Infant Mortality, by Social Class (England and Wales, 1911-1971).

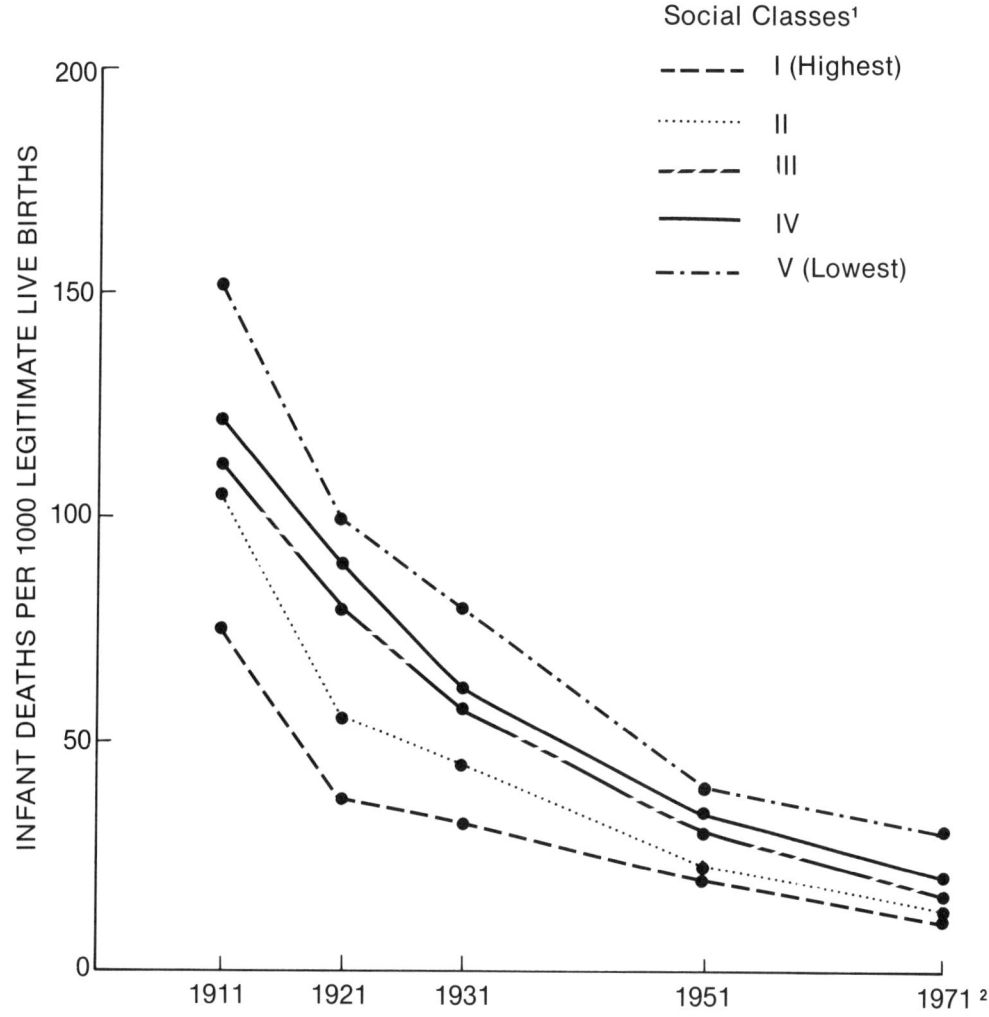

[1] Social class is based on the occupation of the father.
[2] Data for 1971 are for deaths per 1000 live births.
SOURCE: *Occupational Mortality*, Office of Population Censuses and Surveys, Registrar General's decennial supplement for England and Wales, 1970-72, Series DS, No. 1, London, Figure 8.2, p. 174.

Chart B-10 Infant Mortality Rates, by Risk Category,[1] Adequate or Inadequate Medical Care, and Race (New York City, 1968).

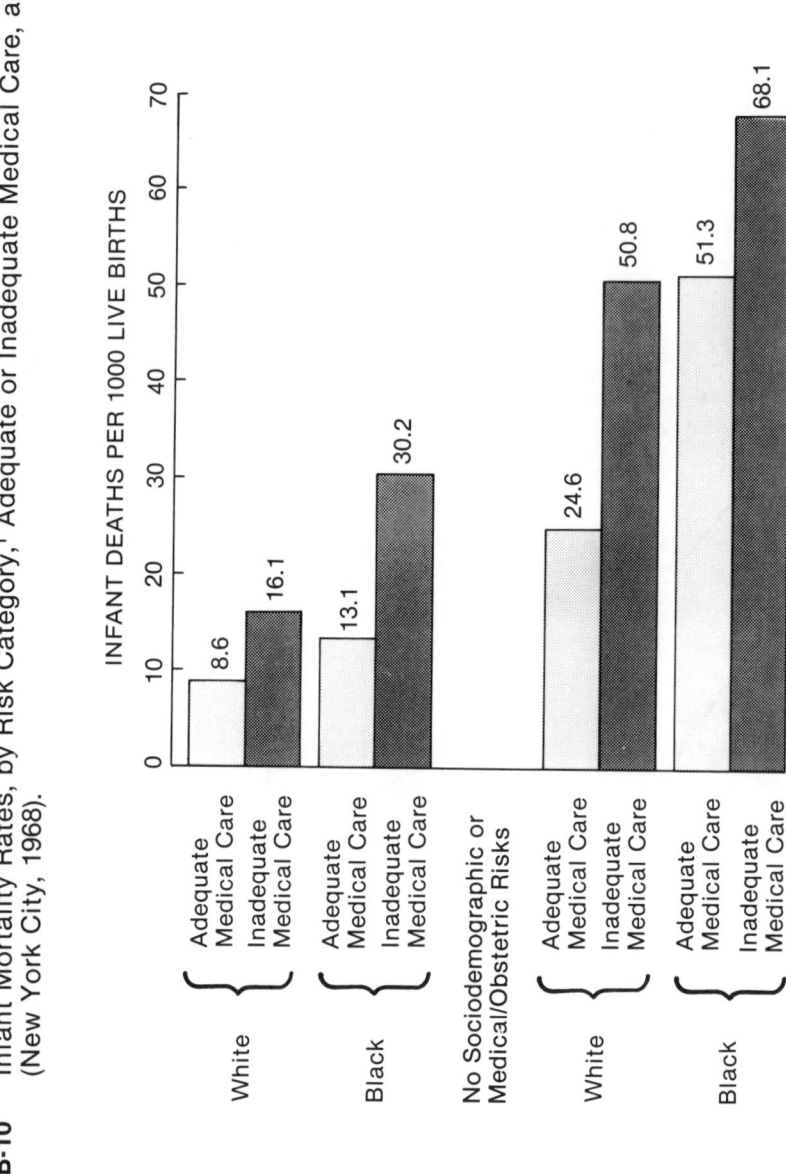

[1]Sociodemographic risks are determined by the age, education, and marital status of the mother. Medical/Obstetric risks are determined by the mother's pregnancy history and by the occurrence of other medical conditions which may have complicated the pregnancy.

SOURCE: Kessner, D.M., et al., *Infant Death: An Analysis by Maternal Risk and Health Care*, Institute of Medicine, National Academy of Sciences, Washington, D.C., 1973, Tables 1 and 2, p. 23.

Chart B-11

Infant Mortality Rates for White Mothers, by Family Income and Mother's Education (U.S.A., 1964-66).

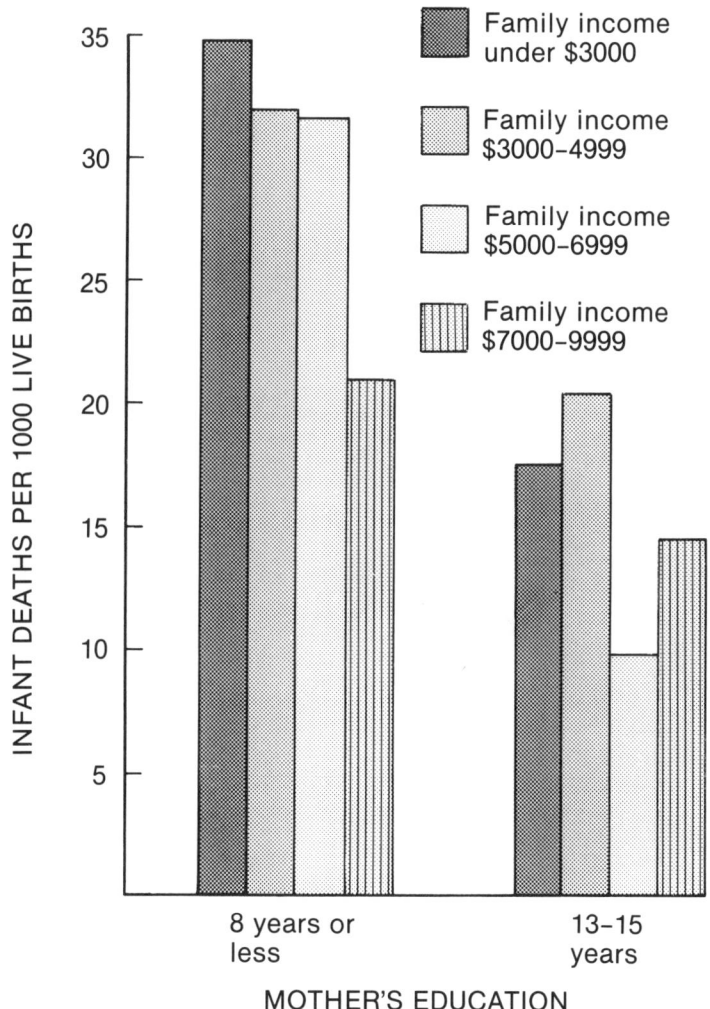

SOURCE: U.S. National Center for Health Statistics, *Infant Mortality Rates: Socioeconomic Factors, United States*, DHEW, Washington, D.C., Series 22, No. 14, March 1972, Table 3, p. 14.

Chart B-12

Percent Distribution of Acute Conditions, by Associated Activity Restriction and Medical Attention (U.S.A., Civilian Non-institutionalized Population, July 1976–June 1977.)

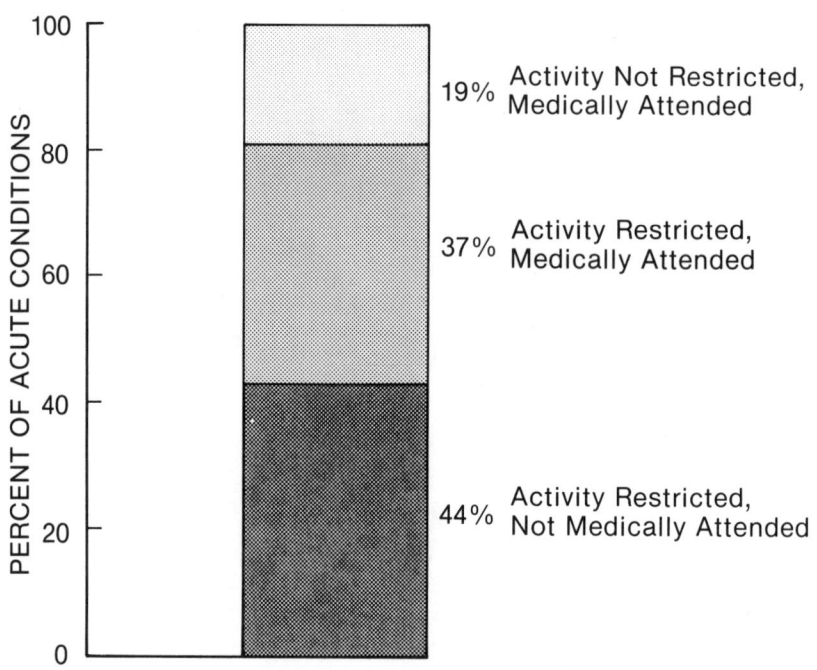

Acute Conditions, Associated Disability and Medical Attention	Incidence Per Person Per Year
All conditions	2.2
Activity not restricted and medically attended	0.4
Activity restricted and medically attended	0.8
Activity restricted and not medically attended	1.0
Days of bed disability	4.2
Days of restricted activity	9.4

SOURCE: U.S. National Center for Health Statistics, *Acute Conditions: Incidence and Associated Disability: United States, July 1976–1977,* Series 10, No. 125, September 1978, Table 1, p. 10, Table 2, p. 11, Table 3, p. 12, and Table 4, p. 13.

Mortality and Morbidity

Chart B-13

Incidence of Acute Conditions, Associated Days of Restricted Activity, and Days of Bed Disability, by Age (U.S.A., Civilian Non-institutionalized Population, July 1976– June 1977).

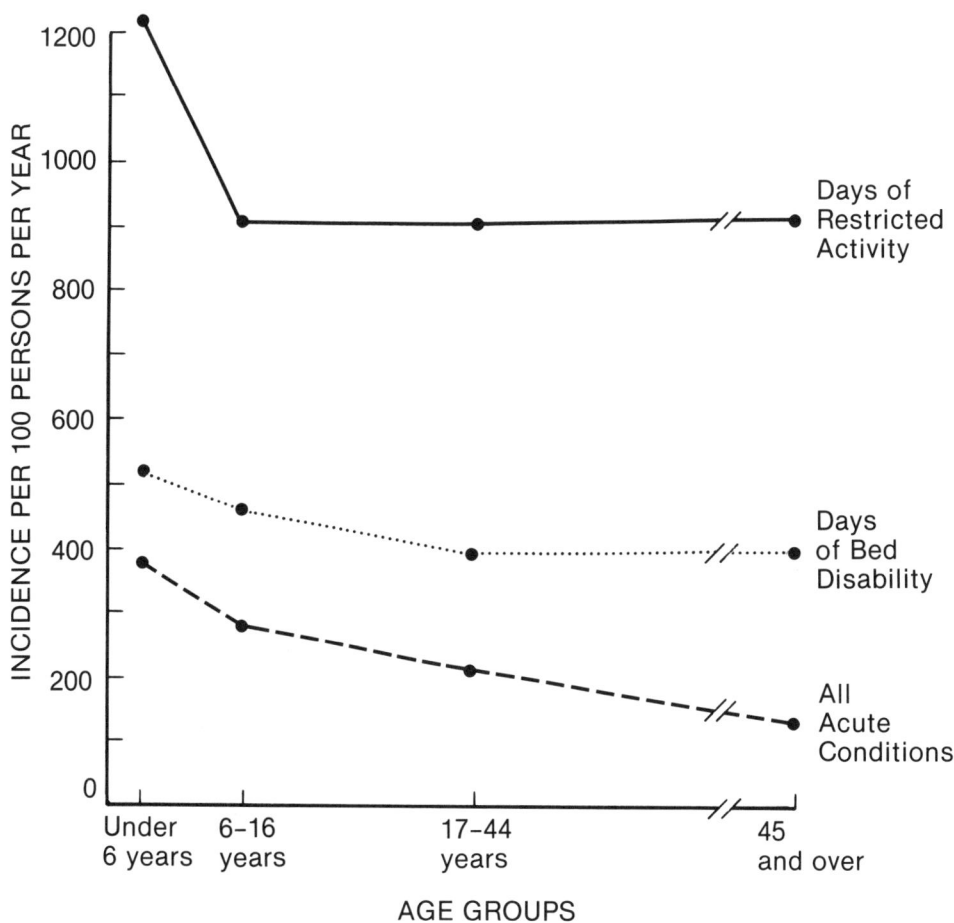

SOURCE: U.S. National Center for Health Statistics, *Acute Conditions: Incidence and Associated Disability: United States, July 1976–1977,* Public Health Service, Hyattsville, Maryland, Series 10, No. 125, September 1978, Table 5, p. 14, Table 6, p. 15, and Table 7, p. 16.

Mortality and Morbidity

Chart B-14

Percent Distribution of Population, by Degree of Chronic Activity Limitation (U.S.A., Civilian Non-institutionalized Population, 1974).

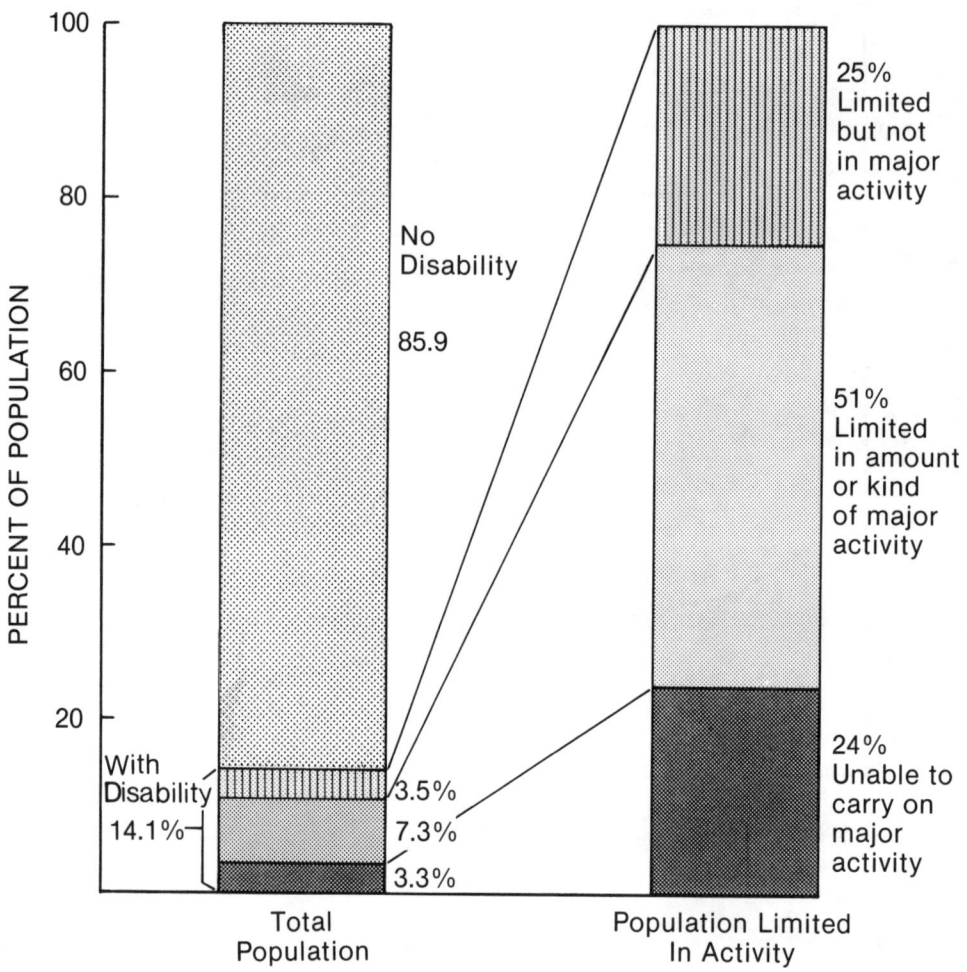

SOURCE: U.S. National Center for Health Statistics, *Limitation of Activity Due to Chronic Conditions: U.S., 1974,* DHEW, Public Health Service, Rockville, Maryland, Series 10, No. III, June 1977, Table 1, p. 14.

Chart B-15

Percent of Population with a Chronic Condition and with Specified Limitations, by Sex and Age (U.S.A., Civilian Non-institutionalized Population, 1977).

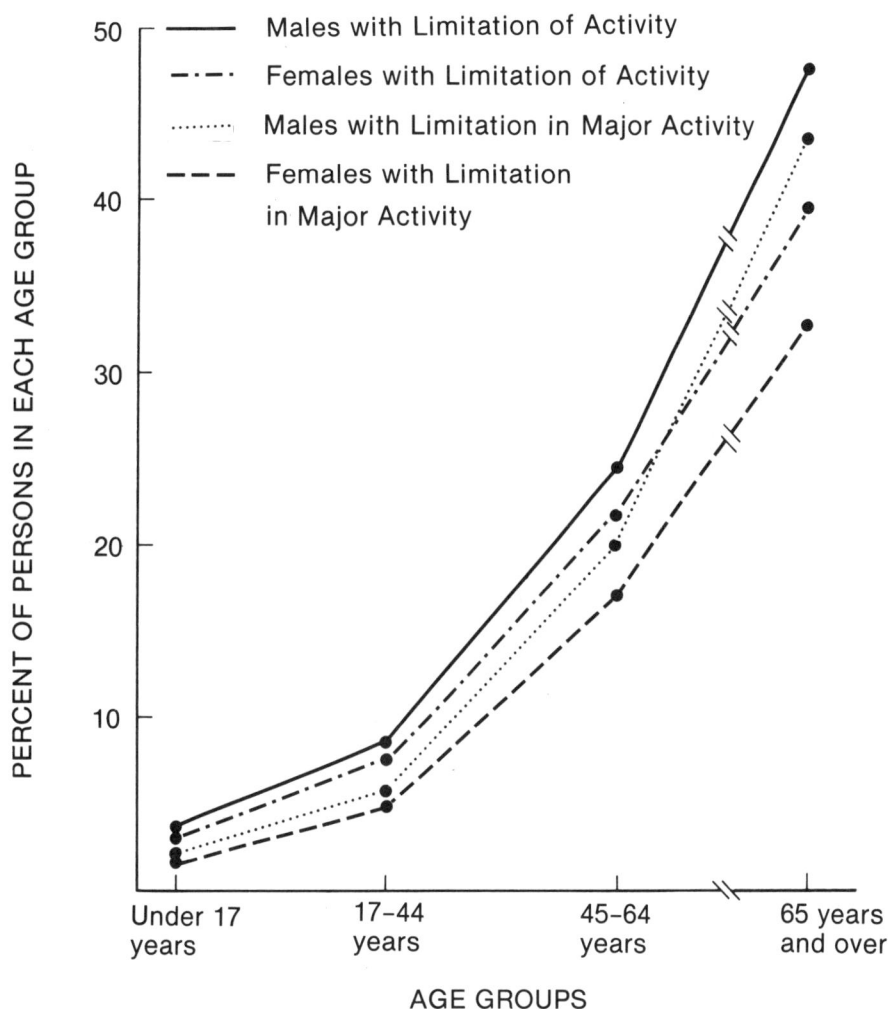

NOTE: "Major Activity" refers to ability to work, keep house, or engage in school or preschool activities.

SOURCE: U.S. National Center for Health Statistics, *Current Estimates From the Health Interview Survey: United States-1977*, DHEW, Public Health Service, Hyattsville, Maryland, Series 10, No. 126, September 1978, Table 14, p. 24.

Chart B-16

Days of Restricted Activity and Bed Disability per Person per Year, by Age and Sex (U.S.A., Civilian Non-institutionalized Population, 1977).

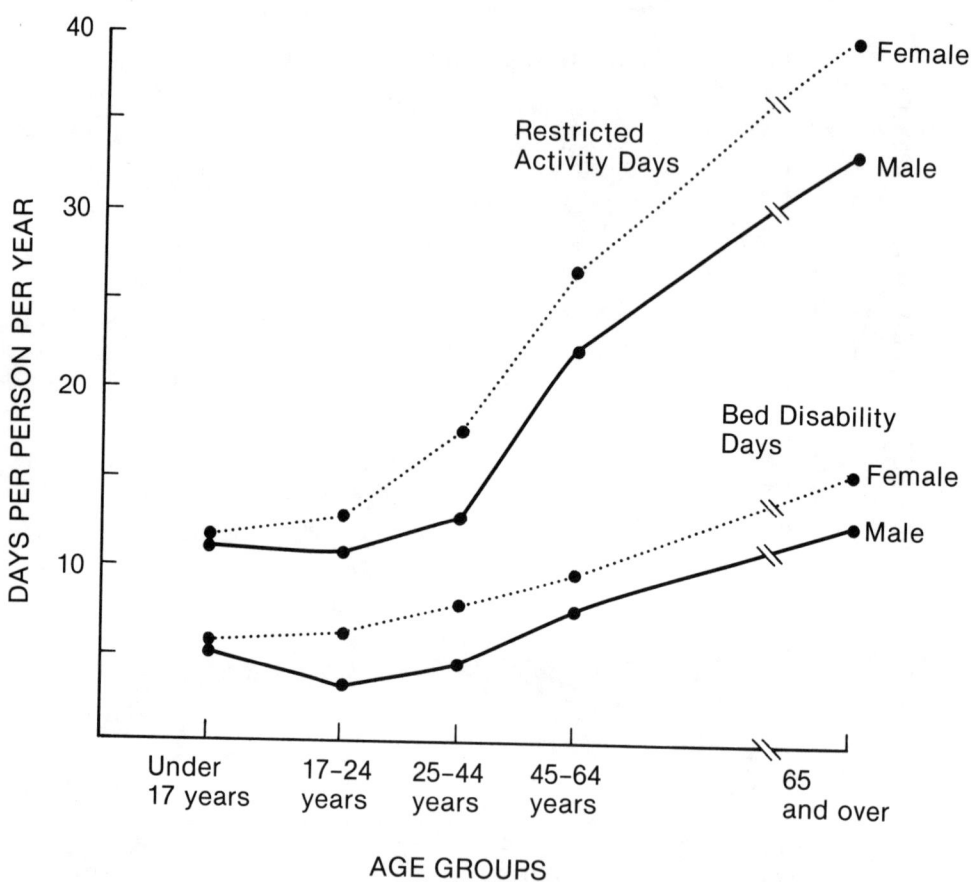

SOURCE: U.S. National Center for Health Statistics, *Current Estimates from the Health Interview Survey: United States, 1977*, DHEW, Public Health Service, Hyattsville, Maryland, Series 10, No. 126, September 1978, Table 12, p. 22.

Mortality and Morbidity

Chart B-17

Restricted Activity and Bed Disability Days per Person per Year, by Family Income (U.S.A., Civilian Non-institutionalized Population, 1975).

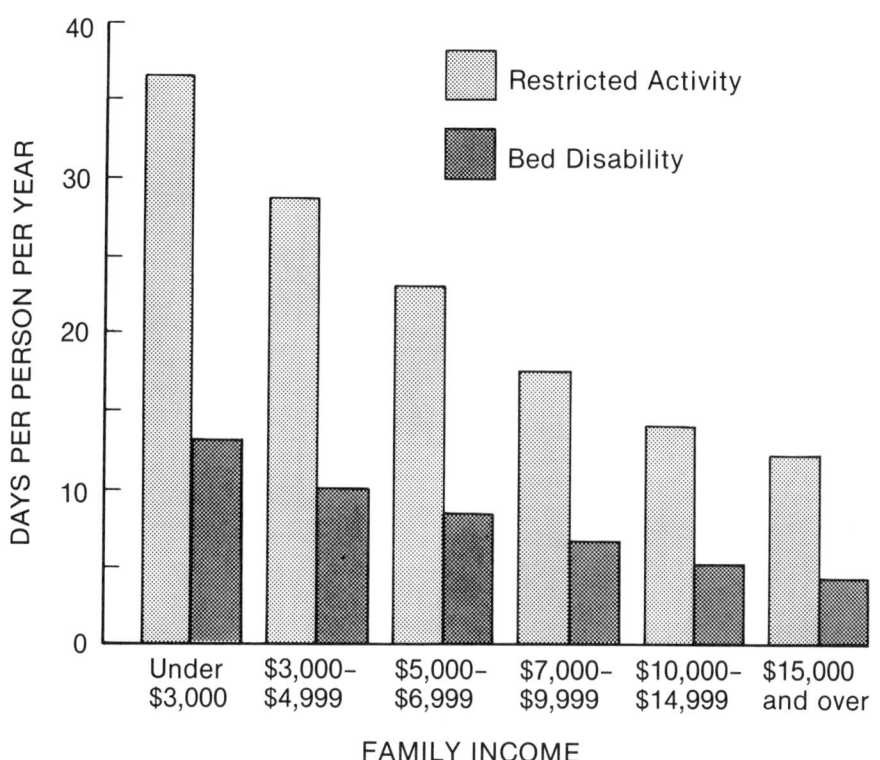

SOURCE: U.S. National Center for Health Statistics, *Disability Days: United States 1975,* Public Health Service, Hyattsville, Maryland, Series 10, No. 118, June 1978, Table H, p. 7.

Chart B-18

Percent of Civilian Non-institutionalized Population with Chronic Conditions Causing Activity Limitation, by Family Income (U.S.A., 1974).

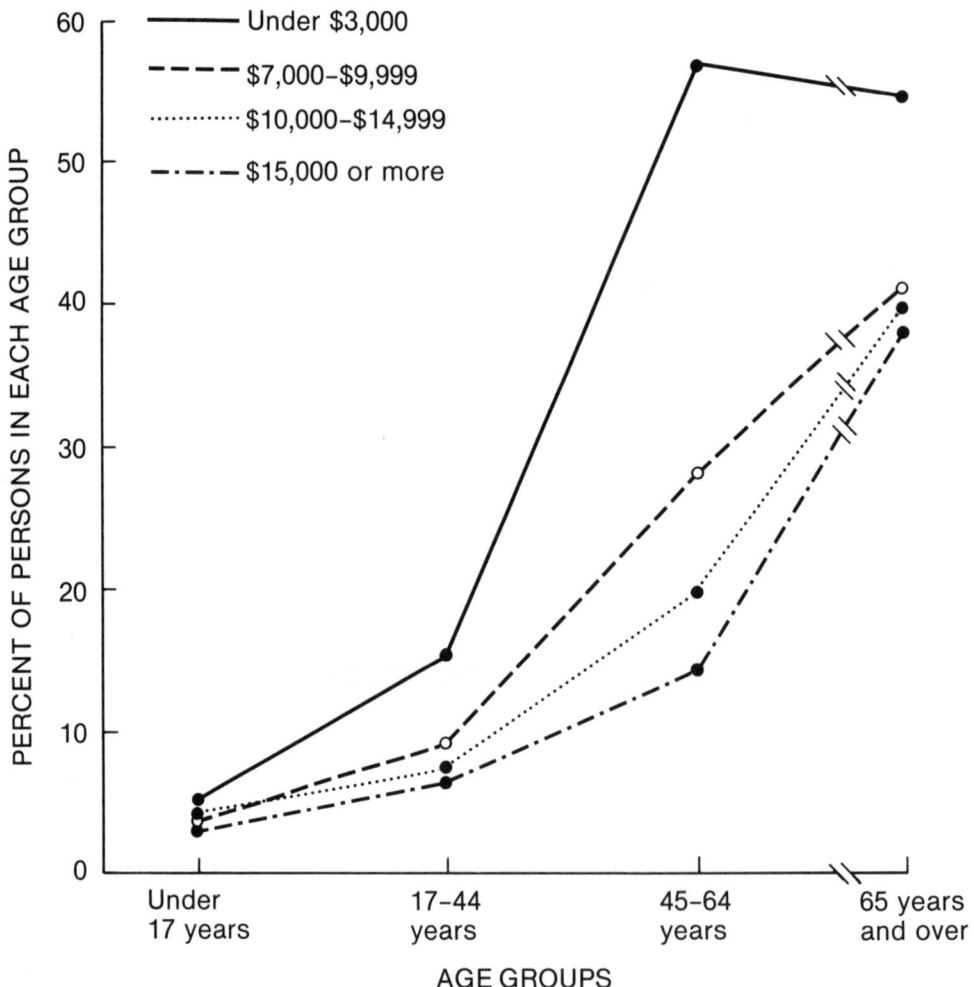

SOURCE: U.S. National Center for Health Statistics, *Limitation of Activity Due to Chronic Conditions: United States, 1974,* Public Health Service, Rockville, Maryland, Series 10, No. 111, June 1977, Table B, p. 5.

SECTION C
Use of Service

Chart C-1

Physician Visits per Person per Year, by Type of Visit (U.S.A., Civilian Non-institutionalized Population, Specified Periods).[1]

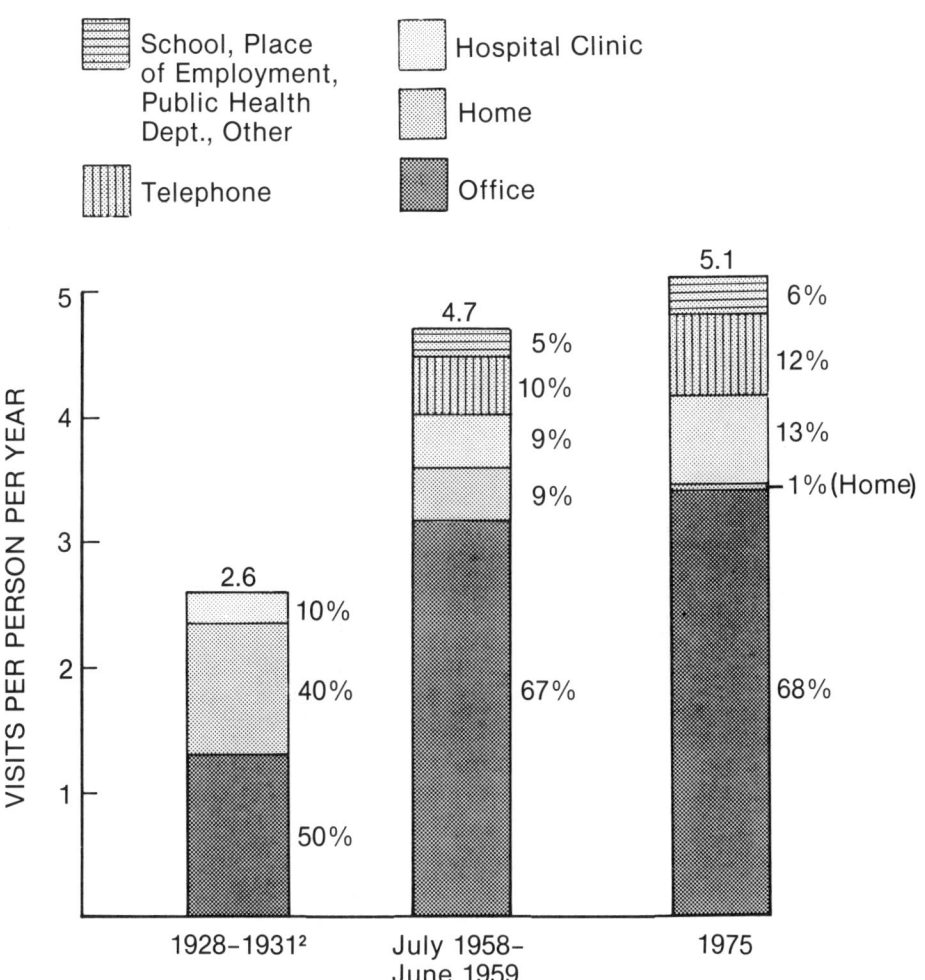

[1]Excludes visits to patients in hospitals. Numbers to the right of bars indicate percent of all visits.

[2]White families only.

SOURCES: For 1928-31: Falk, I.S., M.C. Klem, and N. Sinai, *The Incidence of Illness and the Receipt and Costs of Medical Care Among Representative Family Groups*, Publications of the Committee on Costs of Medical Care, No. 26, Chicago, Illinois, University of Chicago Press, 1933, Table B-27, p. 283; for 1958-59, and 1975: U.S. National Center for Health Statistics, *Physician Visits—Volume and Interval Since Last Visit: U.S. 1975*, Public Health Service, DHEW, Hyattsville, Maryland, Series 10, No. 97, 1975, Table C, p. 9, Table B, p. 5.

Chart C-2

Percent Distribution of Physician Visits, by Place of Visit and Color (U.S.A., Civilian Non-institutionalized Population, 1975).

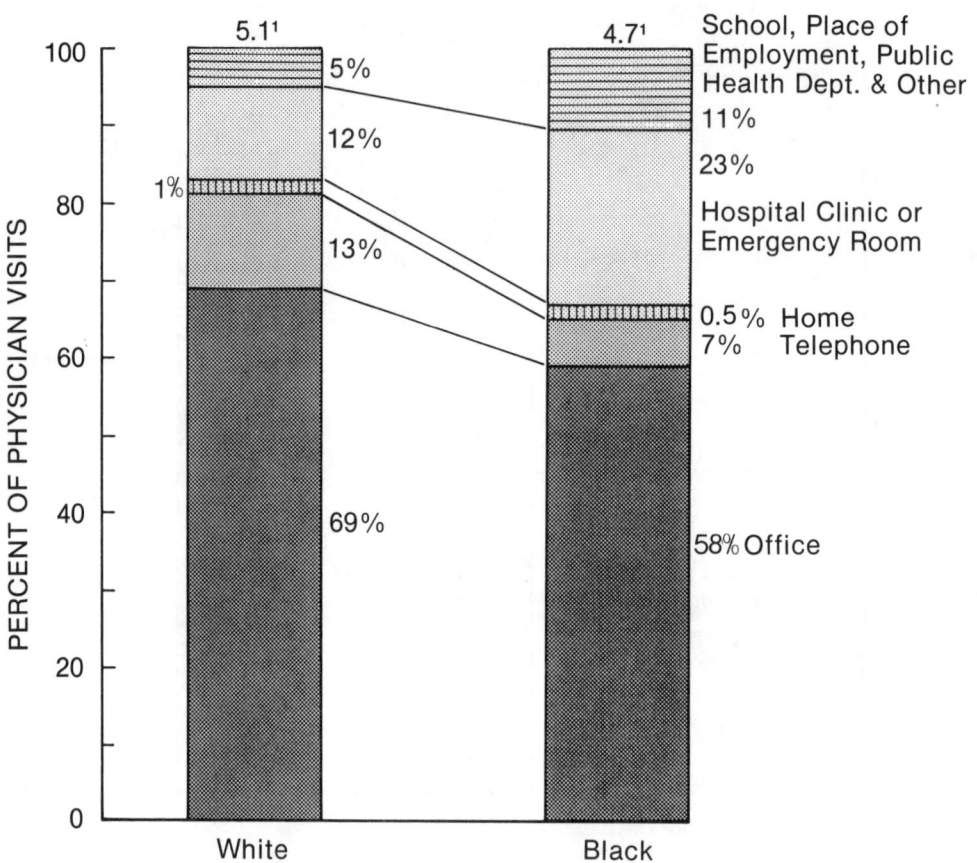

[1]Total number of physician visits per person per year, excluding visits to patients in hospitals.

SOURCE: U.S. National Center for Health Statistics, *Physician Visits, Volume and Interval Since Last Visit: U.S.-1975*, DHEW, Public Health Service, Office of Health Research, Statistics, and Technology, Hyattsville, Maryland, Series 10, No. 128, April 1979, Table 17, p. 31.

Use of Service

Chart C-3

Percent Distribution of Office Visits According to Physician Specialty, by Color of Patient (U.S.A., 1974 and 1977).

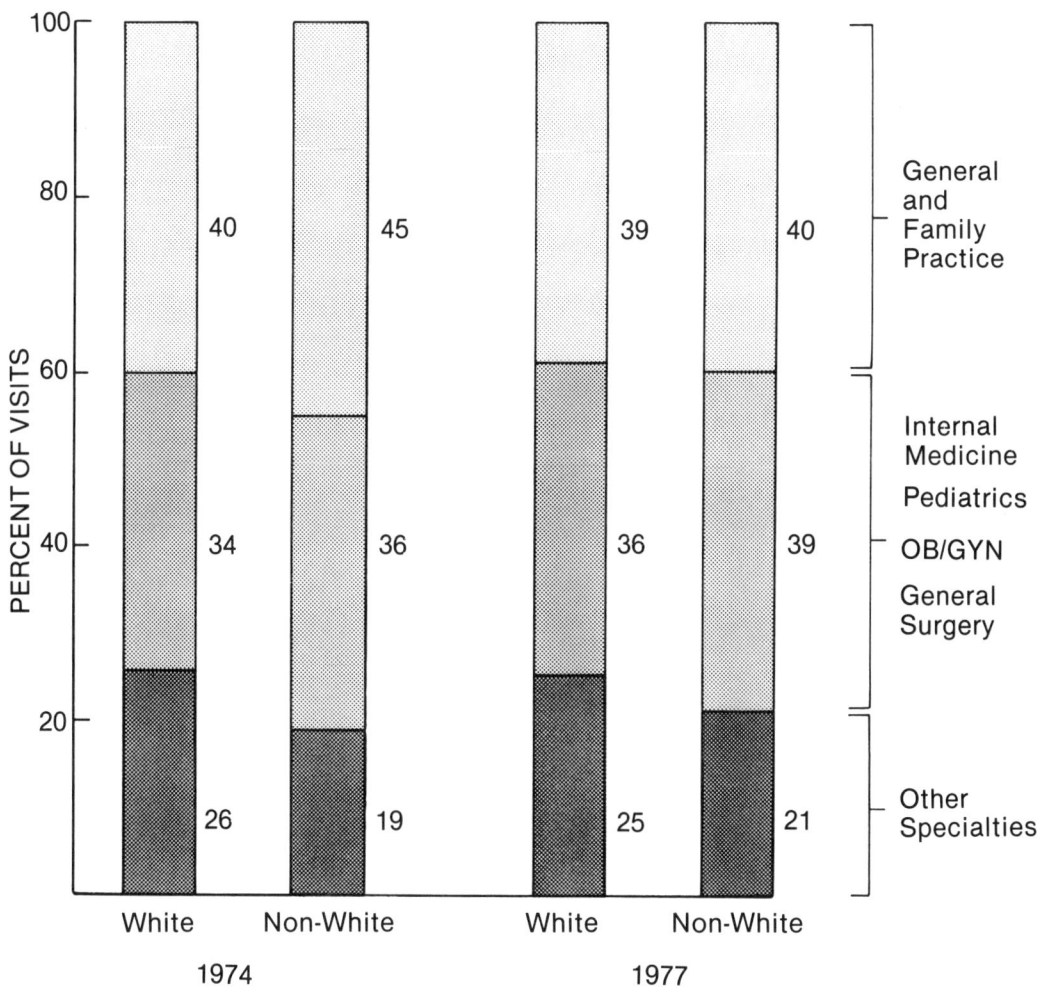

SOURCE: U.S. National Center for Health Statistics, *The National Ambulatory Medical Care Survey, 1977 Summary*, DHEW, Public Health Service, Office of Health Research, Statistics, and Technology, Hyattsville, Maryland, Series 13, No. 44, April 1980, Table 7, p. 21.

Chart C-4

Physician Visits per Person per Year, Excluding Visits to Patients in Hospitals, by Age and Sex
(U.S.A., Civilian Non-institutionalized Population, 1975).

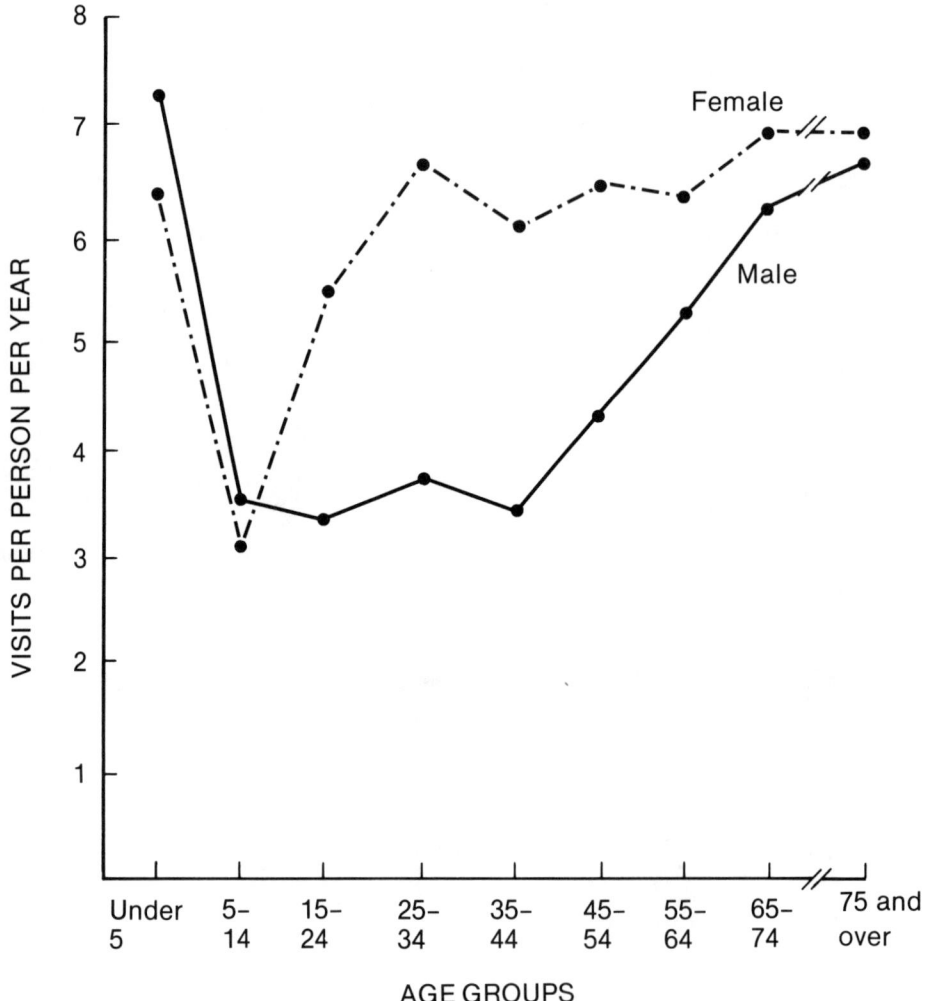

SOURCE: U.S. National Center for Health Statistics, *Physician Visits, Volume and Interval Since Last Visit: U.S., 1975*, DHEW, Public Health Service, Office of Health Research, Statistics, and Technology, Hyattsville, Maryland, Series 10, No. 128, April 1979, Table 11, p. 25.

Use of Service

Chart C-5

Number of Physician Visits in Each Age Group, by Education of Family Head and Residence (U.S.A., Civilian Non-institutionalized Population, 1975).[1]

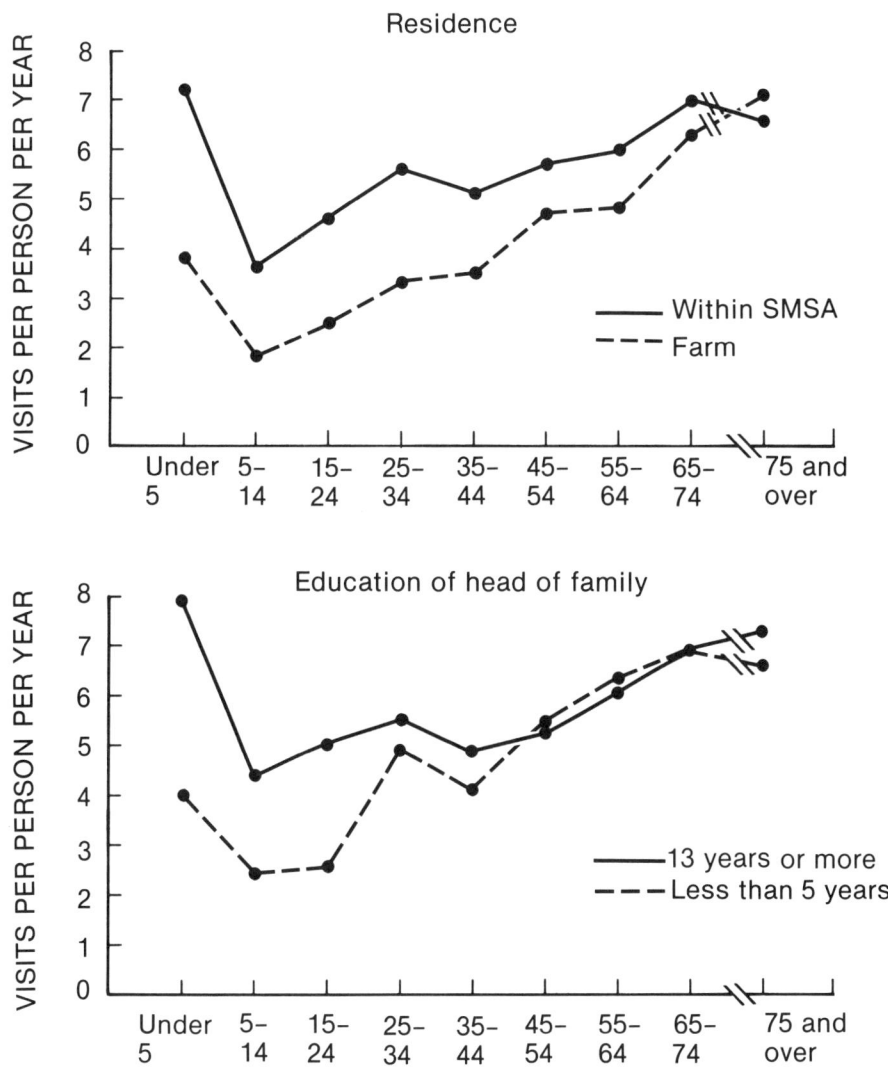

[1] Excludes visits to patients in hospitals.

SOURCE: U.S. National Center for Health Statistics, *Physician Visits—Volume and Interval Since Last Visit: U.S. 1975*, DHEW, Public Health Service, Office of Health Research, Statistics, and Technology, Hyattsville, Maryland, Series 10, No. 128, April 1979, Table 11, p. 25 and Table 4, p. 18.

Use of Service

Chart C-6

Physician Visits per Person per Year, by Age and Income (U.S.A., Civilian Non-institutionalized Population, 1975).[1]

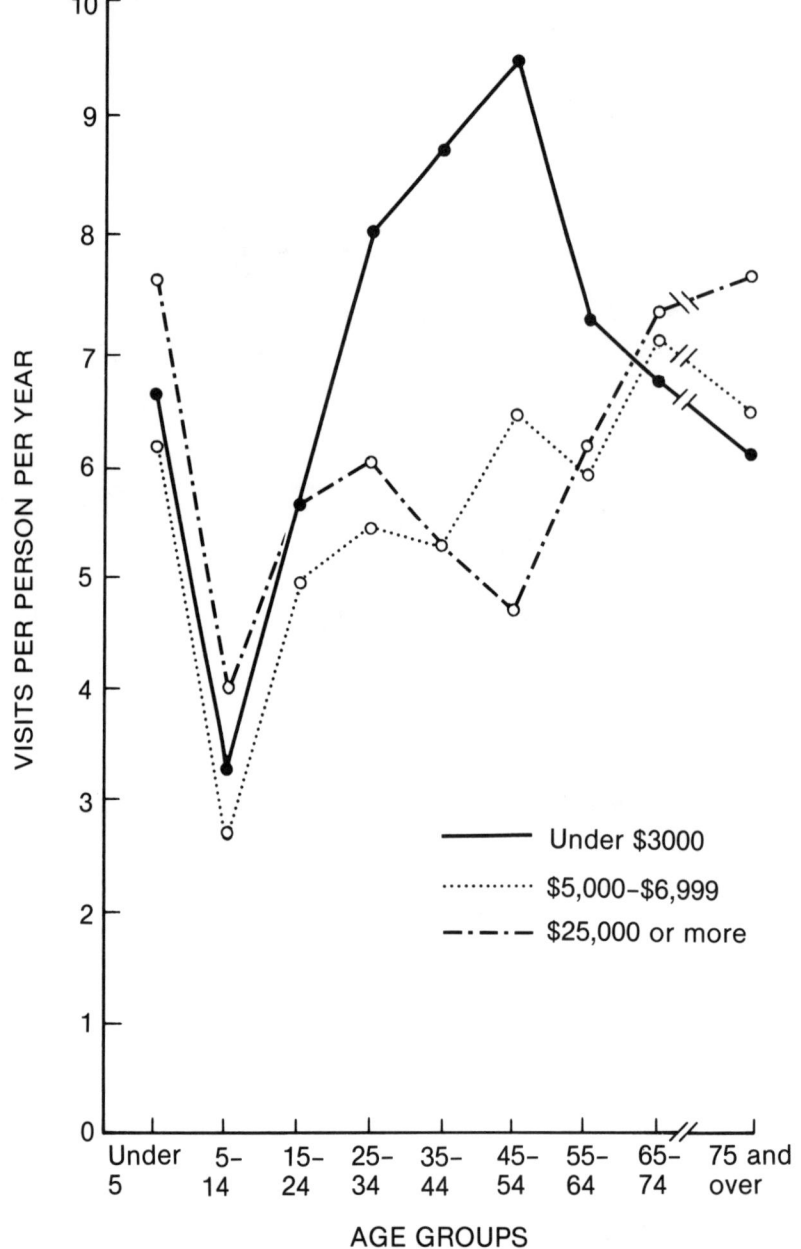

[1]Excludes visits to patients in hospitals.

SOURCE: U.S. National Center for Health Statistics, *Physician Visits, Volume and Interval Since Last Visit: U.S.,1975*, DHEW, Public Health Service, Office of Health Research, Statistics, and Technology, Hyattsville, Maryland, April 1979, Table 7, p. 21.

Use of Service

Chart C-7

Number of Physician Visis per Person per Year, by Family Income, Adjusted to 1967 Dollars (U.S.A., Civilian Non-institutionalized Population, 1964, 1967, 1975).[1]

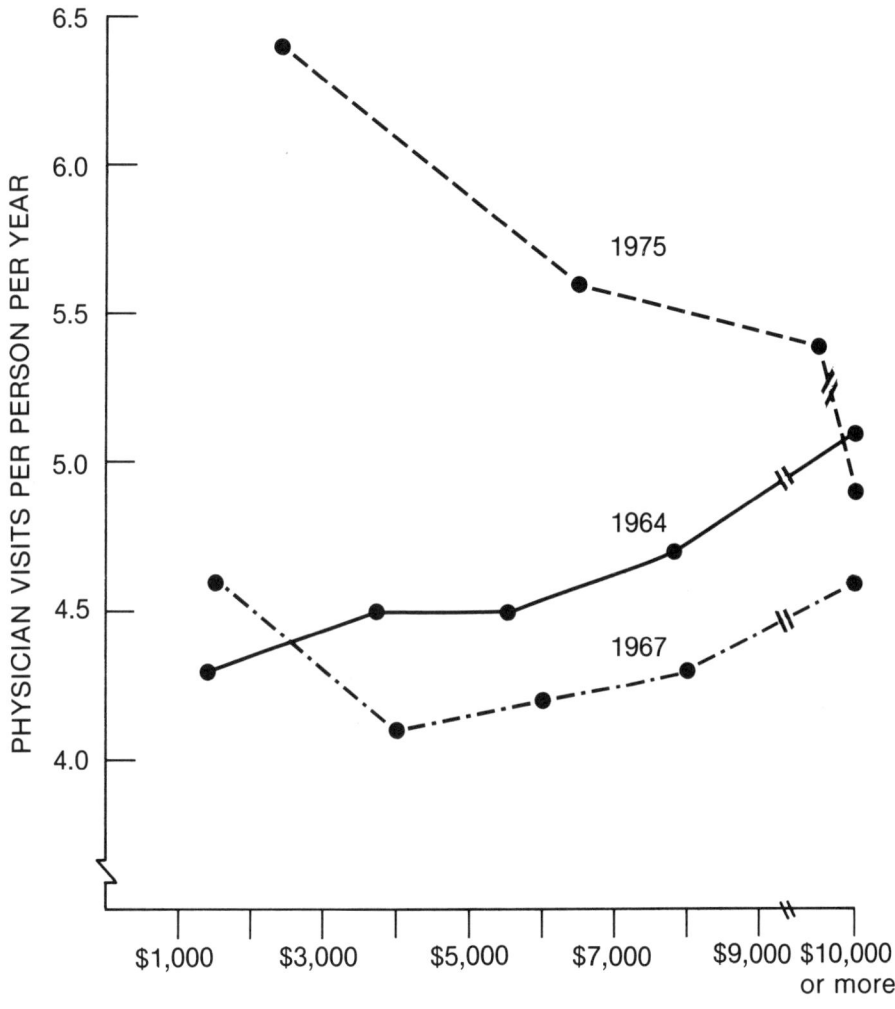

FAMILY INCOME (in 1967 dollars)

[1] Excludes visits to patients in hospitals.

SOURCES: U.S. Department of Commerce, Bureau of the Census, *Statistical Abstract of the U.S., 1978,* Washington, D.C., 1978, Table 792, p. 496; for 1964 and 1967: U.S. National Center for Health Statistics, *Volume of Physician Visits: United States—July 1966-June 1967,* DHEW, Public Health Service, Health Services and Mental Health Administration, Washington, D.C., Series 10, No. 49, November 1968, Table A, p. 3; for 1975: U.S. National Center for Health Statistics, *Physician Visits: Volume and Interval Since Last Visit— United States—1975,* DHEW, Public Health Service, Office of Health Research, Statistics, and Technology, Hyattsville, Maryland, Series 10, No. 128, April 1979, Table 7, p. 21.

Chart C-8

Relative Number of Physician Visits per Person per Year, by Income and Type of Visits (U.S.A., Civilian Non-institutionalized Population, 1975).

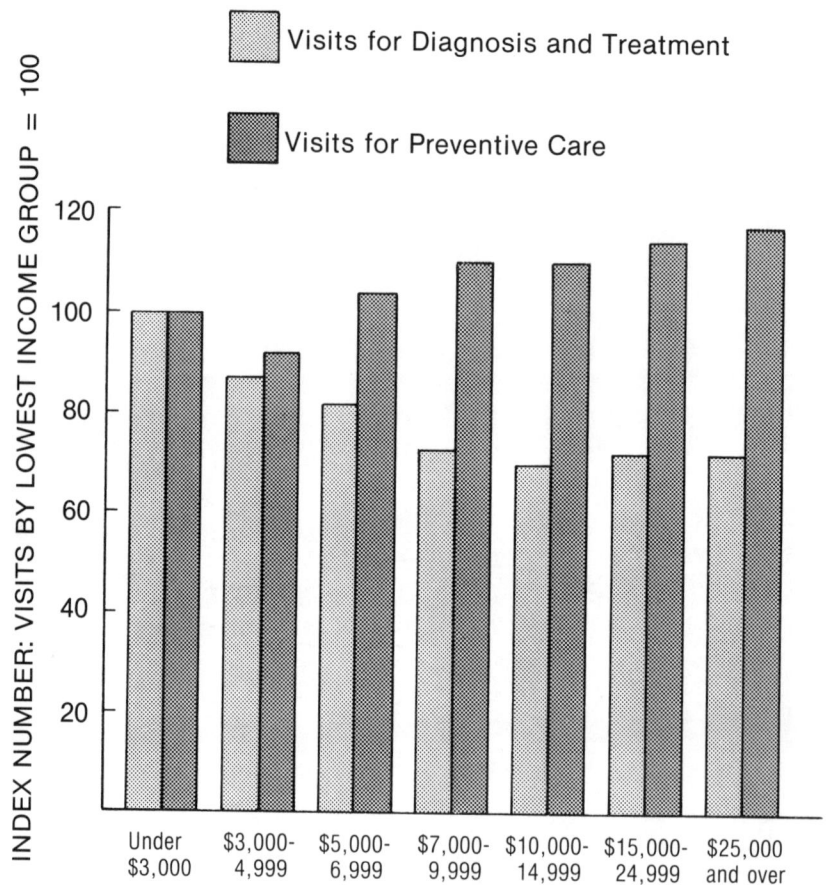

NOTE: Preventive Care visits consist of the following: (a) pre- and post-natal care; (b) routine checkups and checkups for specific purposes such as employment or insurance, in which no diagnosis is made; (c) immunizations provided by a physician or under a physician's supervision; and (d) visits for eye refractions, for preventive services not included in the preceding categories, and visits for which the type of service provided is unknown.

SOURCE: U.S. National Center for Health Statistics, *Physician Visits— Volume and Interval Since Last Visit: U.S. 1975,* DHEW, Public Health Service, Office of Health Research, Statistics, and Technology, Hyattsville, Maryland, Series 10, No. 128, April 1979, Table 3, p. 17 and Table 19, p. 33.

Use of Service

Chart C-9

Percent of Women with Live Births Who Saw a Physician During First Trimester of Pregnancy, by Education (U.S.A., 1953, 1958, 1963, and 1970).

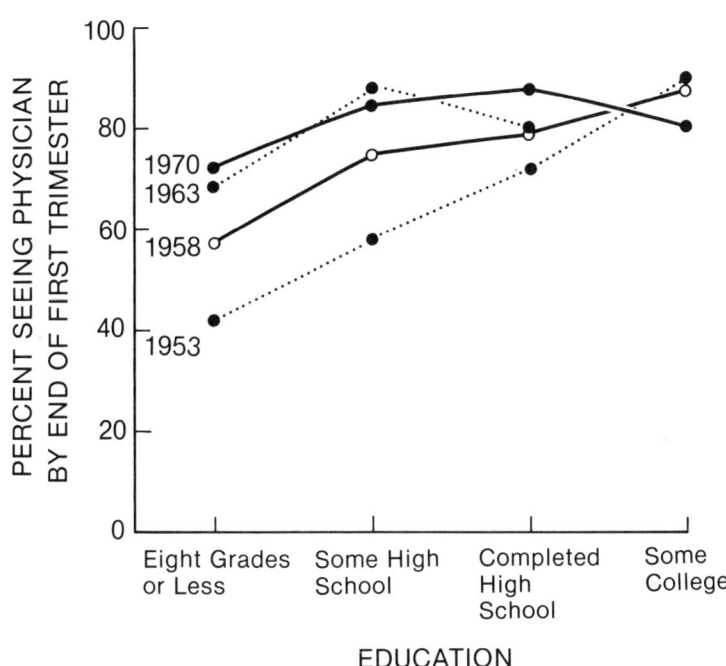

SOURCE: Andersen, Ronald, et al., *Health Service Use: National Trends and Variations*, United States Department of Health, Education and Welfare, October 1972, Table 15, p. 22.

Chart C-10

Percent of Mothers Judged to Have Received Adequate Amounts of Prenatal Care, by Income and Education (One Area of Boston, June 1956).[1]

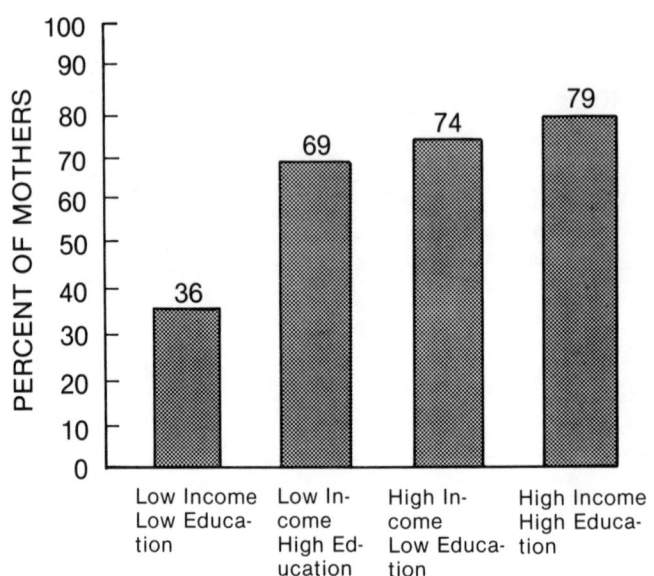

[1] In this study, "high-income" was considered $4000 or over and "high-education" 12 years of schooling or over. There were only 19 mothers in the "high-income," "low-education" group.

SOURCE: Donabedian, A. and L.S. Rosenfeld, "Some Factors Influencing Prenatal Care," *New England Journal of Medicine*, Vol. 265, July 6, 1961, pp. 1–6.

Use of Service

Medical Care Chartbook   45

Chart C-11 Percent Distribution of Single Live Births by Color and Occupational Group of Father and by Source of Delivery Care (New York City, 1955).[1]

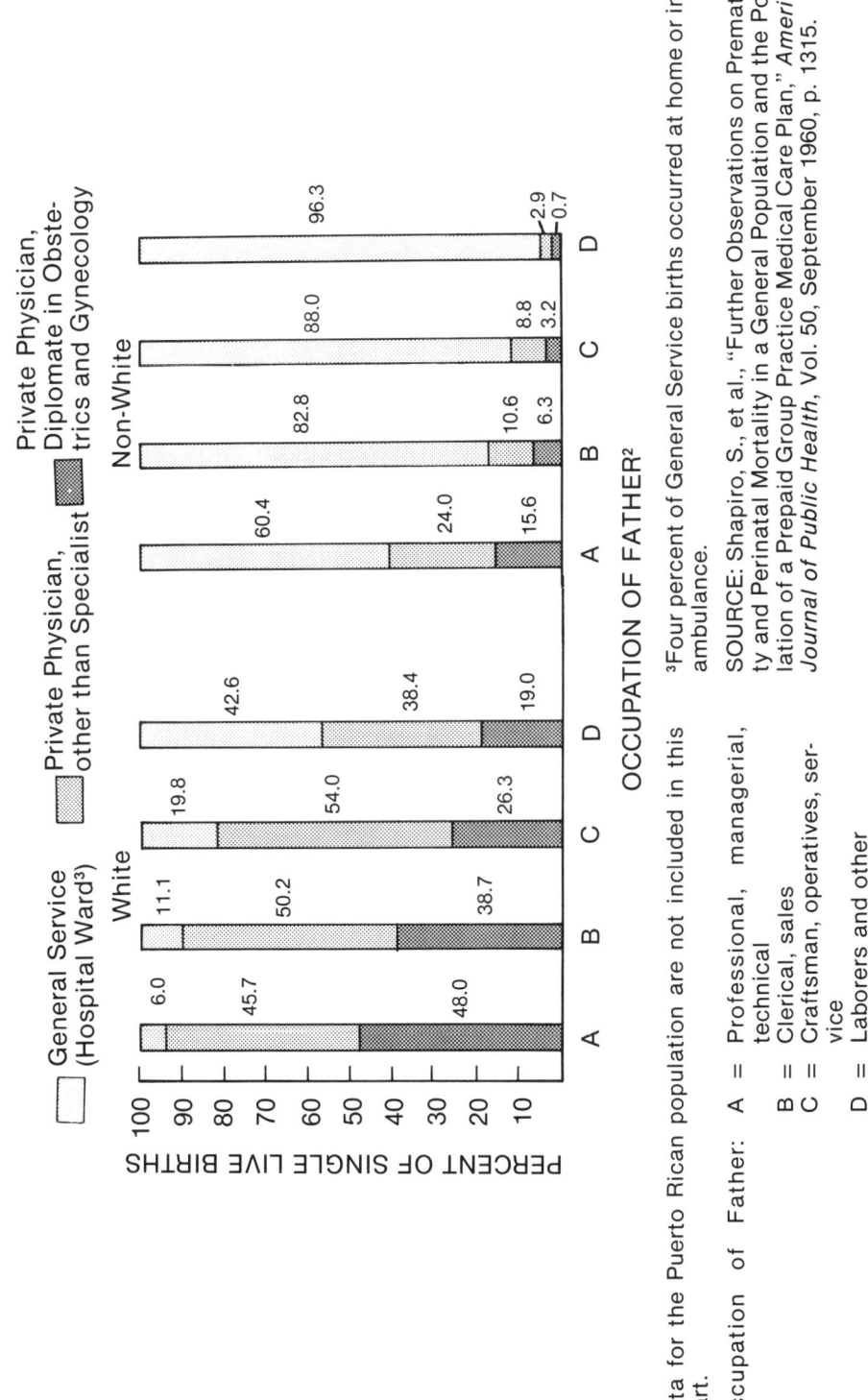

[1] Data for the Puerto Rican population are not included in this chart.

[2] Occupation of Father: A = Professional, managerial, technical
B = Clerical, sales
C = Craftsman, operatives, service
D = Laborers and other

[3] Four percent of General Service births occurred at home or in an ambulance.

SOURCE: Shapiro, S., et al., "Further Observations on Prematurity and Perinatal Mortality in a General Population and the Population of a Prepaid Group Practice Medical Care Plan," *American Journal of Public Health*, Vol. 50, September 1960, p. 1315.

Use of Service

Chart C-12

Opinion of Mothers Concerning the Initiation of Prenatal Care and Their Performance in Actually Receiving Care, by Family Income (Metropolitan Boston, July 1956).[1]

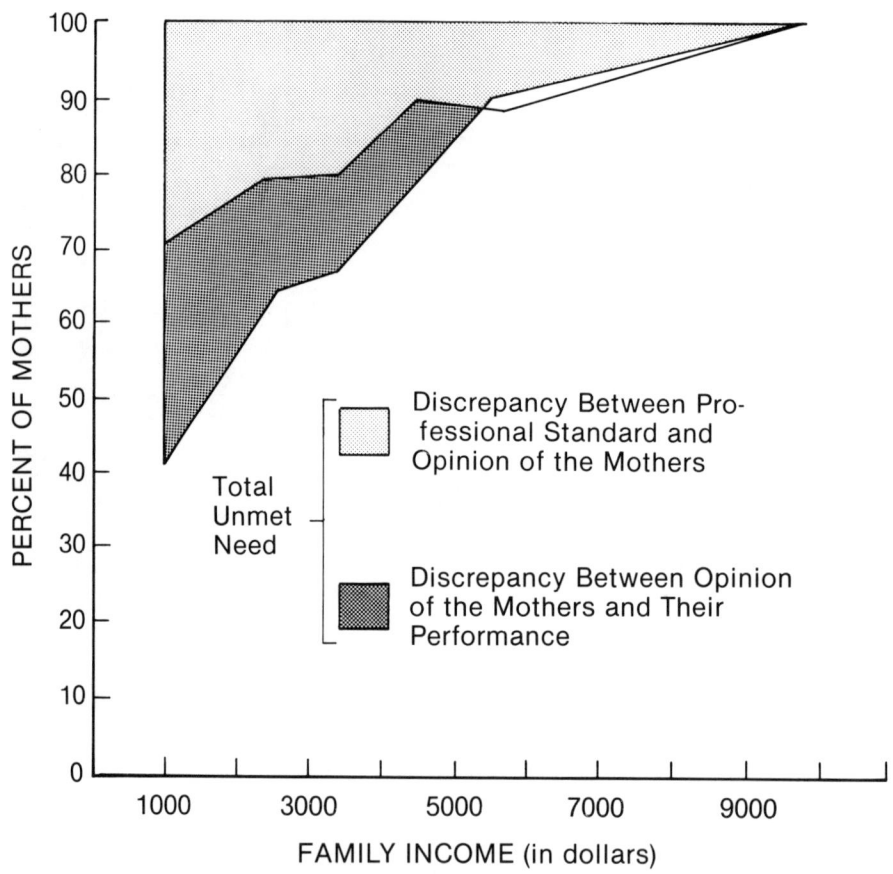

[1]"Opinion" refers to the percentage of mothers expressing the opinion that prenatal visits should start during the first three months of pregnancy; "Performance" refers to the percentage of mothers actually making the first prenatal visit after missing not more than three regular menstrual periods.

NOTE: The slight superiority of performance over opinion in one income group ($5000–$6999) may be an artifact resulting from the different wording of the questions concerning performance and opinion or due to a small number of non-response to one or other of the two questions.

SOURCE: Donabedian, A. and L.S. Rosenfeld, "Some Factors Influencing Prenatal Care," *New England Journal of Medicine*, Vol. 265, July 6, 1971, pp. 1–6.

Use of Service

Chart C-13 Percent of Respondents Who Recognized Specified Symptoms as Requiring Medical Attention and Percent of Respondents Who Received Medical Treatment for Specified Symptoms, by Social Class or Socioeconomic Status of Respondents ("Regionville,"[1] 1946–1950, and Boston, 1956).

Symptoms	Percent Recognizing Symptom as Requiring Medical Attention		Percent Receiving Medical Treatment for Symptom	
	Class I[2]	Class II	Groups IV & V[2]	Groups I & II
Loss of Appetite	57	20	78	68
Persistent Backache	53	19	90	46
Continued Coughing	80	23	57	61
Persistent Joint & Muscle Pains	80	19	72	53
Blood in Stool	98	60	58	42
Blood in Urine	100	69	100	80
Excessive Vaginal Bleeding	92	54	—	—
Swelling of Ankles	77	23	—	—
Loss of Weight	80	21	100	45
Bleeding of Gums	79	20	—	—
Chronic Fatigue	80	19	65	52
Shortness of Breath	77	21	74	54
Persistent Headaches	80	22	56	60
Fainting Spells	80	33	82	56
Pain in Chest	80	31	80	83
Lump in Breast	94	44	—	—
Lump in Abdomen	92	34	—	—

[1] A rural community in New York State.
[2] The "higher" of the two social classes or socioeconomic groupings.

SOURCES: Data on the Recognition of Symptoms: Koos, E.L., *The Health of Regionville*, Columbia University Press, New York, 1954; Data on Treatment by Symptom: Rosenfeld, L. S., J. Katz and A. Donabedian, *Medical Care Needs and Services in the Boston Metropolitan Area*, United Community Services, Boston, 1957.

Chart C-14

Relative Number of Physician Visits of Persons with Limited Activity, and of Bed Disability Days, by Family Income (U.S.A., Civilian Non-institutionalized Population, 1975).[1]

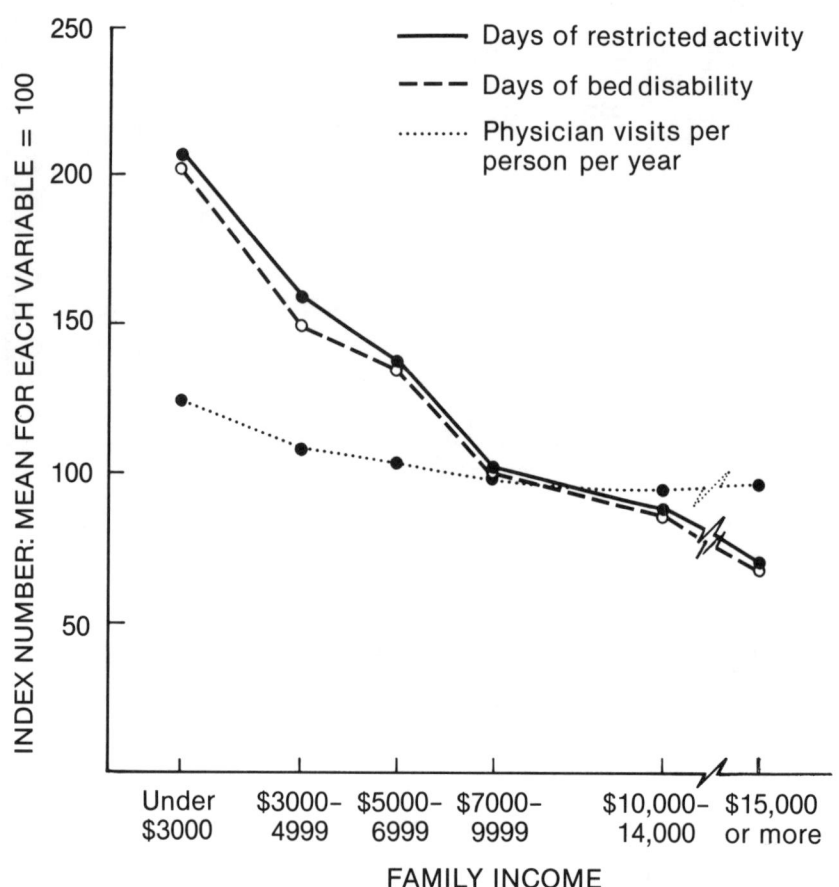

[1]Excludes visits to patients in hospitals.

SOURCES: U.S. National Center for Health Statistics, *Physician Visits, Volume and Interval Since Last Visit: U.S.-1975*, DHEW, Public Health Service. Office of Health Research, Statistics, and Technology, Hyattsville, Maryland, Series 10, No. 128, April 1979, Table 7, p. 21; U.S. National Center for Health Statistics, *Disability Days: U.S.-1975*, DHEW, Public Health Service, Vital and Health Statistics, Hyattsville, Maryland, Series 10, No. 118, June 1978, Table 12, p. 28 and Table 13, p. 29.

Chart C-15

Percent of Families with a Family Doctor and with a Family Dentist, by Social Class ("Regionville"[1], 1946-1950).

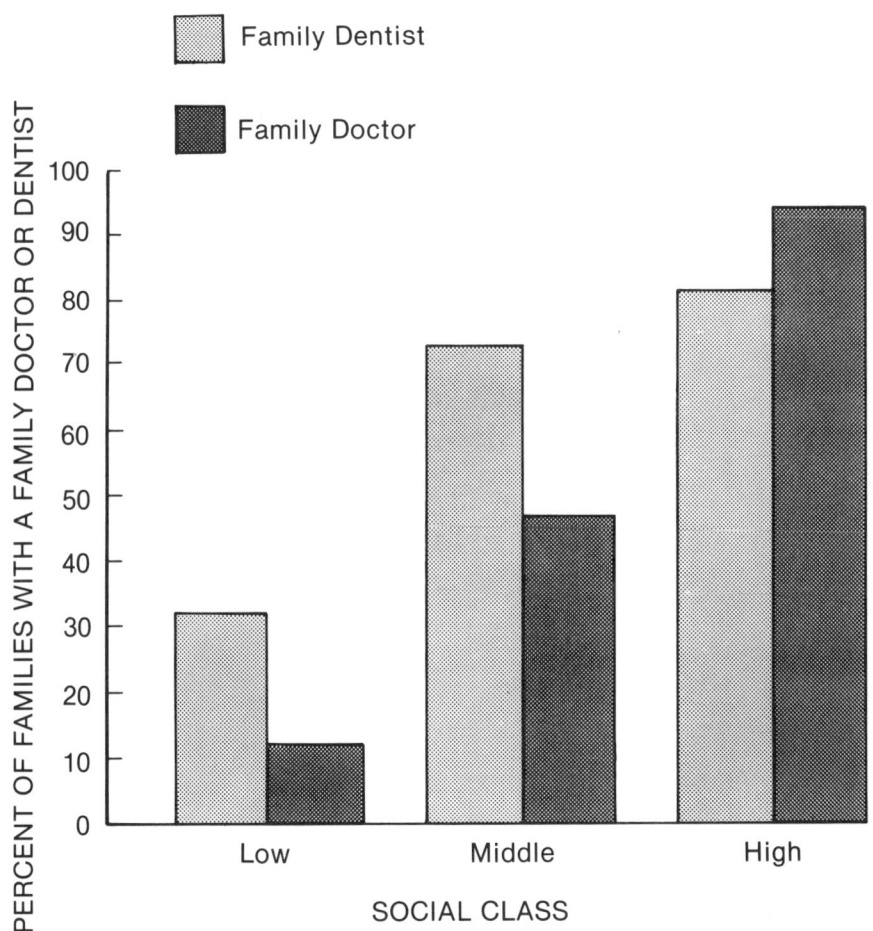

[1] A rural community in New York State.

SOURCE: Koos, E.L., *The Health of Regionville*, Columbia University Press, New York, 1954, Fig. 9, p. 33 and Fig. 15, p. 119.

Chart C-16 Percent Distribution of Patients Suffering from "Neurosis" Who Reported at a Psychiatric Clinic, by Social Class and by Recommendations Concerning Treatment, and Personnel Assigned to Treat the Patient (New Haven, October 1, 1950–September 30, 1951).

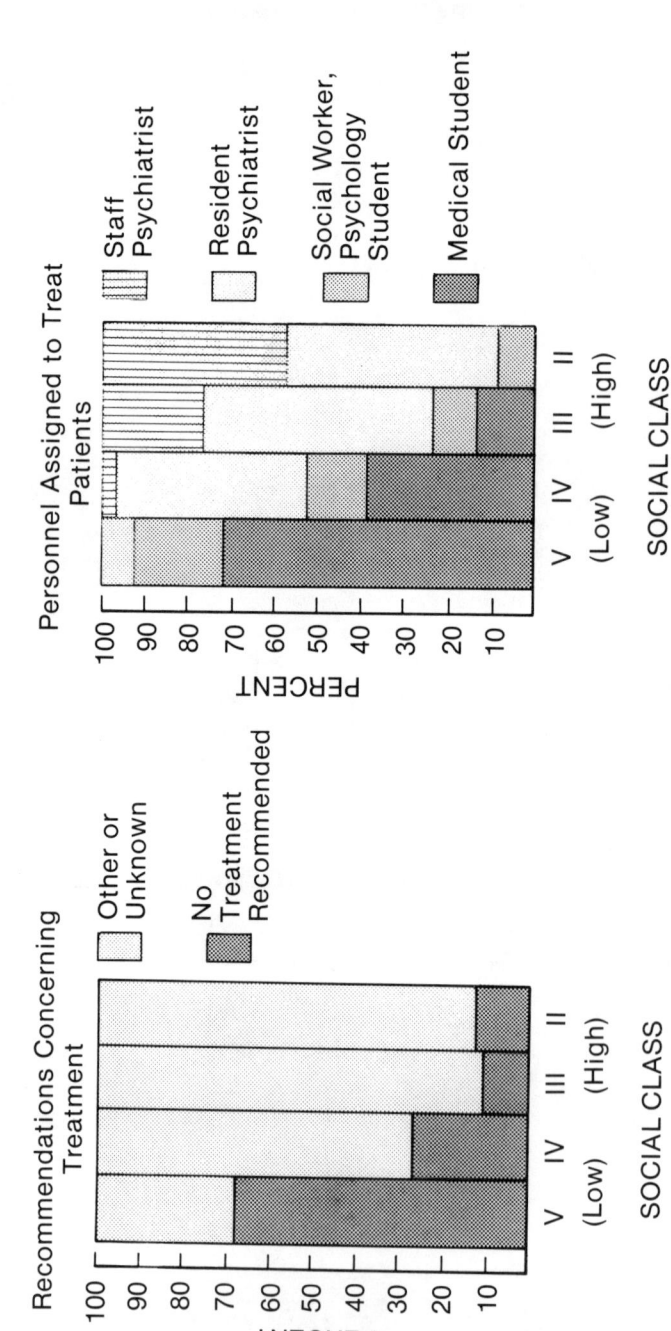

SOURCE: Myers, J. K. and L. Schaffer, "Social Stratification and Psychiatric Practice: A Study of an Outpatient Clinic," *American Sociological Review*, Vol. 19, June 1954, Table 1, p. 308.

Chart C-17

Percent Change in Physician Visits Per 1,000 Ill or Injured, by Sex and Weekly Income of Chief Wage Earner (England and Wales, After National Health Service [1948-1951] Compared to Before [1946-1948]).

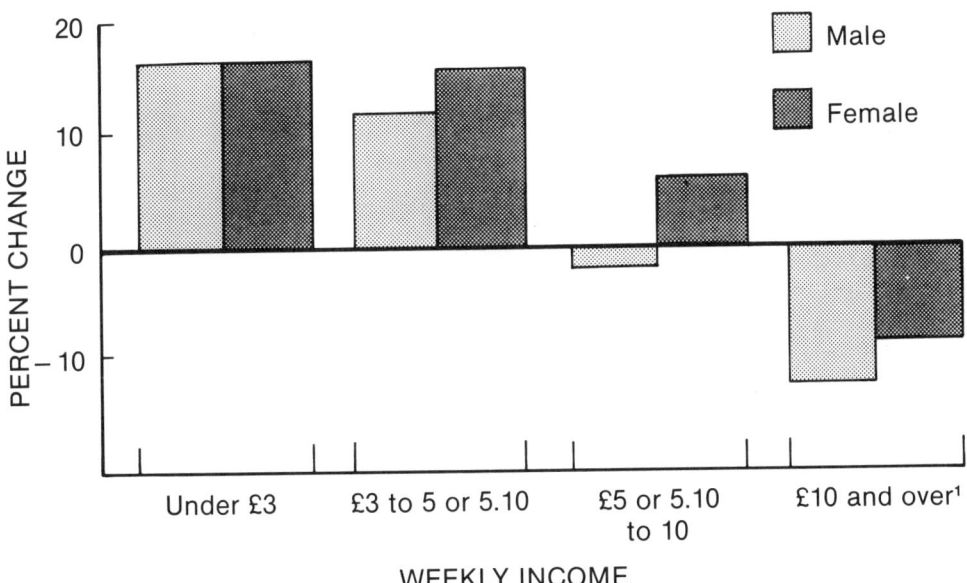

[1]Workers whose income equalled or exceeded £10 per week were not covered to any extent before NHS.

SOURCE: Stewart, W.H. and P.E. Enterline, "Effects of The National Health Service on Physician Utilization and Health in England and Wales," *New England Journal of Medicine*, Vol. 265, December 14, 1961, pp. 1187-1194.

Chart C-18

Percent Change in Number of Visits per 1000 Persons per year to Physician Offices, Emergency Rooms, and Outpatient Departments Before and After the Introduction of Universal Health Insurance in Quebec (Montreal Metropolitan Area, 1970-1974).

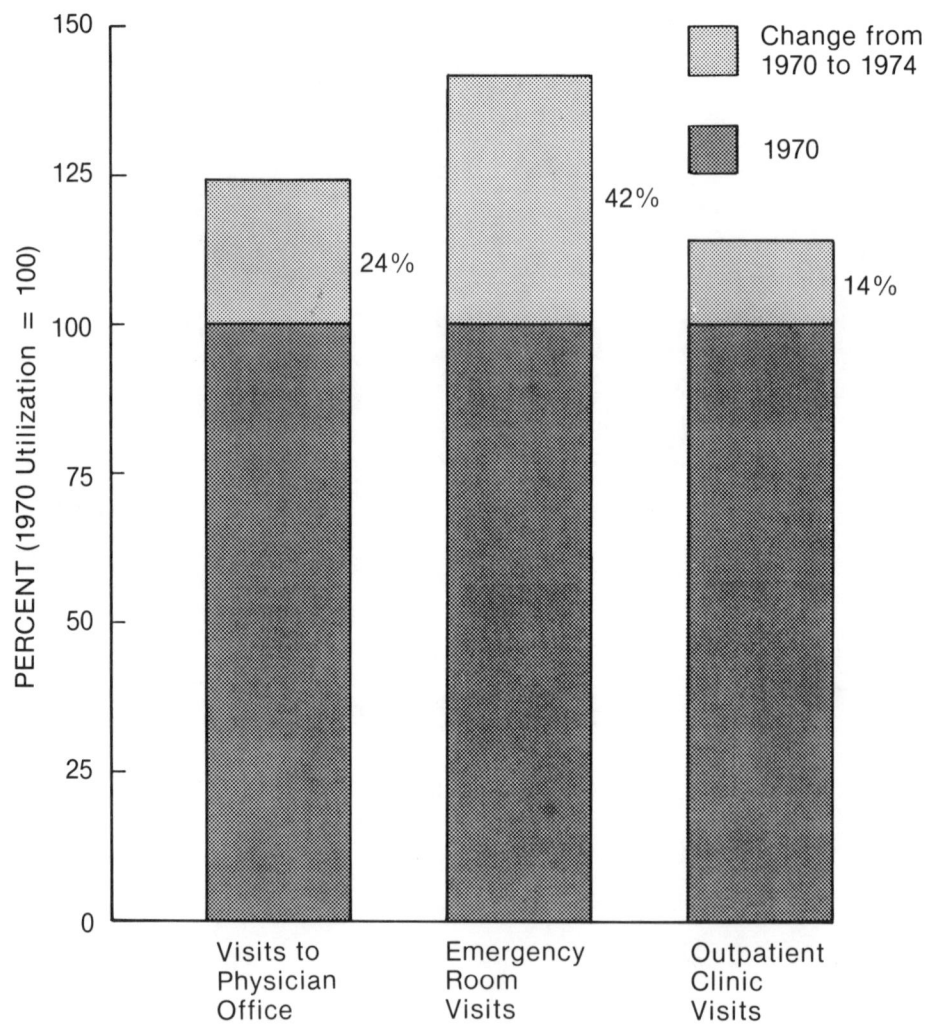

NOTE: Under universal health insurance (Medicare) introduced in Quebec on November 1, 1970, physicians are reimbursed on a fee for service basis directly by the government, and there can be no charge to patients. Services provided in hospital outpatient clinics and emergency rooms are paid in the same manner.

SOURCE: Steinmetz, N. and J.R. Hoey, "Hospital Emergency Room Utilization in Montreal Before and After Medicare," *Medical Care*, February 1978, Vol. XVI, No. 2, Figure 1, p. 135 and text p. 135 and text p. 135 and 138-139.

Use of Service

Chart C-19

Physician Visits per Person per Year, by Family Income Before and After Introduction of Universal Health Insurance
(Montreal Metropolitan Area, Quebec, Canada, Specified Years).[1]

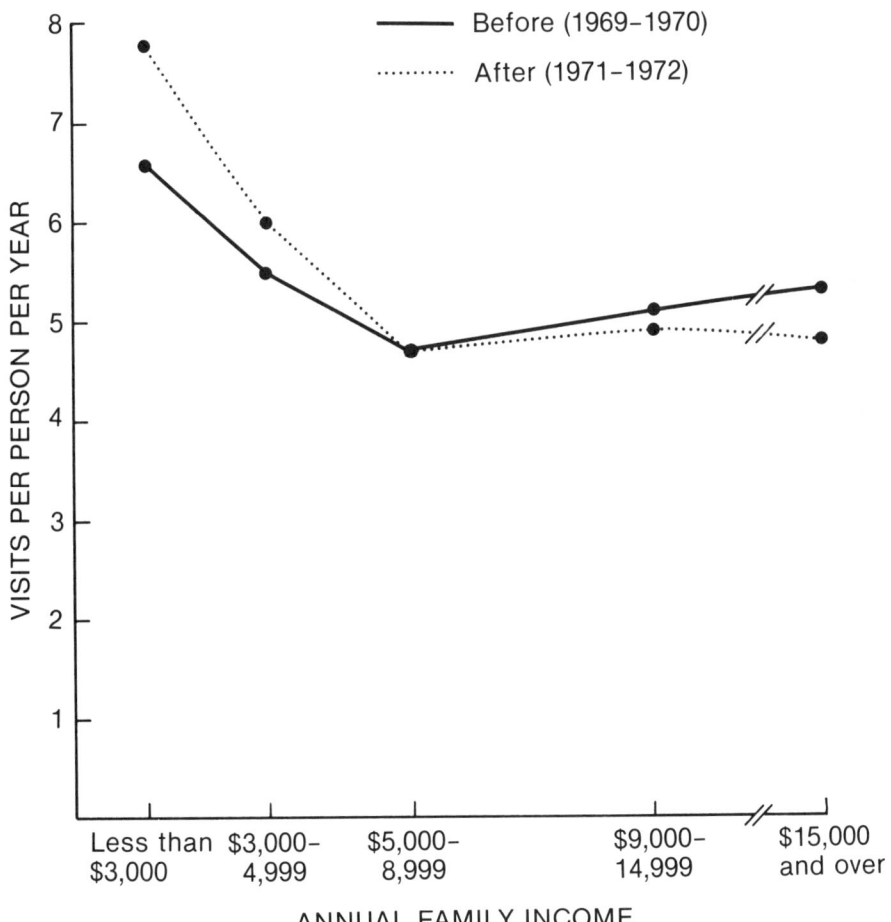

[1]The insurance plan was implemented November 1, 1970 as an addition to pre-existing compulsory hospital insurance. Physician visits exclude inpatient visits and health-department clinic visits.

SOURCE: Enterline, P.E., et al., "The Distribution of Medical Services Before and After 'Free' Medical Care—The Quebec Experience," *New England Journal of Medicine*, Vol. 289, November 29, 1973, Table 2, p. 1175.

Chart C-20

Percent of Women with Specified Types of Visits for Pregnancy, by Family Income, Before and After Introduction of Universal Health Insurance (Quebec, 1972).

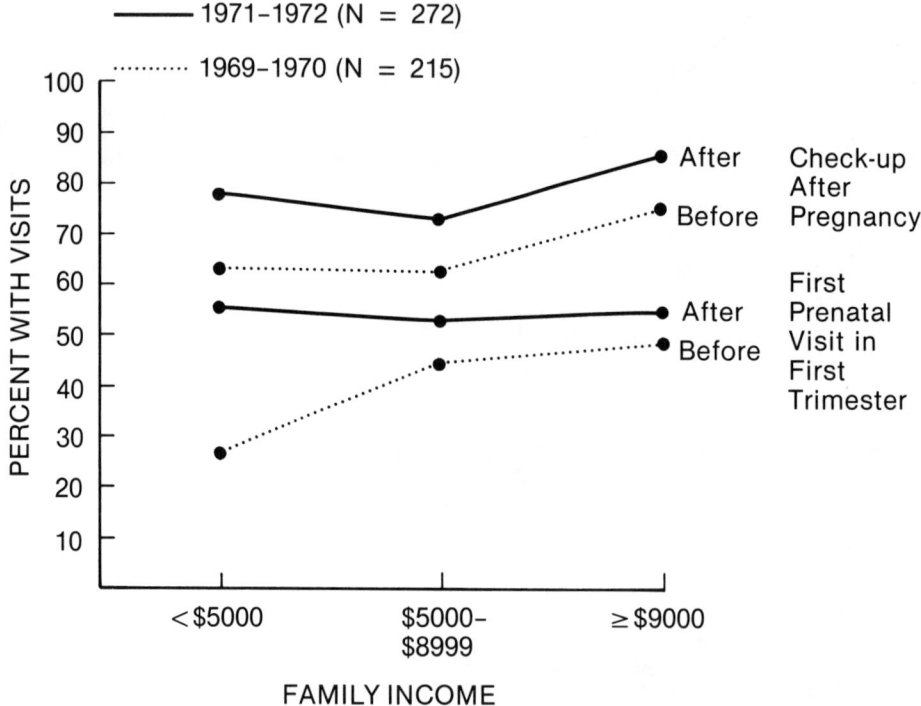

SOURCE: McDonald, A. D., et al., "Effects of Quebec Medicare on Physician Consultation for Selected Symptoms," *New England Journal of Medicine*, Vol. 291, September 26, 1974.

Use of Service

Chart C-21

Percent of Persons Who Consulted a Pharmacist Within the Last Two Weeks About Their Health or Because of an Accident, the Year Before and After the Introduction of Universal Health Insurance Covering Physicians' Services[1], by Family Income (Montreal Metropolitan Area, 1969-70 and 1971-72).

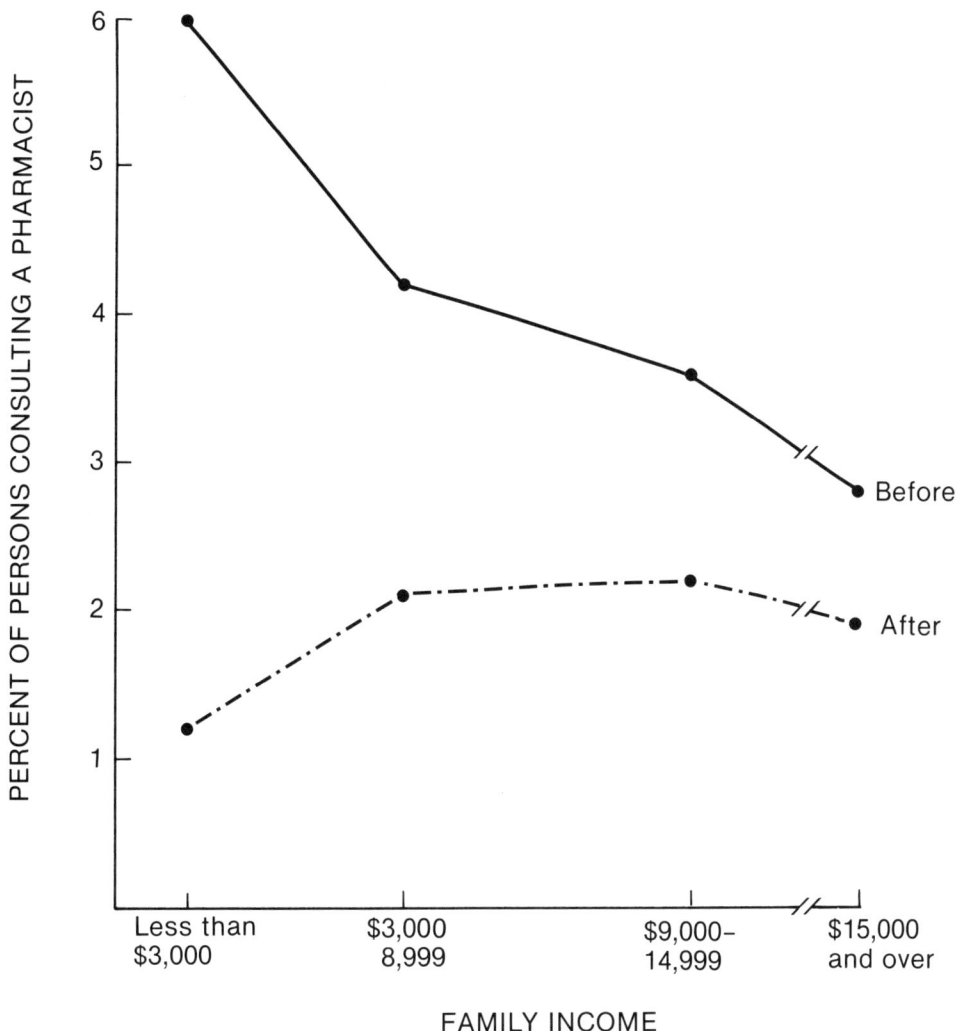

[1]The cost of drugs was not included under the insurance plan.
SOURCE: Ricci, E. M., P. Enterline, and V. Henderson, "Contacts with Pharmacists Before and After "Free" Medical Care—the Quebec Experience," *Medical Care*, Vol. XVI, No. 3, March 1978, Table 3, p. 259.

Use of Service

Chart C-22

Percent of Live Births with Prenatal Care Begun in the First Trimester of Pregnancy, by Color and Specified Population Group (New York, 1955).

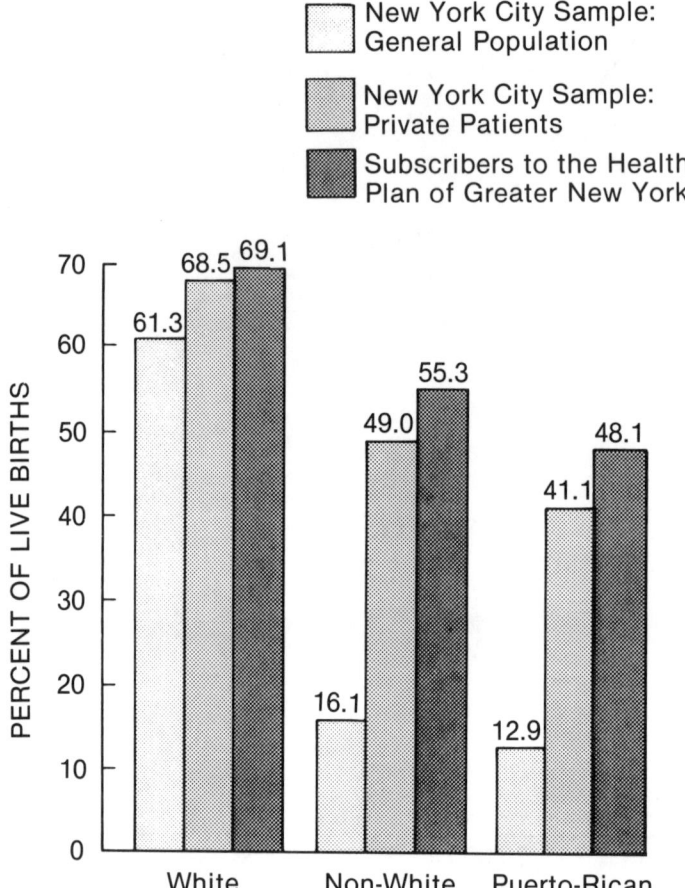

SOURCE: Shapiro, S., L. Weiner, and P. Densen, "Comparison of Prematurity and Perinatal Mortality in a General Population and in the Population of a Prepaid Group Practice Medical Care Plan," *American Journal of Public Health*, Vol. 48, February 1958, p. 175.

Chart C-23

Number of Leucotomy Operations (England and Wales, 1942–1961).

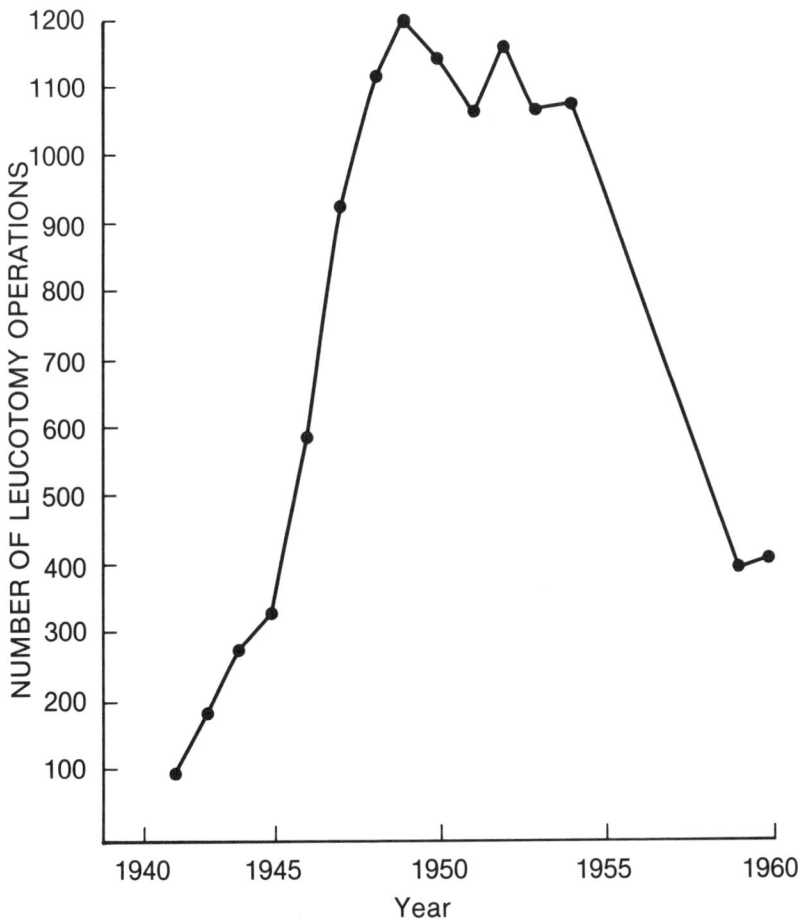

SOURCES: For 1942-1959: Tooth, G. and M. Newton, *Leucotomy in England and Wales 1942-54*, Reports on Public Health and Medical Subjects, No. 104, Ministry of Health, Great Britain, London, 1961; for 1961: Pippard, J., *Journal of Mental Science*, Vol. 108, 1962, p. 250.

Chart C-24 Total and Selected Surgical Operations per 1000 Persons (U.S.A., 1965 and 1977).[1]

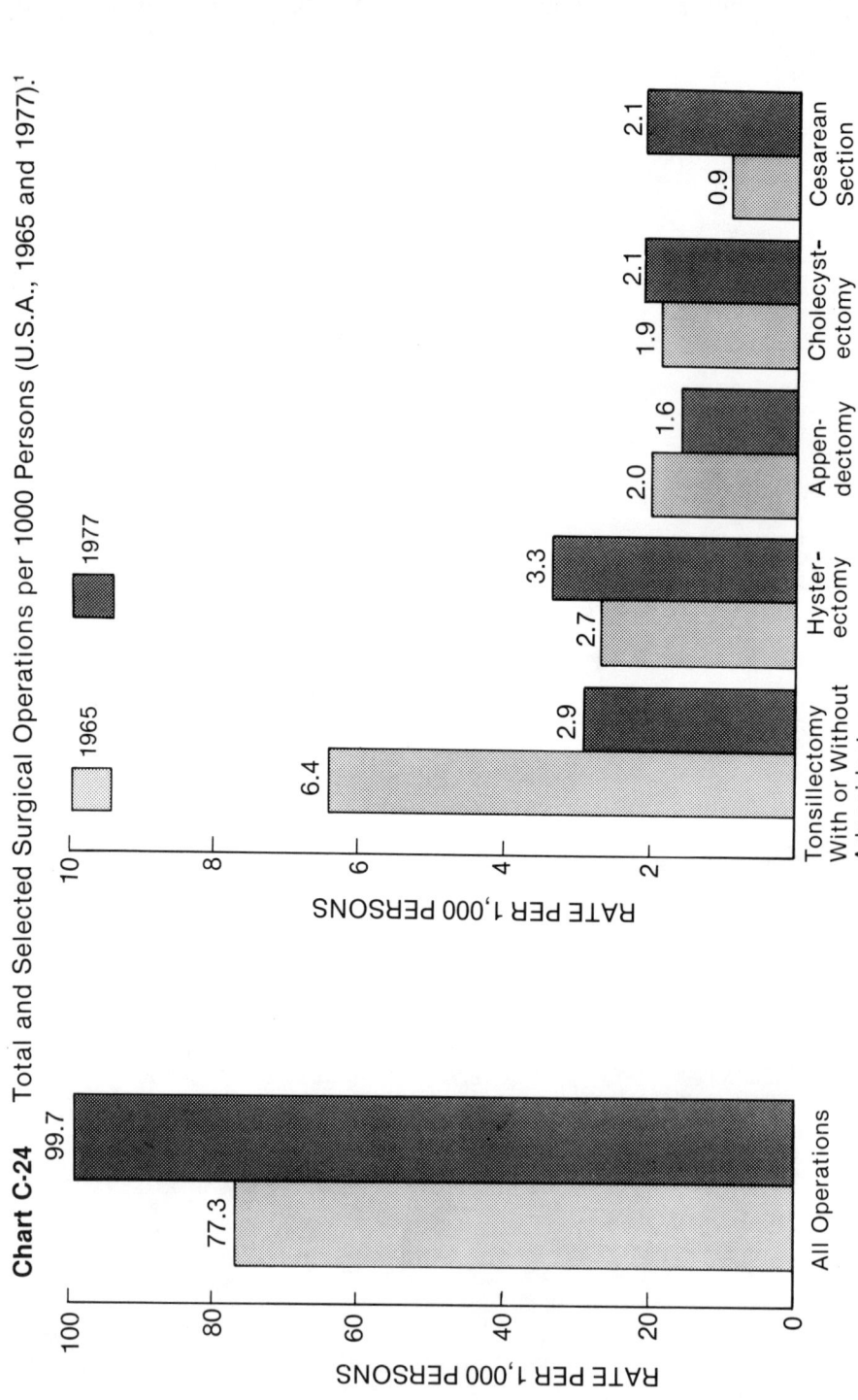

[1]Data are for operations performed in short-stay hospitals.

SOURCES: For 1965: U.S. National Center for Health Statistics, *Surgical Operations in Short-stay Hospitals, U.S.A., 1975*, DHEW, Public Health Service, Hyattsville, Maryland, Series 13, No. 14, April 1978, Table K, p. 10; for 1977: U.S. National Center for Health Statistics, *Utilization of Short-stay Hospitals, United States, 1977*, DHEW, Public Health Service, Hyattsville, Maryland, Series 13, No. 41, March 1979, Table 21, p. 49.

Chart C-25

Relative Supply of Surgeons (1967) and Relative Rates of Specified Surgical Operations for Women (U.S.A., 1965; England and Wales, 1966).

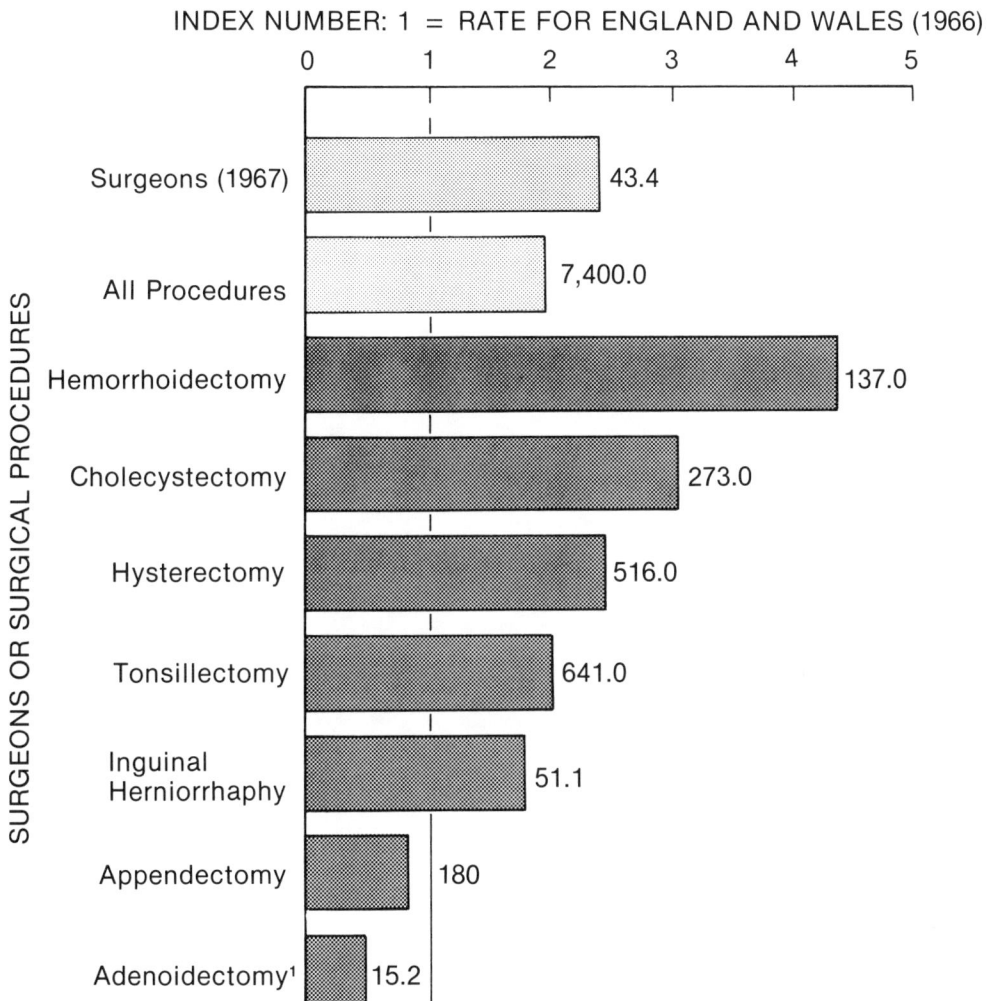

[1]Without tonsillectomy.

NOTE: Numbers to the right of bars are rates per 100,000 in United States.

SOURCE: Bunker, J. P., "Surgical Manpower," *New England Journal of Medicine*, Vol. 282, January 15, 1970, Table 2, p. 137.

Chart C-26

Cumulative Risk of Hysterectomy in Wives of Physicians in Santa Clara County, California, in United States Women, and in Women in the Oxford Area of England.[1]

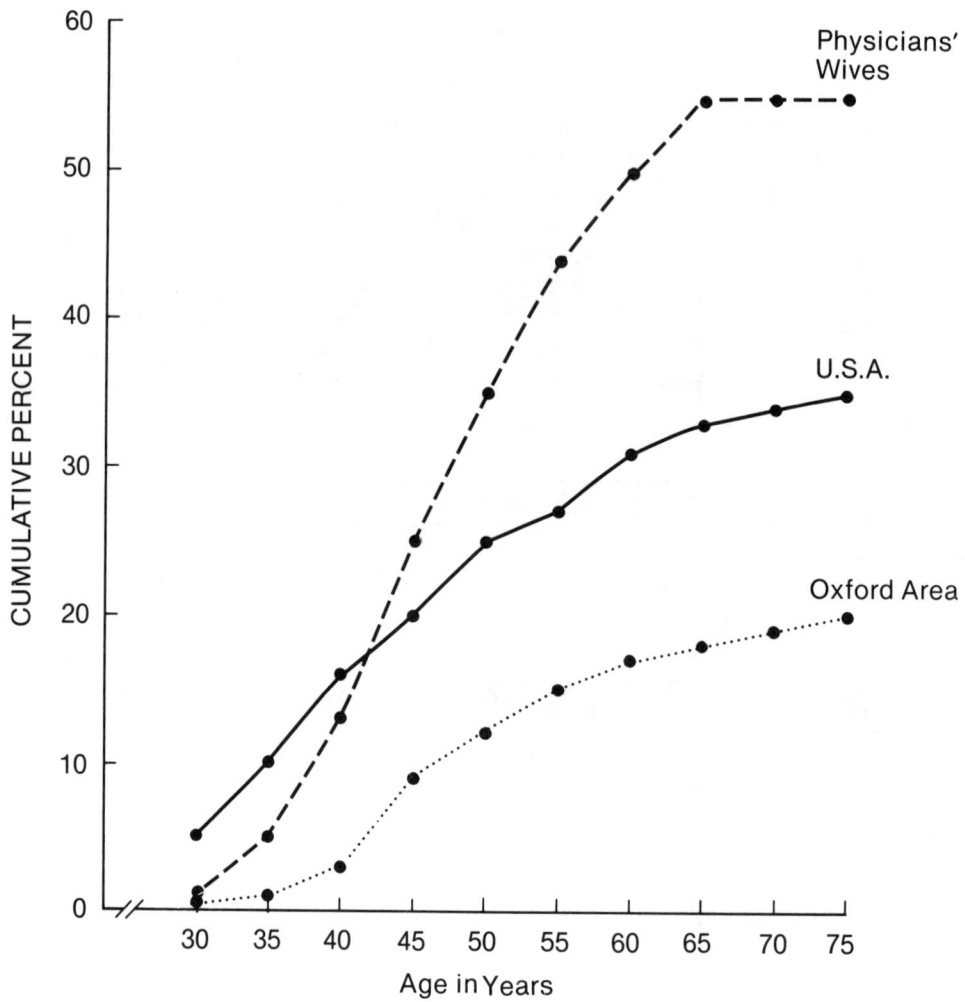

[1]Data on physicians' wives are from life history information; United States data were obtained in 1968; and Oxford data were obtained in 1962–65.

SOURCE: Bunker, J.P. and B.W. Brown, "The Physician-Patient as an Informed Consumer of Surgical Services," *New England Journal of Medicine,* Vol. 290, No. 19, May 9, 1974, Figure 2, p. 1053.

Chart C-27

General Practices by Number of Persons Registered with the Practice and by Use of Service by Those Who are Registered with Each Practice (Three Industrial Towns, England, 1961–1962).

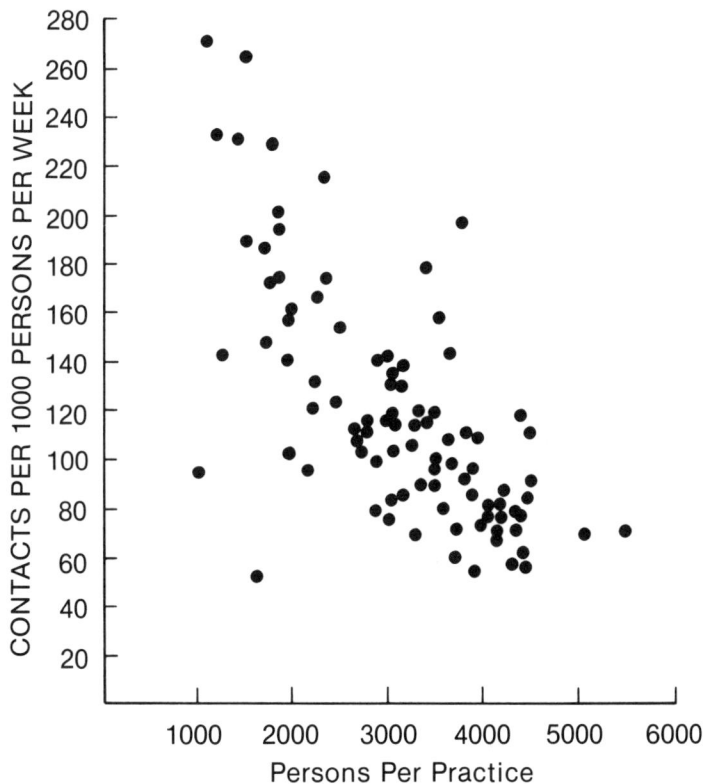

SOURCE: Last, J. M., "Community Demand for Doctors in the Next 10 Years," *British Medical Journal*, Vol. 1, March 22, 1969, pp. 769–772 and data supplied by the author.

Chart C-28

Number of Office Visits Per 1000 Enrollees and per Physician, per Year, by Number of Physicians per 1000 Enrollees, in Kaiser Foundation Health Plan (Portland, Oregon, 1951-1967).

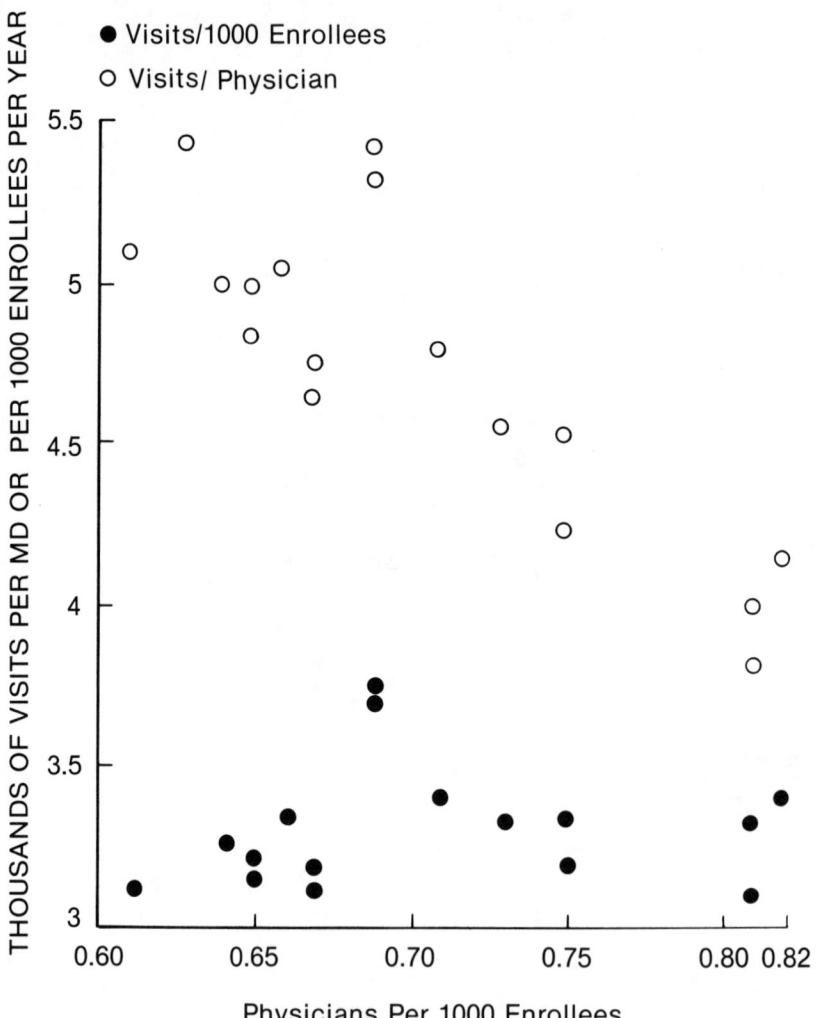

SOURCE: Stevens, Carl, "Physician Supply and National Health Care Goals," *Industrial Relations*, Vol. 10, No. 2, May 1971, Table 4 and Chart 1, pp. 128-130.

Chart C-29

Percent of Variation in Surgical Rates Among Ontario's 49 Counties Accounted for by Differences in Availability of Beds, General Practitioners and Specialists (Ontario, 1974).[1]

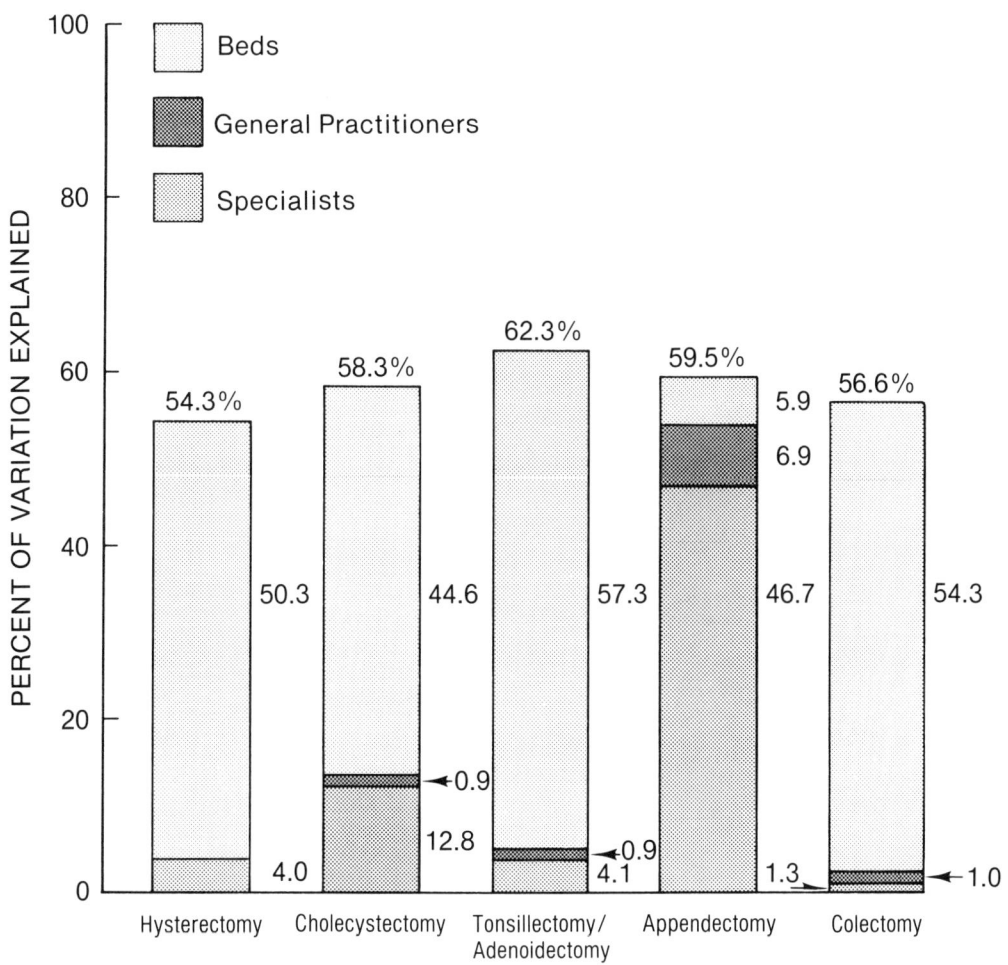

[1]Determined by stepwise multiple linear regression.
SOURCE: Stockwell, Heather and Eugene Vayda, "Variations in Surgery in Ontario," *Medical Care*, Vol. 17, April 1979, Table 3, p. 392.

Chart C-30

Percent of Respondents Expressing Willingness to Travel Specified Distances or More, by Type of Service (A Rural County in Kentucky, June and July, 1968).[1]

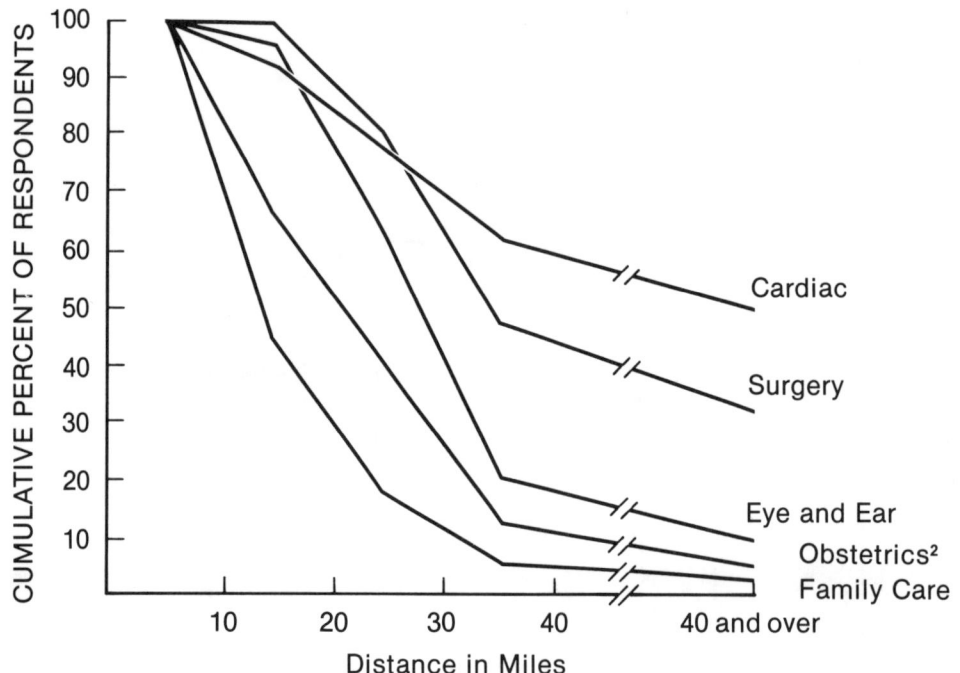

[1]Based on a probability sample of 171 households which constituted about 15 percent of the county's families, with a response rate of 92 percent.

[2]The gradient for obstetric care is very similar to those of x-ray services and dental care. The latter have been omitted to simplify the figure.

SOURCE: Kane, R.L., "Determination of Health Care Priorities and Expectations Among Rural Consumers," *Health Services Research*, Vol. 4, Summer 1969, pp. 142–151.

Use of Service

Chart C-31

Travel Distances the Residents of a Rural Area Considered Reasonable for Obtaining General Medical Care for Routine Illnesses, Maximum Distances They Were Willing to Travel for Such Care, and Actual Distances Traveled, Expressed in Terms of Cumulative Percent of Visits (Franklin and Androscoggin Counties, Maine, 1974).[1]

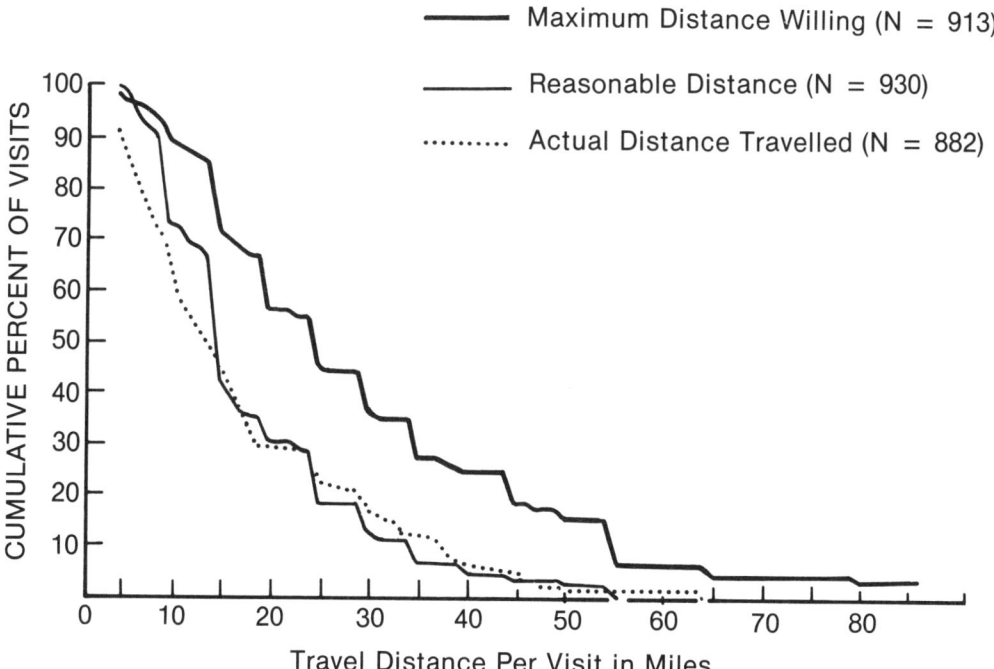

[1] The curves of "reasonable distance" and "maximum distance willing" show the cumulative percent of persons who expressed the corresponding opinions, weighted by the actual number of visits made by those persons during the year preceding the survey.

SOURCE: Shannon, Gary, Joseph Lovett, and Rashid Bashshur, "Travel for Primary Care: Expectation and Performance in a Rural Setting," *Journal of Community Health*, Vol. 5, No. 2, Winter 1979, Figure 4, p. 119.

Use of Service

Chart C-32

Percent of Patients Referred by General Practitioners for Specialist Maternity Care, and Perinatal Mortality Rate in the Practice of Referring Physicians, by Travel Time from the Office of the Referring General Practitioner to the Nearest Specialized Maternity Unit [1] (Oxford Area, England, 1962).

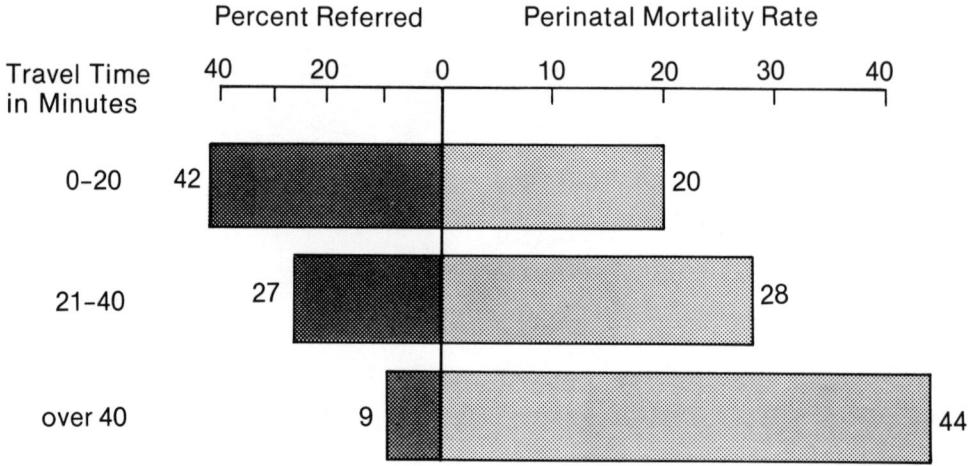

[1]The data shown are for instances in which the travel time from the office of the general practitioner to the nearest specialized maternity unit was longer than the travel time from the office to the nearest general practice maternity unit. When the specialized unit was closer than the general practice unit, referral rates were higher on the average and the perinatal mortality rate lower, and neither was strongly related to the length of travel time.

SOURCE: Hobbs, M.S.T. and E.D. Acheson, "Perinatal Mortality and the Organization of Obstetric Services in the Oxford Area in 1962," *British Medical Journal,* Vol. 1, February 26, 1966, Table 4, p. 502.

Chart C-33 Effects of Liberalized Abortion Law, by Color (New York City, 1965–70 and 1970–71).

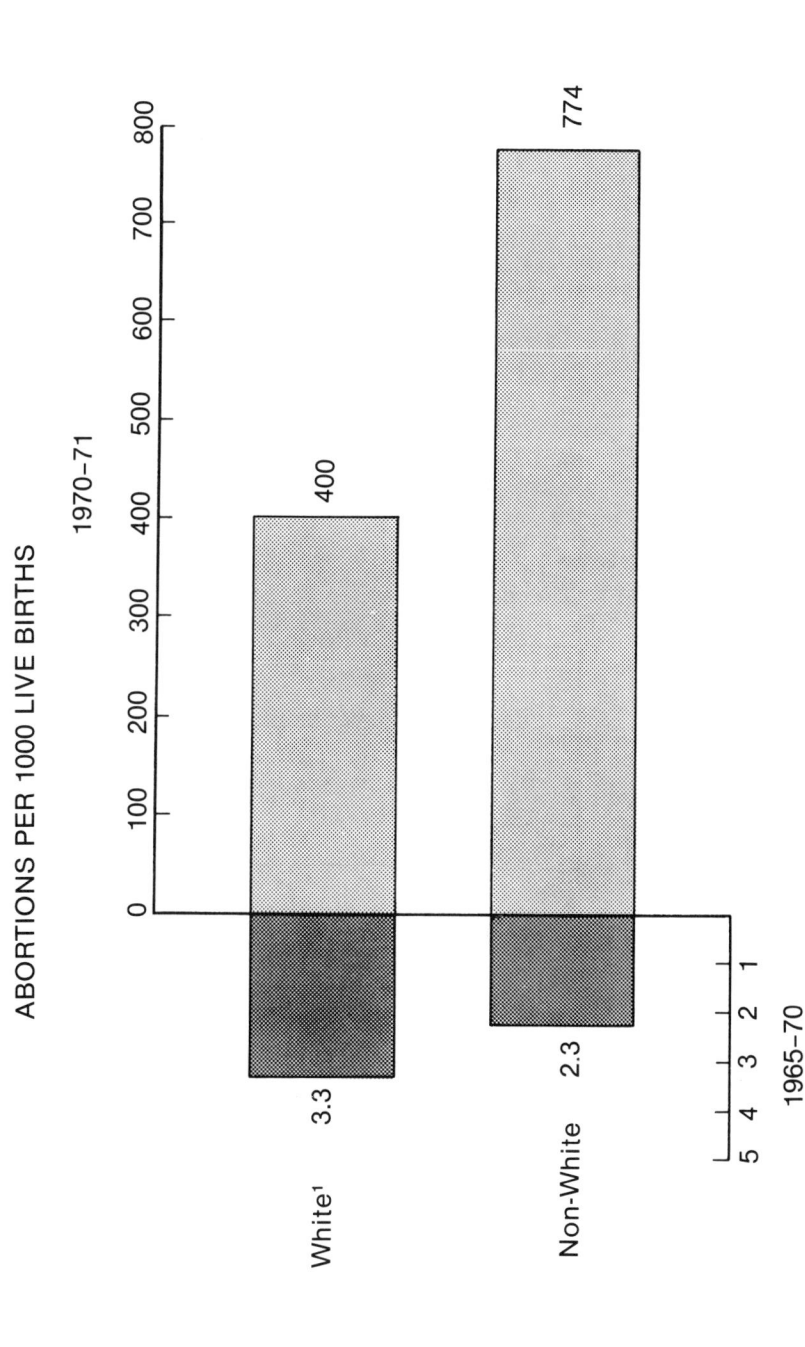

[1]Includes Puerto Ricans.
SOURCE: Tietze, C. and D.A. Dawson, "Induced Abortion: A Factbook," *Reports on Population/Family Planning*, No. 14, December 1973, Table 1, p. 11.

Chart C-34

Percent of Reported Illnesses for Which Medical Care was Received, and Percent of Families Receiving Specified Preventive Medical Services, by Presence of Clinic Facilities (Selected Migrant Worker Camps, Central Valley, California, undated).

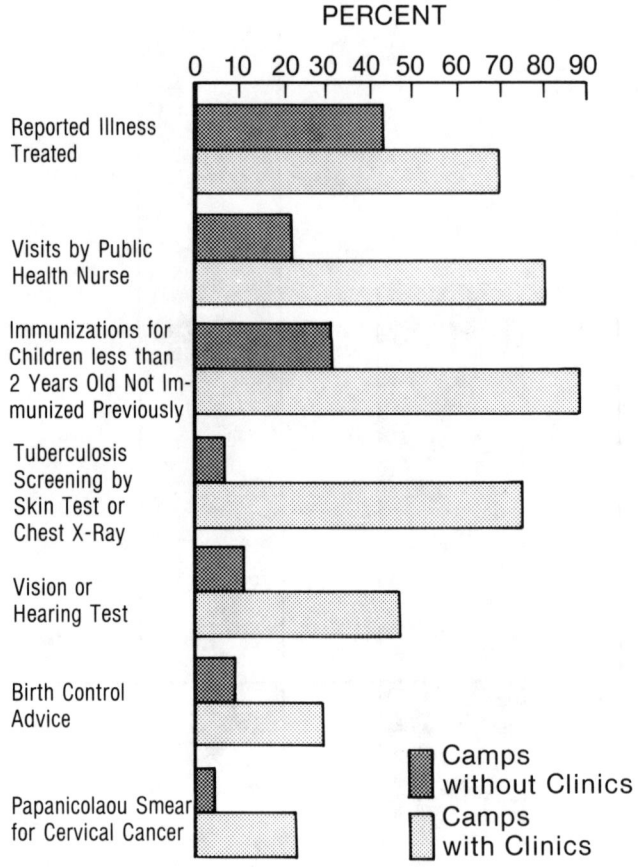

SOURCE: Snyder, H. McC., O. F. Nana, and P. D. Smith, "The Effect of Provision of Medical Facilities on Use by the Migrant Workers of California," *Medical Care*, Vol. 6, September–October 1968, Tables 6 and 8, pp. 394–400.

Use of Service

Chart C-35

Percent of Clinic Patients Referred to Their Physicians Who Kept their Appointment, by Referral Procedure and Patient's Perception of Physician (Chapel Hill, North Carolina, Spring 1961).

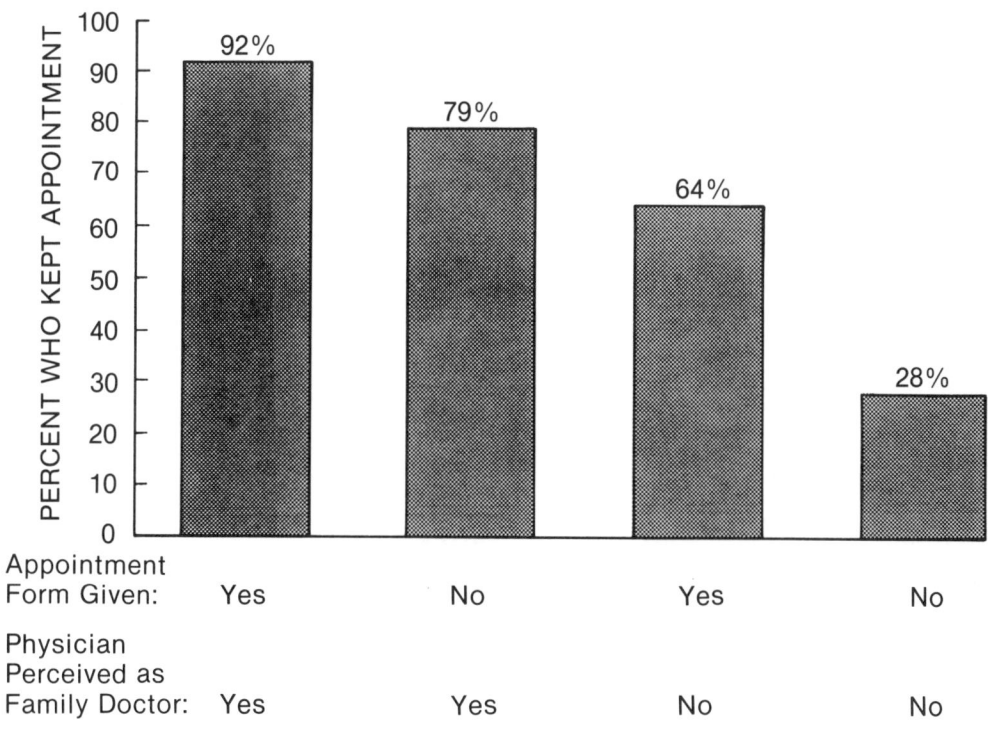

SOURCE: Martin, D.A., "The Disposition of Patients from a Consultant General Medical Clinic: Results of a Controlled Evaluation of an Administrative Procedure," *Journal of Chronic Diseases*, September 1964.

Use of Service

Chart C-36

Percent of Persons Who Reported for Medical Care During the First Year After Receiving an Invitation by the Program to Do So, by Category of Person and Type of Invitation (New York Hospital—Cornell Medical Center, Welfare Medical Care Program, New York City, 1962–1963).

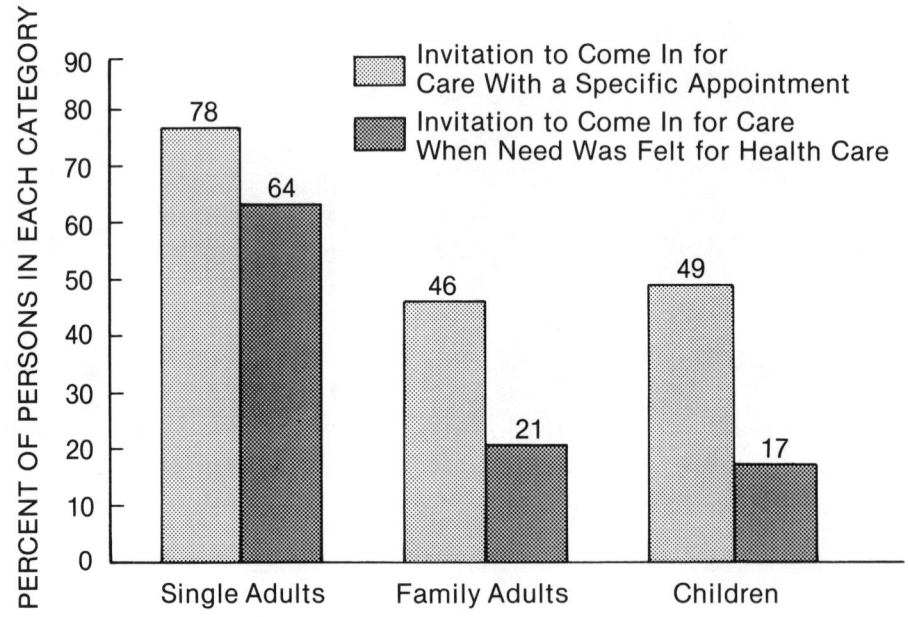

SOURCE: Goodrich, C.H., M. Olendzki, and G.G. Reader, "The New York Hospital—Cornell Medical Center: A Progress Report on an Experiment in Welfare Medical Care," *American Journal of Public Health*, Vol. 55, January 1965, pp. 88–93.

Use of Service

Chart C-37

Geographic Areas by Rates for Non-Obstetrical Surgery and Frequency of Additional Charges Experienced by United Steel Workers Covered by Blue Shield Contracts (U.S.A., July 1, 1957–June 30, 1958).

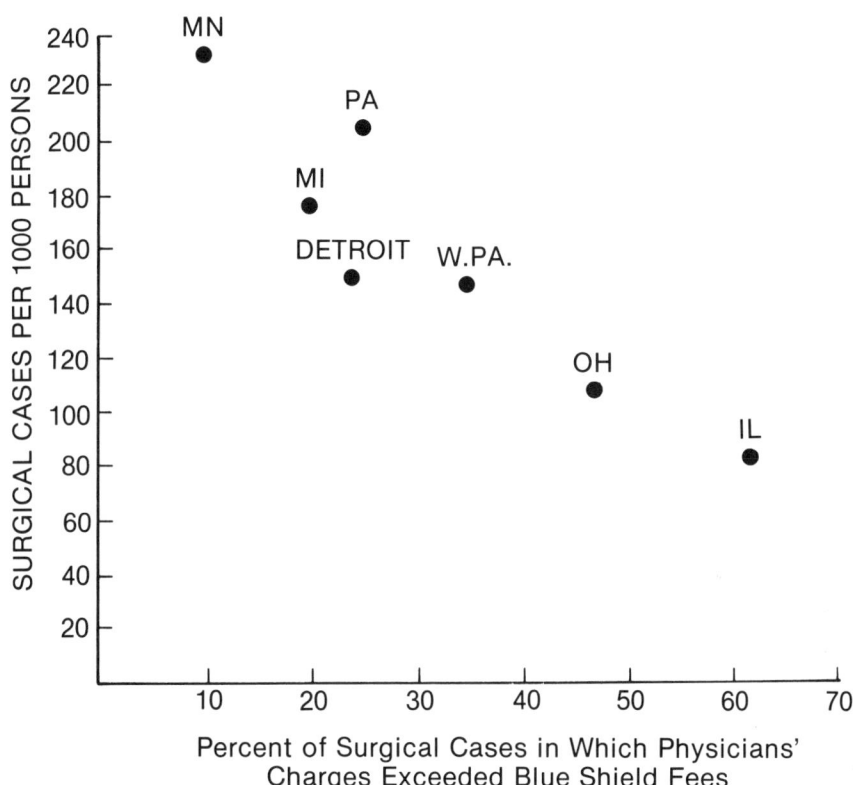

[1]The seven geographic areas represented are (reading from left to right): Minnesota (various areas); Michigan (various areas); Detroit, Michigan; Pennsylvania (Bethlehem and Allentown); Western Pennsylvania; Ohio (Cleveland, Youngstown, etc.); and Illinois (Chicago and nearby).

SOURCE: United Steelworkers of America, Insurance, Pension and Unemployment Benefits Department, *Special Study on the Medical Care Program for Steelworkers and Their Families*, Pittsburgh, Pennsylvania, 1960, p. 75.

Use of Service

Chart C-38

Relative Change in Fees, Number of Visits, and Amount Paid, Related to Change in Method of Payment, Selected Physicians,[1] Medical Care Program for Indigent (Baltimore, January–June 1962 and January–June 1964).

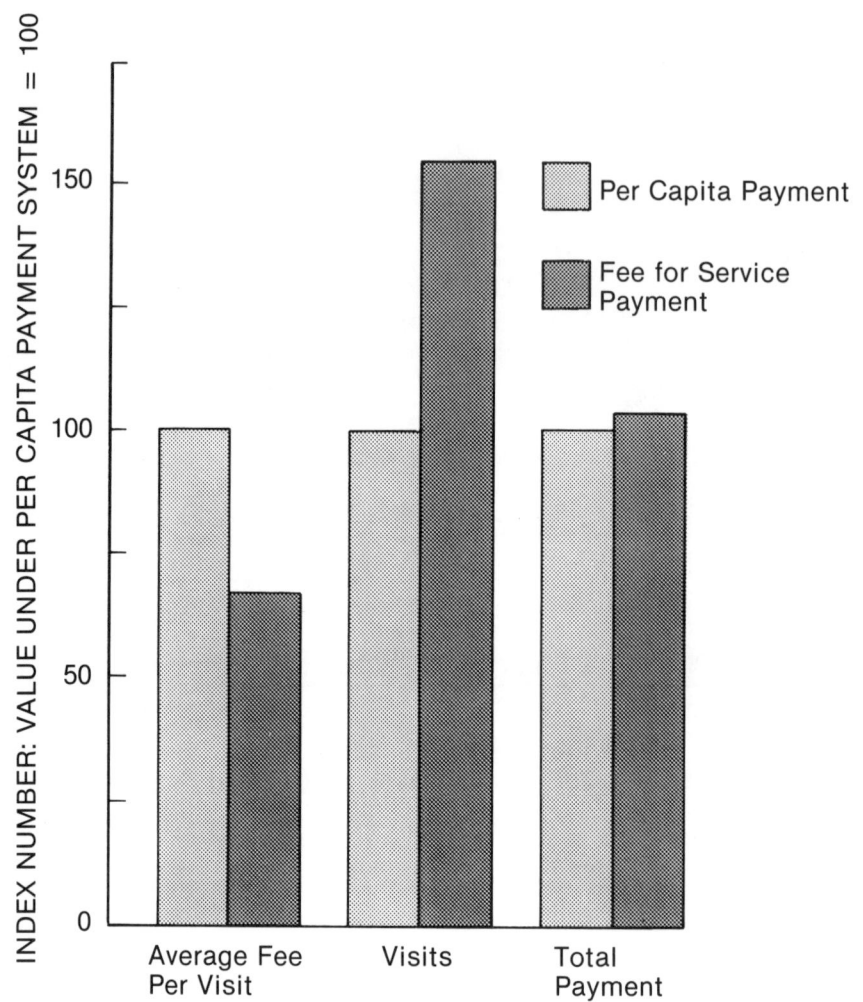

[1] Ten physicians with 1000 or more clients under the Medical Care Program for the Indigent.

SOURCE: Alexander, C.A., "The Effects of Change in Method of Paying Physicians, the Baltimore Experience," *American Journal of Public Health* Vol. 57, No. 8, August 1967, Table 7, p. 1286.

Use of Service

Chart C-39

Percent Distribution of Physician Visits Among Members of a Prepaid Group Practice (Health Insurance Plan of Greater New York, 1956–1957).

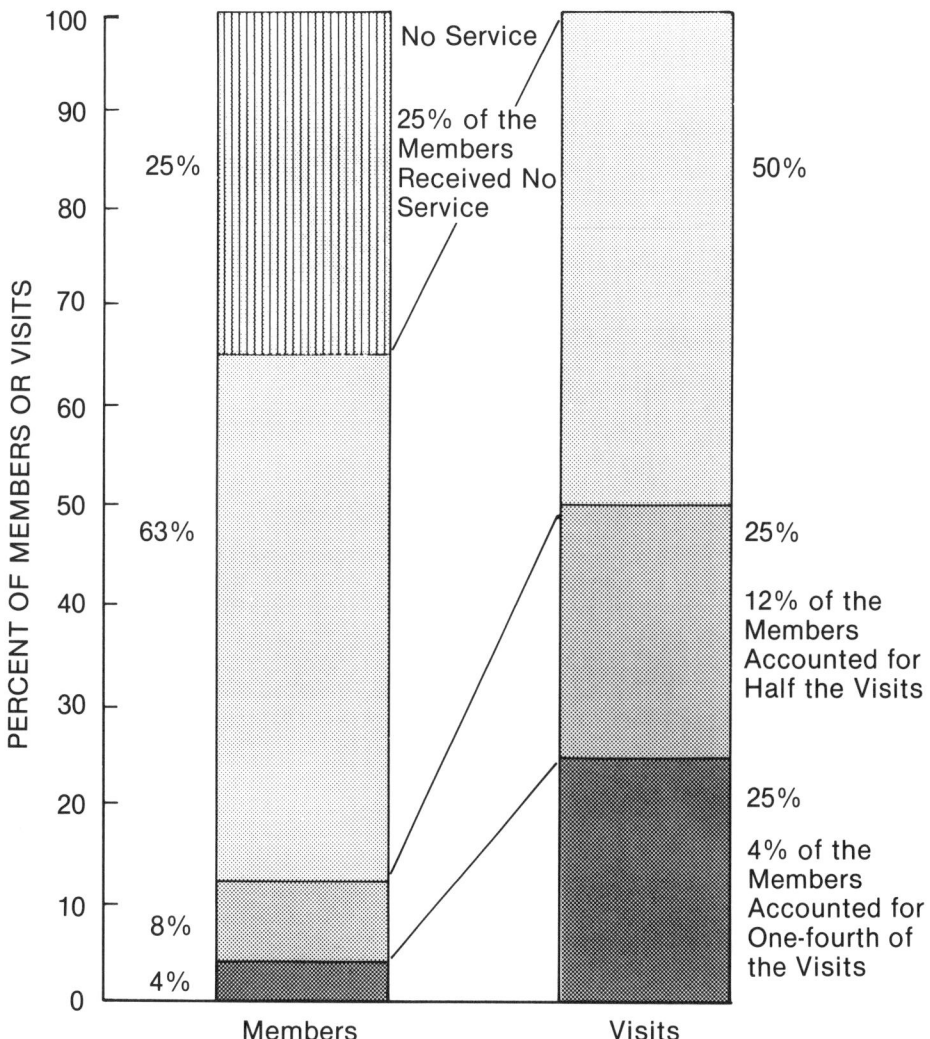

[1]Data based on a 10% sample of subscribers to Health Insurance Plan of Greater New York, who were enrolled throughout the period July 1, 1956–June 30, 1957, and all their dependents enrolled on June 30, 1957.

SOURCE: Densen, P.M., S. Shapiro, and M. Einhorn, "Concerning High and Low Utilizers of Service in a Medical Care Plan, and the Persistence of Utilization Levels Over a Three-Year Period," *Milbank Memorial Fund Quarterly*, Vol. 37, July 1959, p. 219.

Chart C-40

Percent Distribution of Members and of Outpatients Visits, by Number of Visits per Member in a Prepaid Group Practice (Community Health Association,[1] Detroit, 1970-71).

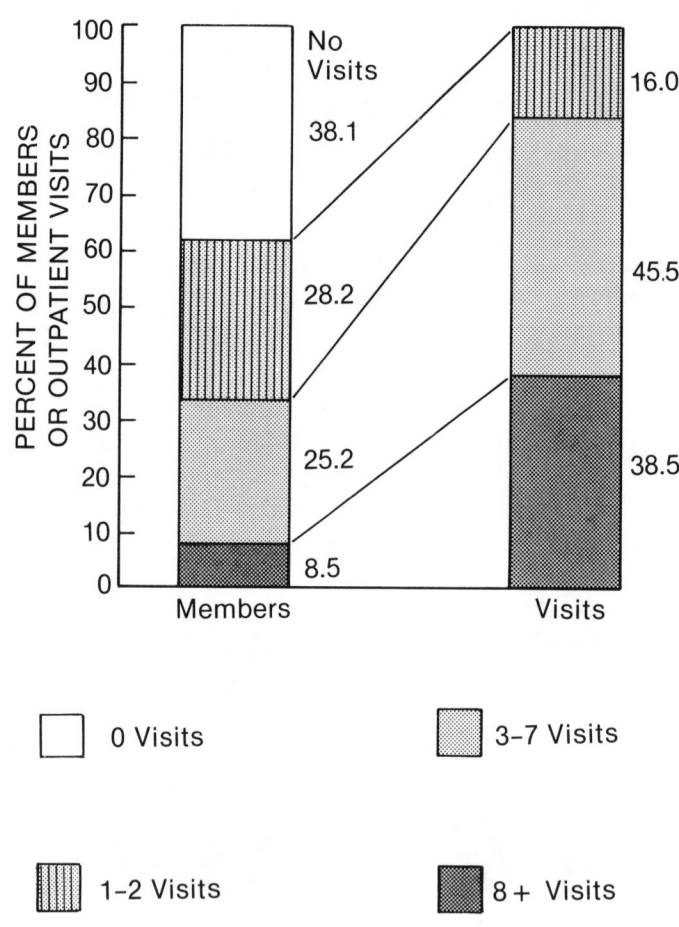

[1]A hospital-based prepaid group practice.
SOURCE: *CHA 1961-1971*, Community Health Association of Detroit, Detroit, 1972, Table 9, p. 10.

Use of Service

Chart C-41

Percent Distribution of Members and of Claims, by Number of Claims per Member in a Comprehensive Individual Practice Plan (Group Health Insurance, Inc., New York, 1964).

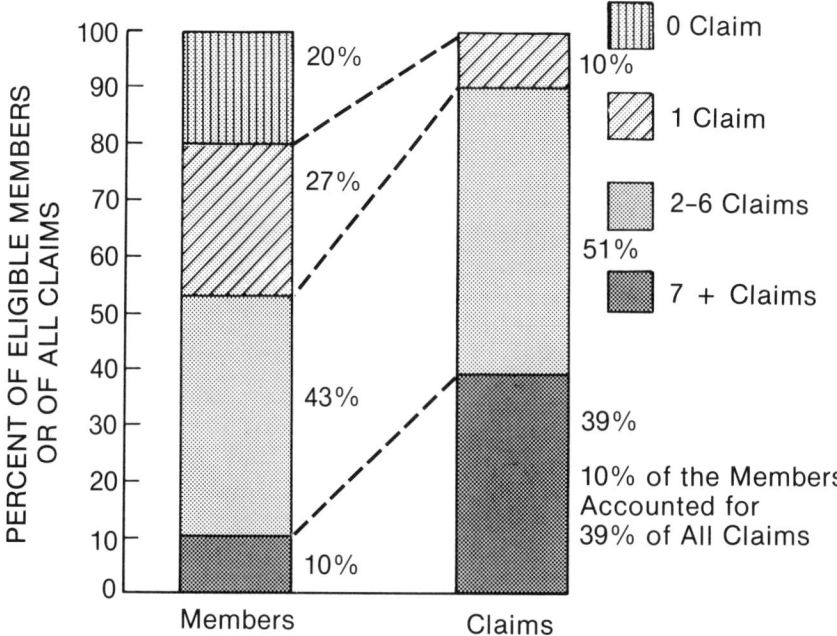

SOURCE: Avnet, Helen Hershfield, *Physician Service Patterns and Illness Rates*, Group Health Insurance, Inc., New York, 1967, Table 32, p. 93.

Chart C-42

Dental and Physician Visits per Person per Year, by Age and Sex (U.S.A., Civilian Non-institutionalized Population, 1977).

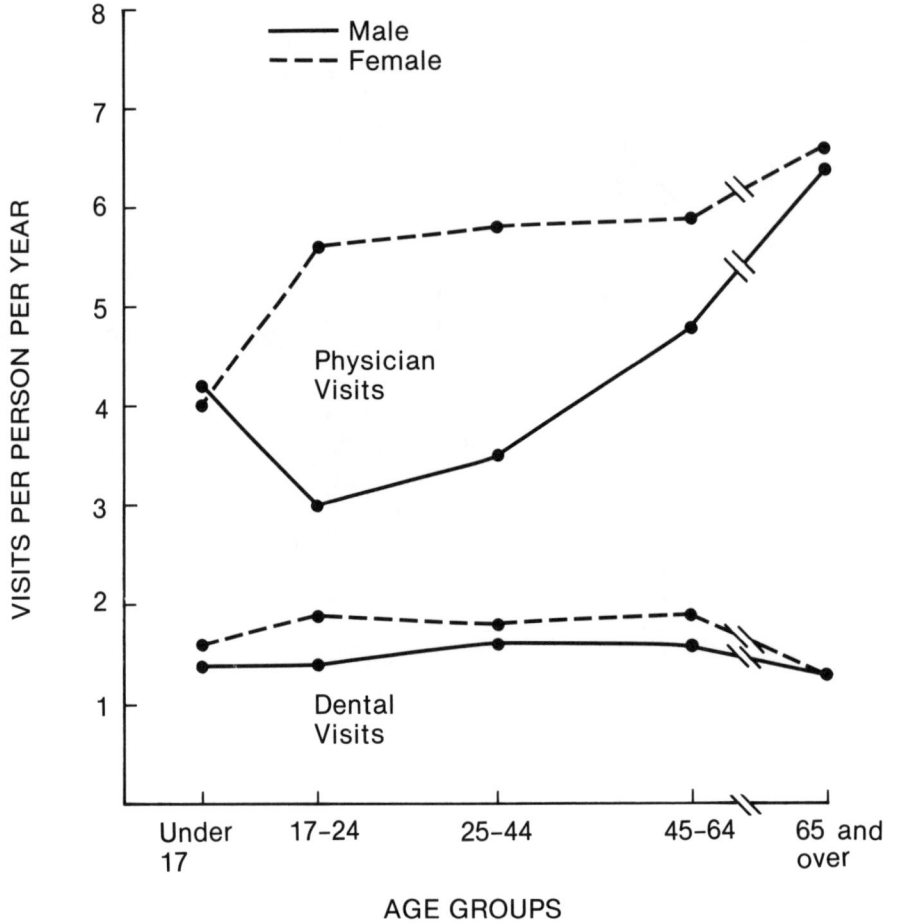

SOURCE: U.S. National Center for Health Statistics, *Current Estimates from the Health Interview Survey: U.S., 1977*, Public Health Service, Office of Health Research, Statistics, and Technology, Hyattsville, Maryland, Series 10, No. 126, Table 20, p. 30 and Table 18, p. 28.

Use of Service

Chart C-43

Percent of Persons, by Age Groups and Time Elapsed Since Last Visit to a Physician and a Dentist (U.S.A., Civilian Non-institutionalized Population, 1977).

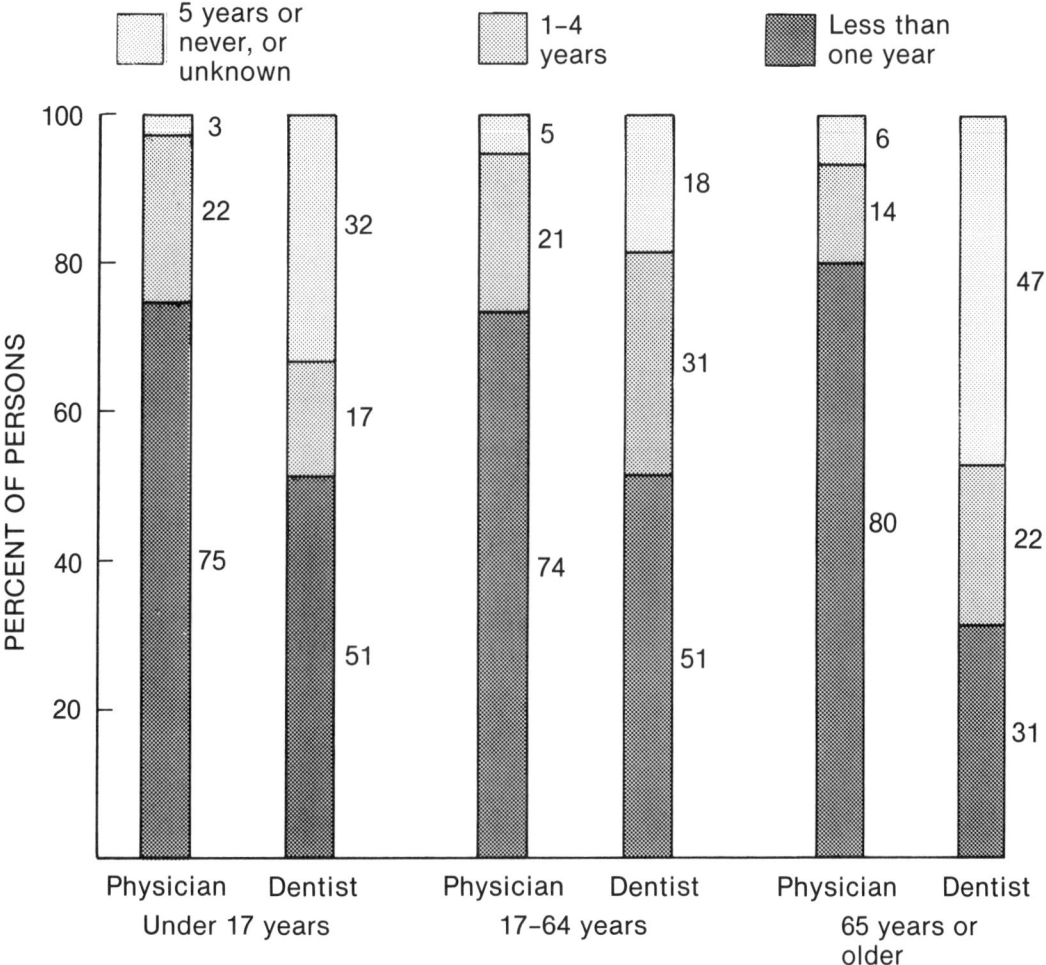

SOURCE: U.S. National Center for Health Statistics, *Current Estimates from the Health Interview Survey: U.S., 1977,* Public Health Service, Office of Health Research, Statistics, and Technology, Hyattsville, Maryland, Series 10, No. 126, September 1978, Table 19, p. 29 and Table 21, p. 31.

Chart C-44 Relative Frequency of Physician and Dental Visits, by Family Income, Residence, and Color (U.S.A., Physicians, 1975; Dentists, 1978).

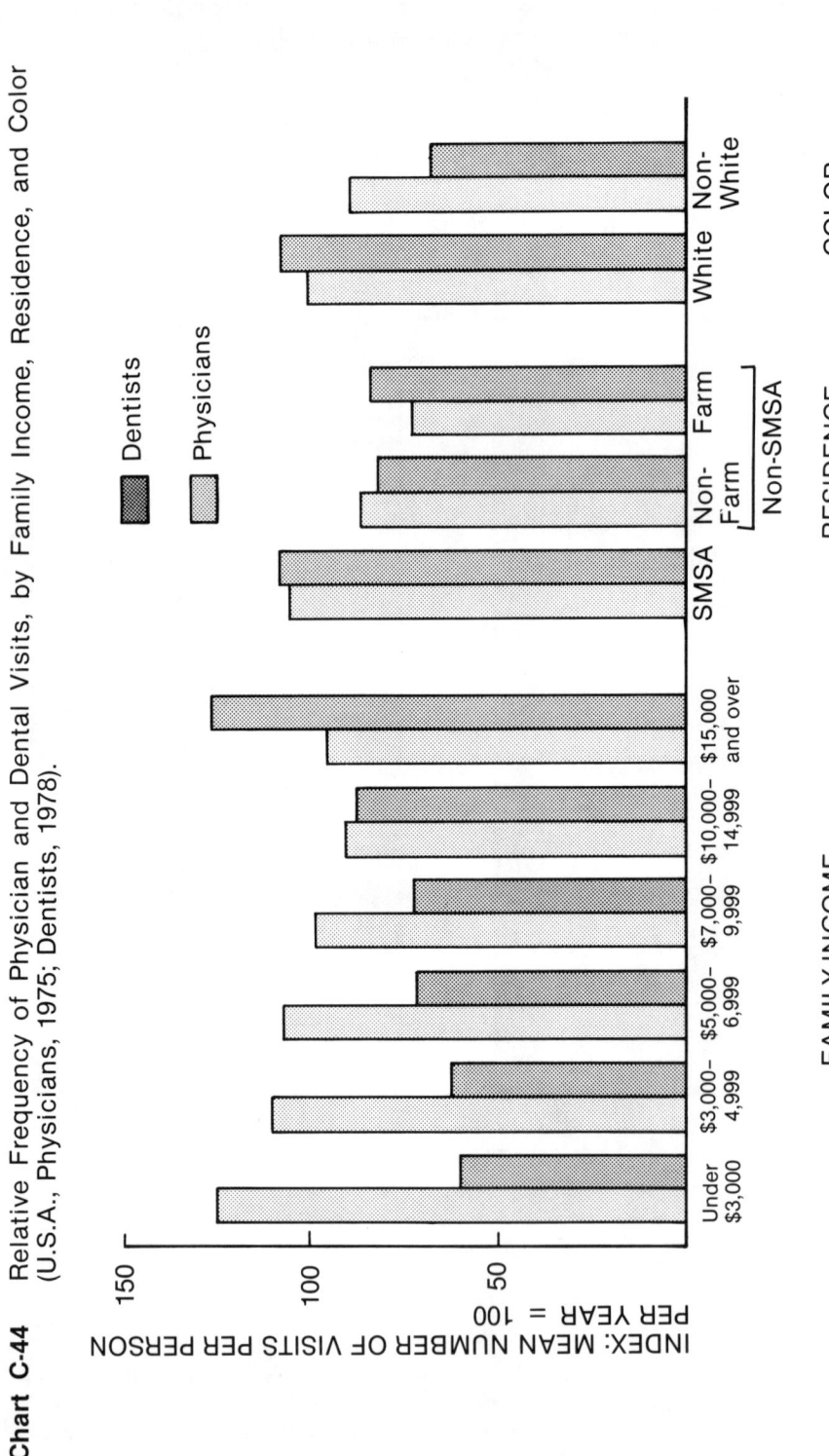

SOURCES: For physicians: National Center for Health Statistics, *Physician Visits: Volume and Interval Since Last Visit, U.S.—1975*, Public Health Service, Office of Health Research, Statistics and Technology, Hyattsville, Maryland, April 1979, Table 7, p. 21, and Table 23, p. 9; for dentists: Tabulation received from Illness and Disability Statistics Branch, Division of Health Interview Statistics, Office of Health Policy, Research, and Statistics, U.S. National Center for Health Statistics.

Chart C-45

Percent of Dental Visits During Which an Extraction was Performed, by Education of Family Head, Color, and Geographic Area (U.S.A., July 1963–June 1964).

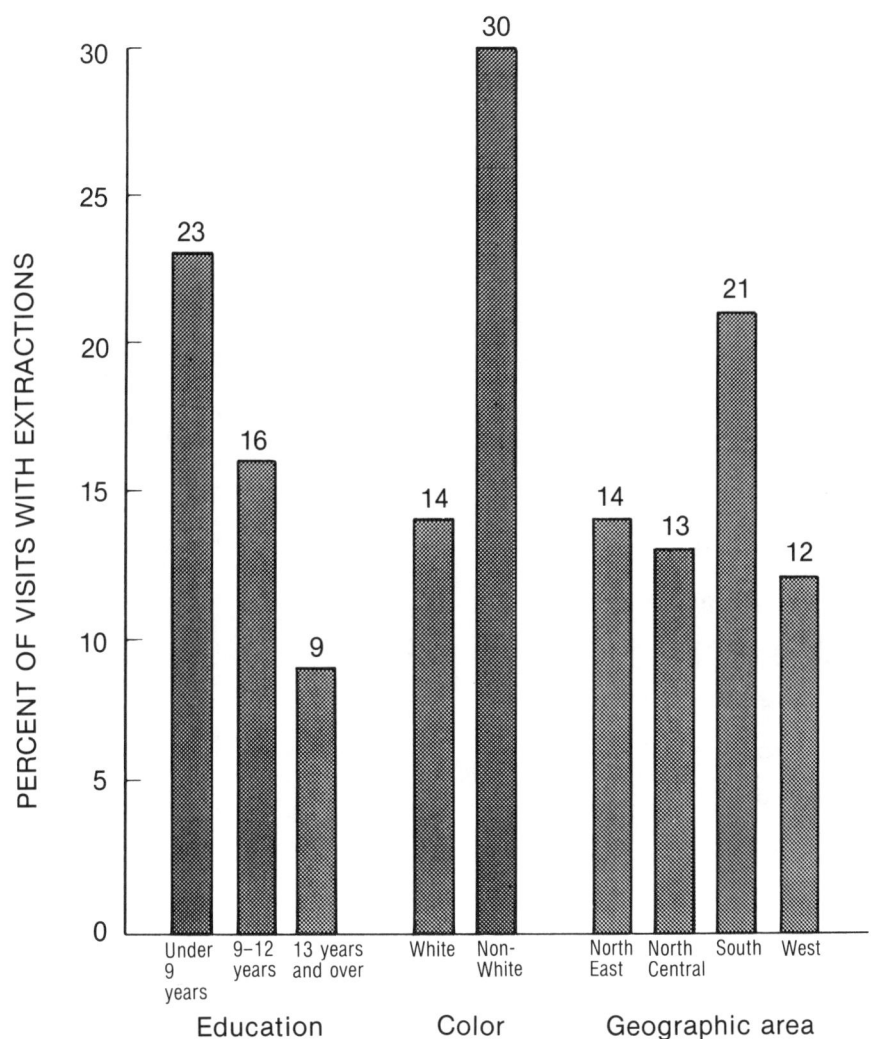

SOURCE: U.S. National Center for Health Statistics, *Volume of Dental Visits: United States, July 1963–June 1964,* Public Health Service, Washington, D.C., Series 10, No. 23, October 1965, Table 14, p. 29, Table 18, p. 33, and Table 21, p. 36.

Use of Service

Chart C-46 General Hospital Beds and Admissions per 1000 Persons and Average Length of Stay (Selected Countries and Specified Years).

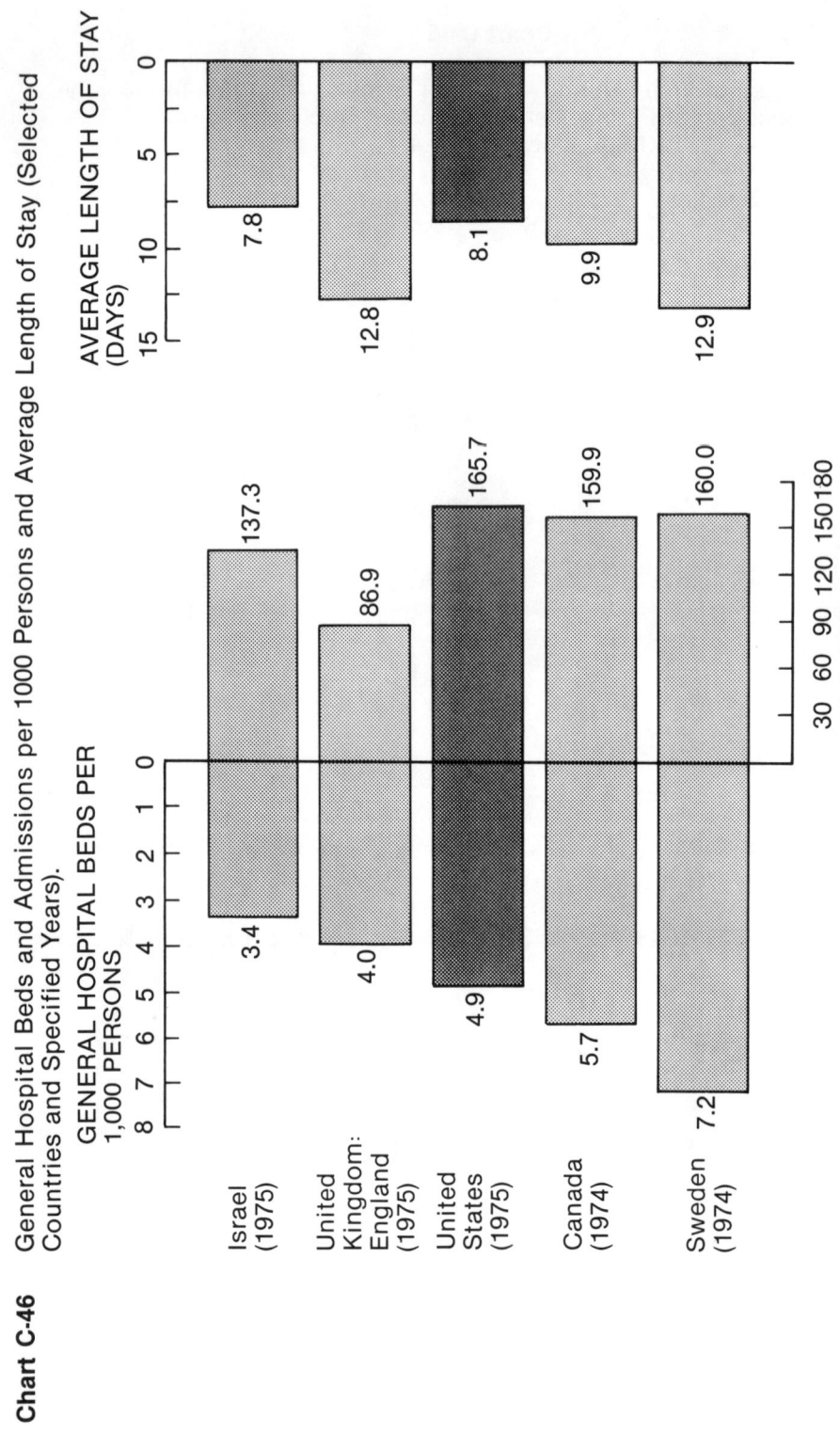

SOURCE: World Health Organization, *World Health Statistics Annual, 1977*, Vol. 111, *Health Personnel and Hospital Establishments*, Geneva, Switzerland, 1977, Table 4.2, pp. 196–202.

Chart C-47

Utilization of General Hospitals[1] (U.S.A., Selected Years, 1928-1978).

Year	Admissions Per 1000 Persons Per Year	Hospital Days Per 1000 Persons Per Year	Average Length of Stay[2]
1928[3]	58.6	746	12.7
1946	98.3	896	9.1
1950	110.5	900	8.1
1955	117.2	912	7.8
1960	128.9	977	7.6
1965	138.2	1073	7.8
1970	145.1	1190	8.2
1975	159.4	1291	8.1
1978	161.1	1288	8.0

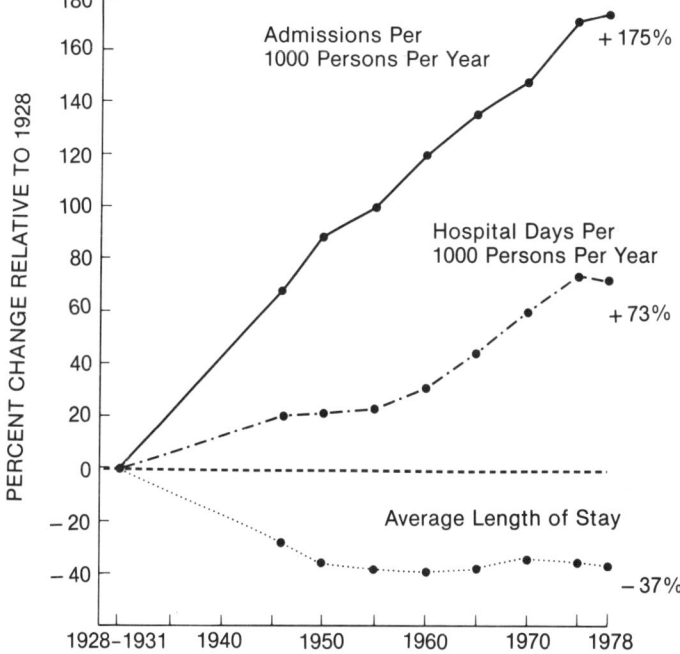

[1]For 1928, this definition includes all hospitals except TB and psychiatric hospitals; for 1946-1978, it includes all non-federal, short-term general and other special hospitals listed by the American Hospital Association.

[2]Figures for average length of stay prior to 1970 include short-term psychiatric and TB hospitals. After 1970, those hospitals are excluded from those figures. In 1978, short-term TB hospitals had 1,895 admissions and short-term psychiatric hospitals had 20,834 admissions.

[3]1928 data are from a sample study in 17 states and the District of Columbia conducted from February 1928 through May 1931. Data for 1946-1978 are nationwide data.

SOURCES: For 1928: Falk, I.S., M.C. Klem, and N. Sinai, *The Incidence of Illness and the Receipt and Costs of Medical Care Among Representative Family Groups*, Committee on the Costs of Medical Care, No. 26, January 1933, Appendix Table B-27, p. 283; for 1946-1970: "Hospital Statistics," *Hospitals*, Guide Issue 45, August 1971, Part 2, Table 1, pp. 460-462; for 1971-1978: *Hospital Statistics*, Annual editions, American Hospital Association, Table 2A, pp. 8-9; for population, 1928-1978: U.S. Department of Commerce, Bureau of the Census, *Statistical Abstract of the U.S., 1978*, Washington, D.C., 1979.

Use of Service

Chart C-48

Hospital Days per 1000 Persons per Year, in Short-Stay Non-Federal Hospitals, by Age and Sex (U.S.A., Civilian Non-institutionalized Population, 1976).

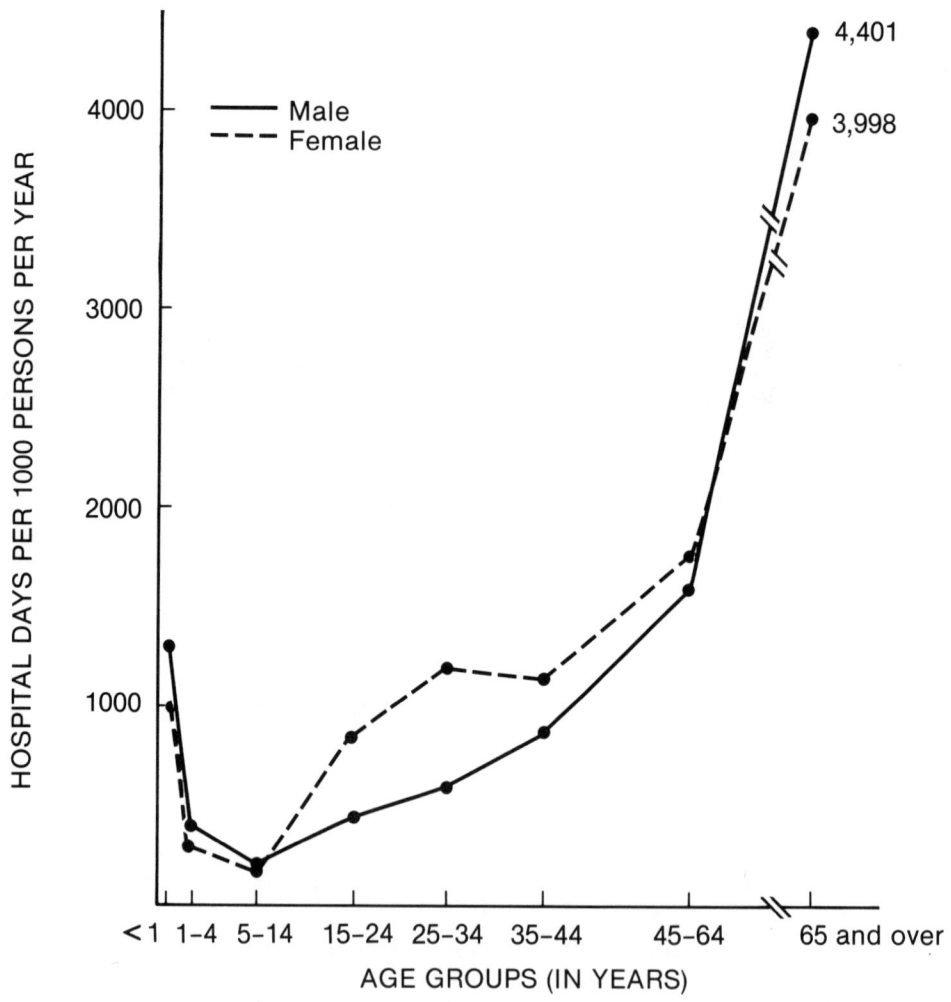

SOURCE: U.S. Department of Commerce, Bureau of the Census, *Statistical Abstract of the United States, 1978,* Washington, D.C., 1978, Table 170, p. 112.

Use of Service

Chart C-49

Relative Utilization Rates in Short-Term General Hospitals, by Age of Patient (U.S.A., 1977).

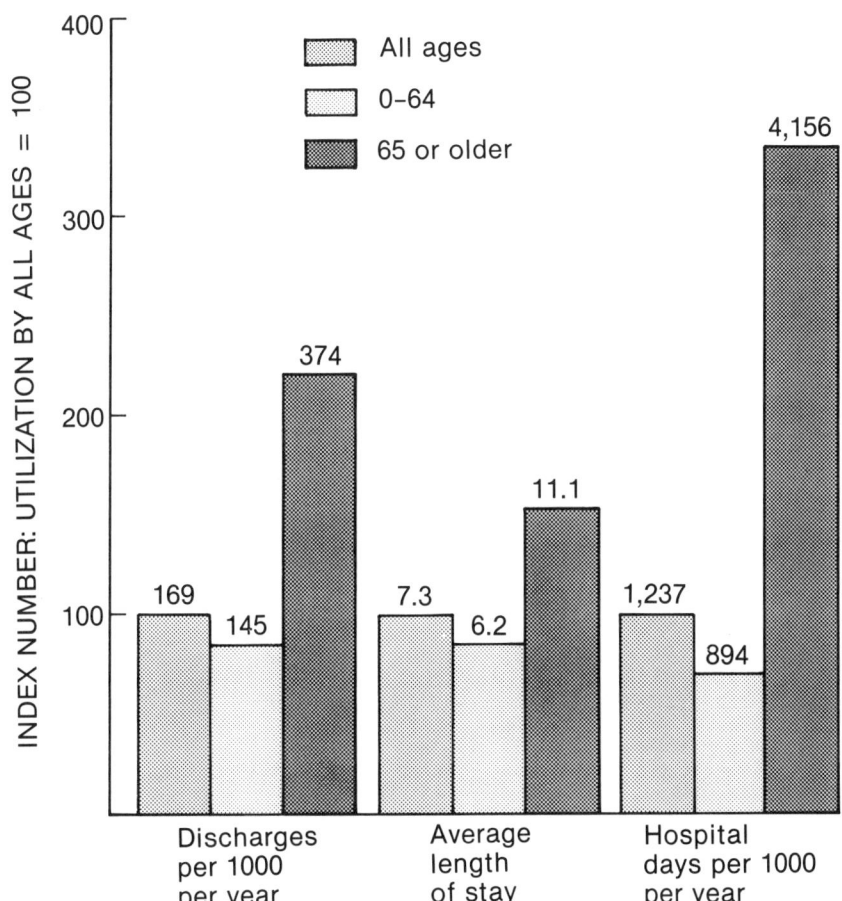

NOTE: Numbers above bars refer to actual data as distinct from index number.
SOURCE: U.S. National Center for Health Statistics, *Vital and Health Statistics,* DHEW, Public Health Service, Office of Health Research, Statistics, and Technology, Hyattsville, Maryland, Series 13, No. 41, March 1979, Table 2, p. 21, Table 11, p. 57, Table 8, p. 31, and Table 3, p. 23.

Use of Service

Chart C-50

Percent Change in Rates of Admission Per 100,000 Persons to Four Regional State Psychiatric Hospitals Following an Administrative Desegregation Order, by Color and by Specified Diagnosis (Maryland, July 1, 1961–December 31, 1962 and January 1, 1963–June 30, 1964).

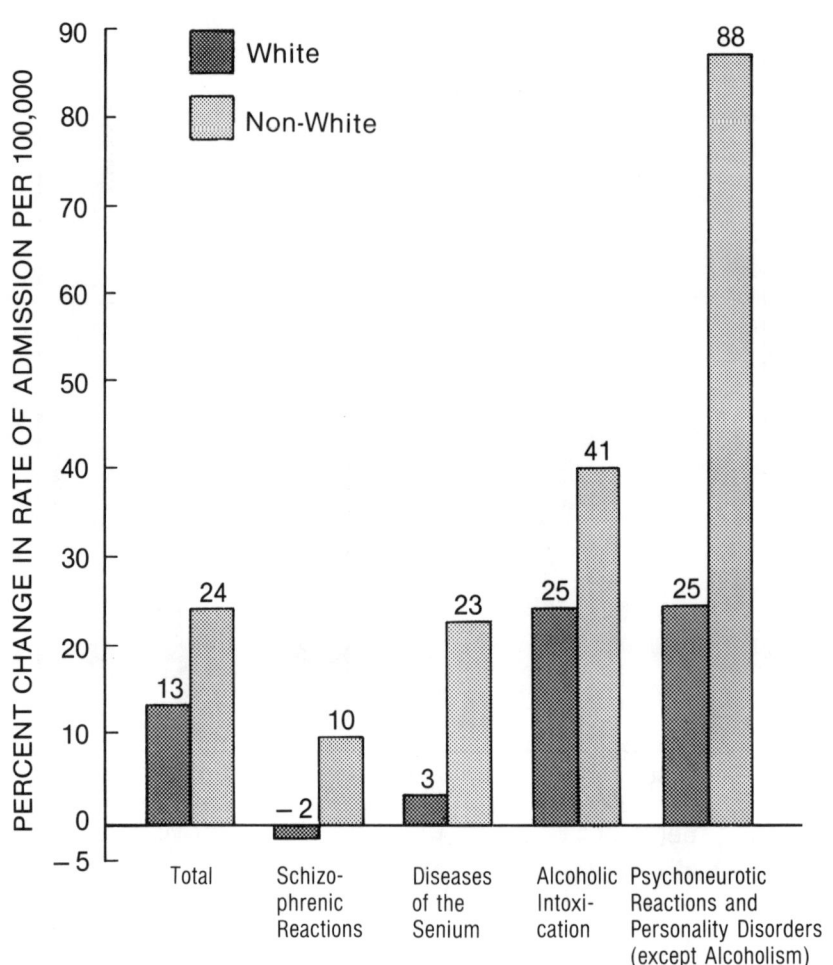

SOURCE: Gorwitz, Kurt and Frances Jean Warthen, "Effects of Desegregation of a State Hospital System on Rates of Treated Mental Illness," *HSMHA Health Reports*, Vol. 86, No. 1, January 1971, Table 4, p. 42.

Chart C-51 Utilization of Short-stay Hospitals, by Geographic Area (U.S.A., 1977).

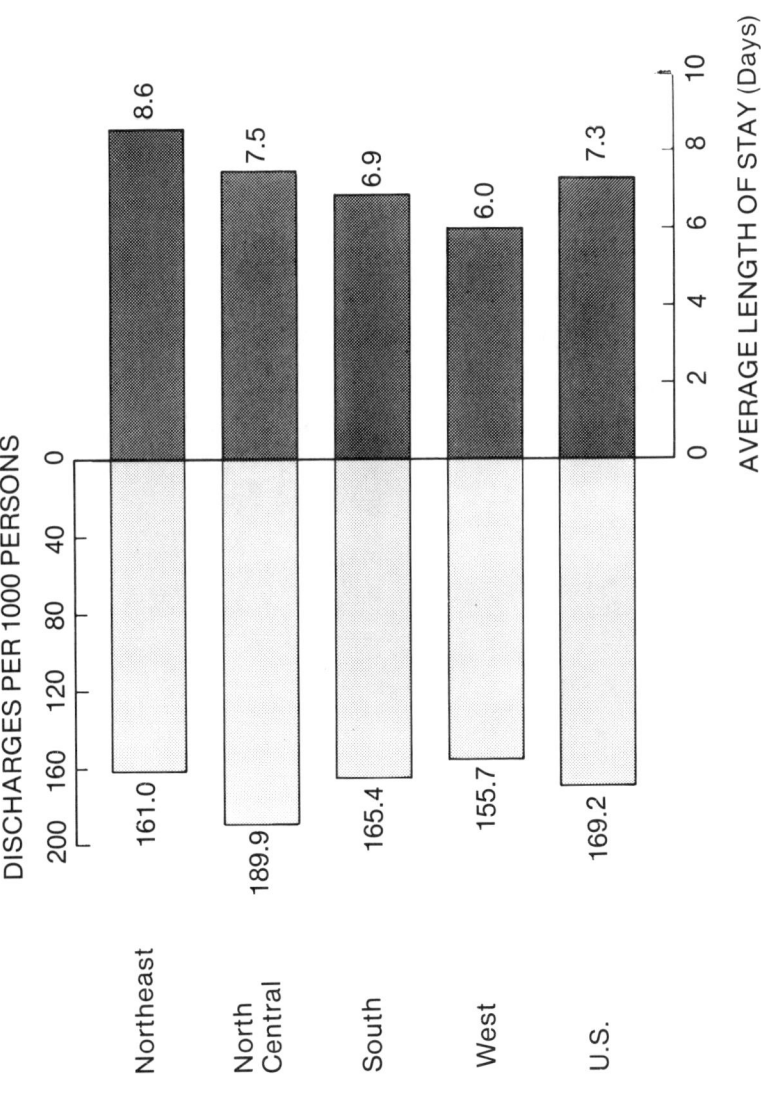

SOURCE: U.S. National Center for Health Statistics, *Utilization of Short-stay Hospitals, Annual Summary of the United States, 1977*, DHEW, Public Health Service, Office of Health Research, Statistics, and Technology, Hyattsville, Maryland, Series 13, No. 41, March 1979, Table 8, p. 31 and Table 9, p. 32.

Chart C-52

Days of Hospital Care per 1000 Persons per Year, Excluding Newborns, in Saskatchewan, Canada, and U.S.A. (1946–1975).[1]

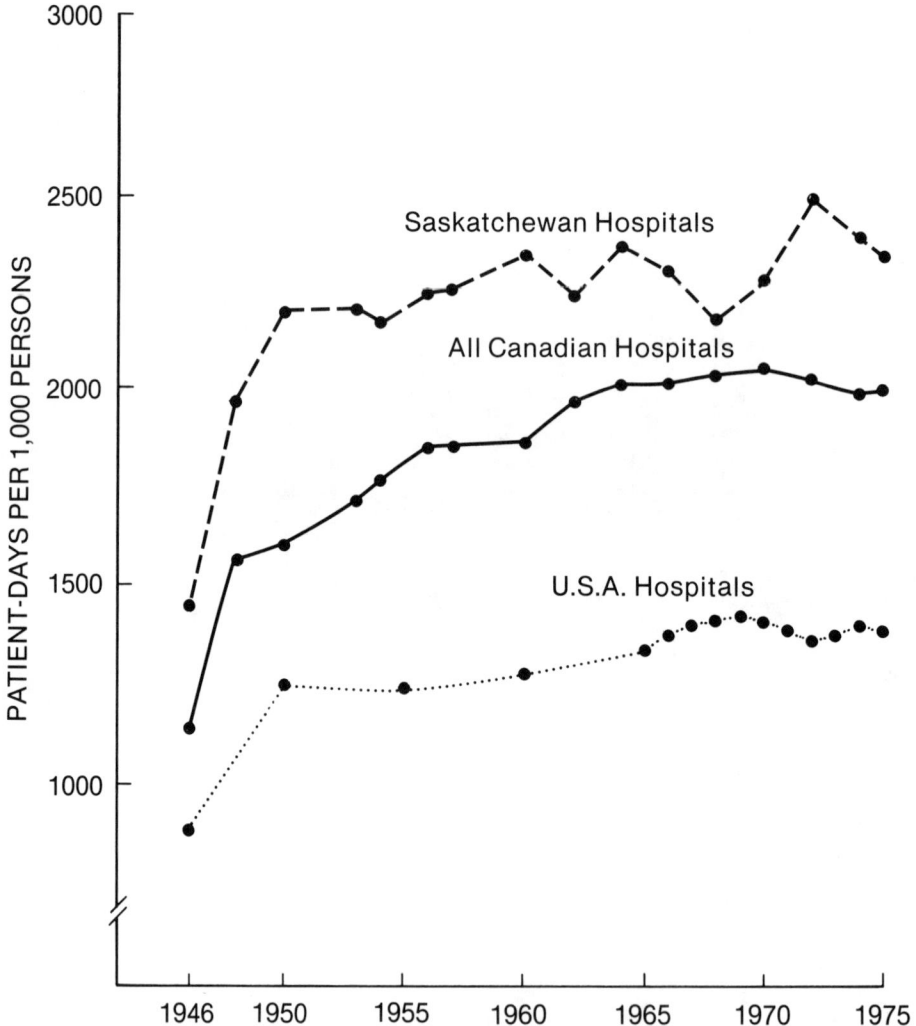

[1]Data for 1946 exclude all federal hospitals. Data for 1948–1975 include public, private, and federal hospitals for Saskatchewan and Canada, and federal and non-federal short-term general and other special hospitals for the United States.

NOTE: The Saskatchewan Hospital Services Plan, a government-sponsored compulsory program of hospital care insurance covering all residents of the province, went into effect in 1947.

SOURCES: For Canada and Saskatchewan: Dominion Bureau of Statistics, Bureau of Trade and Commerce, *Annual Report of Hospitals,* 1946, 1947, 1948, 1950; Dominion Bureau of Statistics, Health and Welfare Division, *Hospital Statistics,* Vol. 1, 1953, 1954, 1956, 1957, 1964, 1968; Statistics Canada, *Hospital Statistics,* Vol. 1, Hospital Beds, 1972, 1975; for U.S.A.: *Hospital Statistics, 1979 Edition,* American Hospital Association, Table 1, pp. 4–5.

Use of Service

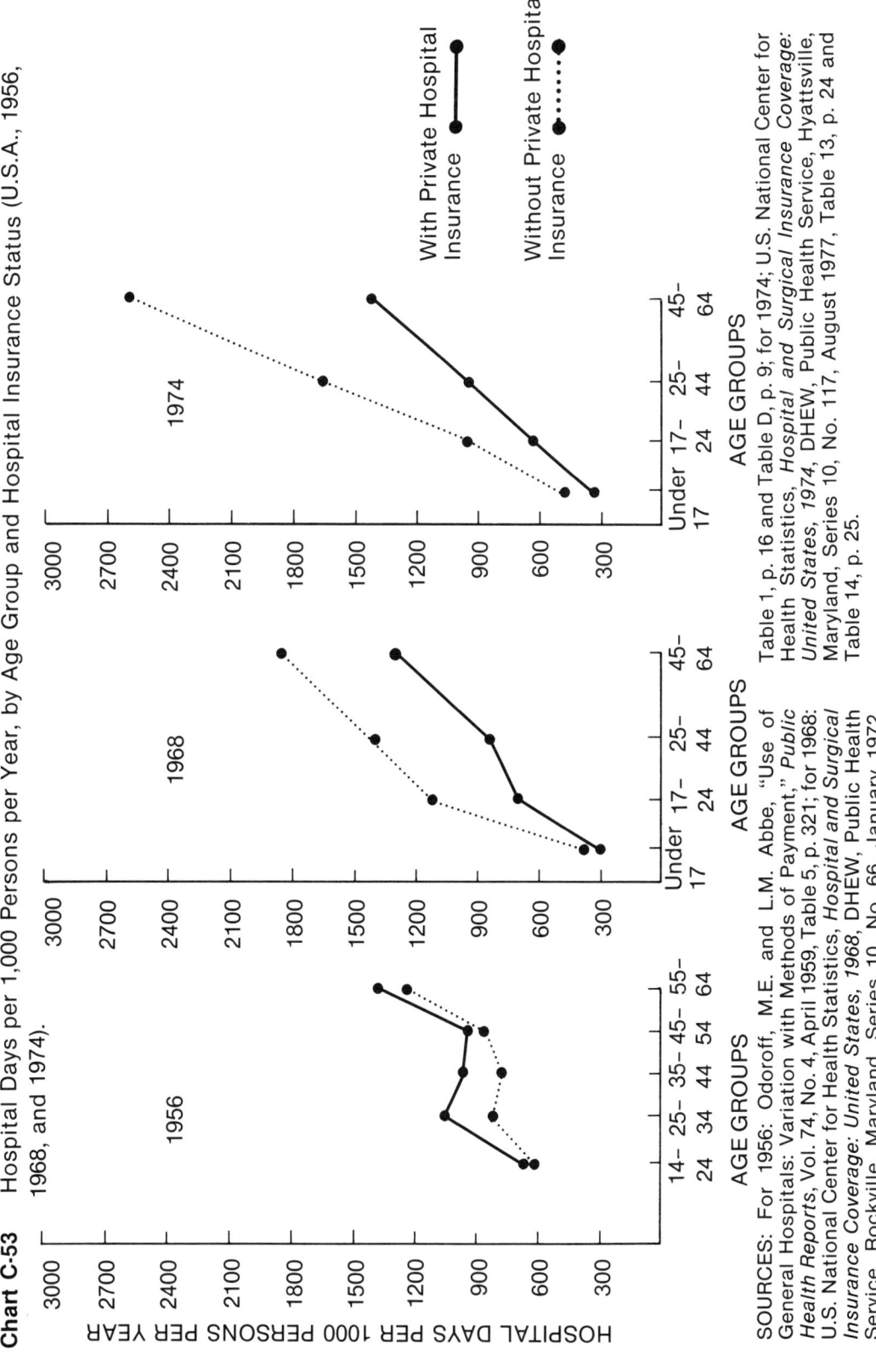

Chart C-53 Hospital Days per 1,000 Persons per Year, by Age Group and Hospital Insurance Status (U.S.A., 1956, 1968, and 1974).

SOURCES: For 1956: Odoroff, M.E. and L.M. Abbe, "Use of General Hospitals: Variation with Methods of Payment," *Public Health Reports*, Vol. 74, No. 4, April 1959, Table 5, p. 321; for 1968: U.S. National Center for Health Statistics, *Hospital and Surgical Insurance Coverage: United States, 1968*, DHEW, Public Health Service, Rockville, Maryland, Series 10, No. 66, January 1972, Table 1, p. 16 and Table D, p. 9; for 1974: U.S. National Center for Health Statistics, *Hospital and Surgical Insurance Coverage: United States, 1974*, DHEW, Public Health Service, Hyattsville, Maryland, Series 10, No. 117, August 1977, Table 13, p. 24 and Table 14, p. 25.

Use of Service

Chart C-54

Percent of Persons Under Age 65 with Short-stay Hospital Episodes in the Past Year, by Private Insurance Status and Income (U.S.A., Civilian Non-institutionalized Population, 1974).

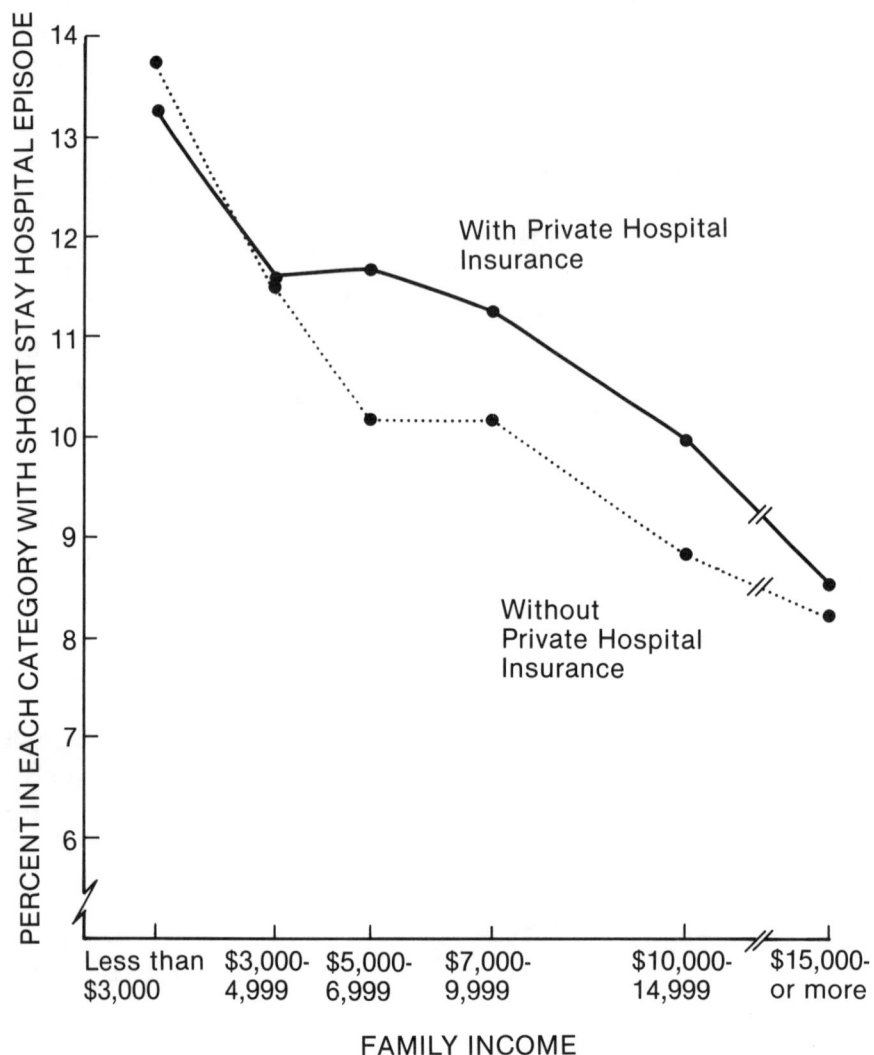

SOURCE: U.S. National Center for Health Statistics, *Hospitals and Surgical Insurance Coverage–United States, 1974,* DHEW, Public Health Service, Office of Health Research, Statistics, and Technology, Hyattsville, Maryland, Series 10, No. 117, August 1977, Table 13, p. 24.

Chart C-55 Days in Short-term Hospitals per 1000 Persons per Year, by Family Income and Private Hospital Insurance Status, for Persons Under Age 65 (U.S.A., 1956 and 1974).

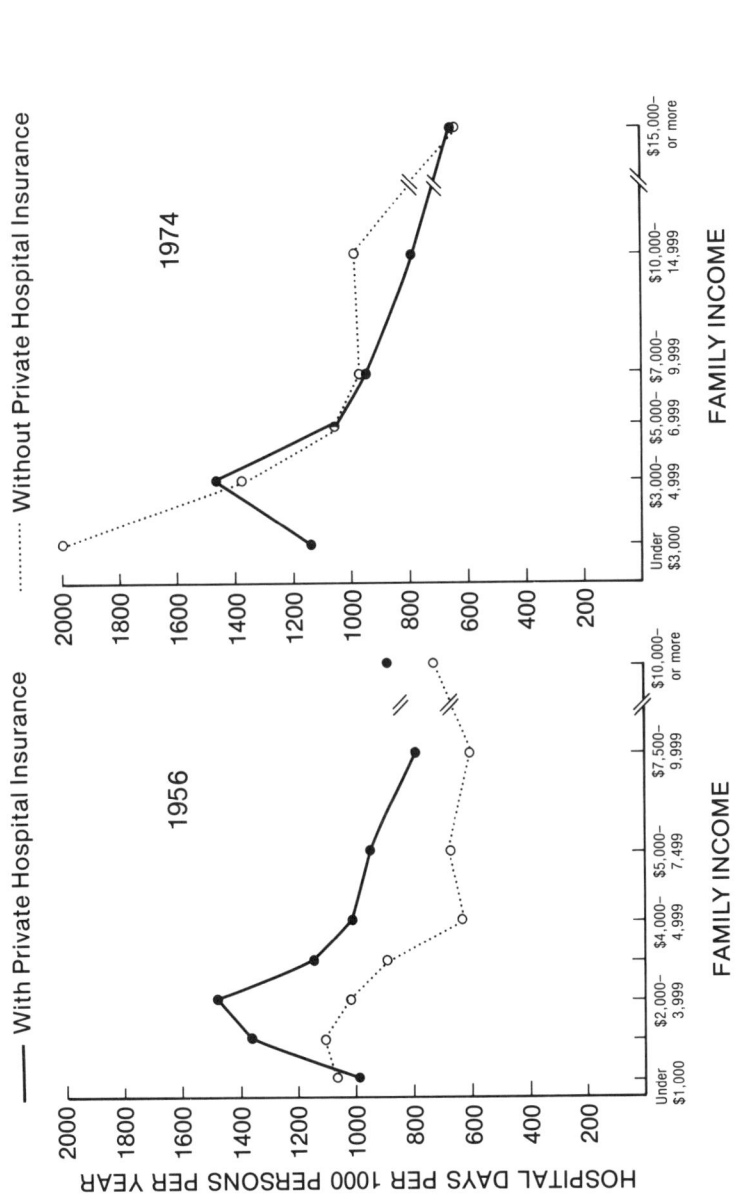

SOURCES: For 1956: U.S. Department of Health, Education, and Welfare, *Public Health Reports*, Public Health Service, Vol. 74, No. 4, April 1959, Table 7, p. 323; for 1974: U.S. National Center for Health Statistics, *Hospital and Surgical Insurance Coverage-United States, 1974*, DHEW, Public Health Service, Office of Health Research, Statistics, and Technology, Hyattsville, Maryland, Series 10, No. 117, August 1977, Table 13, p. 24 and Table 14, p. 25.

Chart C-56

Relative Utilization of Selected Services, by Multiple Insurance Status (U.S.A., 1963).

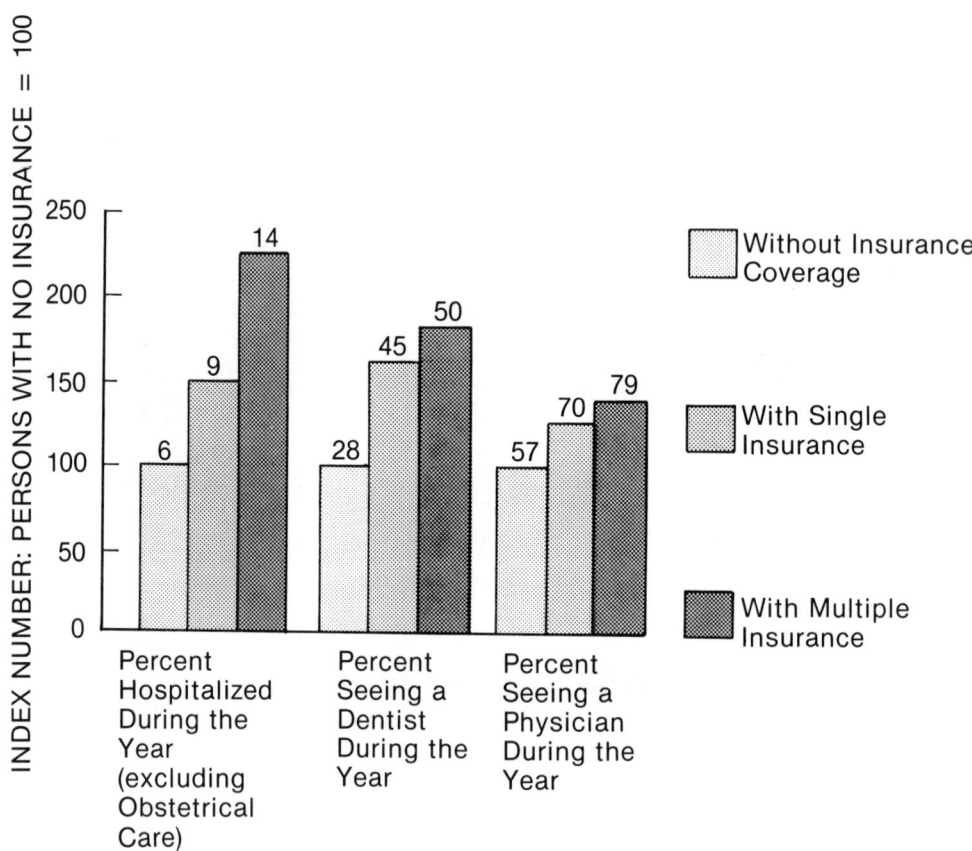

NOTE: Actual values are shown above bars.

SOURCE: Andersen, R. and D.C. Riedel, *People and Their Hospital Insurance*, University of Chicago, Center for Health Administration Studies, Chicago, 1967, Research Series 23, Table 9, p. 22.

Use of Service

Chart C-57

Percent of Hospital Patients Who Stayed in the Hospital for Longer and Shorter Times than Considered Necessary, by Source of Payment of Hospital Expenses (Patients with 17 Selected Diagnoses, Michigan Hospitals, 1958).

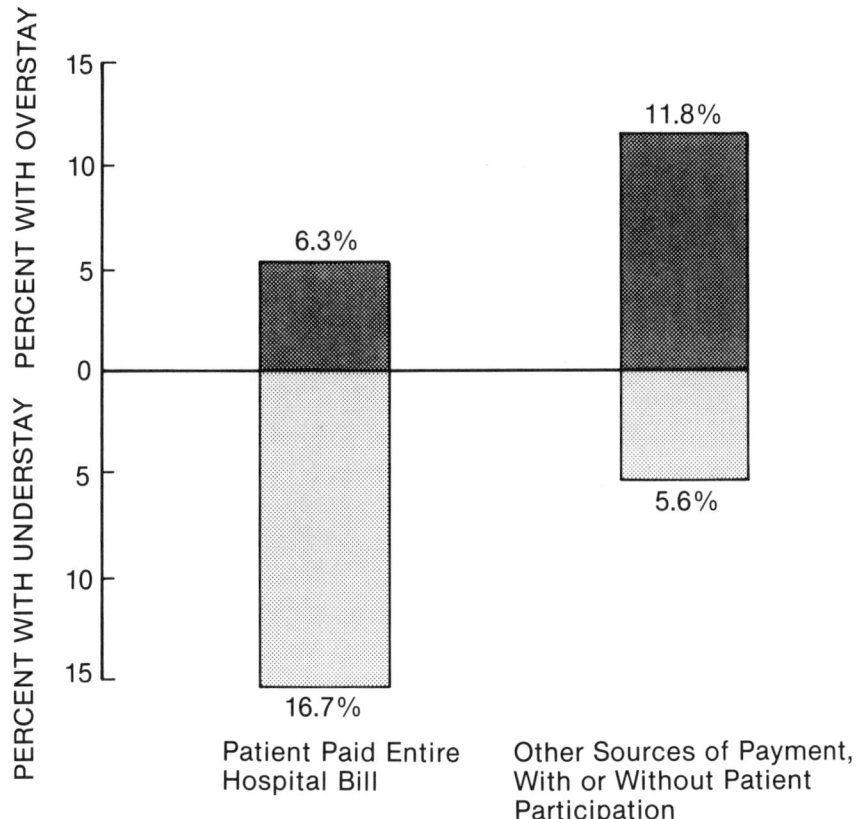

SOURCE: McNerney, W.J., et al., *Hospital and Medical Economics—A Study of Population, Services, Costs, Methods of Payment, and Controls*, Hospital Research and Education Trust, Chicago, 1962, Table 221, p. 490.

Use of Service

Chart C-58

Percent Distribution of Hospital Stays and of Hospital Days, by Appropriateness of Admission and of Stay[1], Sample of Discharges in 16 Diagnostic Categories, 22 Non-Federal, Short-term Hospitals (Hawaii, 1968).

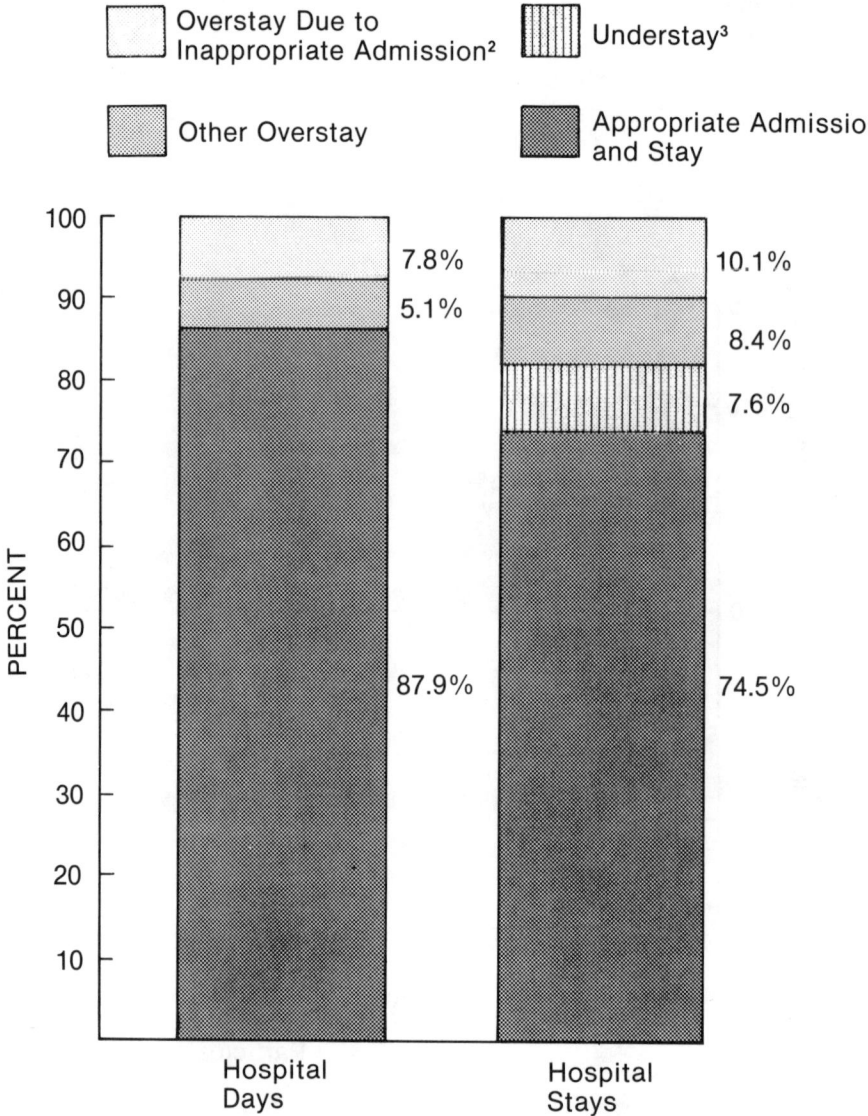

[1]Judged according to criteria for each diagnosis formulated by panels of "outstanding practitioners" in Hawaii.

[2]Entire stay of inappropriately admitted cases considered to be "overstay."

[3]The category of "understay" is not represented in "hospital days." Days of understay would have to be added to hospital days actually experienced.

SOURCE: Payne, B.C. and T.F. Lyons, *Method of Evaluating and Improving Medical Care Quality: Episode of Illness Study*, Ann Arbor: School of Medicine, The University of Michigan, February 1972, pp. 39–43.

Use of Service

Chart C-59

Relative Hospital Admission Rates for Specified Diagnoses (Selected Localities,[1] Saskatchewan, Canada, 1956).

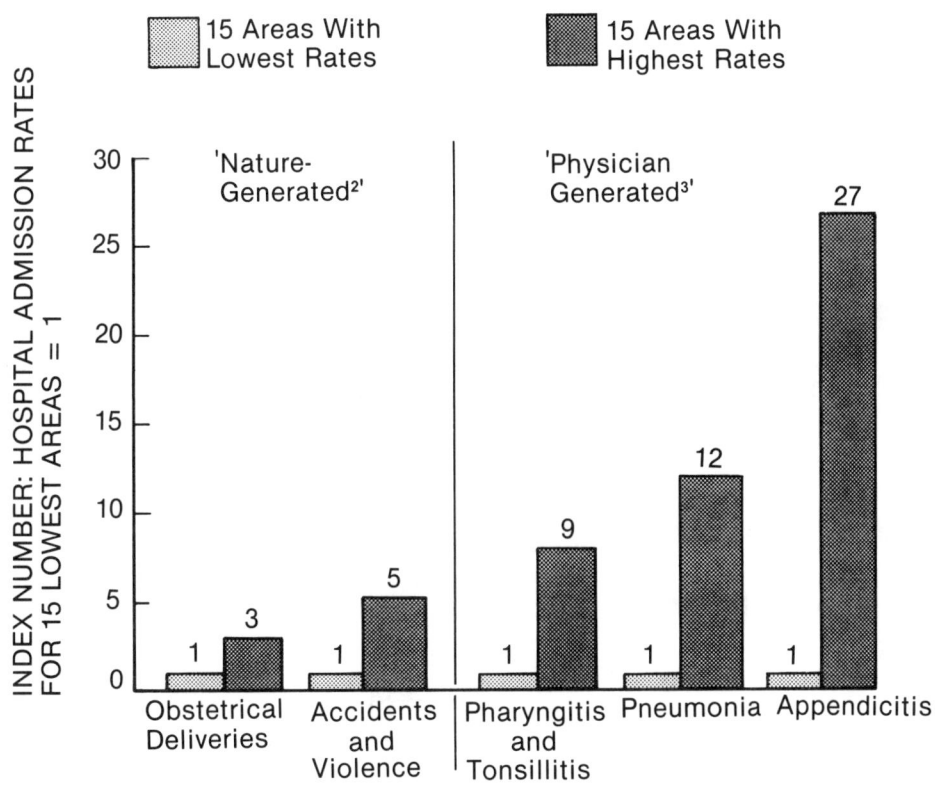

[1] 15 places with highest rates and 15 places with lowest rates among a total of 310 localities.

[2] 'Nature-generated' includes conditions in which an outside event largely determines the need for hospitalization.

[3] 'Physician-generated' includes conditions in which a relatively refined medical or surgical diagnosis determines whether or not the patient should be hospitalized.

SOURCE: Roemer, M.I., "How Medical Judgment Affects Hospital Admissions," *Modern Hospital*, Vol. 49, April 1960, p. 112.

Chart C-60

Utilization Changes of a General Hospital Associated With an Increase in its Bed Capacity (A County in Upstate New York, 1957–1959).

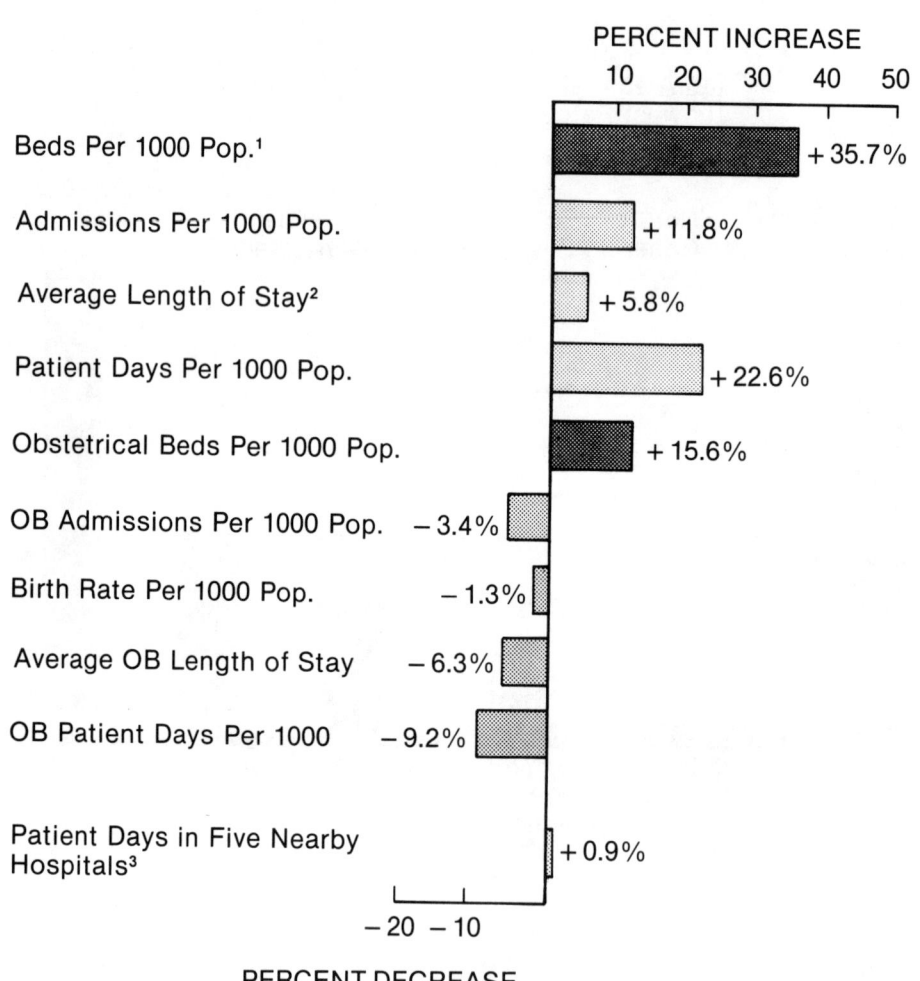

[1] Including 12 beds in a proprietary hospital serving the same county.

[2] Of 53 diagnostic categories, length of stay was increased in 40 and reduced in 13.

[3] Patient-days were increased in three hospitals and reduced in two with a range of +7.2% to −2.2%.

SOURCE: Roemer, M.I., "Bed Supply and Hospital Utilization: A Natural Experiment," *Hospitals*, Vol. 35, November 1, 1961, pp. 36–42.

Use of Service

Chart C-61

Percent Distribution of Short-term Hospital Stays and Hospital Admissions (U.S.A., 1977).

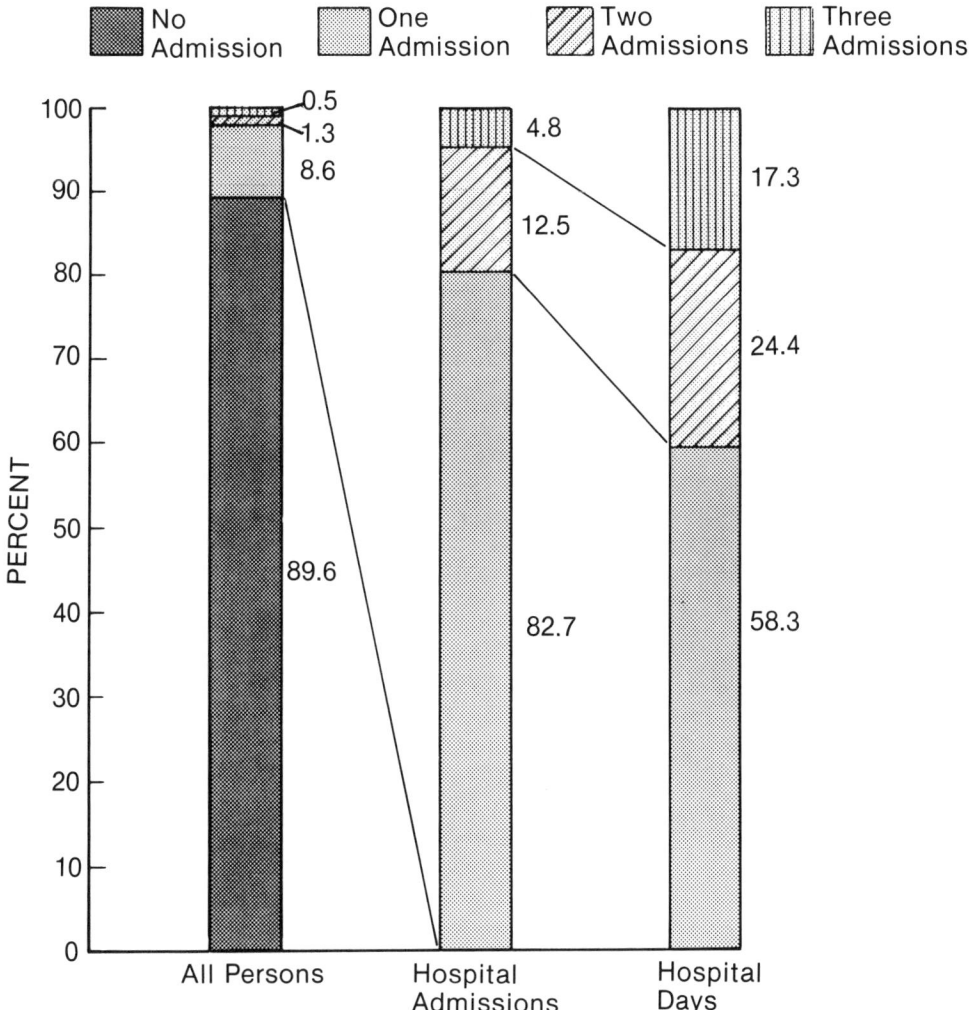

SOURCE: U.S. National Center for Health Statistics, *Current Estimates from the Health Interview Survey: U.S. 1977,* Public Health Service, Office of Health Research, Statistics, and Technology, Hyattsville, Maryland, Series 10, No. 126, September 1978, Table 16, p. 26 and Table 17, p. 27.

Chart C-62

Reduction in Medical Care Utilization by High-Utilizers of Services Following Psychiatric Intervention (Kaiser Foundation Health Plan, California, 1959–1964).

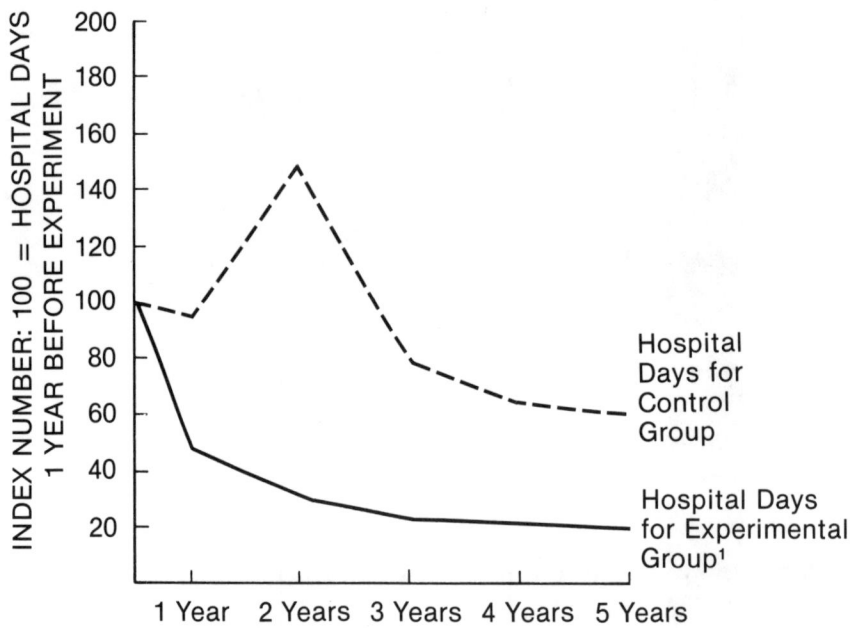

TIME AFTER PSYCHIATRIC INTERVENTION

[1] Of the 152 patients in the experimental group, 80 were seen for one interview only, 41 were seen for two to eight interviews (mean of 6.2), defined as "brief therapy," and 31 were seen for nine or more interviews (mean of 33.9), defined as "long term therapy."

SOURCE: Follette, William and Nicholas A. Cummings, "Psychiatric Services and Medical Utilization in a Prepaid Health Plan Setting," *Medical Care*, Vol. 1, January–February 1967, Table 7, p. 31.

Use of Service

Chart C-63

Percent Distribution of Persons 3 Years of Age and Over Who Were Examined for Corrective Lenses in the Previous 2 Years, by Source of Prescription and Years in School of the Head of the Family (U.S.A., Civilian Noninstitutionalized Population, July 1965–June 1966).

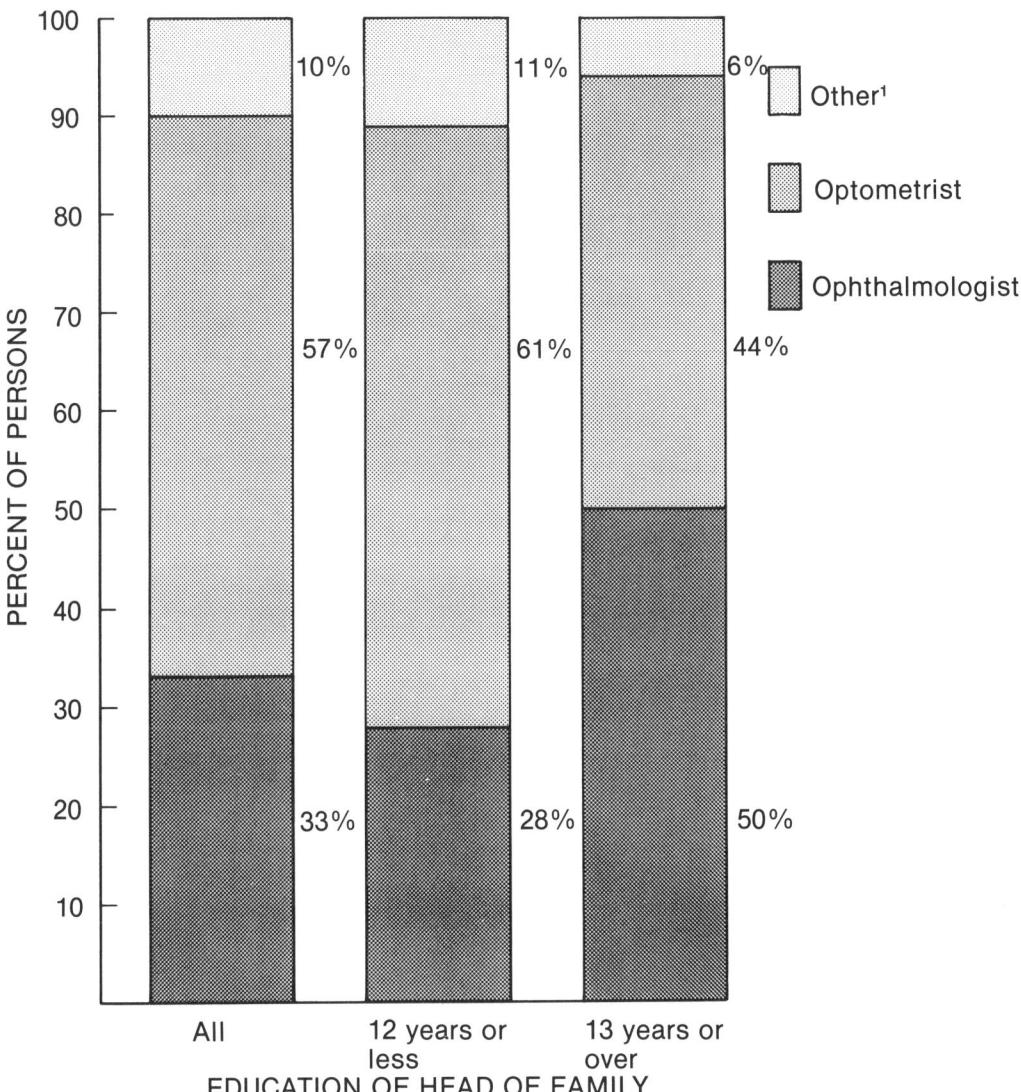

[1] Includes unknown source of optical prescription amounting to about 8.9 percent of the entire sample.

NOTE: Partial verification suggested that "the respondents' inability to distinguish between ophthalmologists and optometrists is not a major reporting problem."

SOURCE: U.S. National Center for Health Statistics, *Characteristics of Persons With Corrective Lenses: United States, July 1965–June 1966*, Public Health Service, Washington, D.C., Series 10, No. 53, June 1969, Table 18, p. 35.

Chart C-64

Percent of Population Who Received Services from Selected Practitioners During Year Prior to Interview, by Family Income (U.S.A., Civilian Non-institutionalized Population, 1974).

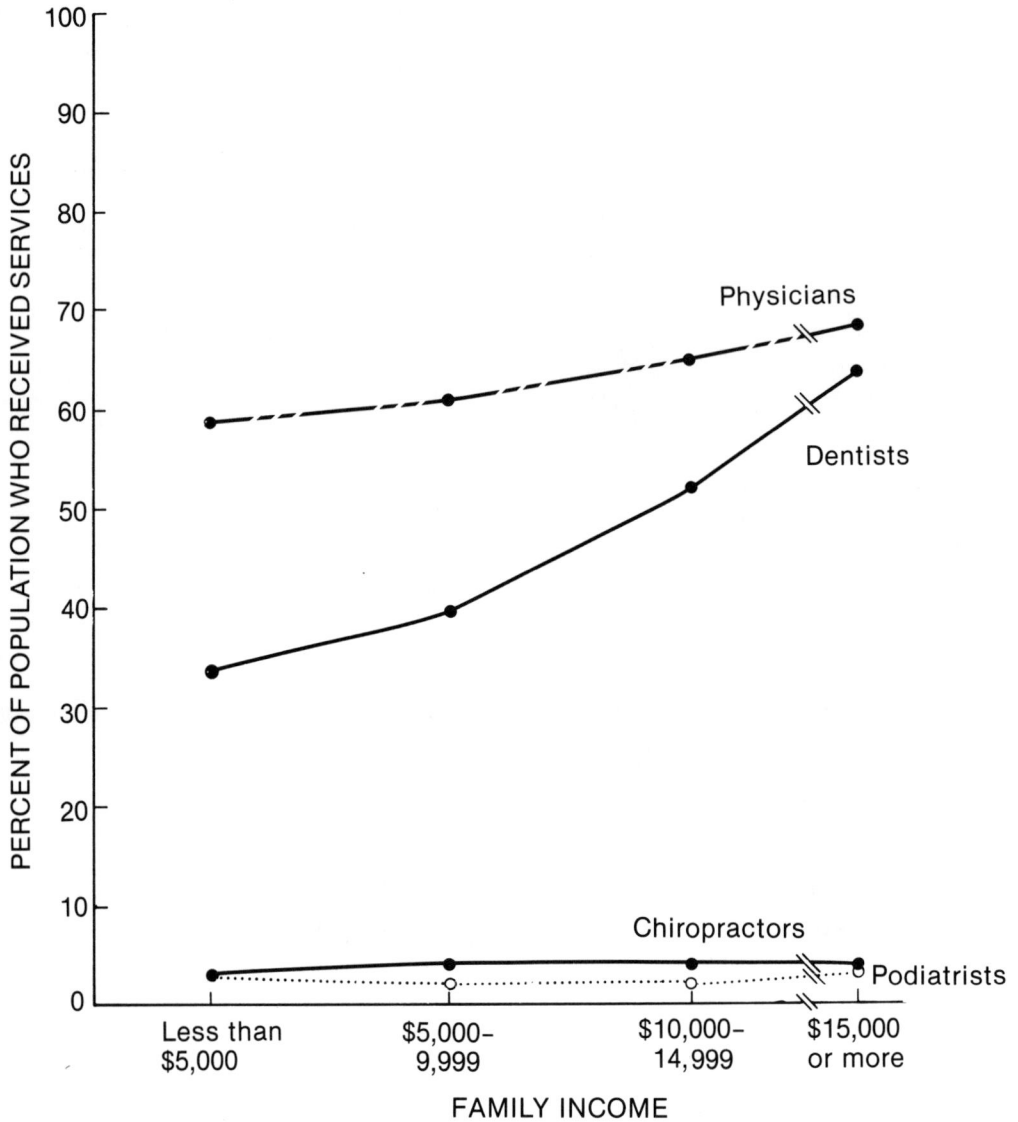

SOURCE: U.S. National Center for Health Statistics, *Health, United States, 1978*, DHEW, Public Health Service, Office of the Assistant Secretary for Health, Hyattsville, Maryland, December 1978, Table 93, p. 295.

Use of Service

Chart C-65 Average Number of Prescribed Drugs Purchased per Person per Year, by Selected Characteristics and Age (U.S.A., 1973).

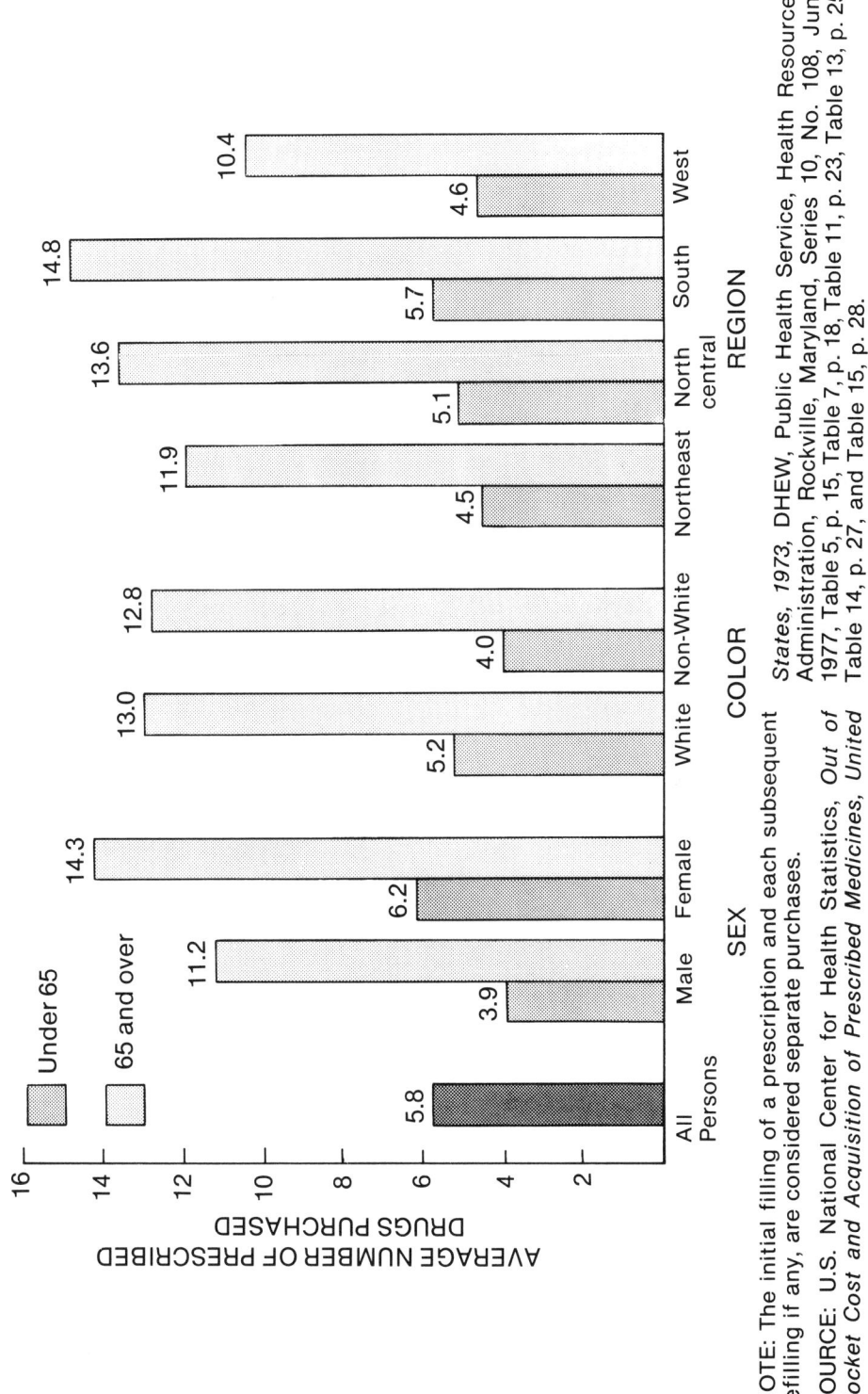

NOTE: The initial filling of a prescription and each subsequent refilling if any, are considered separate purchases.

SOURCE: U.S. National Center for Health Statistics, *Out of Pocket Cost and Acquisition of Prescribed Medicines, United States, 1973*, DHEW, Public Health Service, Health Resources Administration, Rockville, Maryland, Series 10, No. 108, June 1977, Table 5, p. 15, Table 7, p. 18, Table 11, p. 23, Table 13, p. 25, Table 14, p. 27, and Table 15, p. 28.

SECTION D
Costs and Expenditures

Glossary of Selected Terms Used in Section D

National health expenditures are the amounts spent for all health services and supplies and health-related research and construction activities consumed in the United States during a specific time period.

Health services and supplies expenditures are outlays for goods and services relating directly to patient care plus expenses for administering health insurance programs and for government public health activities. This category is equivalent to total national health expenditures minus expenditures for research and construction.

Personal health care expenditures are outlays for goods and services relating directly to patient care. The expenditures in this category are total national health expenditures minus expenditures for research and construction, expenses for administering health insurance programs, and expenditures for government public health activities.

Out-of-pocket expenses are amounts paid directly by the individual or family member exclusive of any part paid by insurance, other person, or agency.

Private expenditures are outlays for services provided or paid for by nongovernmental sources — consumers, insurance companies, private industry, and philanthropic organizations.

Public expenditures are outlays for services provided or paid for by Federal, State, and local government agencies or expenditures required by governmental action (such as workmen's compensation insurance payments).

Chart D-1

Percent Distribution of Medical Care Costs and of Wages Lost Due to Morbidity and Illness-Related Mortality (U.S.A., 1963 and Fiscal year 1975).

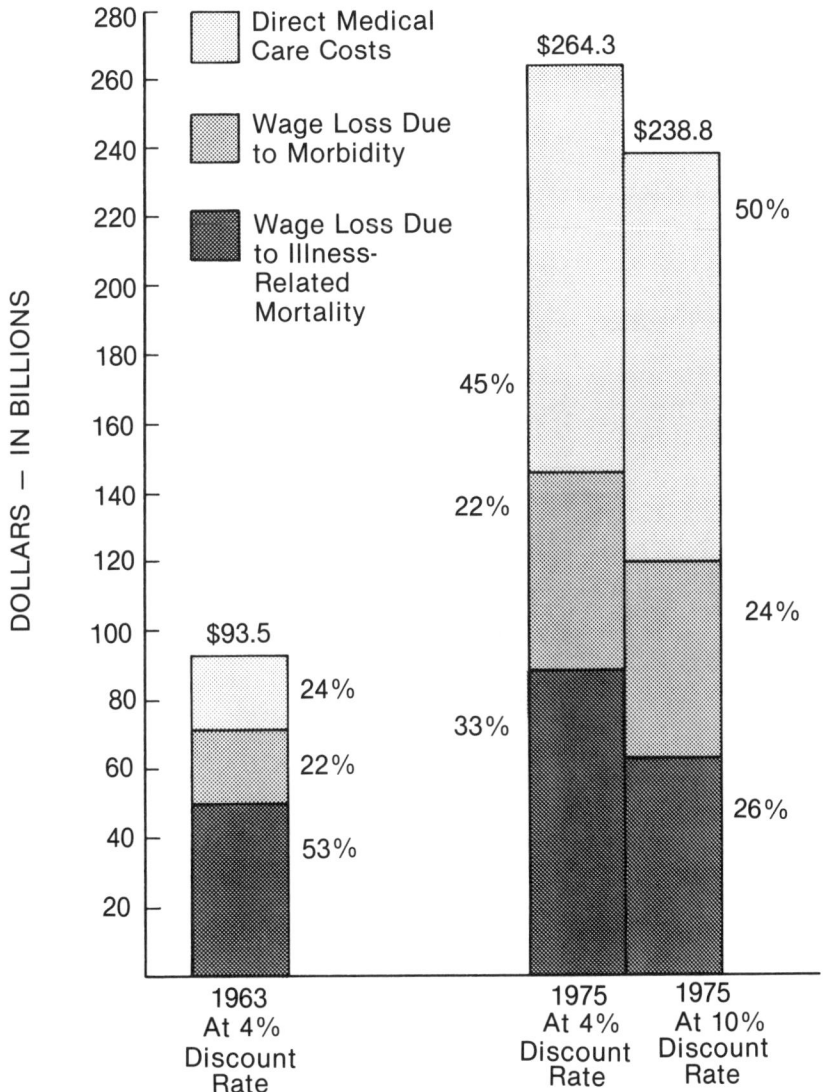

[1]1963 excludes $4.3 billion for drugs and drug sundries. 1975 includes drugs and sundries.

SOURCES: For 1963: Cooper, B.S. and D.P. Rice, "The Economic Cost of Illness Revisited," *Social Security Bulletin,* Vol. 39, No. 2, February 1976, Table 8, p. 31; for 1975: Berk, A., L. Paringer, and S.J. Mushlin, "The Economic Cost of Illness; Fiscal 1975," *Medical Care,* Vol. 16, No. 9, September 1978, Table 1, p. 785, Table 2, p. 786, Table 3, p. 787, and Table 5, p. 789.

Costs and Expenditures

Chart D-2

Direct and Indirect Cost of Selected Illnesses[1] (U.S.A., 1975).

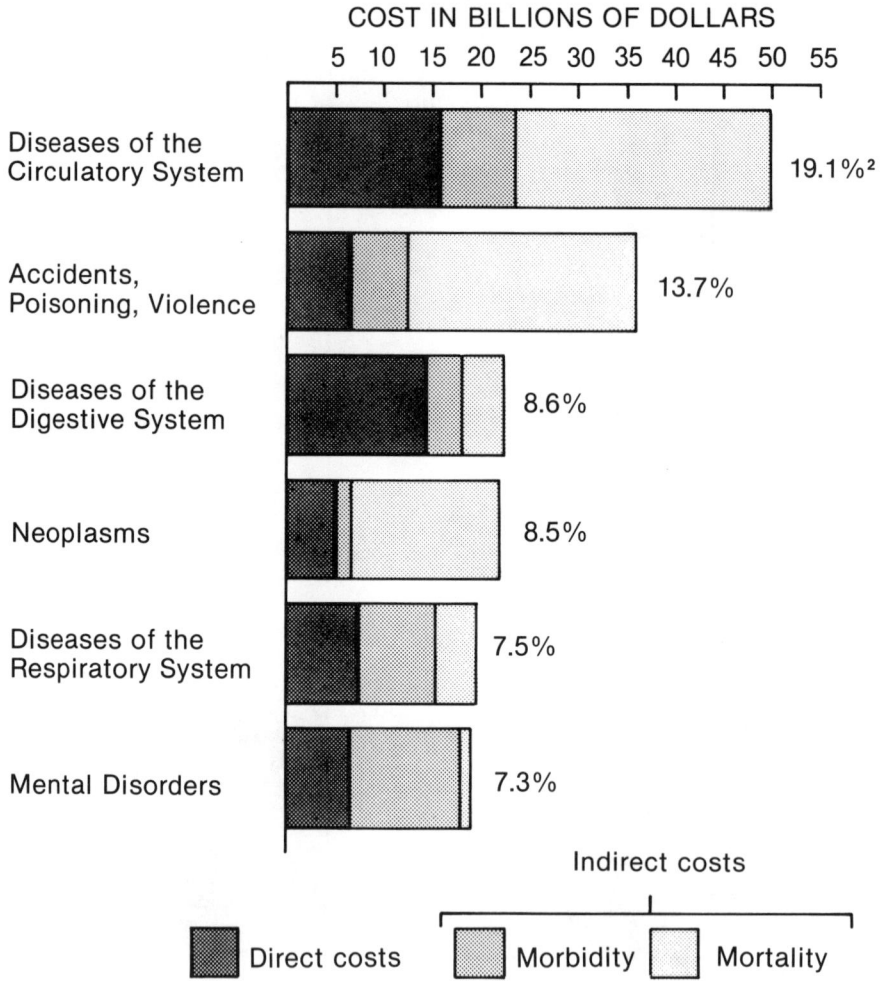

[1]Six most costly diagnoses on the basis of total economic costs for 1975 with lost future earnings discounted at 4%.

[2]Percent of total economic costs ($264.3 billion for 1975).

SOURCE: Berk, A., L. Paringer, and S. J. Mushkin, "The Economic Cost of Illness, Fiscal 1975," *Medical Care*, Vol. 16, No. 9, September 1978, Table 2, p. 786.

Costs and Expenditures

Chart D-3 Present Value of Lifetime Earnings, Discounted at 6 Percent and 10 Percent, by Age and Sex (U.S.A., Fiscal 1975).

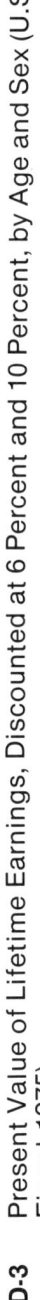

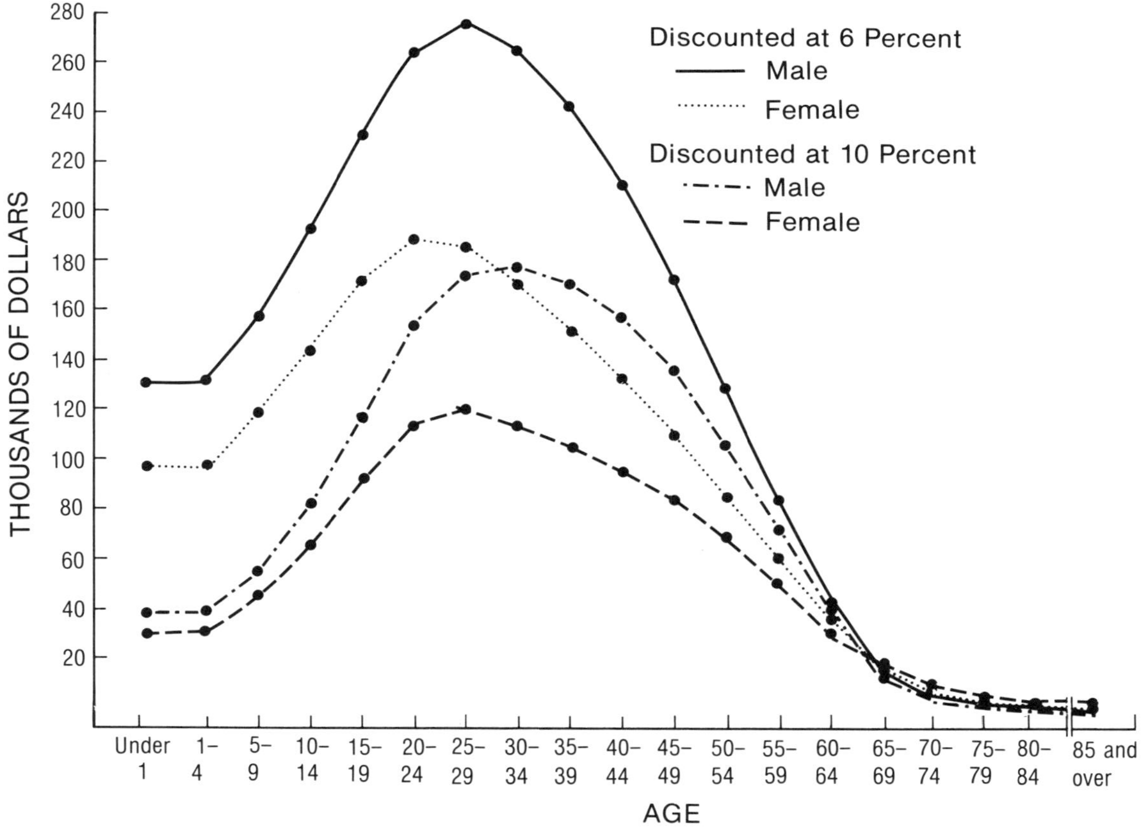

SOURCE: Rice, D. and T. Hodgson, "Social and Economic Implications of Cancer in the United States," paper presented to the Expert Committee on Cancer Statistics of the World Health Organization and International Agency for Research on Cancer in Madrid, Spain, June 20-26, 1978.

Chart D-4

Expenditures for Defense, Health, and Education as a Percent of Gross National Product (U.S.A., Selected Fiscal Years, 1950–1977).

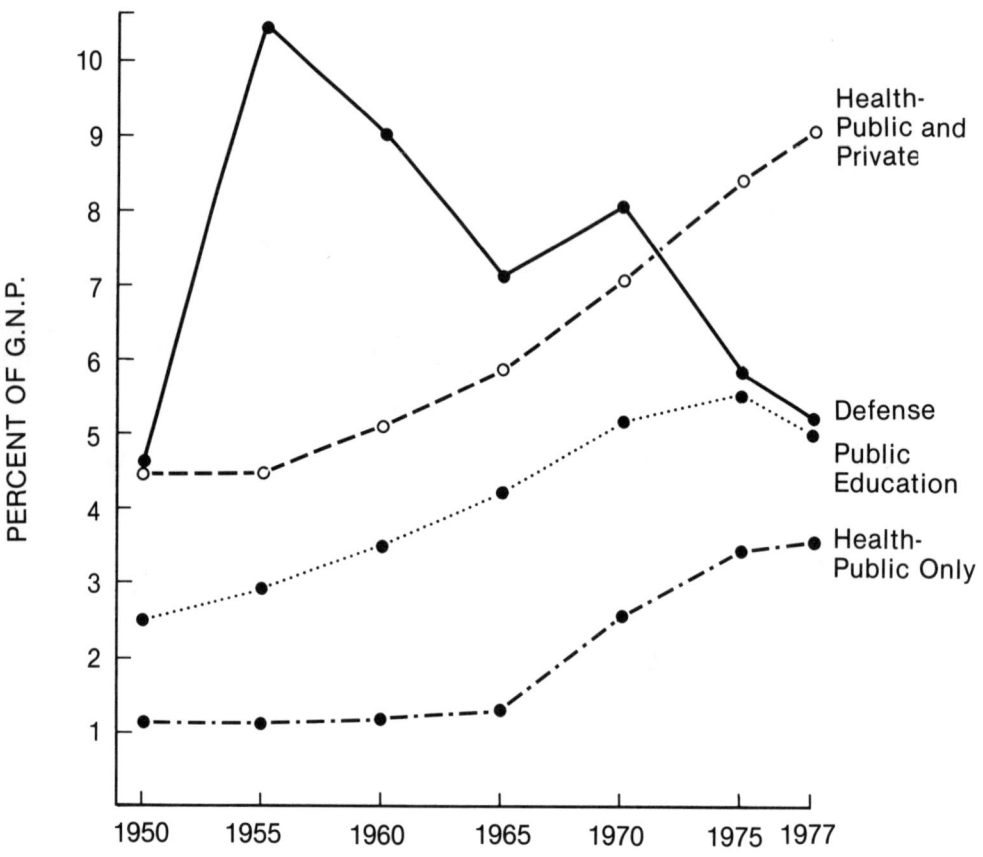

SOURCES: For defense: U.S. Department of Commerce, Bureau of the Census, *Statistical Abstract of the United States: 1978*, Washington, D.C., 1978, Table 584, p. 370; for education and public expenditures for health: McMillan, A., "Social Welfare Expenditures Under Public Programs, Fiscal year 1977," *Social Security Bulletin*, June 1979, Vol. 42, No. 6, Table 3, p. 10; for health expenditure-total, public and private: Gibson, R.M., and C.R. Fisher, "National Health Expenditures, Fiscal Year 1977," *Social Security Bulletin*, July 1978, Vol. 41, No. 7, Table 1, p. 5.

Costs and Expenditures

Chart D-5

Percent Distribution of National Expenditures for Education and Health and for Selected Categories within Health, by Public and Private Sources (U.S.A., 1977).

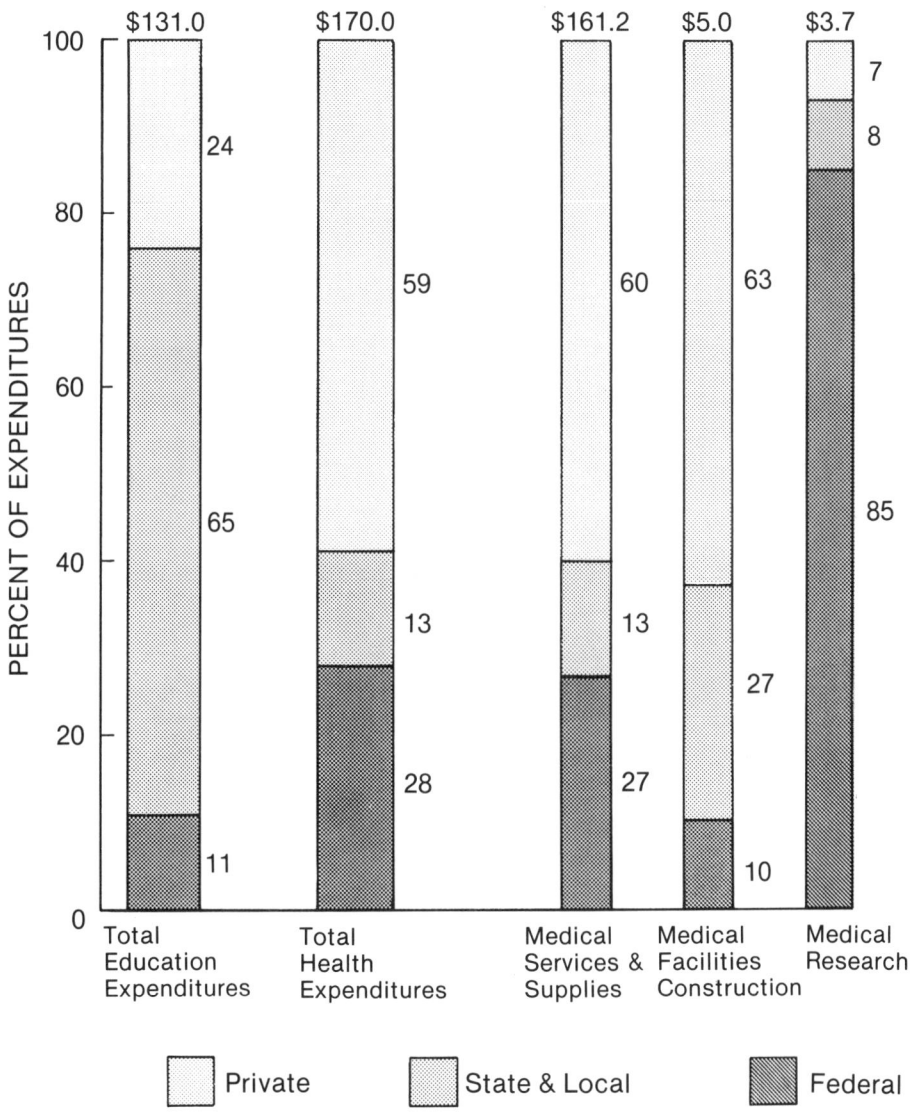

NOTE: Dollar amounts above bars are in billions.

SOURCES: For health: Gibson, Robert M., "National Health Expenditures, 1978," *Health Care Financing Review*, Summer 1979, Vol. 1, Issue 1, Table 4, p. 25; for education: McMillan, Anna, "Social Welfare Expenditures Under Public Programs, Fiscal Year 1977," *Social Security Bulletin*, Vol. 42, June 1979, p. 8.

Chart D-6

National Health Care Expenditures as Percent of Gross National Product (Selected Countries, 1960-1976).

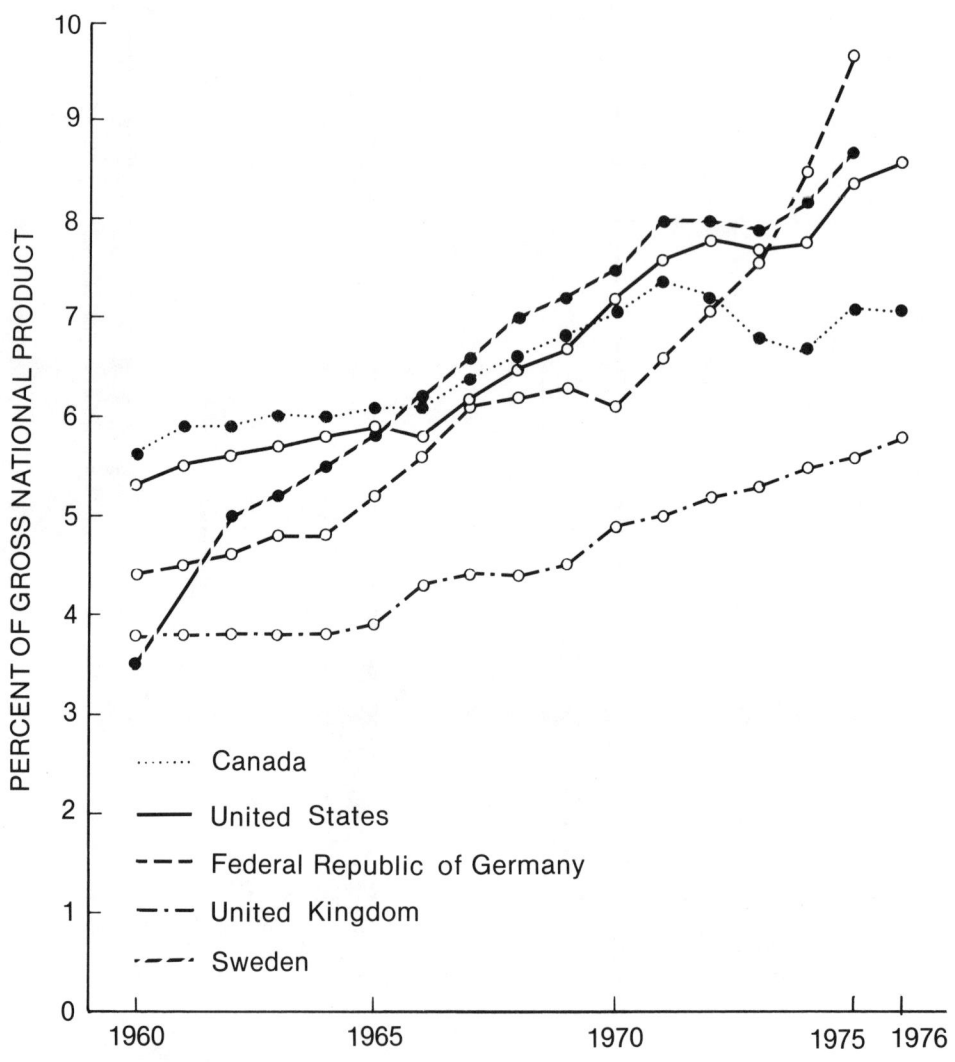

SOURCE: Simanis, Joseph G. and J. R. Coleman, "Health Care Expenditures in Nine Industrialized Countries, 1960-76," *Social Security Bulletin*, Vol. 43, No. 1, January 1980, Table 1, p. 5.

Costs and Expenditures

Chart D-7

Expenditures for Health Services as a Percent of Gross National Product, 1975, and Average Annual Increase in Health Expenditures, 1970–1975 (Selected Countries).

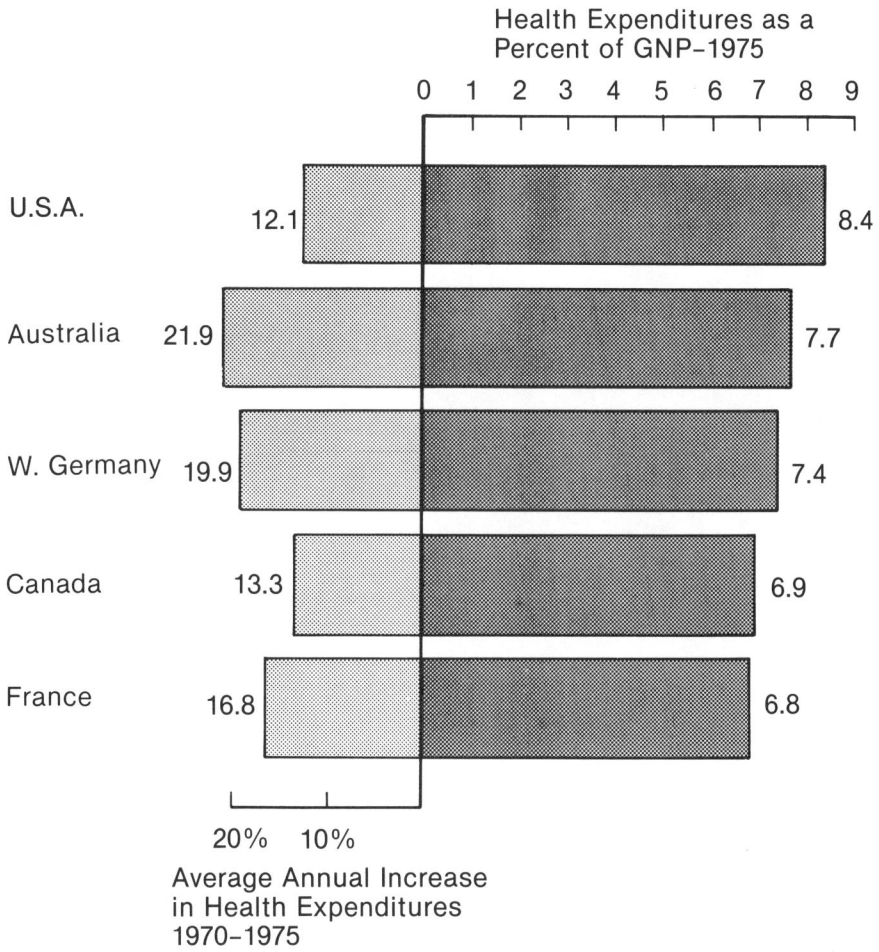

SOURCE: Reinhart, U.E., "Can the United States Learn From Foreign Medical Insurance Systems?", *Hospital Progress*, Vol. 59, No. 11, November 1978, Table 1, p. 60.

Chart D-8 National Health Expenditures, by Private and Public Sources of Funds (U.S.A., 1929–1978).

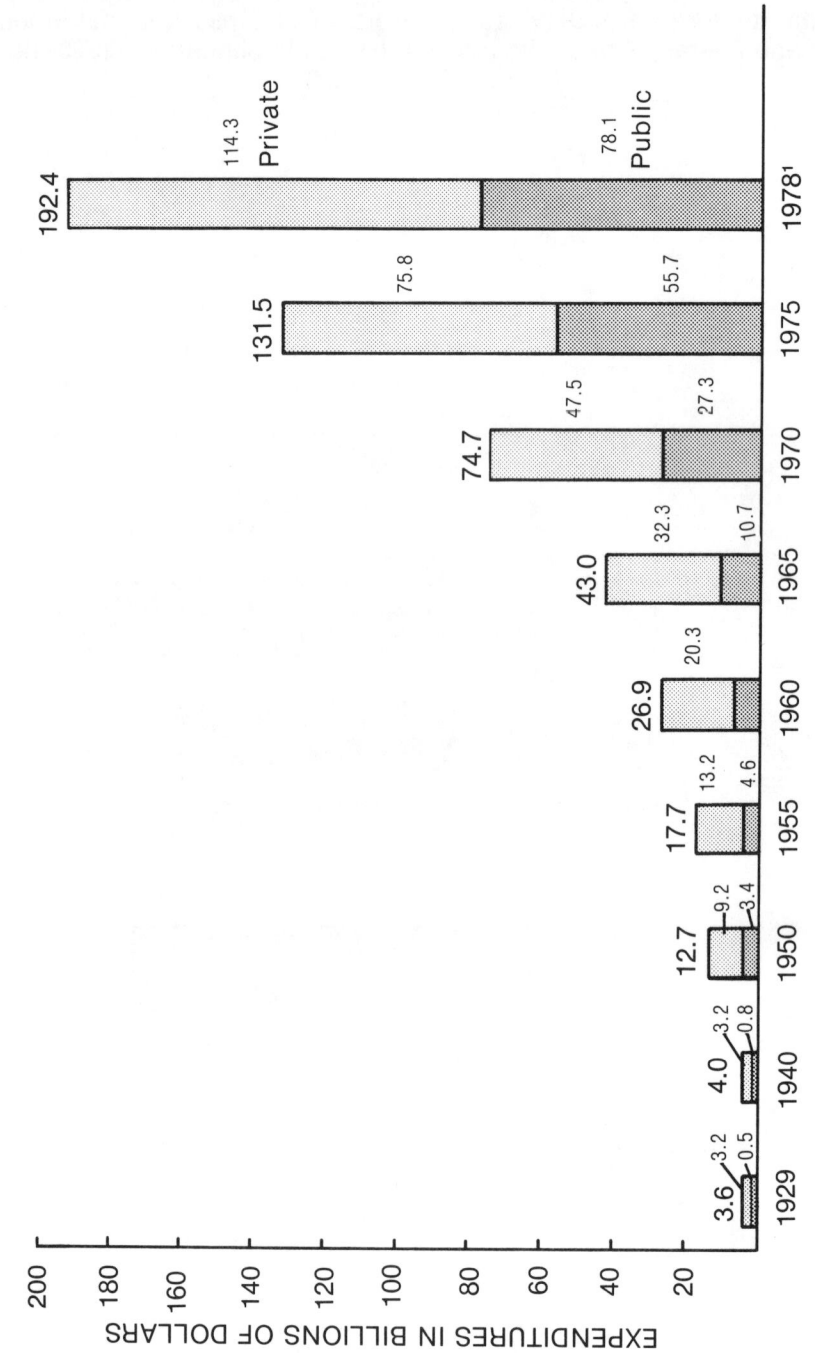

[1]Preliminary estimate
SOURCE: Gibson, R.M., "National Health Expenditures, 1978," *Health Care Financing Review*, DHEW, Vol. 1, Issue 1, Summer 1979, Table 7, p. 32.

Chart D-9

Percent Distribution of National Health Expenditures, by Category of Expenditure, and by Source of Funds (U.S.A., 1978).[1]

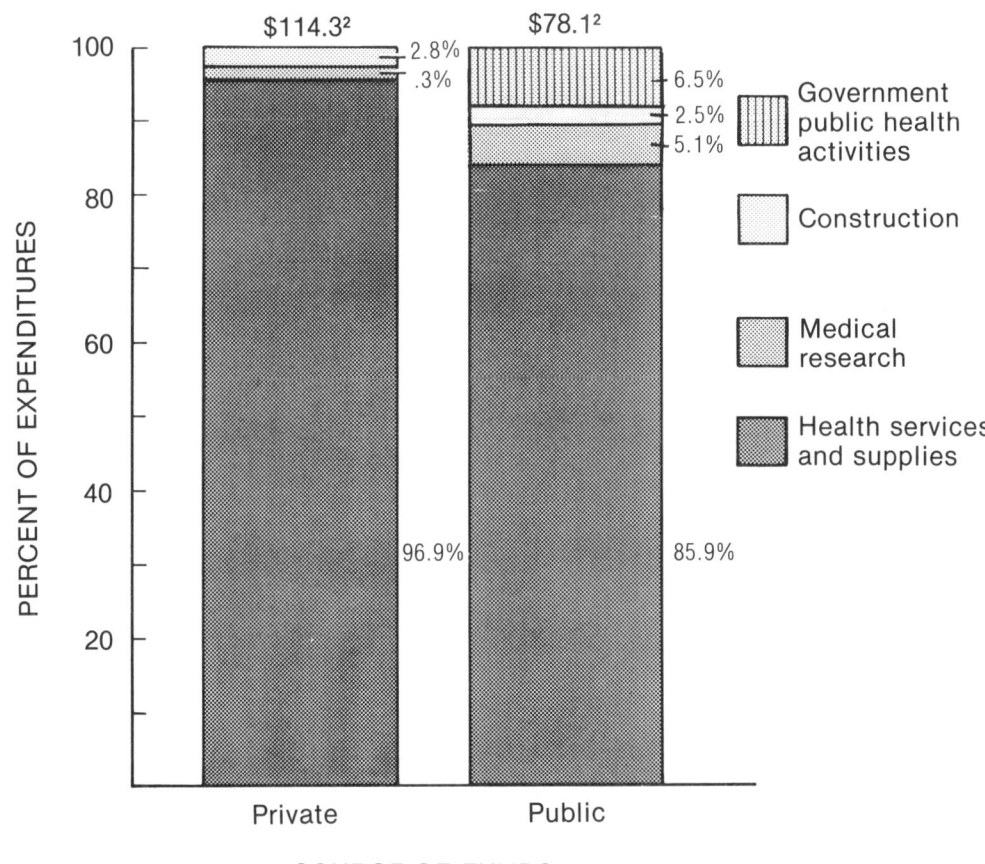

[1] Estimate.
[2] In billions of dollars.
SOURCE: Gibson, R.M., "National Health Expenditures 1978", *Health Care Financing Review,* Summer 1979, Table 4, p. 25.

Chart D-10

Percent Distribution of National Health Expenditures, by Private and Public Sources of Funds (U.S.A., Selected Years, 1929-1978).

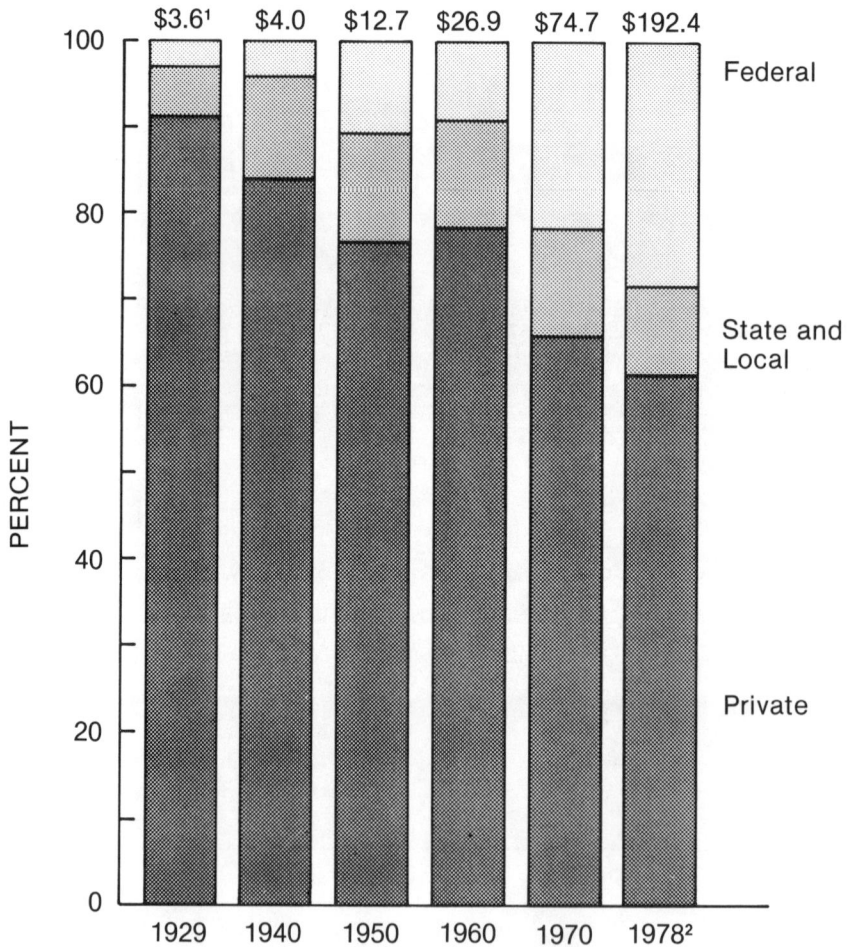

[1] In billions of dollars.

[2] Preliminary estimate.

SOURCE: Gibson, R.M., "National Health Expenditures, 1978," *Health Care Financing Review*, Vol. 1, Issue 1, Summer 1979, Table 1, p. 22 and Table 7, p. 32.

Costs and Expenditures

Chart D-11

Percent Distribution of Health Expenditures for Health Services and Supplies, by Type of Expenditure (U.S.A., Selected Years, 1929-1978).

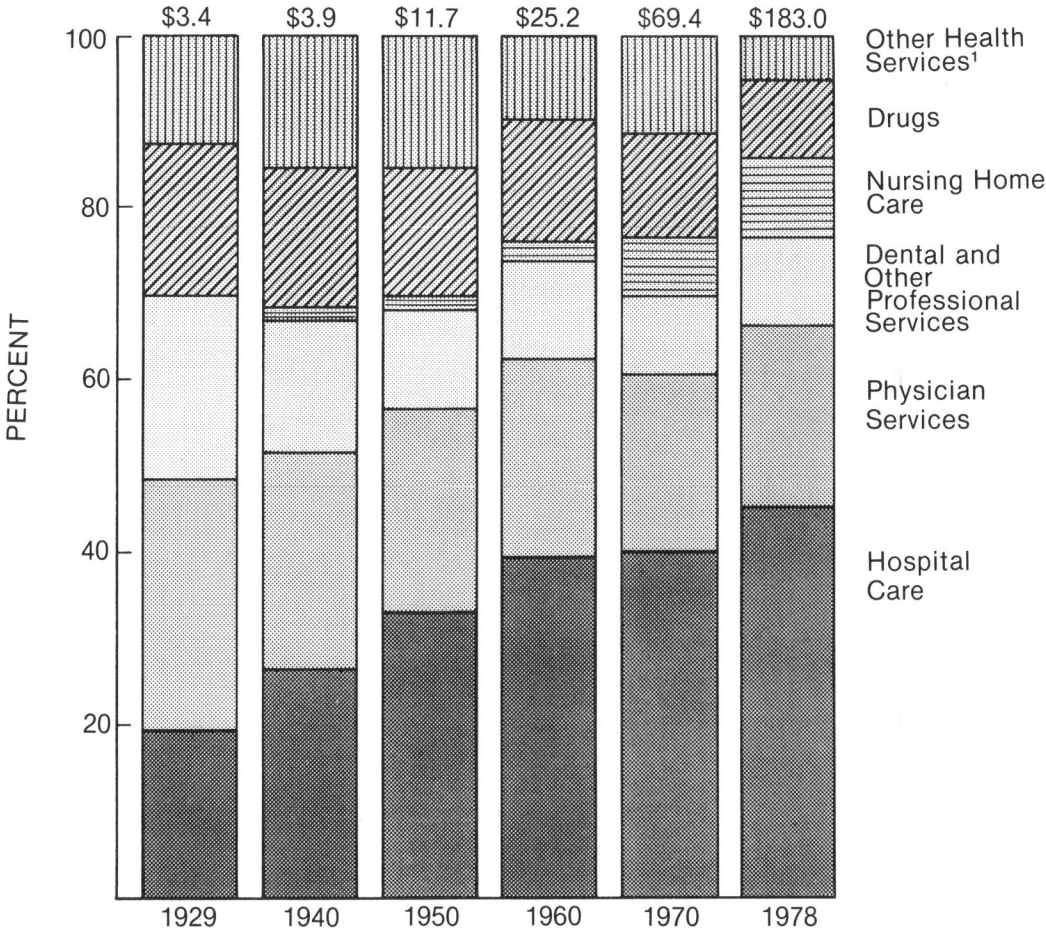

[1]Other health services includes: public program expenditures for health services not classified as to type of service covered; industrial inplant services; school health services; and medical activities in federal units other than hospitals.

NOTE: Numbers above bars are total expenditures for health services and supplies, in billions of dollars.

SOURCES: Gibson, Robert M., "National Health Expenditures, 1978," *Health Care Financing Review*, Vol. 1., Issue 1, Summer 1979, Table 3, pp. 23-24.

Chart D-12 Public Expenditures for Health Services and Supplies, by Program (U.S.A., 1966 and 1978).

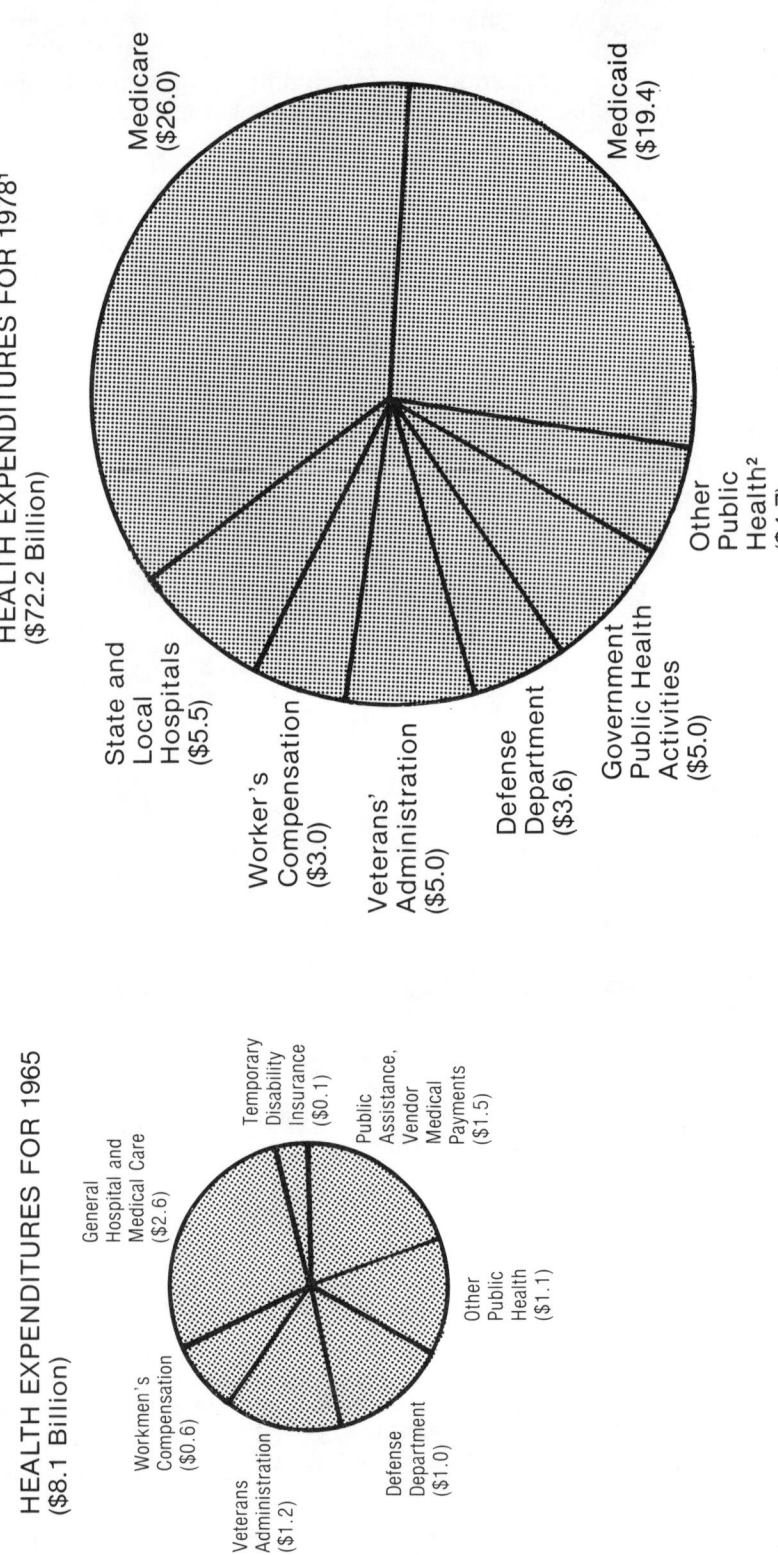

HEALTH EXPENDITURES FOR 1978[1]
($72.2 Billion)

- Medicare ($26.0)
- Medicaid ($19.4)
- Other Public Health[2] ($4.7)
- Government Public Health Activities ($5.0)
- Defense Department ($3.6)
- Veterans' Administration ($5.0)
- Worker's Compensation ($3.0)
- State and Local Hospitals ($5.5)

HEALTH EXPENDITURES FOR 1965
($8.1 Billion)

- General Hospital and Medical Care ($2.6)
- Temporary Disability Insurance ($0.1)
- Public Assistance, Vendor Medical Payments ($1.5)
- Other Public Health ($1.1)
- Defense Department ($1.0)
- Veterans Administration ($1.2)
- Workmen's Compensation ($0.6)

[1]Estimate.

[2]Includes expenditures for maternal and child health, vocational rehabilitation, temporary disability, alcoholism, drug abuse, mental health, and school health.

SOURCES: For 1965: Rice, D.P. and B.S. Cooper, "National Health Expenditures, 1950–67," *Social Security Bulletin*, January 1969, Table 4, p. 11; for 1978: Gibson, Robert M., "National Health Expenditures, 1978," *Health Care Financing Review*, Vol. 1, No. 1, Summer 1979, Table 6, p. 29.

Chart D-13 Percent Distribution of Personal Health Care Expenditures by Direct and Third Party Payments (U.S.A., Selected Years, 1950–1978).

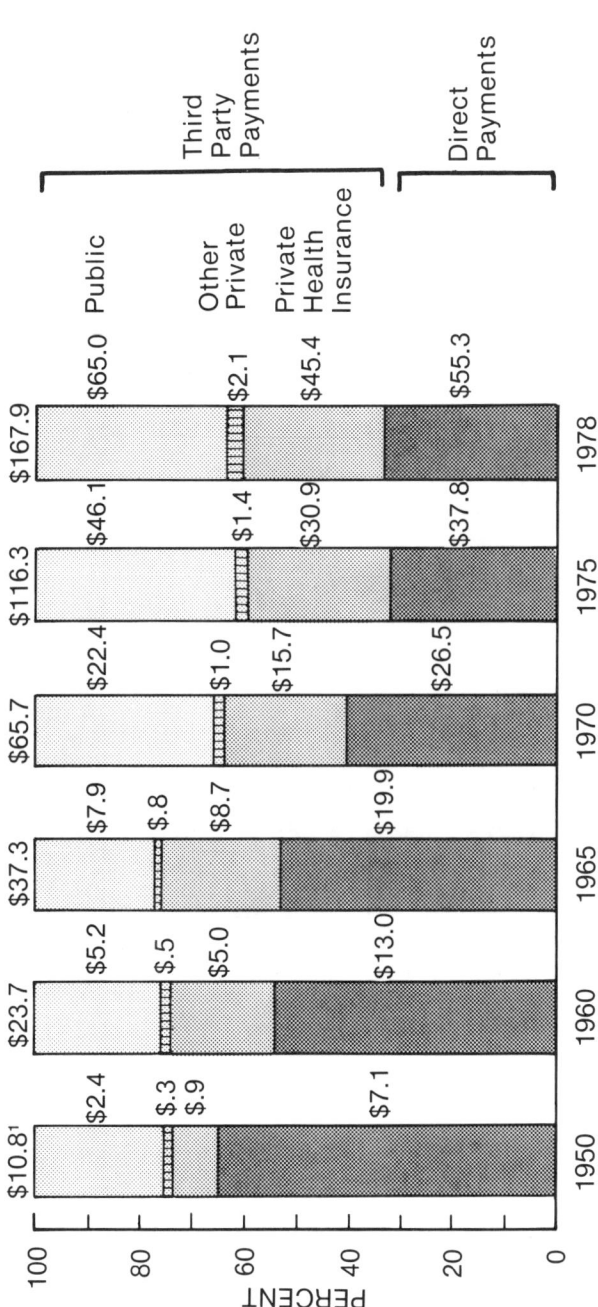

[1]Total expenditures in billions of dollars; includes all expenditures other than expenses for prepayment and administration, for government public health activities, and for expenditures of private voluntary agencies for other health services.

SOURCE: Gibson, R.M., "National Health Expenditures, 1978," *Health Care Financing Review*, DHEW, Vol. 1, Issue 1, Summer 1979, Table 7, p. 32.

Chart D-14

Components of Increases in Expenditures for Personal Health Care from 1950 to 1960, 1960 to 1970, and 1970 to 1978 (U.S.A.).[1]

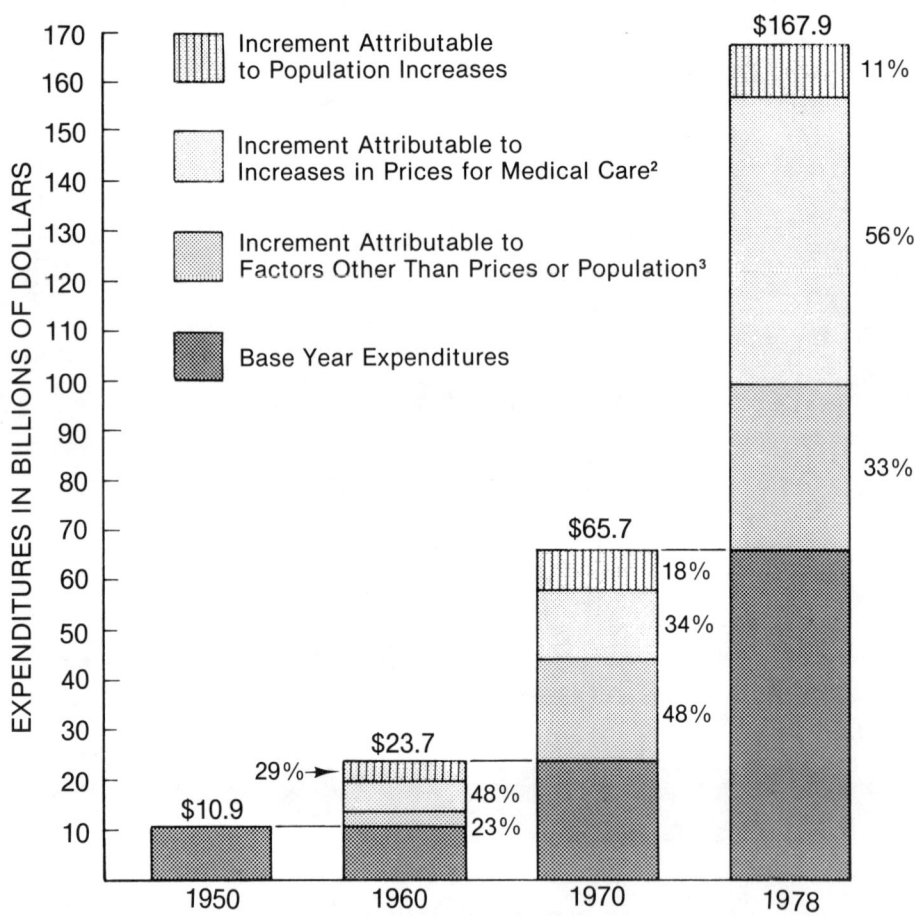

[1]Includes all expenditures for health services and supplies other than (a) expenses for prepayment and administration and (b) expenditures for government public health activities.

[2]As reflected in the Medical Care component of the Consumer Price Index.

[3]Includes increases in expenditures due to higher rates in the use of services and the introduction of new services and techniques.

NOTE: The figures to the right of bars represent the percent of the total increment that corresponds to each component.

SOURCES: Prepared by John R.C. Wheeler and Leon Wyszewianski, The University of Michigan, June 1980, based on information on expenditures and population in Gibson, Robert M., "National Health Expenditures, 1978," *Health Care Financing Review*, Summer 1979, p.21 and Table 7, p.32; data on the Consumer Price Index were obtained from *Statistical Abstract of the United States, 1979*, U.S. Department of Commerce, Bureau of the Census, Washington, D.C., 1979, Table 790, p.483.

Costs and Expenditures

Chart D-15

Percent Increase in Medical Care and Other Major Components in the Consumer Price Index (U.S.A., 1950–1978).

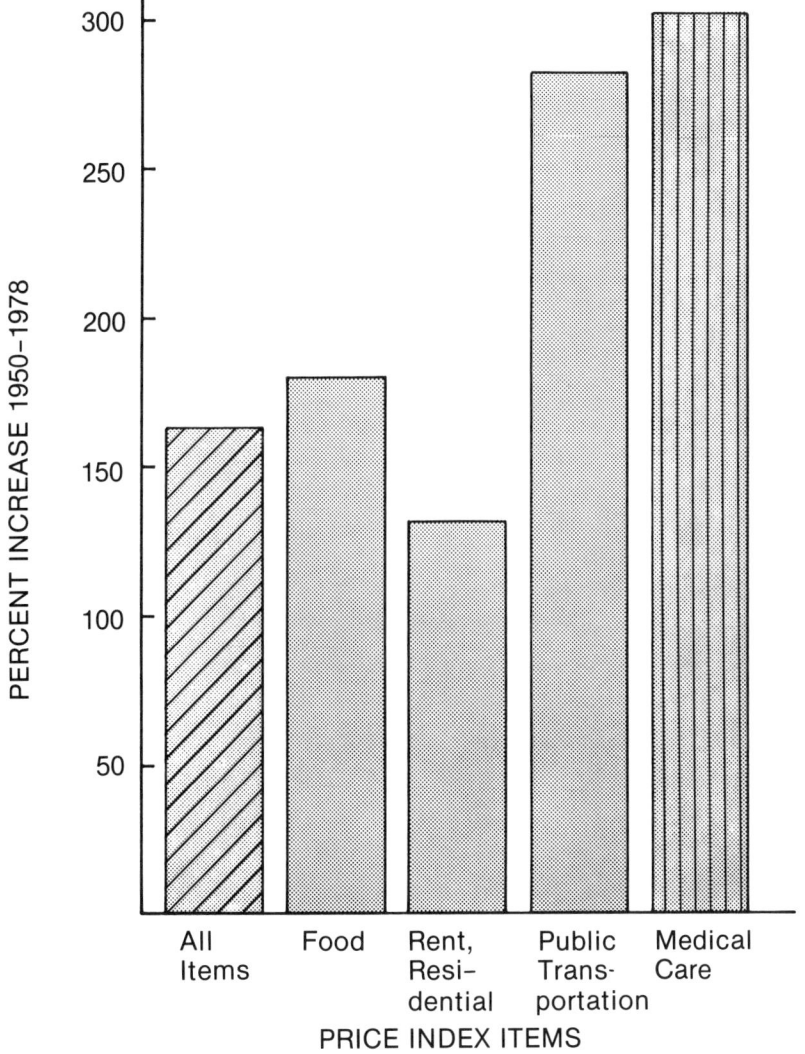

SOURCE: U.S. Department of Commerce, Bureau of the Census, *Statistical Abstract of the United States: 1978,* Washington, D.C., 1978, Table 792, p. 490.

Chart D-16

Relative Change in Selected Components of the Medical Care Price Index
(U.S.A., Selected Years, 1960–1978).

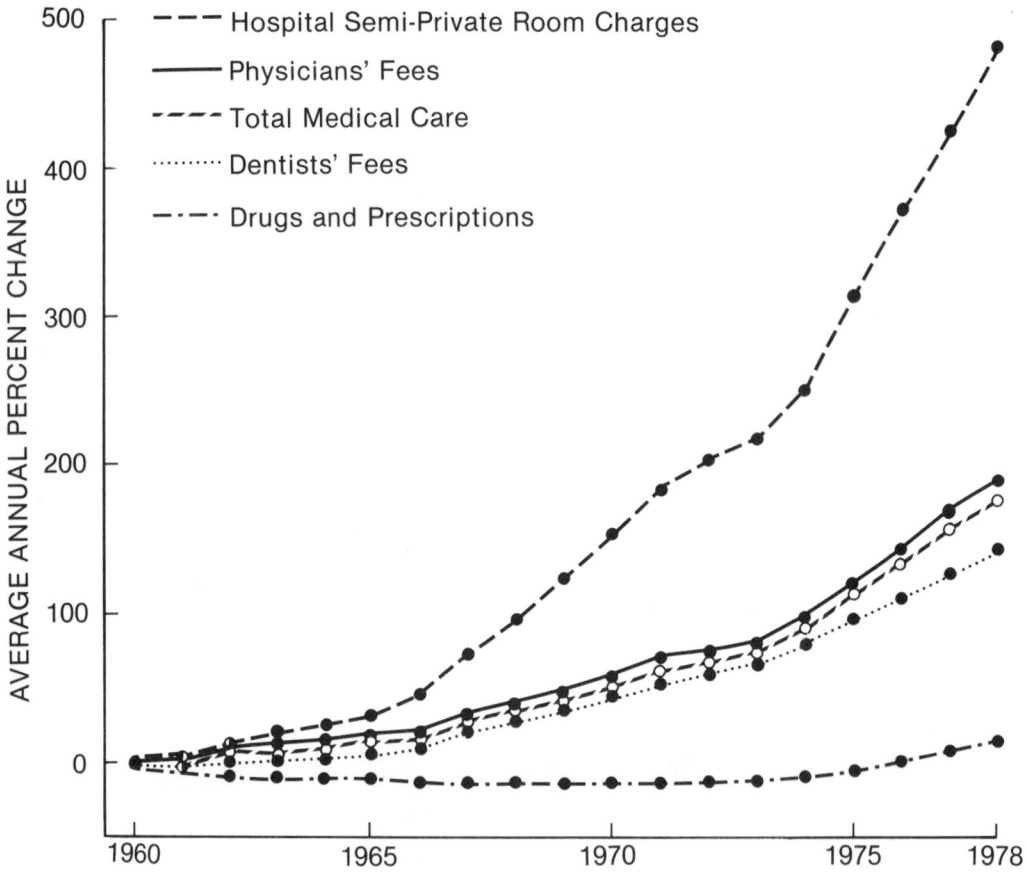

NOTE: The prescription drug component of the Medical Care Price Index was revised in 1977 to include a larger sample of drugs. However, the component continues to include a stable set of drugs over time. As a result it tends to reflect the decreases in the price of drugs that frequently occur in the years following the initial introduction of brand-name drugs, while it tends not to reflect increases in drug costs attributable to newly introduced, higher-priced brand-name products.

SOURCES: For 1960–1977: *National Health Insurance Report*, Vol. 9, No. 2, January 15, 1979, p. 7; for 1978: U.S. Department of Commerce, Bureau of the Census, *Statistical Abstract of the U.S., 1978*, Washington, D.C., 1978, Table 141, p. 99; and Health Care Financing Administration, *Health Care Financing Trends*, Vol. 1, No. 2, Winter 1980, Table C-1, p. 10.

Chart D-17

Percent Change in Hospital Costs for Non-federal, Short-term General and Other Special Hospitals (U.S.A., 1950–1978).

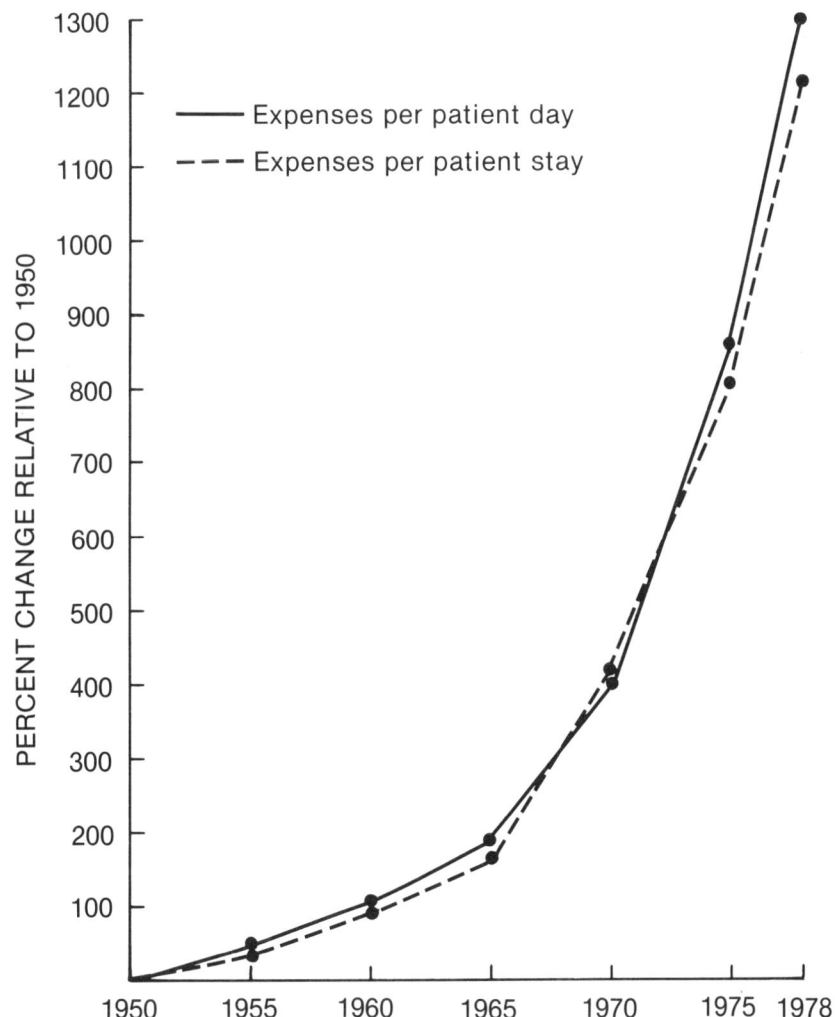

SOURCE: *The American Hospital Association Guide to the Health Care Field: 1979 Edition*, American Hospital Association, Table 1, p. A-7.

Costs and Expenditures

Chart D-18

Average Annual Percent Increase in the Consumer Price Index for All Items and Selected Medical Care Items, Before, During, and After the Economic Stabilization Program[1] (U.S.A., 1968-1978).

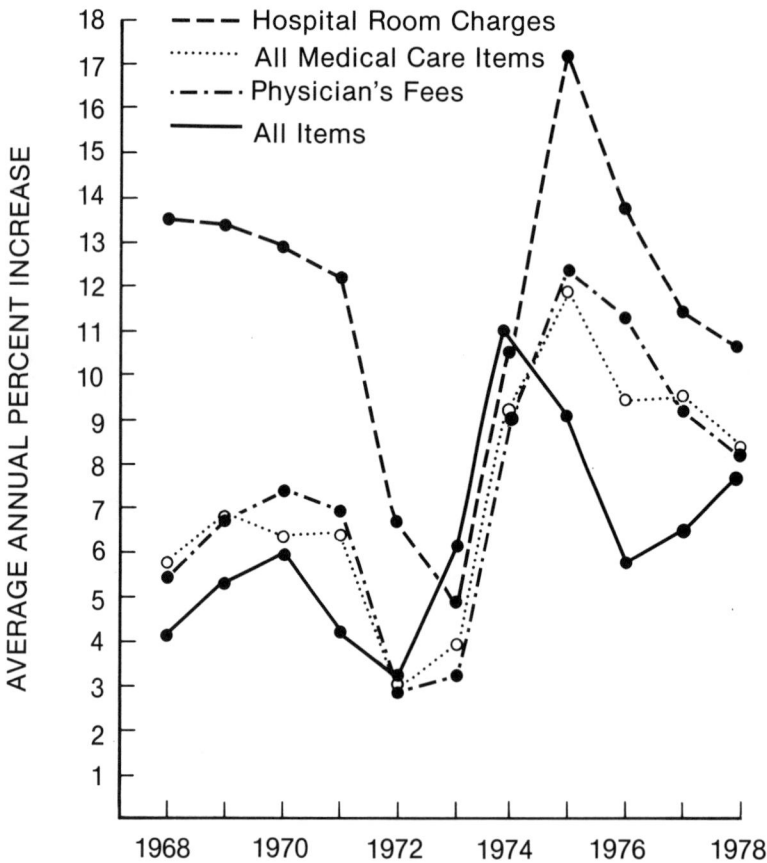

[1]The Economic Stabilization Program was in effect from August 1971 through April 1974.

SOURCES: U.S. Department of Commerce, Bureau of the Census, *Statistical Abstract of the United States, 1978*, Washington, D.C., 1978, Table 782, p. 483 and Table 141, p. 99; for 1978: Bureau of Labor Statistics, *Monthly Labor Review*, No. 23, Consumer Price Index for All Urban Consumers and revised Consumer Price Index for Urban Wage Earners and Clerical Workers, U.S. City Average, Vol. 101, September 1978, Table 9, p. 97, and Vol. 102, March 1979, Table 3, p. 97.

Costs and Expenditures

Chart D-19 Average Charge Per Day of Hospitalization in Short-stay Hospitals, by Bed Size and Length of Stay (U.S.A., 1970).

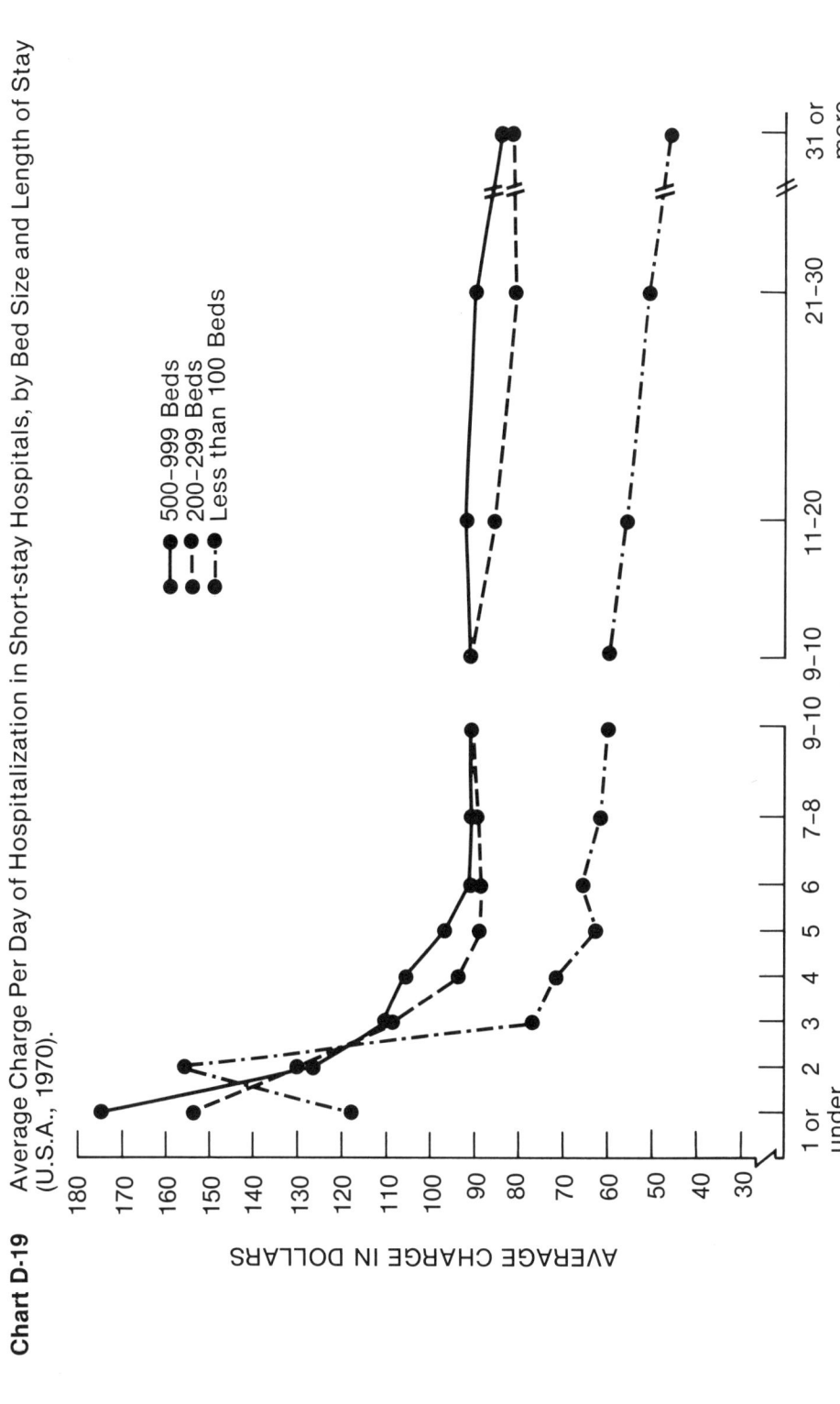

SOURCE: U.S. National Center for Health Statistics, Data from the National Health Survey, *Patient Charges in Short-Stay Hospitals, United States—1968–1970*, DHEW, Health Resources Administration, Rockville, Maryland, Series 13, No. 15, May 1974, Table 8, p. 26.

Chart D-20

Percent Change in Disposable Personal Income and in Out-of-Pocket Health Expenses (U.S.A., 1950–1977).

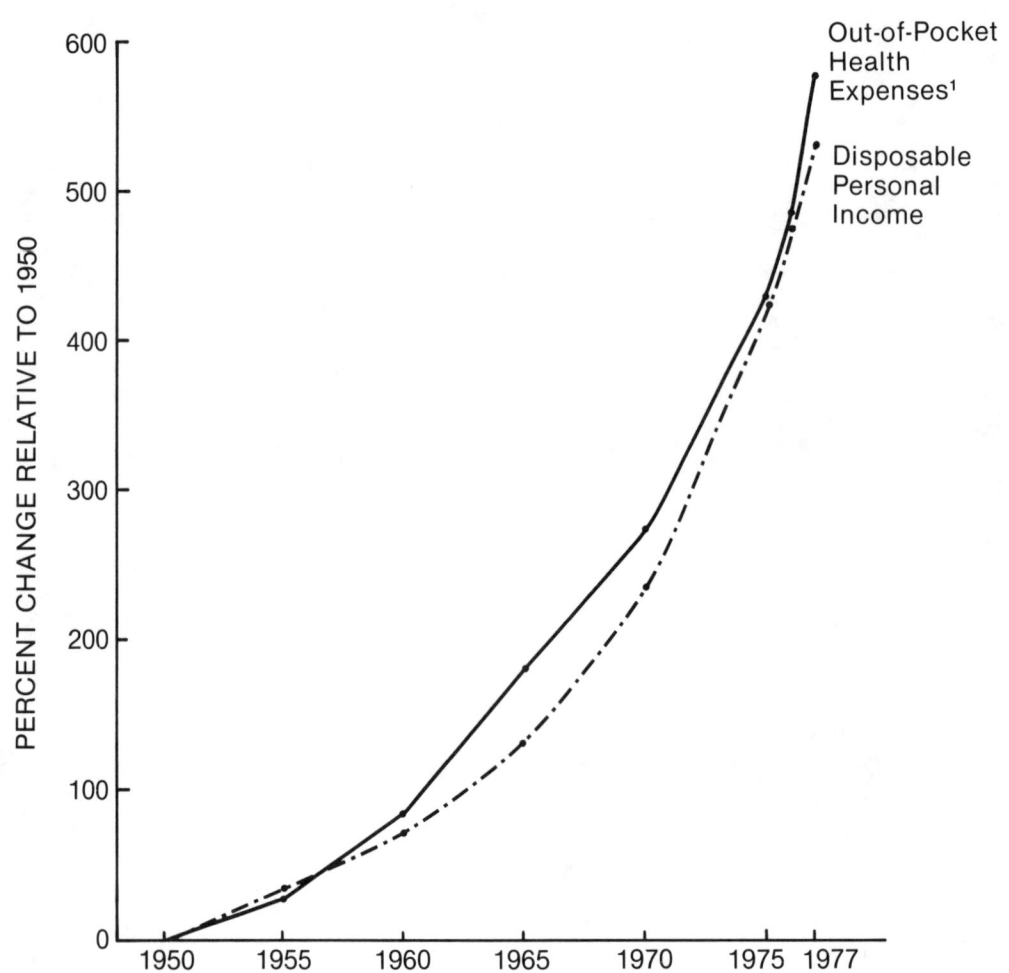

[1]Excludes payments for Medicare or private health insurance premiums, but includes deductible and coinsurance amounts.

SOURCES: For out-of-pocket expenses: Gibson, R.M., "National Health Expenditures, 1978," *Health Care Financing Review*, Summer 1979, Table 7, p. 32; for disposable income: *Health Insurance Institute Source Book of Health Insurance Data, 1978–1979*, Washington, D.C., The Institute, 1979, Table 5.13, p. 54.

Costs and Expenditures

Chart D-21

The Consumer Dollar: Distribution of Personal Consumption Expenditures, by Product (U.S.A., 1977).

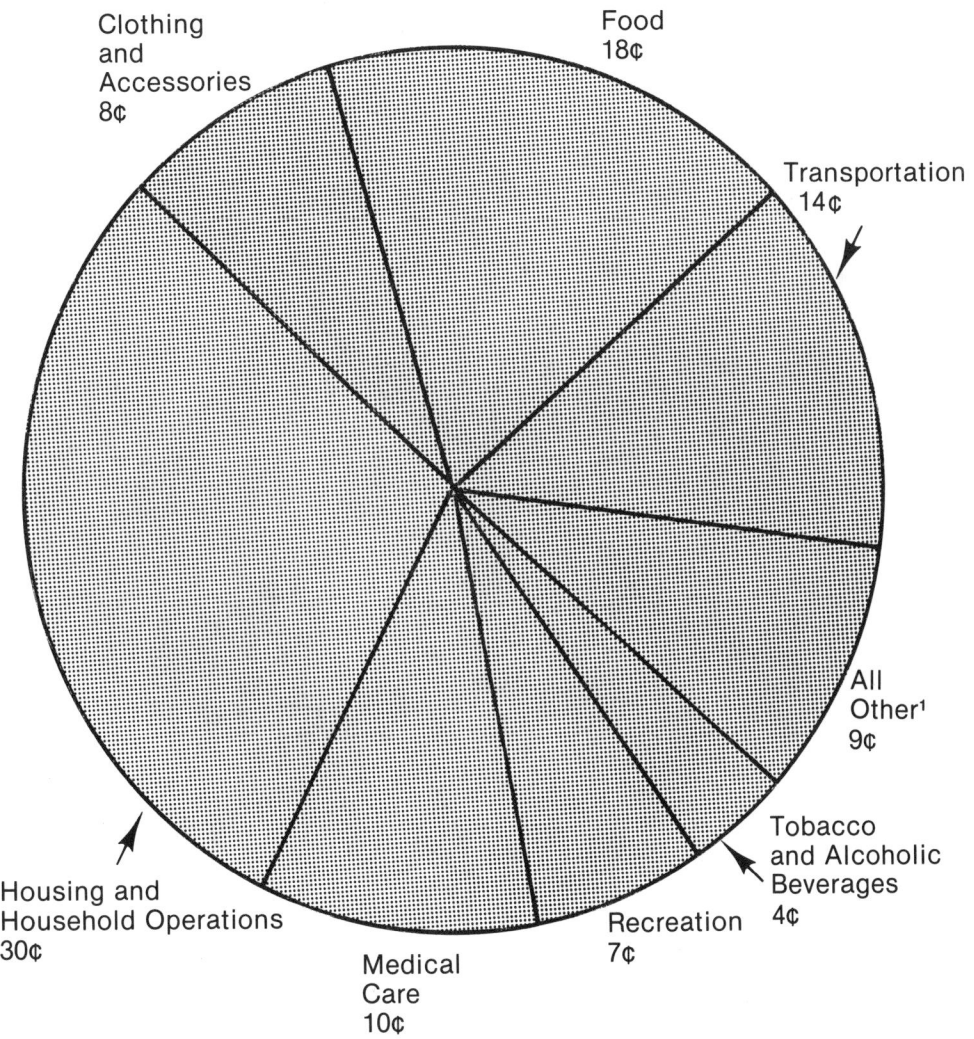

[1] Includes expenditures for personal business (5¢), private education and research (1.5¢), and personal care (1.4¢).

SOURCE: U.S. Department of Commerce, Bureau of the Census, *Statistical Abstract of the United States: 1978,* Washington, D.C., Table 717, p. 444.

Chart D-22 The Medical Care Dollar: Percent Distribution of Private Consumer Expenditures for Health Services and Supplies, by Type of Expenditure (U.S.A., 1960, 1970, and 1978).

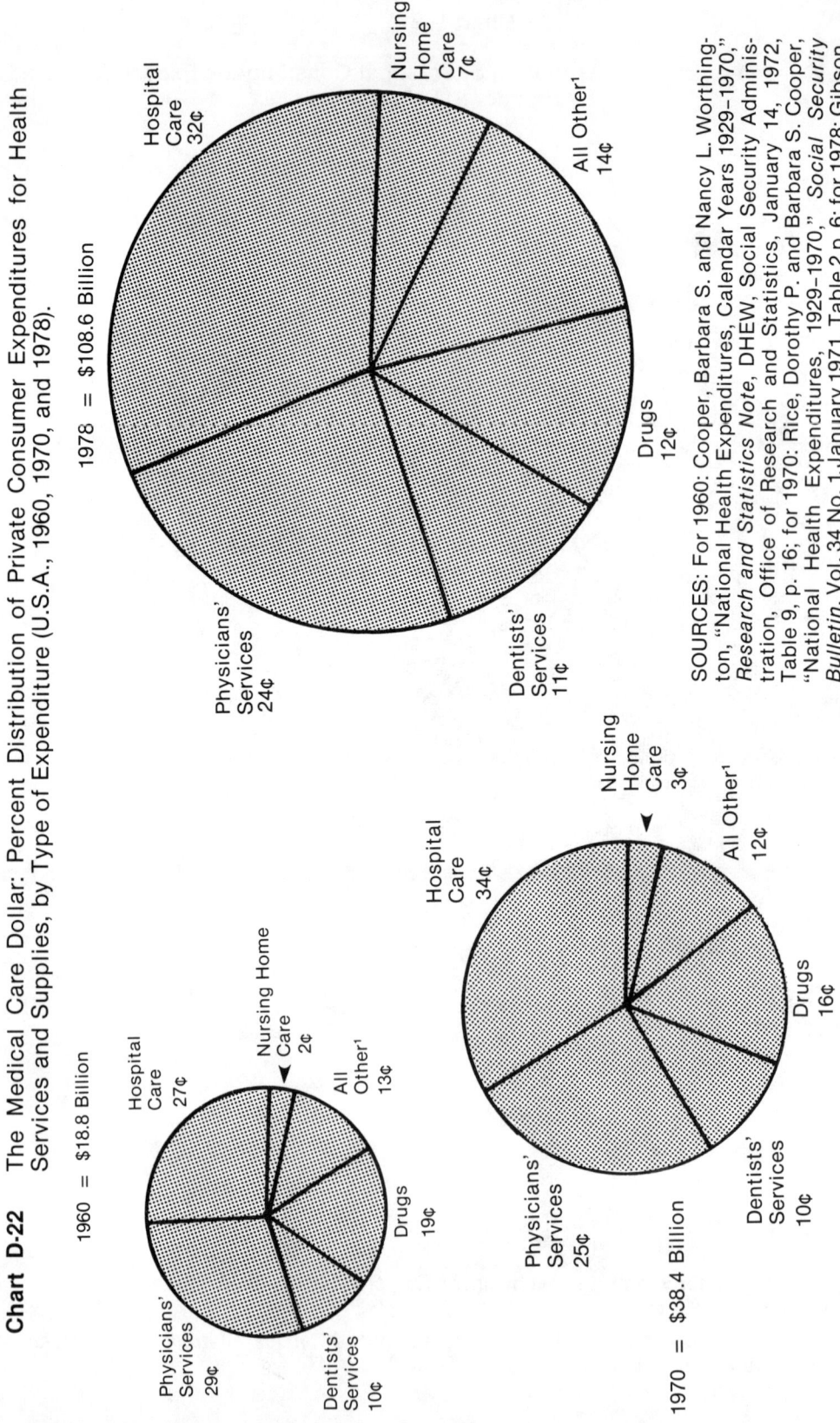

[1] "All Other" includes eyeglasses and appliances, expenses for prepayment, and other professional services.

SOURCES: For 1960: Cooper, Barbara S. and Nancy L. Worthington, "National Health Expenditures, Calendar Years 1929-1970," *Research and Statistics Note*, DHEW, Social Security Administration, Office of Research and Statistics, January 14, 1972, Table 9, p. 16; for 1970: Rice, Dorothy P. and Barbara S. Cooper, "National Health Expenditures, 1929-1970," *Social Security Bulletin*, Vol. 34 No. 1, January 1971, Table 2, p. 6; for 1978: Gibson, R.M., "National Health Expenditures, 1978," *Health Care Financing Review*, Vol. 1, Issue 1, Summer 1979, Table 4, p. 25 and Table 7, p. 32.

Chart D-23

Percent Distribution of Total Families and Unrelated Individuals, and of Their Total Out-of-Pocket Health Expenses, by Level of Expense (U.S.A., Civilian Non-institutionalized Population, 1975).

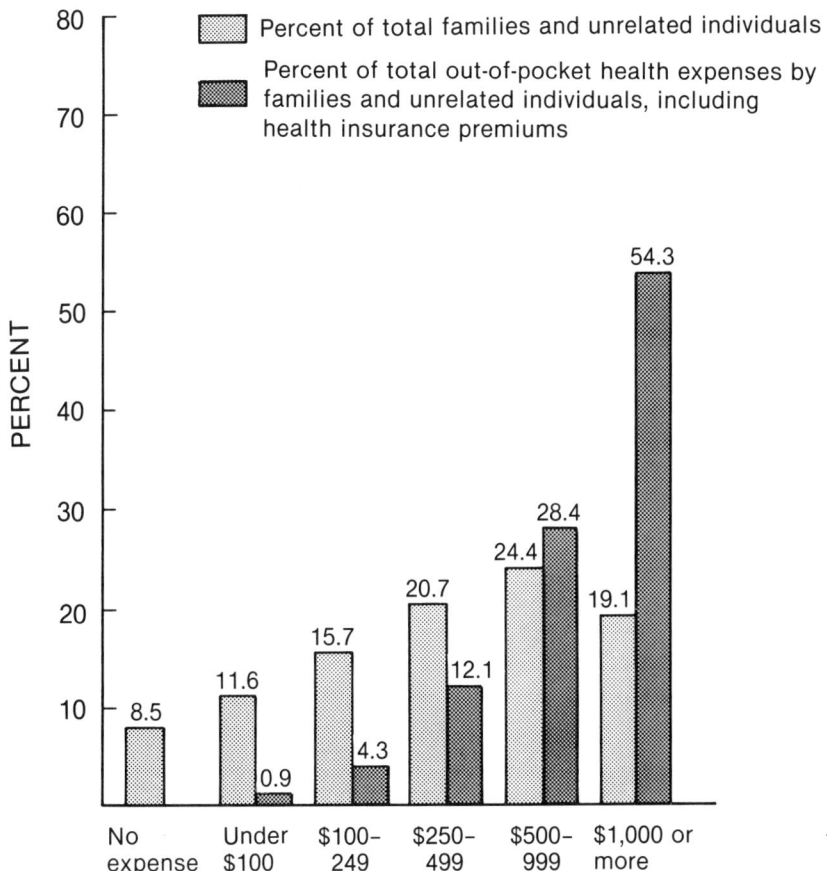

SOURCE: U.S. National Center for Health Statistics, *Family Out-of-Pocket Health Expenses: United States, 1975,* DHEW, Public Health Service, Office of Health Research, Statistics, and Technology, Hyattsville, Maryland, Series 10, No. 127, March 1979, Table 2, p. 20.

Chart D-24 Out-of-Pocket Health Expenses, Including Health Insurance Premiums, per Family per Year, and as a Percent of Family Income, by Income (U.S.A., Civilian Non-institutionalized Population, 1975).

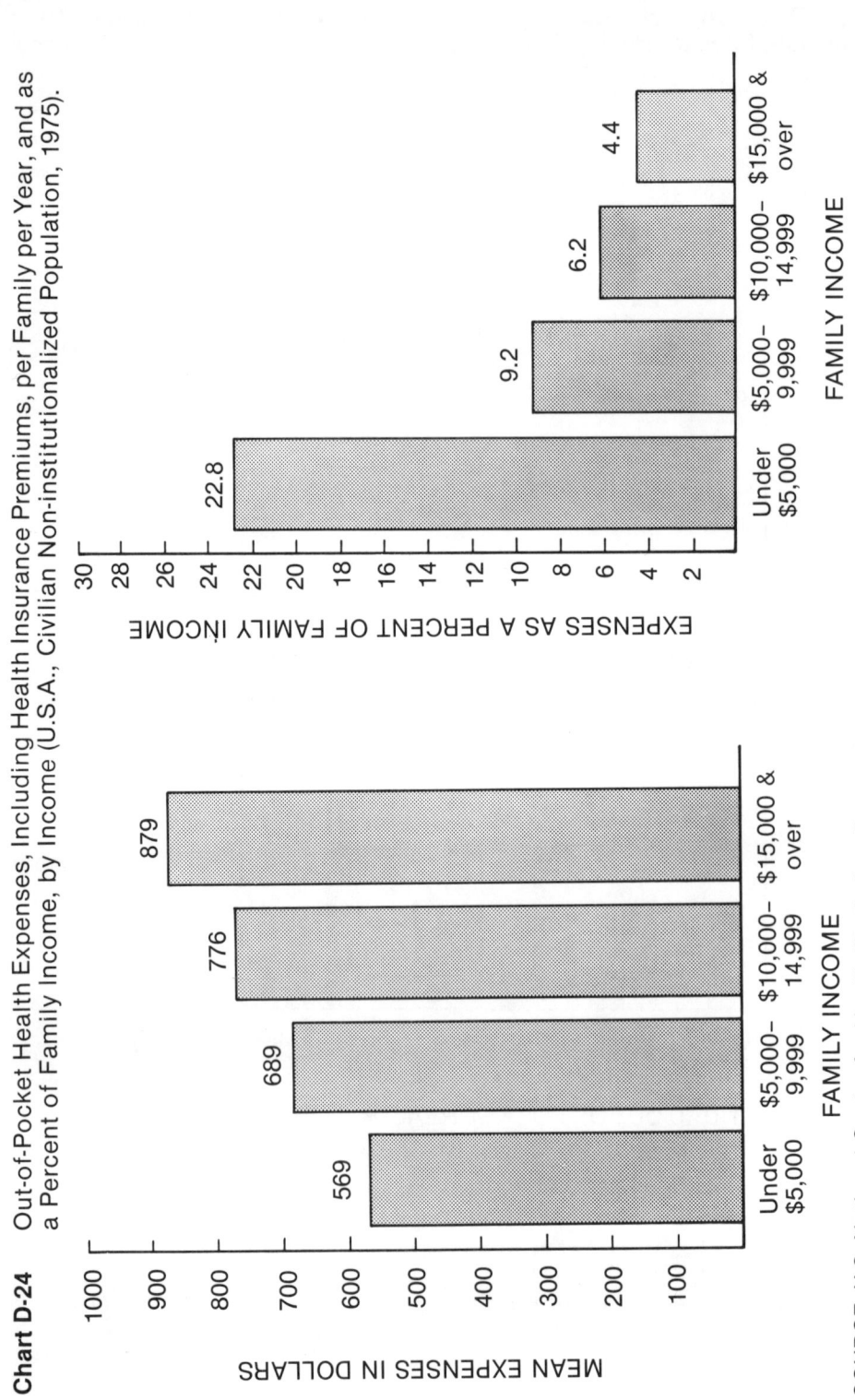

SOURCE: U.S. National Center for Health Statistics, *Family Out-of-Pocket Health Expenses, United States, 1975*, DHEW, Public Health Service, Office of Health Research, Statistics, and Technology, Hyattsville, Maryland, Series 10, No. 127, March 1979, Table H, p.11.

Costs and Expenditures

Chart D-25

Out-of-Pocket Health Expenses, by Family Income and Type of Expense (U.S.A., Civilian Non-institutionalized Population, 1975).

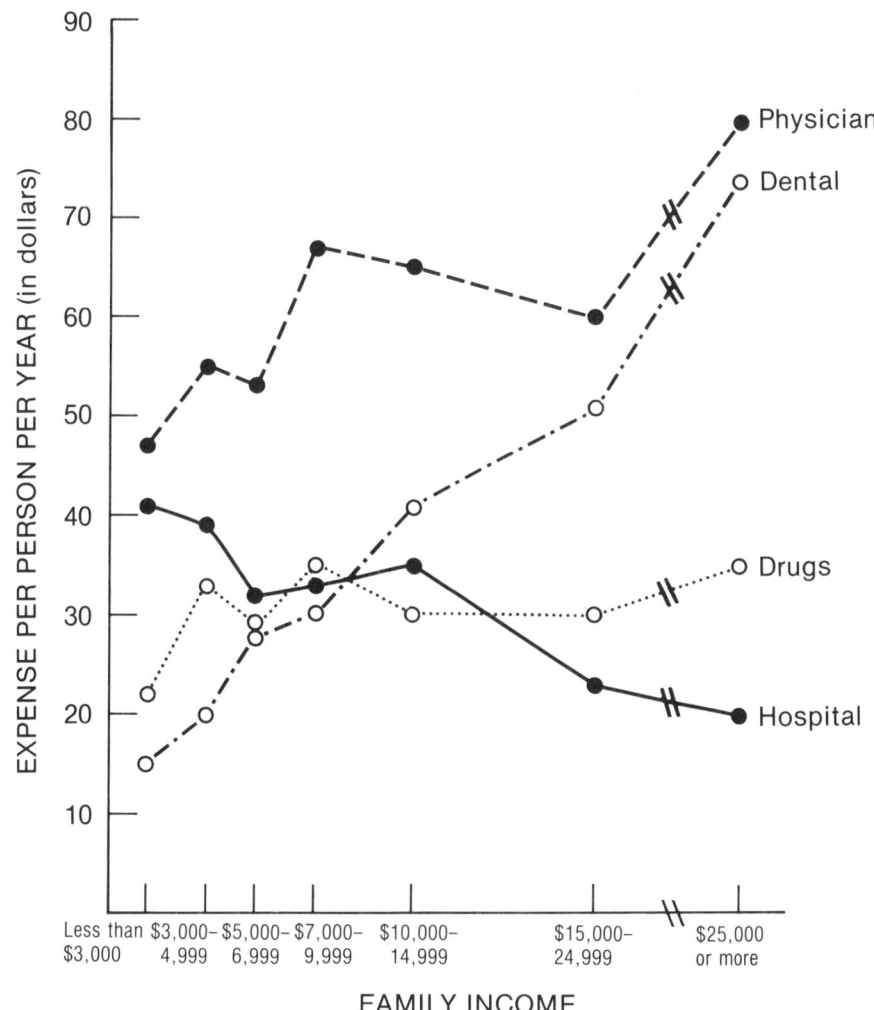

SOURCE: U.S. National Center for Health Statistics, *Personal Out-of-Pocket Health Expenses: United States, 1975,* DHEW, Public Health Service, Office of Health Research, Statistics, and Technology, Hyattsville, Maryland, Series 10, No. 122, November 1978, Table E, p. 10.

Chart D-26

Relative Change in Per Capita Out-of-Pocket Payments for Personal Health Care, by Two Age Groups (U.S.A., Selected Years, 1970–1978).

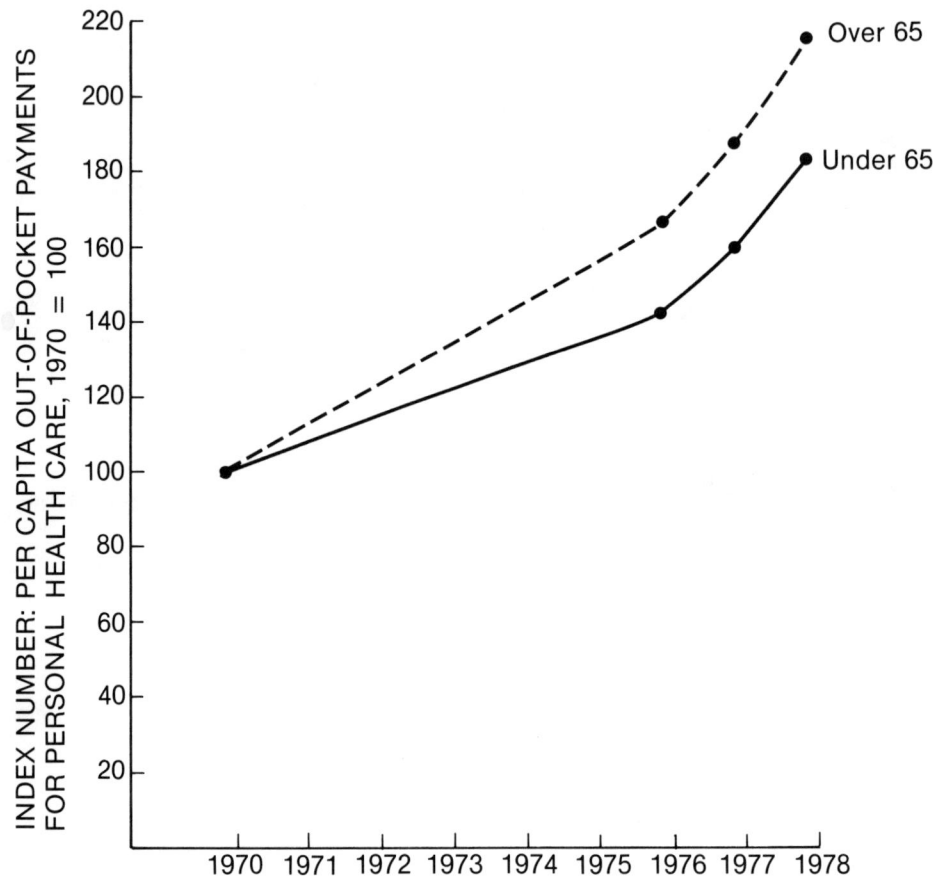

SOURCE: Data provided by Charles Fisher, Office of Policy, Planning, and Research, Financial and Actuarial Analyses, Health Care Financing Administration, June 1980.

Costs and Expenditures

Chart D-27

Percent Distribution of Expenditures for Personal Health Care, by Type of Expenditure and Age (U.S.A., Fiscal 1977).

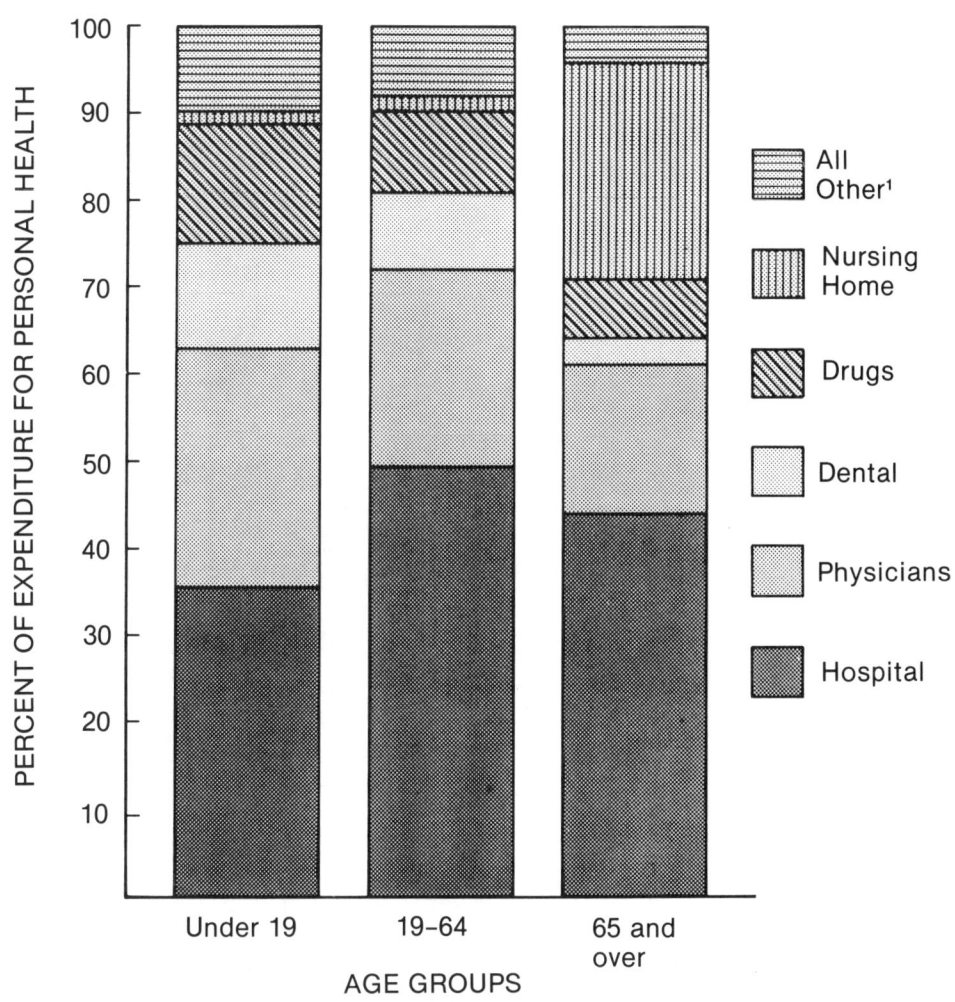

[1]Includes other professional services, eyeglasses and appliances, and other health services.

SOURCE: Gibson, C.M. and C.R. Fisher, "Age Differences in Health Care Spending, Fiscal Year 1977," *Social Security Bulletin*, Vol. 42, No. 1, January 1979, Table 1, p. 5.

Chart D-28 Out-of-Pocket Expense for Prescribed Medicine per Person per Year, by Population Groups of Specified Characteristics (U.S.A., Civilian Non-institutionalized Population, 1973).

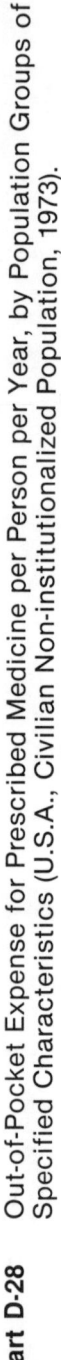

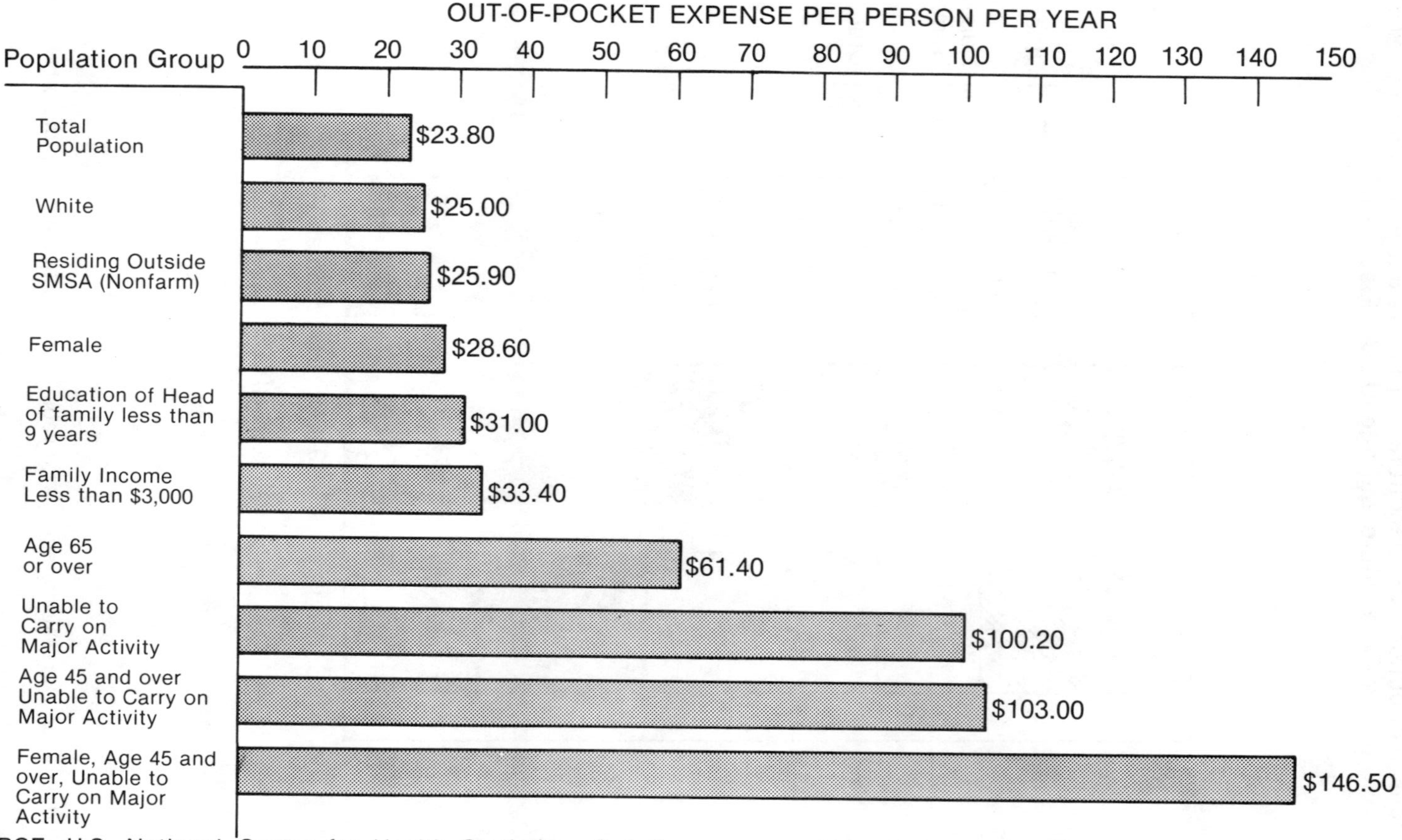
OUT-OF-POCKET EXPENSE PER PERSON PER YEAR
Population Group
0
10
20
30
40
50
60
70
80
90
100
110
120
130
140
150
Total Population
$23.80
White
$25.00
Residing Outside SMSA (Nonfarm)
$25.90
Female
$28.60
Education of Head of family less than 9 years
$31.00
Family Income Less than $3,000
$33.40
Age 65 or over
$61.40
Unable to Carry on Major Activity
$100.20
Age 45 and over Unable to Carry on Major Activity
$103.00
Female, Age 45 and over, Unable to Carry on Major Activity
$146.50

SOURCE: U.S. National Center for Health Statistics, *Out-of-Pocket Cost and Acquisition of Prescribed Medicines, United States, 1973,* DHEW, Health Resources Administration, Rockville, Maryland, Series 10, No. 108, June 1977, Table 1, p. 10, Table 2, p. 12, and Table 3, p. 13.

Chart D-29 Number of Total New Pharmaceutical Products and of Newly Synthesized Drugs Introduced Each Year (U.S.A., 1960–1979).

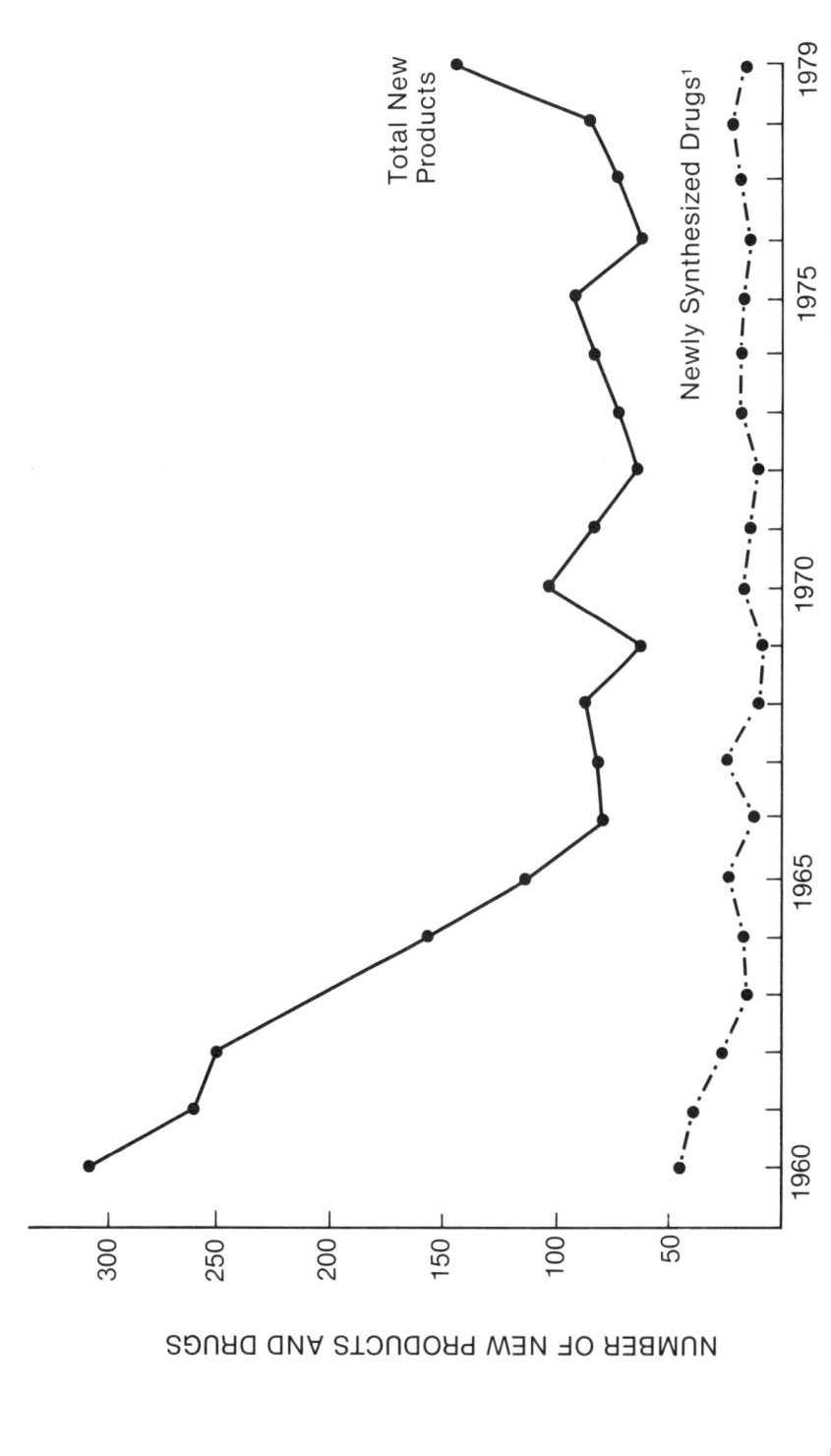

[1] Products which are new single chemical agents not previously known, including new salts.

SOURCES: For 1960–1974: Fulda, T., *Prescription Drug Data Summary, 1974*, DHEW, Social Security Administration, Office of Research and Statistics, Washington, D.C., 1976, Table III-8, p. 30; for 1975–1979: de Haen, Paul, *New Product Survey*, Vol. 26, Micromedex, Englewood, Colorado, 1980.

Chart D-30 Wholesale Prices of Selected Brand Name Drug Products as Multiples of Prices of Chemically Equivalent Unbranded (Generic) Drug Products (U.S.A., 1980).

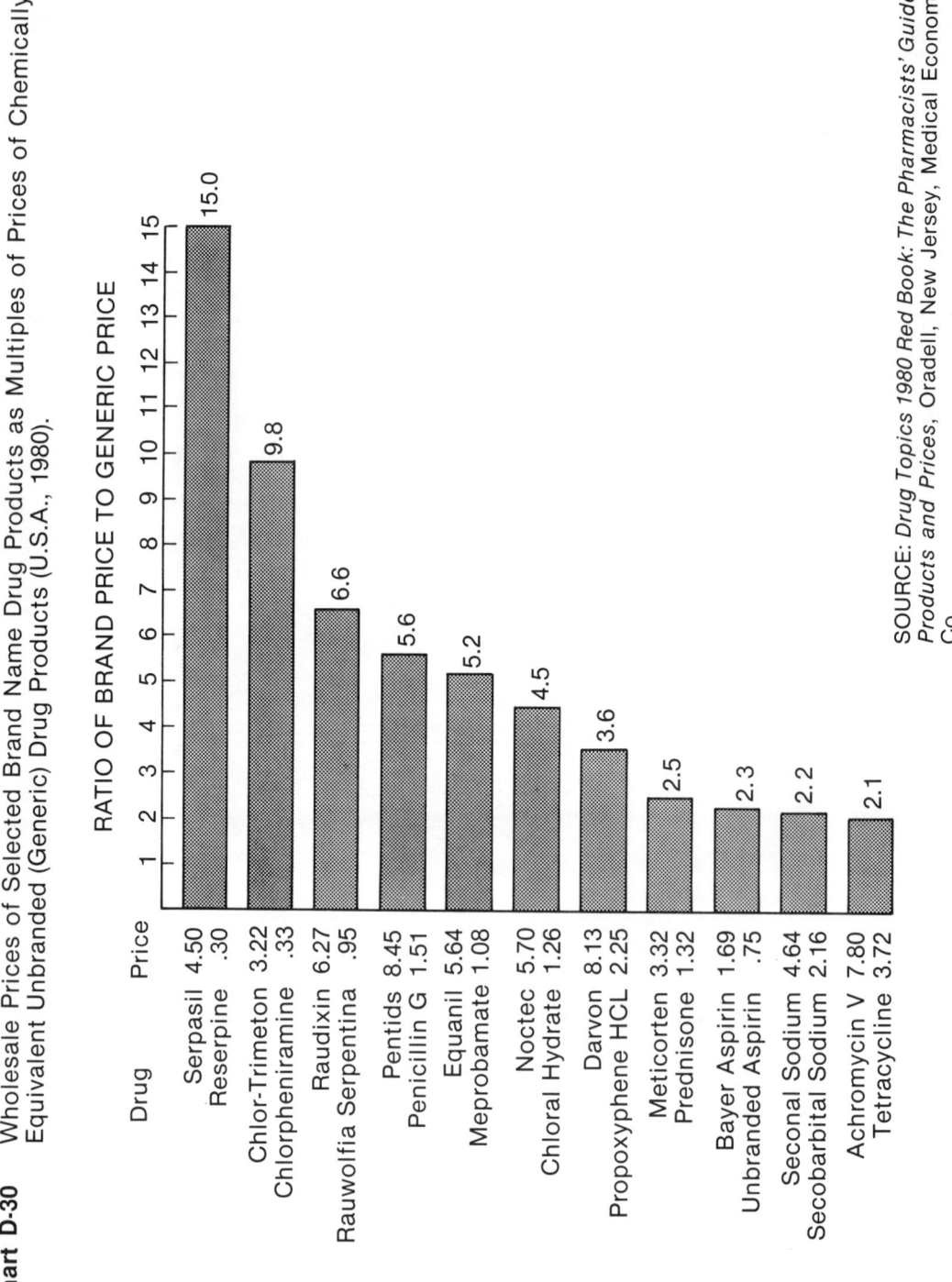

SOURCE: *Drug Topics 1980 Red Book: The Pharmacists' Guide to Products and Prices*, Oradell, New Jersey, Medical Economics Co.

Chart D-31

Percent Distribution of New Prescriptions by Availability of the Prescribed Drug Product from One or More Manufacturers, by Extent to Which the Substitution of the Product Was permitted and Took Place, and Percent Distribution of Associated Costs and of Potential and Actual Savings (Michigan, April 1, 1977–March 31, 1978).

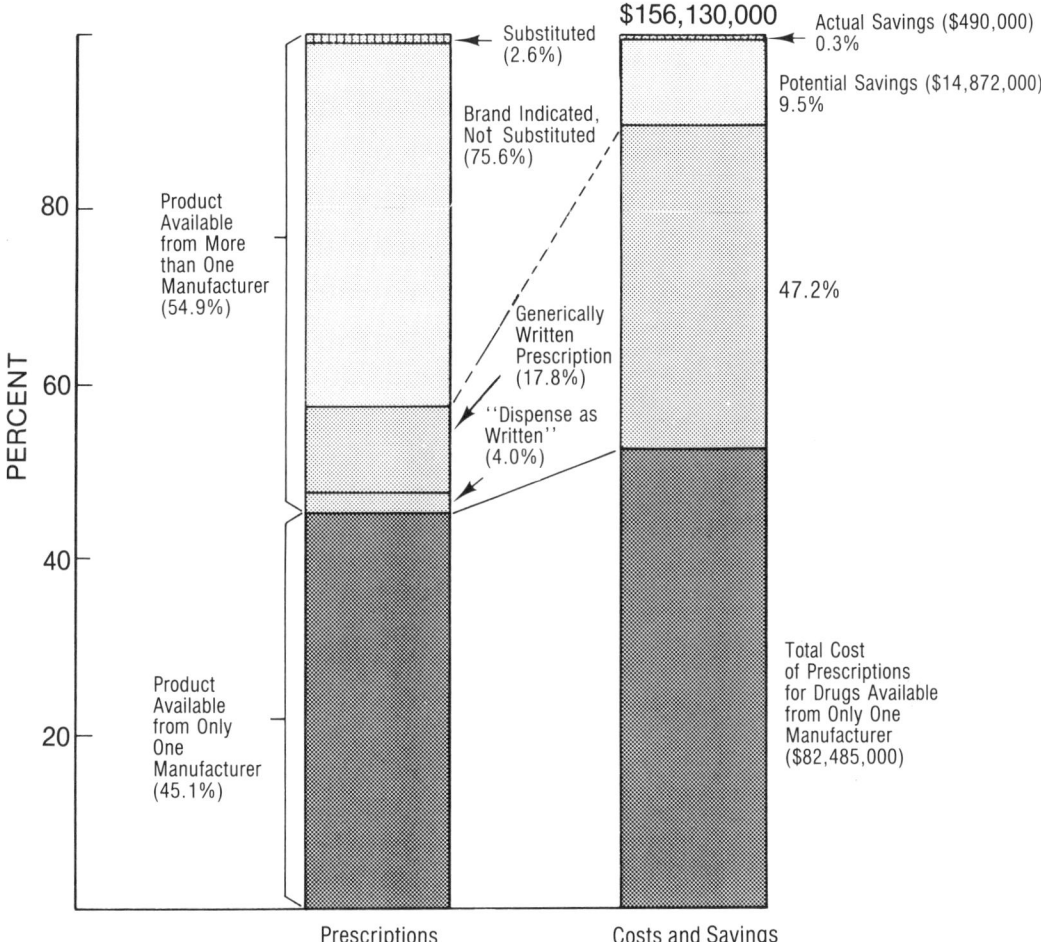

NOTE: The data shown are based on a sample of 15,000 new prescriptions filled in community pharmacies in Michigan. A drug product selection law went into effect on April 1, 1976 in Michigan permitting a pharmacist to substitute a generic equivalent for the drug prescribed, so long as neither the client nor the physician oppose such substitution, and provided that the drug substituted is less costly than the prescribed drug. Costs and savings shown are estimates for the state of Michigan for one year.

SOURCES: Goldberg, T., "Cost Implications of Drug Product Selection Legislation," Presented at the Invitational Dissemination Workshop on Drug Product Selection, Detroit, Michigan, April 13 and 14, 1978; Wayne State University Generic Drug Study Group, "Testimony on Drug Product Selection Legislation before the Special Committee of the Michigan House of Representatives, Lansing, Michigan, October 29, 1979,";DeVito, Carolee, et. al., "The Effects of Drug Product Selection Legislation in Michigan and Wisconsin: Review After Three Years of Operation," Presented at the 127th Annual Meeting of the American Pharmaceutical Association, Washington, D.C., April 22, 1980.

Chart D-32

Average Net Profits after Taxes as a Percent of Net Stockholders' Equity, U.S. Drug Manufacturers and All U.S. Manufacturing Corporations (U.S.A., Selected Years, 1960–1978).

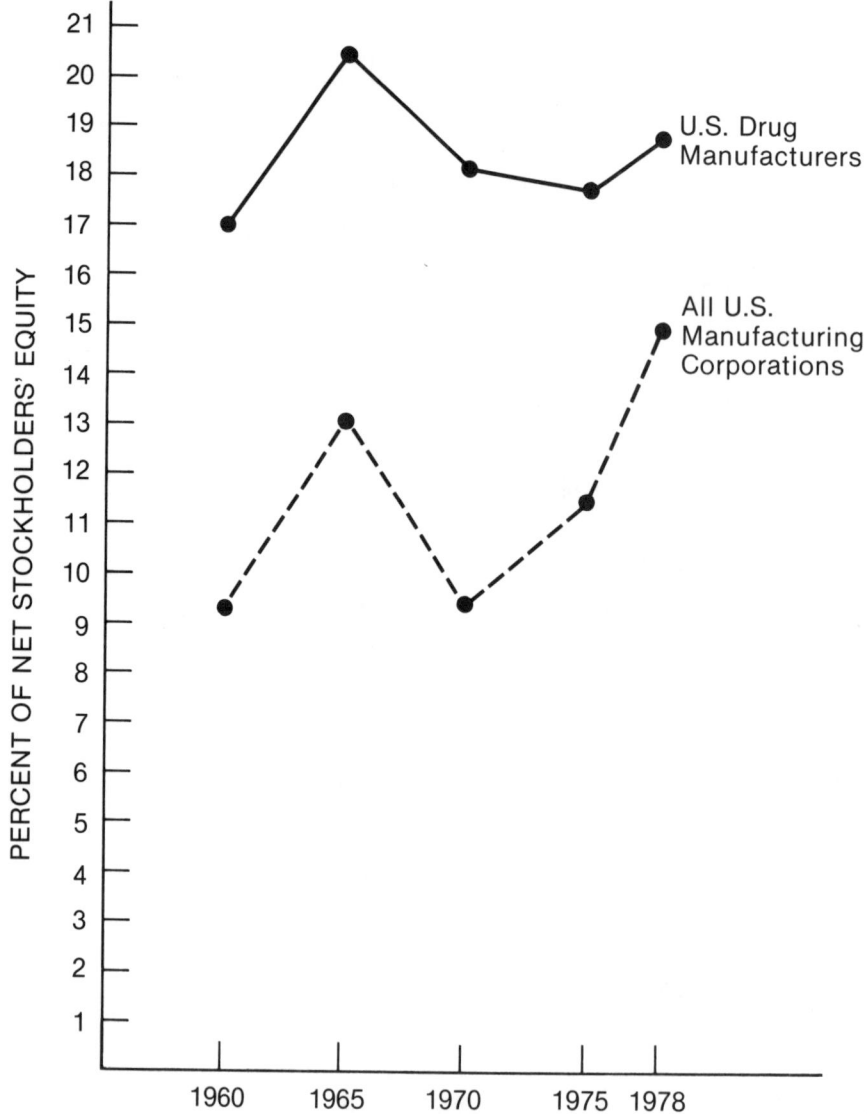

NOTE: "Stockholders' equity" refers to the portion of assets on which stockholders have a claim, as distinguished from assets on which creditors have a claim. *Net* stockholders' equity is defined as the average of beginning and end of year stockholders' equity.

SOURCES: For 1960–1970: Fulda, T.R., *Prescription Drug Data Summary, 1974,* DHEW, Social Security Administration, Office of Research and Statistics, 1976, Table III-9, p. 31; for 1975–1978: Calculated from the Federal Trade Commission–Securities and Exchange Commission, *Quarterly Financial Report for Manufacturing, Mining, and Trade Corporations,* Washington, D.C.

Costs and Expenditures

SECTION E
Health Personnel

Chart E-1

Physicians per 100,000 Persons for Continents and Selected Countries.

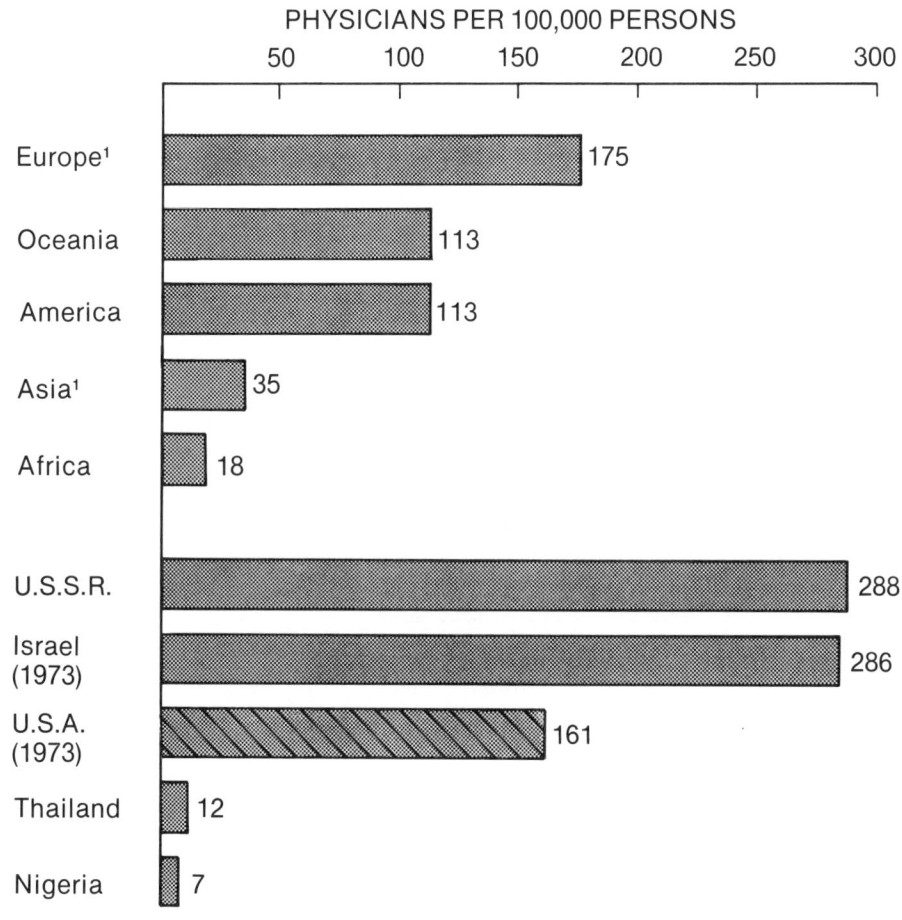

	Physicians per 100,000 Persons
Europe[1]	175
Oceania	113
America	113
Asia[1]	35
Africa	18
U.S.S.R.	288
Israel (1973)	286
U.S.A. (1973)	161
Thailand	12
Nigeria	7

[1]Excludes U.S.S.R.

NOTE: Data for continents are for 1977. Data for countries are for 1975, unless otherwise indicated.

SOURCES: For continents: World Health Organization, *World Health Statistics: Vital Statistics and Causes of Death*, Geneva, Switzerland, 1979, Table 3, p. 10; for countries: World Health Organization, *World Health Statistics Report*, Vol. 30, No. 2, 1977, Table 2, pp. 166-171; and World Health Organization, *World Health Statistics Report*, Vol. 29, No. 3, 1976; Table 2, pp. 132-139.

Health Personnel

Chart E-2

Number of Physicians per 100,000 Persons (Selected Countries, 1973-1975).

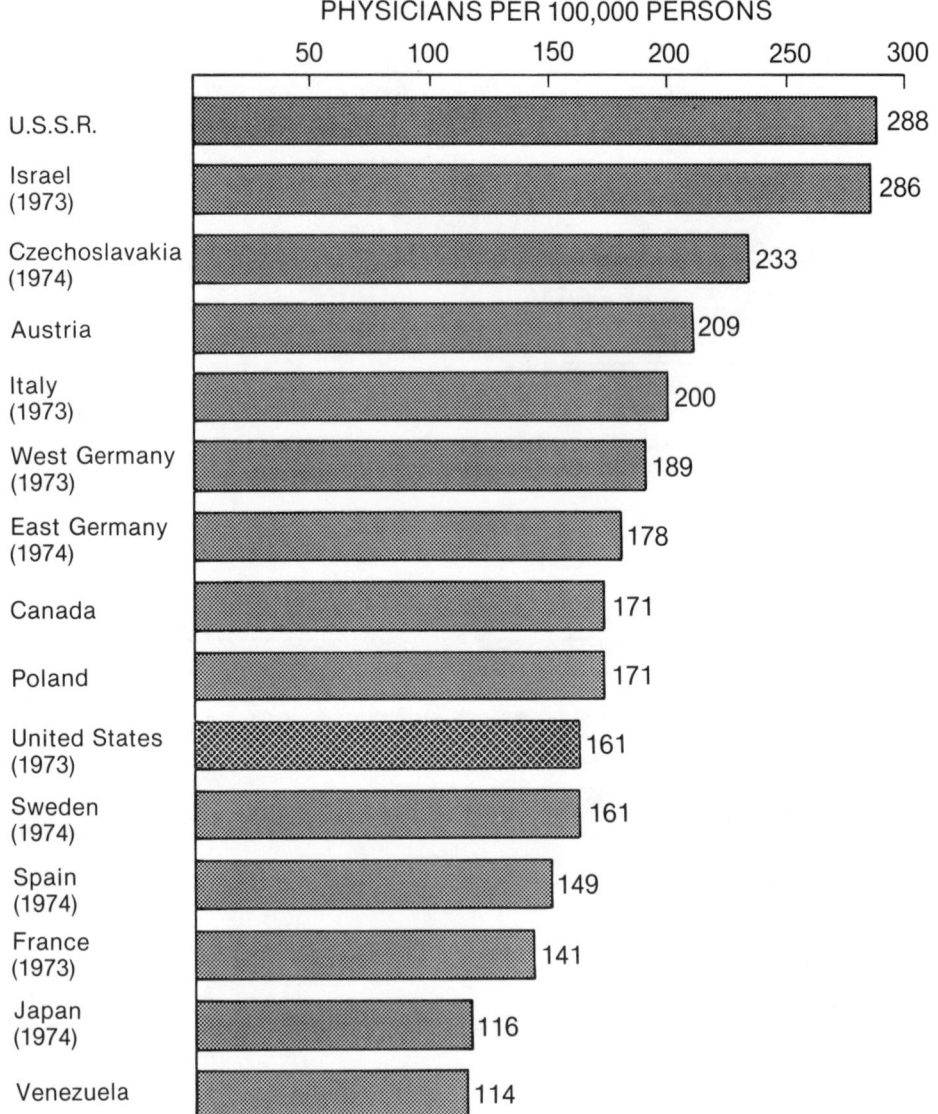

Country	Physicians per 100,000 Persons
U.S.S.R.	288
Israel (1973)	286
Czechoslavakia (1974)	233
Austria	209
Italy (1973)	200
West Germany (1973)	189
East Germany (1974)	178
Canada	171
Poland	171
United States (1973)	161
Sweden (1974)	161
Spain (1974)	149
France (1973)	141
Japan (1974)	116
Venezuela	114

NOTE: Data are for 1975 unless otherwise indicated.

SOURCES: World Health Organization, *World Health Statistics Report*, Vol. 30, No. 2, 1977, Table 2, pp. 166-171 and World Health Organization, *World Health Statistics Report*, Vol. 29, No. 3, 1976, Table 2, pp. 132-139.

Chart E-3

Number of Physicians and of All Other Health Personnel (U.S.A., Selected Years, 1900–1978).

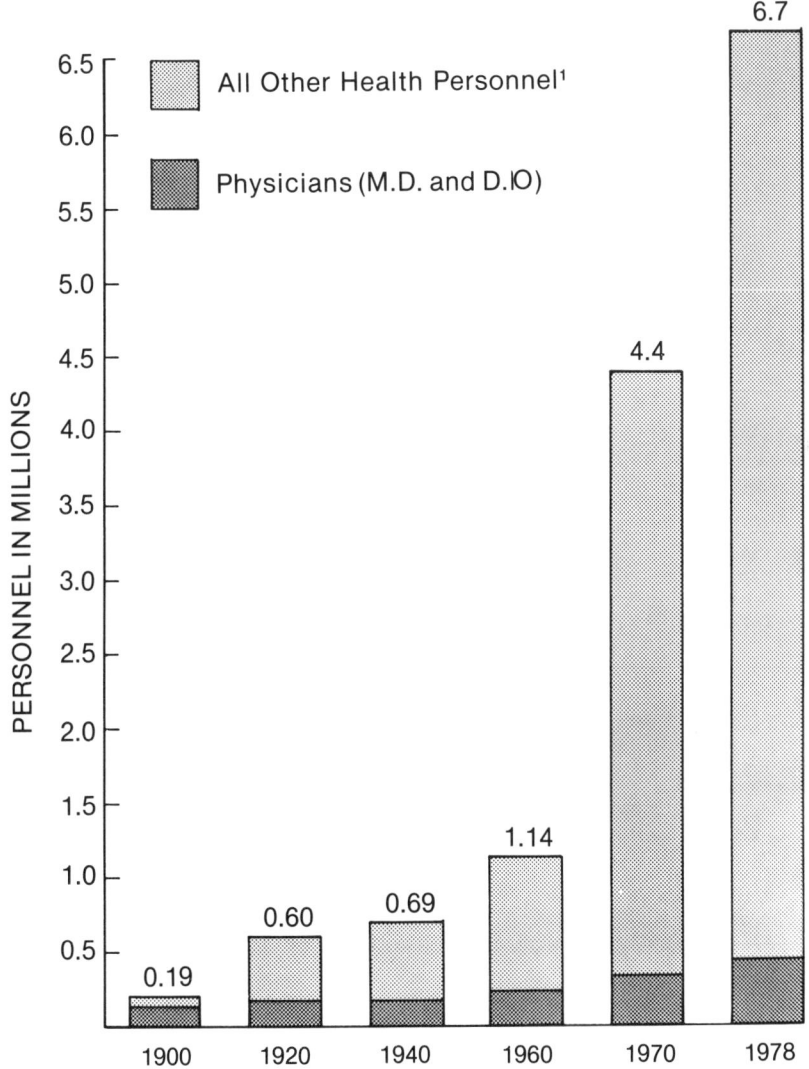

[1]Includes persons with special training and education designed to help them function in a health setting. Data for 1970 and 1978 are based on a somewhat broader definition of "other health personnel" than data for 1960.

SOURCES: For 1900–1960: *Chartbook on Health Status and Health Manpower*, Public Health Service, Division of Public Health Methods, Washington, D.C., 1961, p. 30; for 1970: U.S. National Center for Health Statistics, *Health Resources Statistics, 1970–71*, DHEW, Public Health Service, Washington, D.C., 1971, Table 1, p. 8; for 1978: U.S. Department of Health, Education, and Welfare, *Health, United States, 1979*, Public Health Service, Office of Health Research, Statistics, and Technology, Hyattsville, Maryland, 1980, p. 151.

Chart E-4

Number of Physicians,[1] Dentists, and Registered Nurses per 100,000 Persons (U.S.A., 1900–1976 and Projections for Physicians for 1980 and 1990).

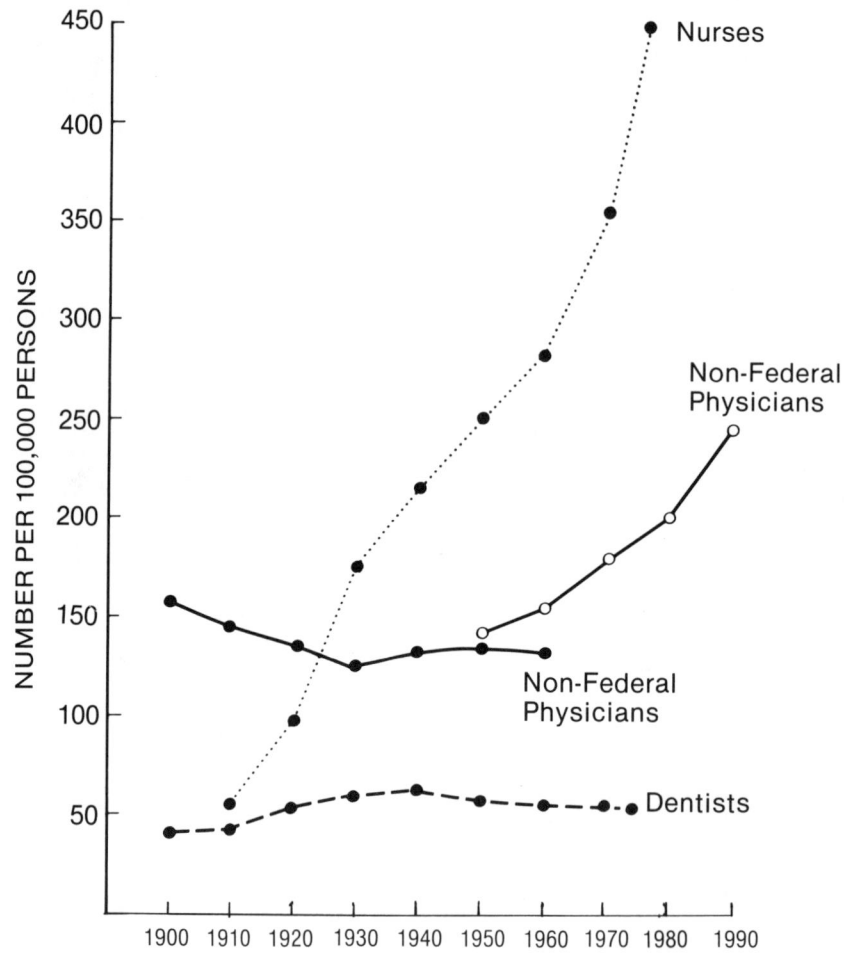

[1]Includes M.D.'s and D.O.'s. In 1963 the convention for computing physician-population ratios was changed, resulting in an increase in the ratio. Data using the new convention were available beginning in 1950.

SOURCES: U.S. Department of Health, Education, and Welfare, *Health Education and Welfare Trends, 1964, Part 1, National Trends,* Washington, D.C., 1965, p.26; U.S. National Center for Health Statistics, *Health Resources Statistics, 1971,* DHEW, Public Health Service, Rockville, Maryland, 1972, Table 37, p.76; U.S. National Center for Health Statistics, *Health, United States, 1978,* DHEW Public Health Service, Health Resources Administration, Hyattsville, Maryland, 1978, Table 129, p.344. U.S. National Center for Health Statistics, *Health Resources Statistics, 1976–1977,* DHEW, Public Health Service, Office of Health Research, Statistics, and Technology, Hyattsville, Maryland, 1979, Table 103, p.168; U.S. National Center for Health Statistics, *Health, United States, 1979,* DHEW, Public Health Service, Hyattsville, Maryland, 1979, Table 49, p.157.

Chart E-5

Physician — Population Ratios, by Geographic Area and Selected States (U.S.A., 1978).

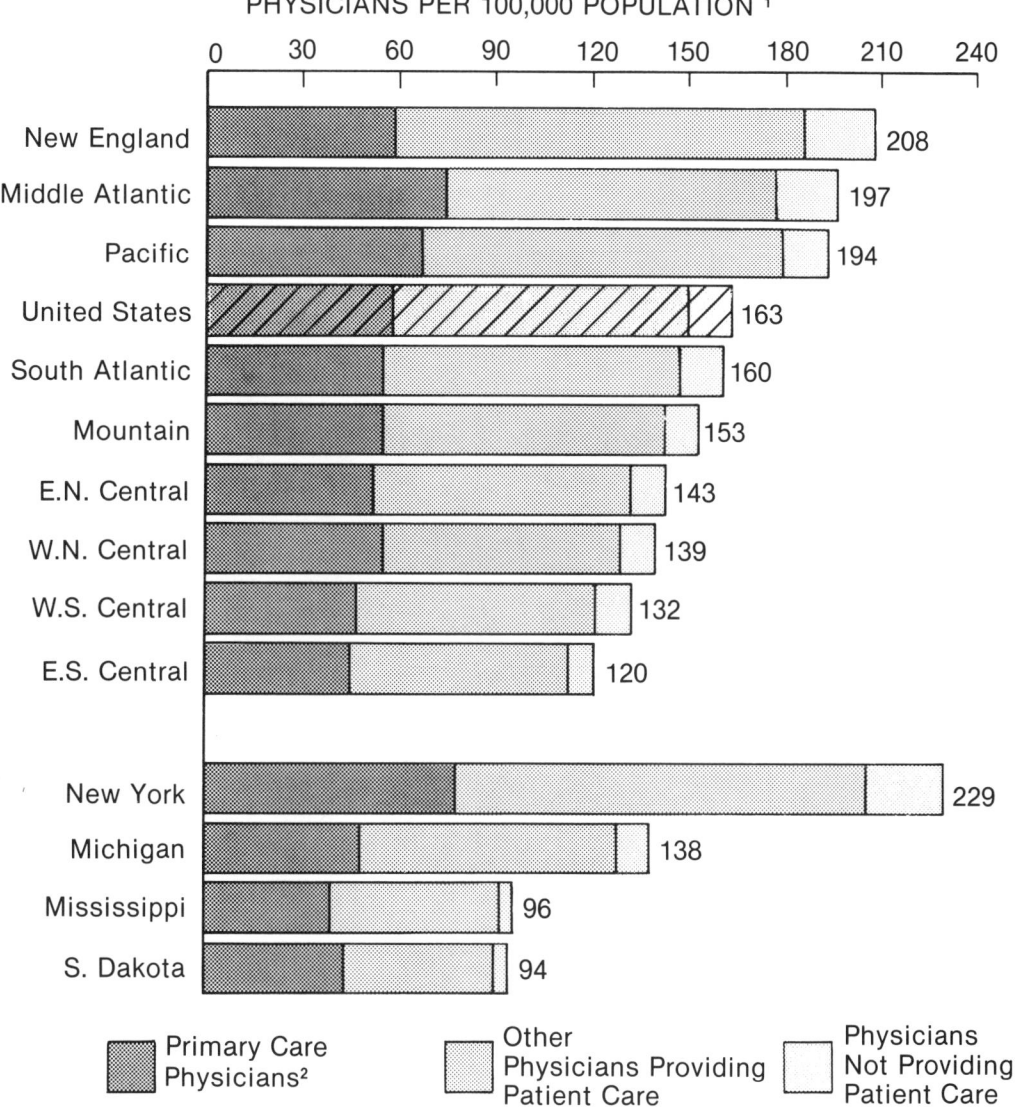

[1]Includes physicians in residency training; excludes physicians working for the federal government, osteopathic physicians, and inactive physicians.

[2]Physicians in family practice, general practice, internal medicine, and pediatrics.

SOURCE: American Medical Association, *Physician Distribution and Medical Licensure in the U.S., 1978*, Center for Health Services Research and Development, Department of Statistical Analysis, 1979, Table G, p. 23, Table 6, p. 74, Table 7, p. 79, Table 8, pp. 80-88, and Table 9, pp. 92-146.

Chart E-6 Physician-Population Ratios, by Type of Practice and Type of Area (U.S.A., 1978).[1]

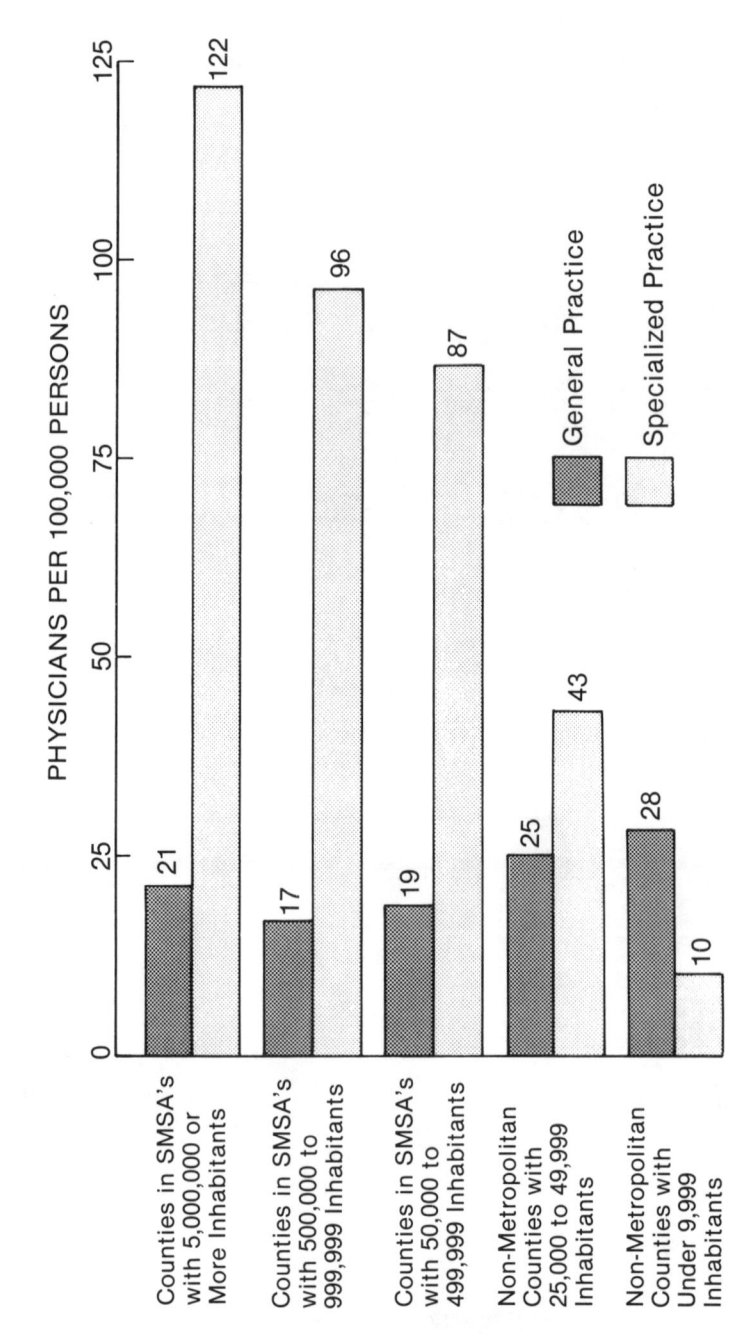

[1]Includes only physicians in active practice, not hospital-based. Excludes physicians working for the federal government and osteopathic physicians.

SOURCE: American Medical Association, *Physician Distribution and Medical Licensure in the U.S., 1978*, Center for Health Services Research and Development, Department of Statistical Analysis, 1979, Table E, p. 15 and Table O, p. 34.

Health Personnel

Medical Care Chartbook 145

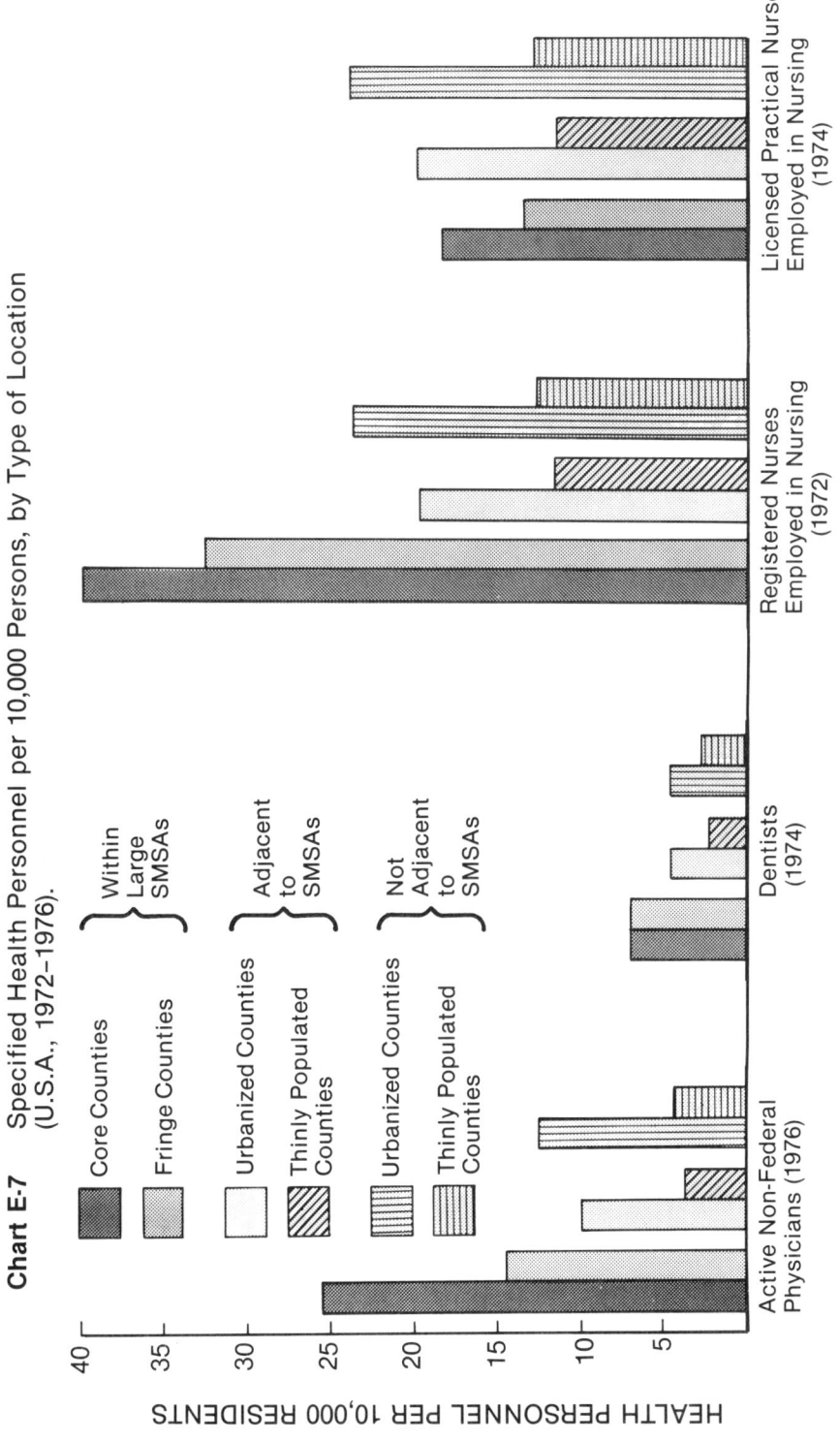

Chart E-7 Specified Health Personnel per 10,000 Persons, by Type of Location (U.S.A., 1972–1976).

SOURCE: U.S. National Center for Health Statistics, *Health, United States, 1978*, DHEW, Public Health Service, Health Resources Administration, Hyattsville, Maryland, 1978, Table 12a, p. 344.

Health Personnel

Chart E-8

States by Physician-Population Ratios[1] and by per Capita Personal Income (U.S.A., 1977).

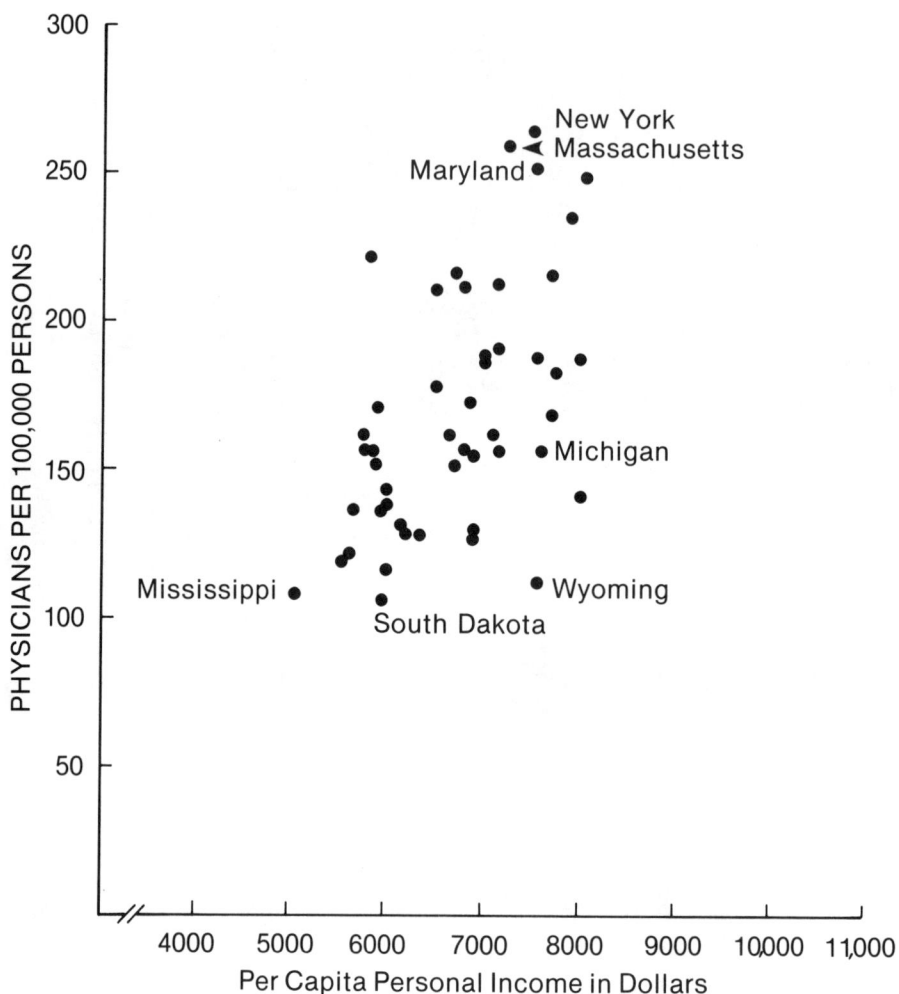

[1]Includes only active non-federal physicians.

SOURCES: U.S. Department of Commerce, Bureau of the Census, *Statistical Abstract of the United States, 1978*, Washington, D.C., 1978, Table 725, p. 449; American Medical Association, *Physician Distribution and Medical Licensure in the U.S., 1978*, Center for Health Services Research and Development, 1979, Table G, p. 23.

Chart E-9 Physicians in Private Practice per 100,000 Persons and Relative Supply of Physicians by Specialty Status, "Poverty" and "Non-Poverty" Areas (Chicago, 1966).[1]

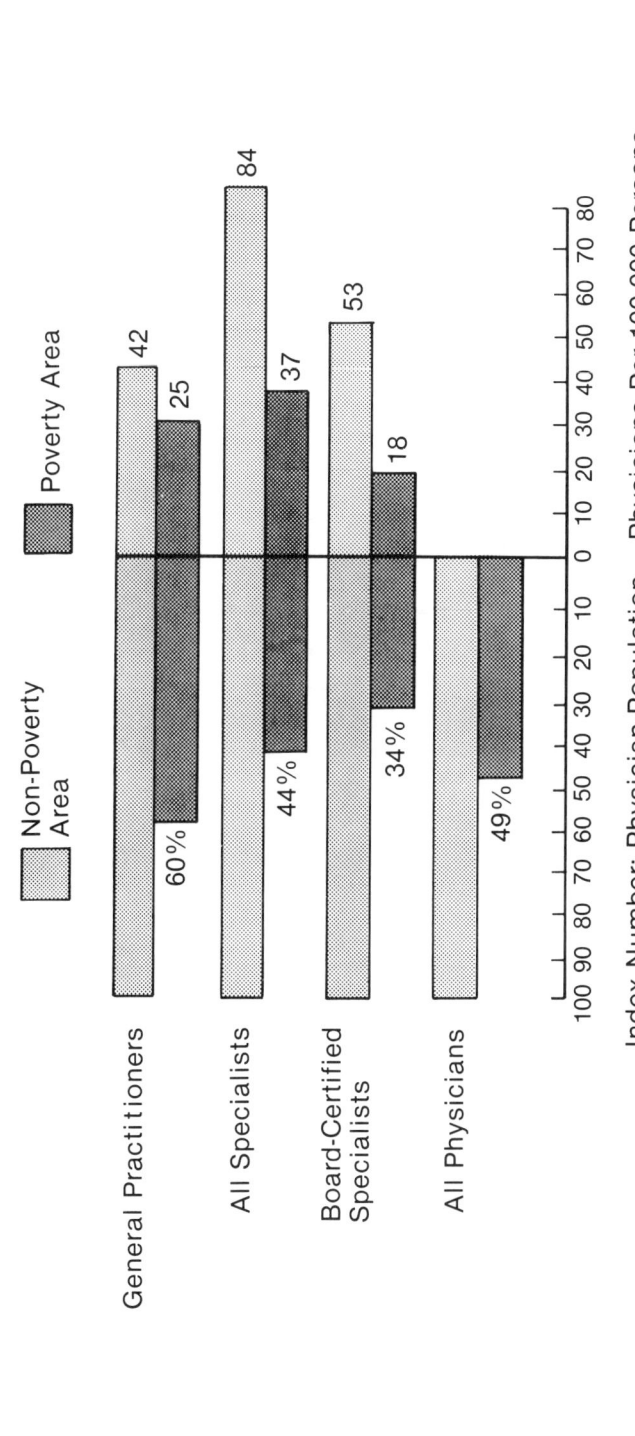

[1] "Poverty" and "Non-Poverty" areas were delineated by aggregating census tracts using as criteria income, education, housing, unemployment, proportion on welfare and juvenile delinquency.

SOURCE: Chicago Board of Health, *Chicago Board of Health Medical Report*, 1966.

Health Personnel

Chart E-10

Relative Physician-Population Ratios by Specialty, in Groups of Census Tracts Arrayed by Socio-economic Status[1] (Boston and Brookline, Massachusetts, 1940 and 1961).

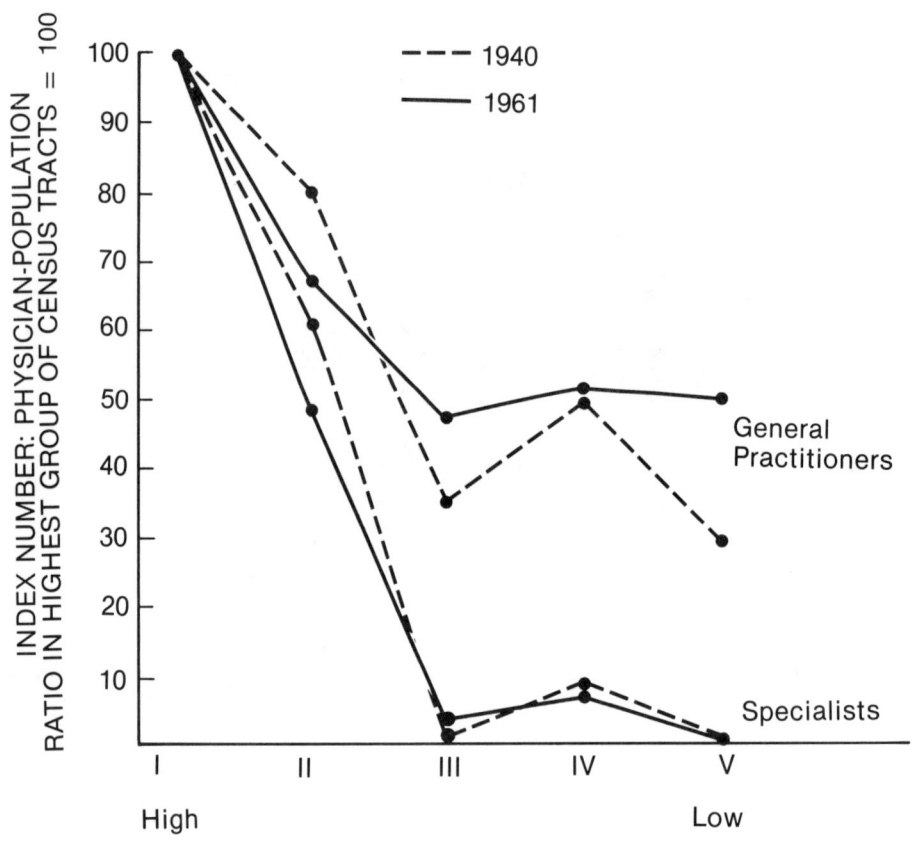

[1]Census tracts are arrayed by rank on a combined score of income, education and occupation, and divided into 5 groups of approximately equal population. The numerator of the physician-population ratio is the number of physicians whose offices are located in the specified census tracts *excluding* physicians with addresses in hospitals or medical schools and those not usually involved in clinical practice.

SOURCE: Dorsey, Joseph L., "Physician Distribution in Boston and Brookline, 1940 and 1961," *Medical Care.* Vol. 7, No. 6, November–December 1969, Figure 2, p. 433, Figure 3, p. 433, and Figure 5, p. 434.

Health Personnel

Chart E-11 Geographic Areas, by Physician-Population Ratios, by Limitation of Activity of Residents, and by Personal Income (U.S.A., 1965–1967).[1]

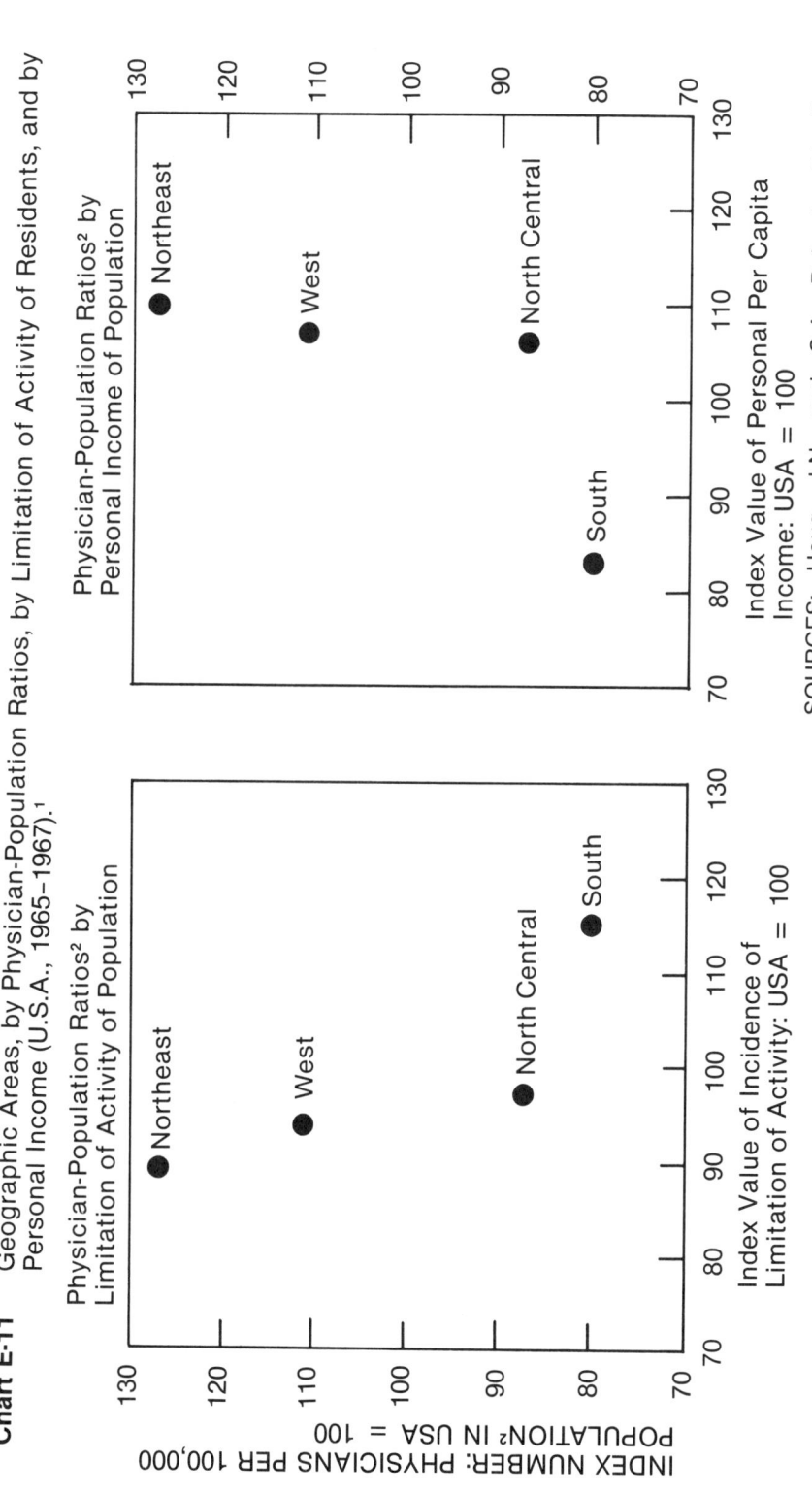

SOURCES: Haug, J.N. and G.A. Roback, *Distribution of Physicians, Hospitals, and Hospital Beds in the United States, 1967*, American Medical Association, Chicago, 1968, Table 10, pp. 124–127; U.S. National Center for Health Statistics, *Chronic Conditions and Limitations of Activity and Mobility: United States, July 1965–June 1967*, Public Health Service, Series 10, No. 61, Washington, D.C., January 1971, Table 27, p. 45.

[1] Data for limitation of activity are for 1965–1967. Physician-population ratios are for 1967. Income data are for 1966. Population data used as the base for per capita figures are for January 1, 1967.

[2] Excludes federal physicians and osteopathic physicians.

Chart E-12 Geographic Areas, by Physician-Population Ratios, by Limitation of Activity of Residents, and by Personal Income (U.S.A., 1976 and 1977).[1]

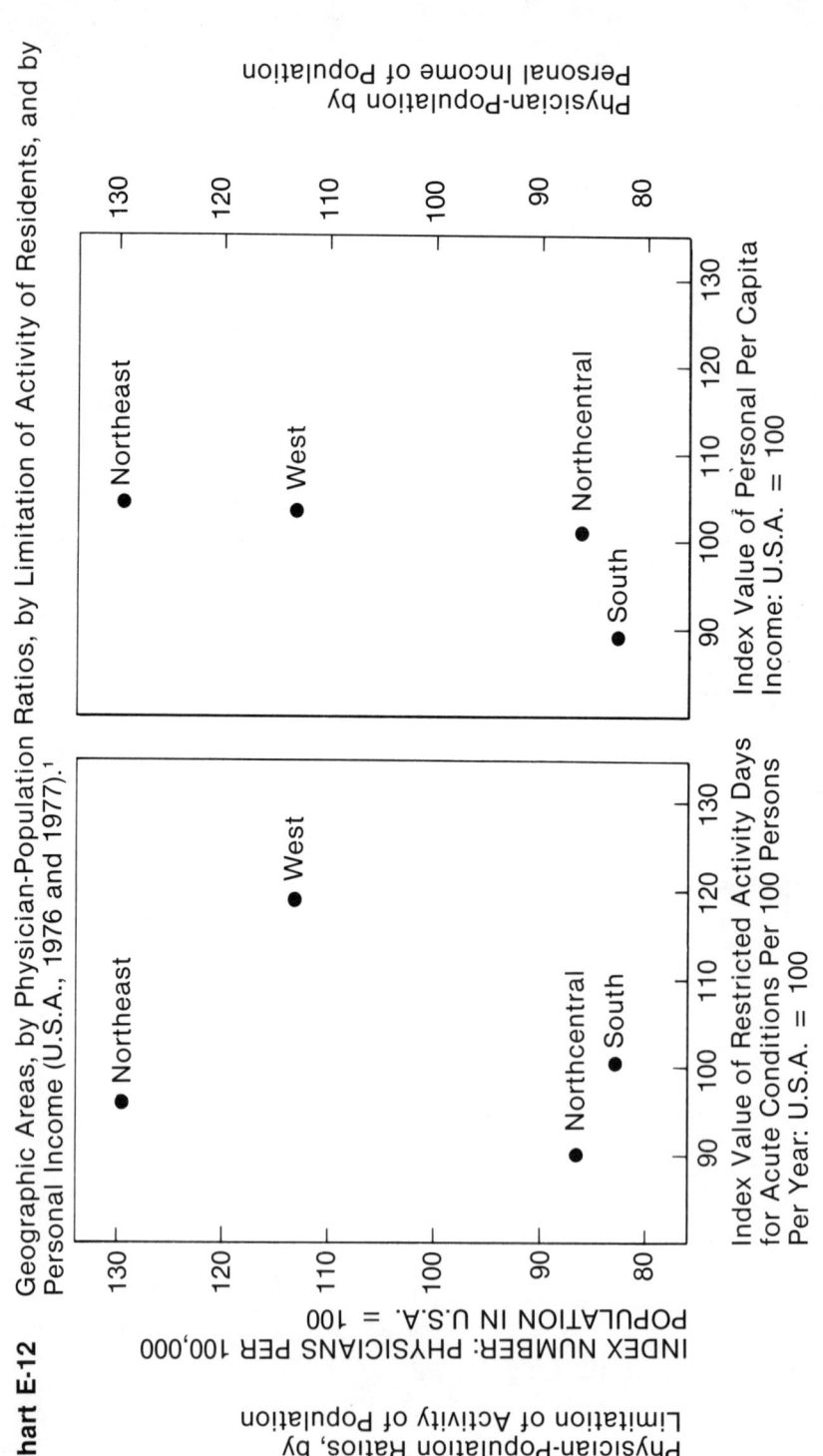

[1] Physician-population ratios are for 1976. Per capita income and restricted activity days are for 1977.

[2] Excludes federal physicians and osteopathic physicians.

SOURCES: For per capita income: U.S. Department of Commerce, Bureau of the Census, *Statistical Abstract of the United States, 1978*, Washington, D.C., 1978, Table 752, p. 449; for disability days: U.S. National Center for Health Statistics, *Acute Conditions, Incidence and Associated Disability, United States, July 1976–June 1977*, Public Health Service, Hyattsville, Maryland, September 1978, Table 18, p. 27; for physician-population ratios: U.S. National Center for Health Statistics, *Health, United States, 1978*, DHEW, Public Health Service, Hyattsville, Maryland, December 1978, Table 27, p. 342.

Chart E-13 Relative Number of Medical Schools, Medical Students, Women Medical Students, Medical Graduates, and Women Medical Graduates (U.S.A., Selected Years, 1949–1978).

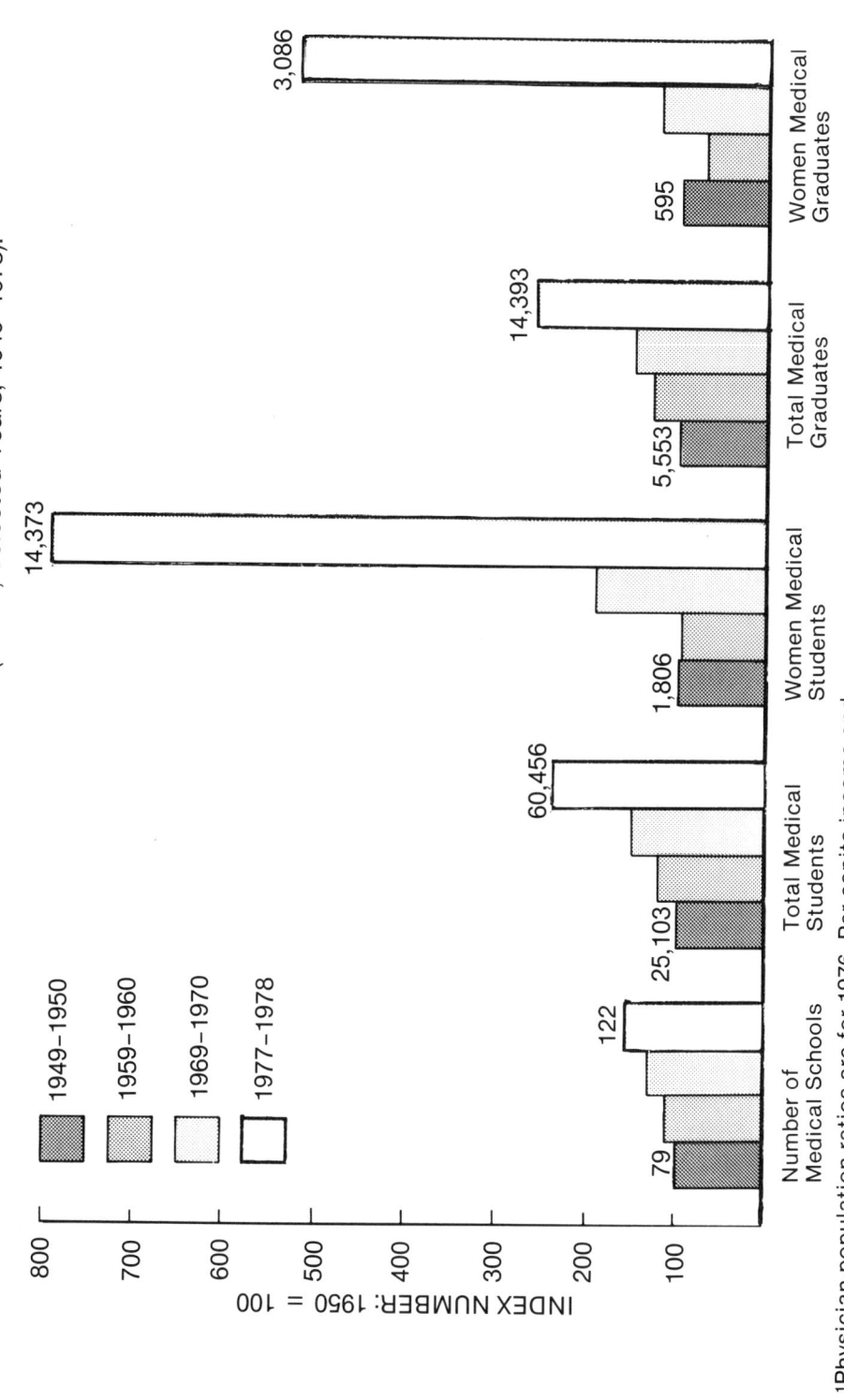

SOURCE: Haug, James N. and Kathleen Kuntzman, *Socio-Economic Factbook for Surgery, 1979*, American College of Surgeons, 1979, Table 1, p. 8.

[1]Physician-population ratios are for 1976. Per capita income and restricted activity days are for 1977.

NOTE: Numbers on top of bars represent actual values for the specific category.

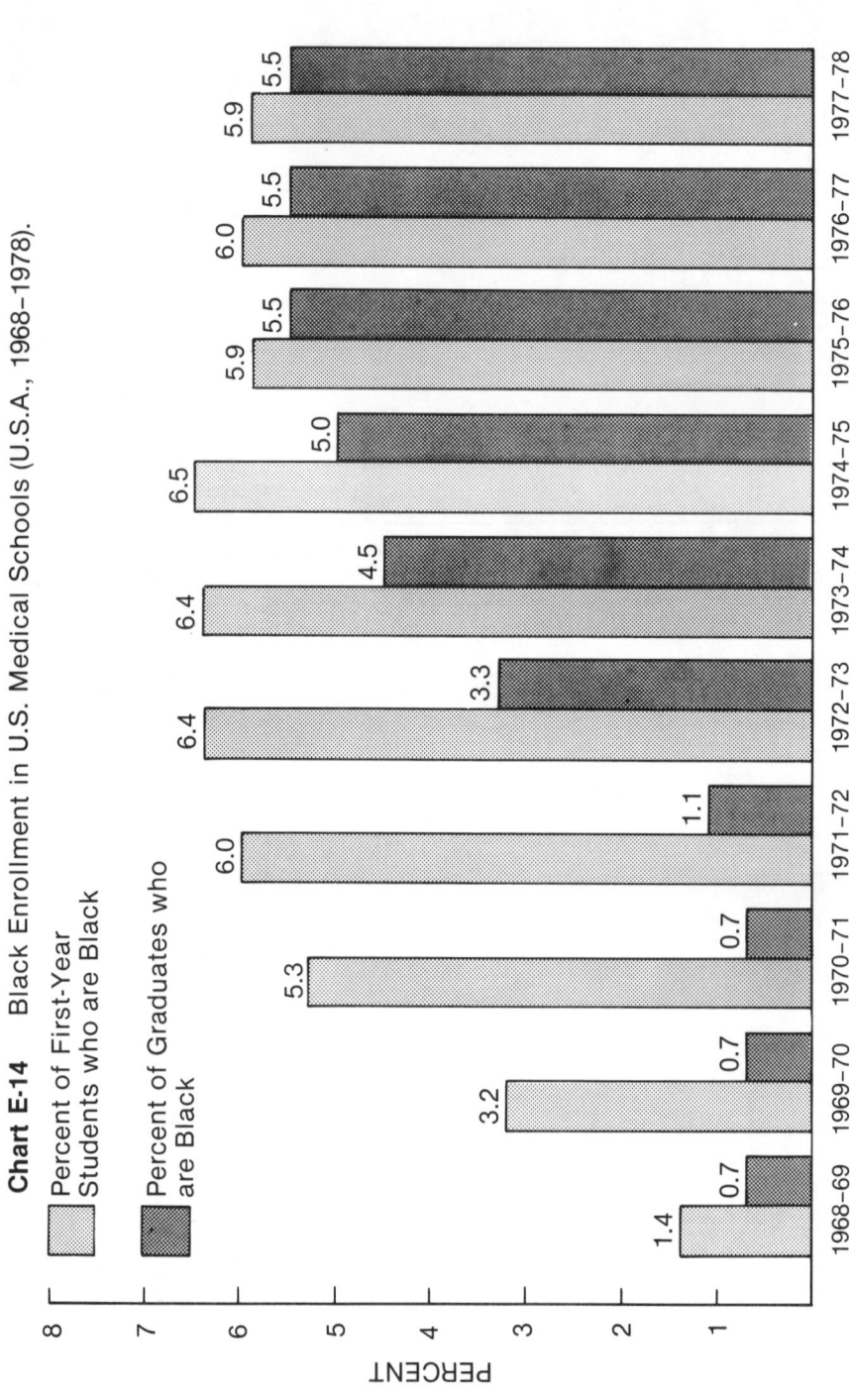

Chart E-14 Black Enrollment in U.S. Medical Schools (U.S.A., 1968–1978).

NOTE: 1968–1972 data exclude Howard, Meharry, and University of Puerto Rico. 1972–1977 data exclude University of Puerto Rico.

SOURCES: "Medical Education in the United States, 1971–72," *Journal of the American Medical Association*, Vol. 222, No. 8, November 20, 1972, Table 22, p. 983; "Medical Education in the United States, 1973–1974," *Journal of the American Medical Association*, Vol. 231, January 1975, Table 13, p. 18; "Medical Education in the United States, 1976–77," *Journal of the American Medical Association*, Vol. 238, No. 26, December 26, 1977, Table 12, p. 2772; "Medical Education in the United States, 1977–78," *Journal of the American Medical Association*, Vol. 240, No. 26, December 22, 1978, Table 11, p. 2824.

Medical Care Chartbook

Chart E-15

Percent of Medical School Applicants Accepted (U.S.A., Selected Years, 1950–1978).

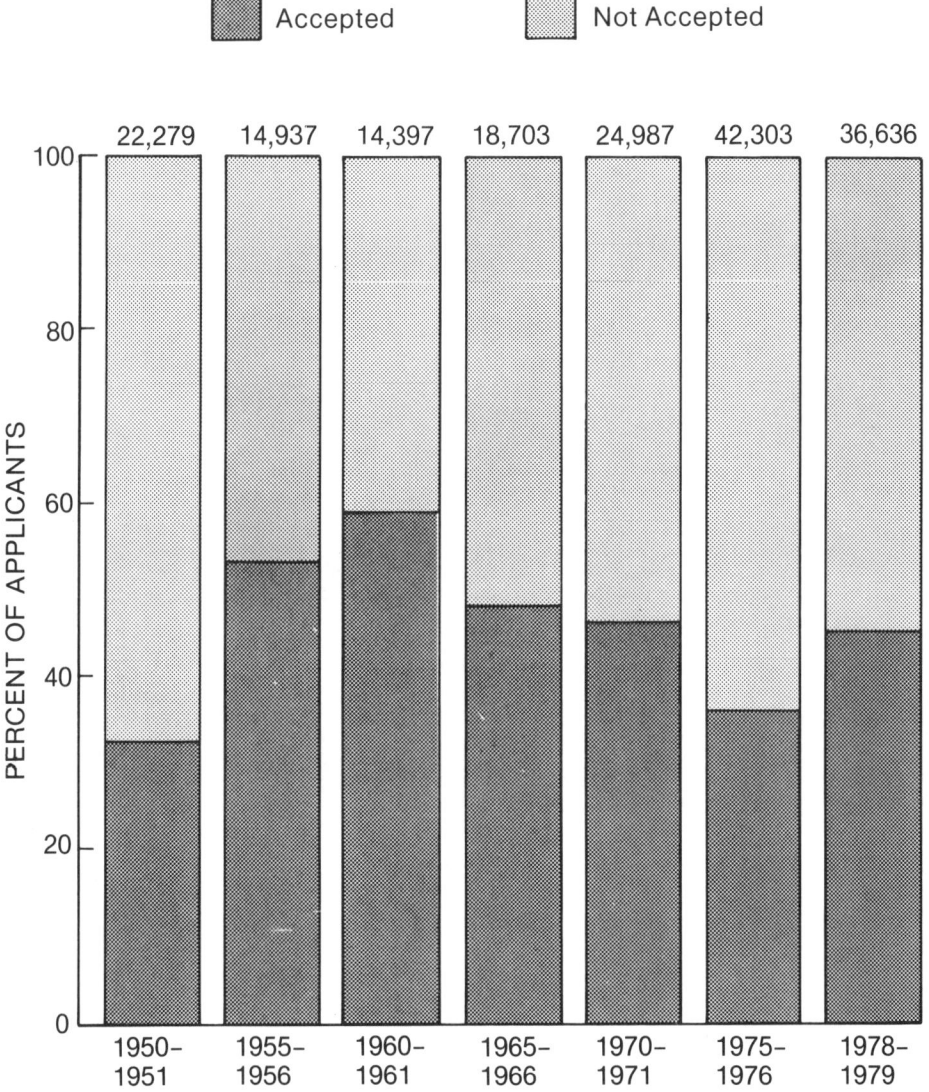

NOTE: Numbers above bars are actual number of persons who applied to one or more medical schools.

SOURCES: For 1950-51: "Medical Education in the United States, 1964-1965," *Journal of the American Medical Association,* Vol. 194, No. 7, November 15, 1965, Table 10, p. 163; for 1955-1976: "Medical Education in the United States, 1975-1976," *Journal of the American Medical Association,* Vol. 236, No. 26, December 27, 1976, Table 8, p. 2961; for 1978-1979: "Medical Education in the United States, 1978-1979," *Journal of the American Medical Association,* Vol. 243, No. 9, March 7, 1980, Table 5, p. 852.

Health Personnel

Chart E-16 Percent Distribution of Families of Medical School Applicants, Families of Applicants Accepted to Medical School, and of All Families, by Family Income (U.S.A., 1976–1977).

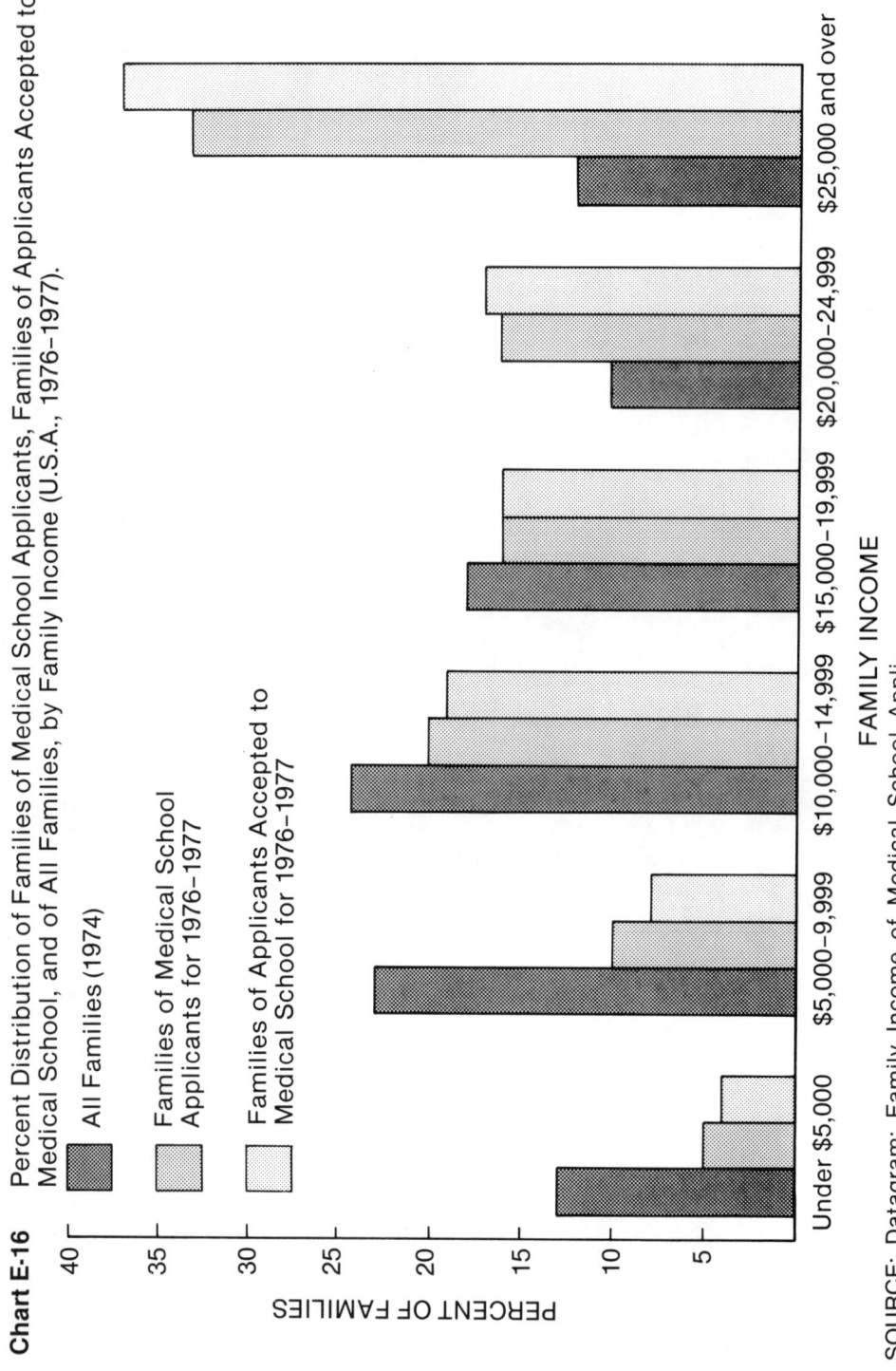

SOURCE: Datagram: Family Income of Medical School Applicants and Acceptees and of College Students, *Journal of Medical Education*, Vol. 52, November 1977, Table 1, p. 949.

Chart E-17

Number of Residencies, Internships, and Graduates of United States Medical Schools (U.S.A., Selected Years, 1940–1977).

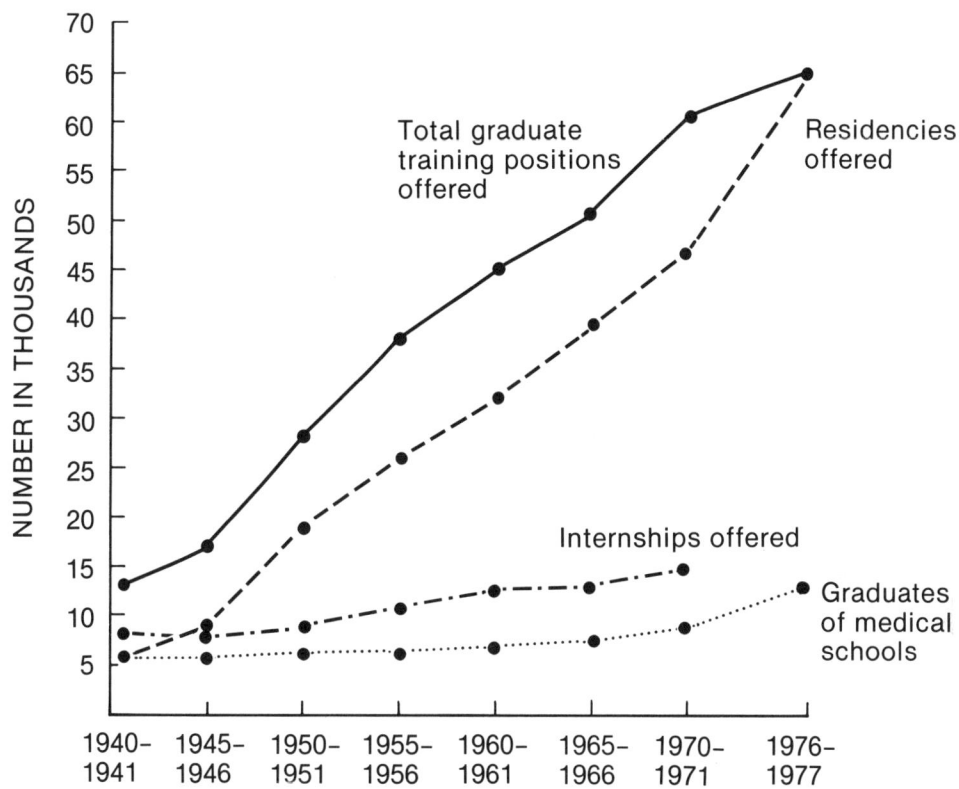

NOTE: The number of residencies exceeds that of internships because the latter continue for several years. For 1976–1977, figures are not given in the internship category due to the change in designation of the first year of graduate training from internship to residency.

SOURCES: "Medical Education in the U.S.," *Journal of the American Medical Association*, Vol. 240, No. 26, December 22, 1978, Table 6, p. 2822; for 1976–1977: *Directory of Residency Training Programs*, (accredited by the Liaison Committee on Graduate Medical Education), Table 14, p. 14.

Chart E-18

Percent of All Medical Residents and of Women Residents in Selected Specialties (U.S.A., 1978–1979).

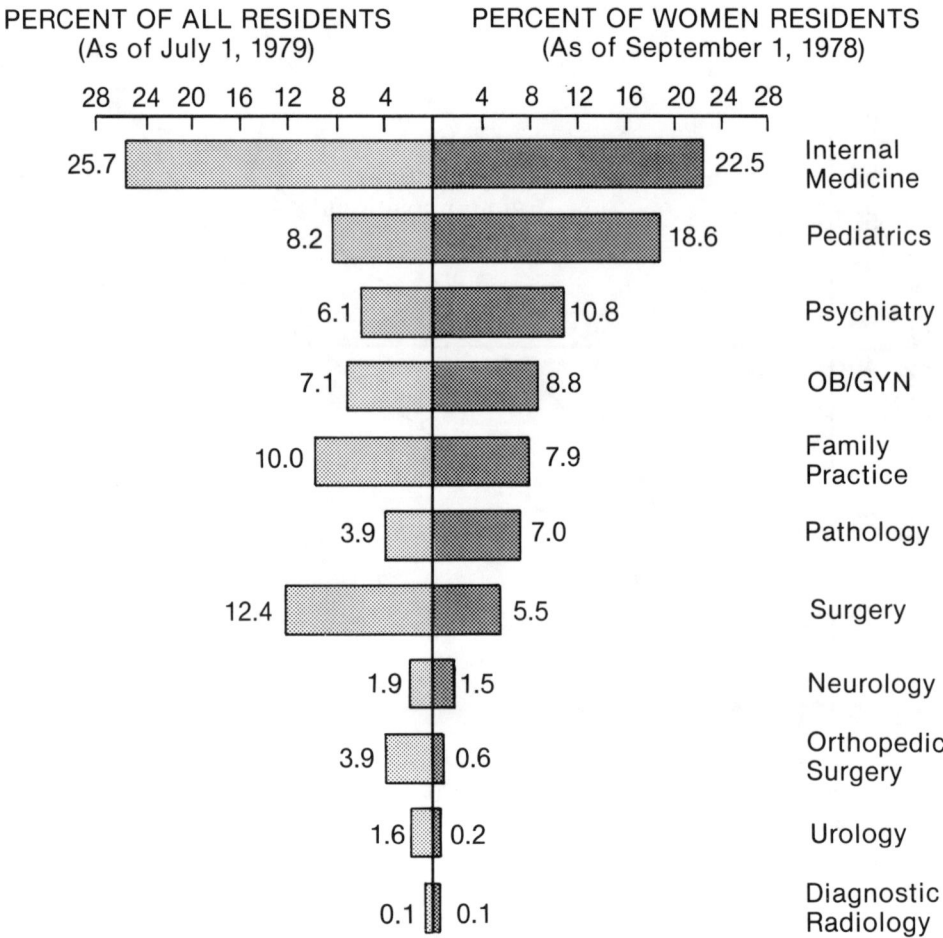

SOURCE: "Medical Education in the United States, 1978–1979," *Journal of the American Medical Association,* Vol. 243, No. 9, March 7, 1980, Table 5, p. 872 and Table 11, p. 877.

Health Personnel

Chart E-19

Percent Distribution of Residencies Vacant and Filled by Medical Graduates from U.S. and Canadian Schools and by Foreign Medical School Graduates (U.S.A., Selected Years, 1950-1977).

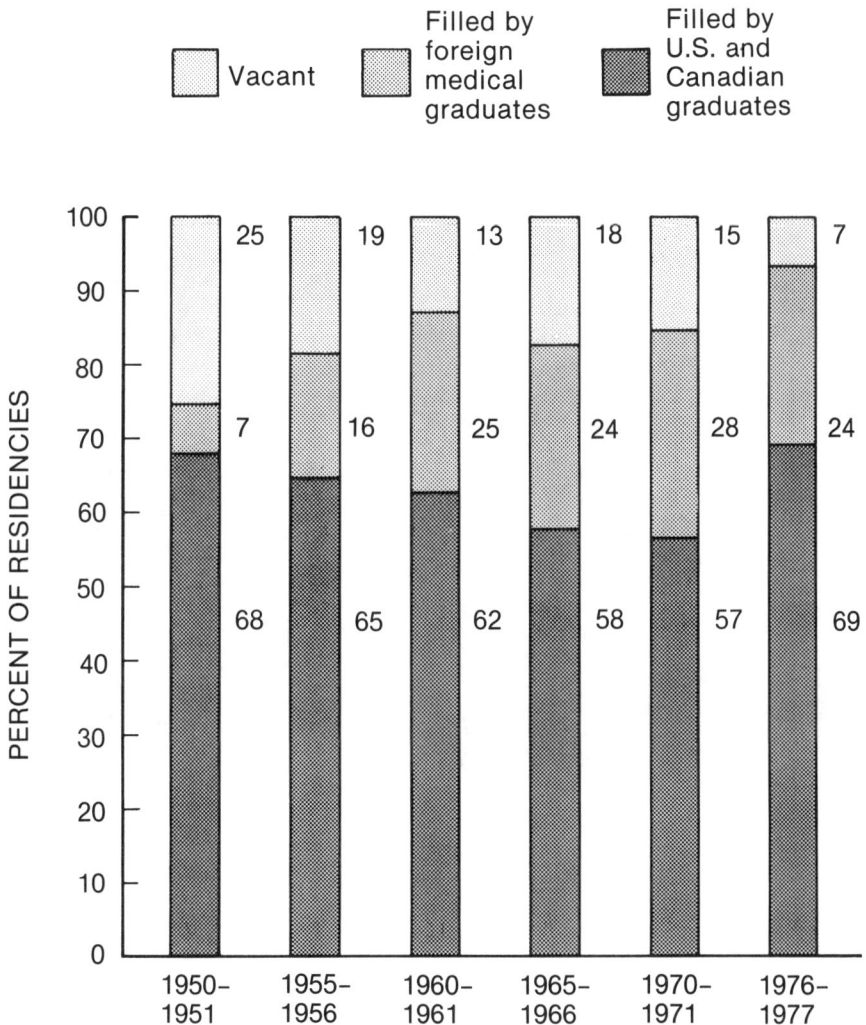

SOURCES: For 1950-1966: "Medical Education in the United States, 1965-1966," *Journal of the American Medical Association*, Vol. 198, November 21, 1966, Table 26, p. 29; for 1970-1971: Ruhe, C.A.W., et al., *Directory of Approved Internships and Residencies*, American Medical Association, Chicago, 1971, Table 10, p. 9; for 1976-1977: *Directory of Residency Training Programs*, (accredited by the Liaison Committee on Graduate Medical Education), Table 14, p. 14.

Health Personnel

Chart E-20

Percent of Internships and Residencies Filled by Graduates of Foreign Medical Schools[1] and Percent of Total Initial Licentiates Who are Graduates of Foreign Medical Schools (U.S.A., 1950–1978).

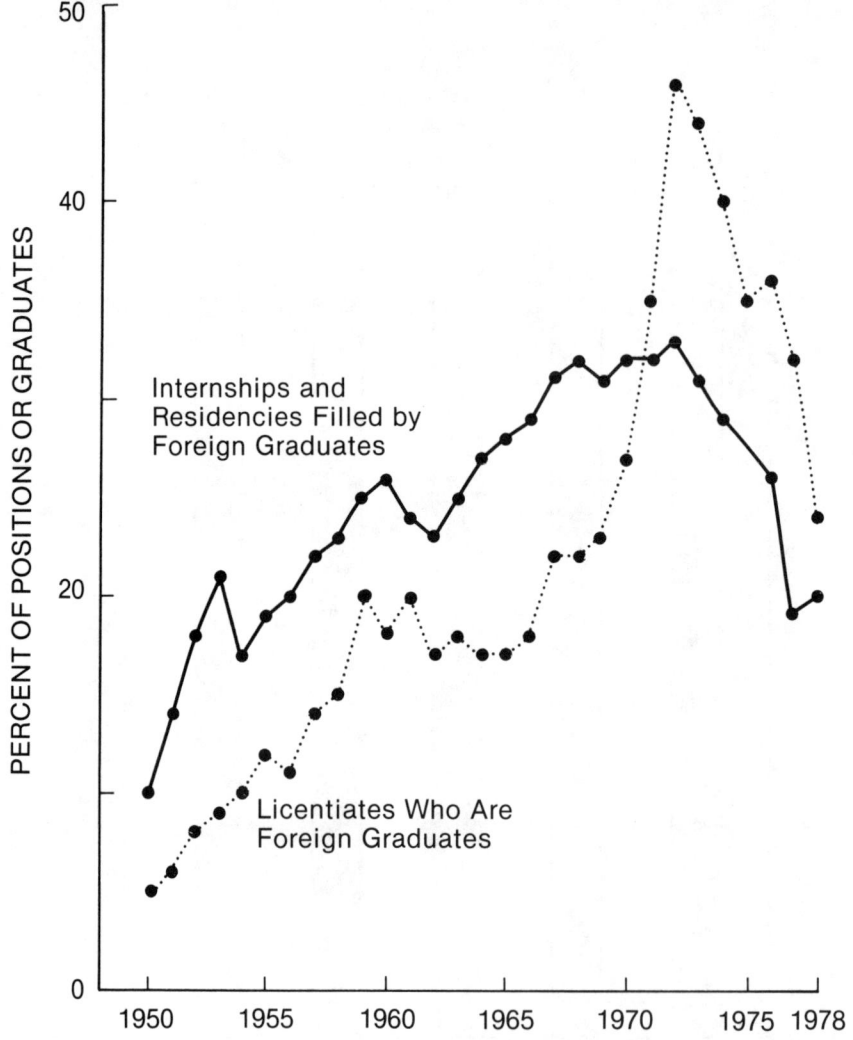

[1] Excludes graduates of Canadian medical schools.

SOURCES: For 1950–1974: "Medical Education in the United States, 1975–76," *Journal of the American Medical Association*, Vol. 236, No. 26, December 27, 1976, Table 29, p. 2991; for 1975 and 1976: "Medical Education in the United States, 1976–1977," *Journal of the American Medical Association*, Vol. 238, No. 26, December 26, 1977, Table 3, p. 2782 and Table 7, p. 2785; for 1977: "Medical Education in the United States, 1977–78," *Journal of the American Medical Association*, Vol. 240, No. 6, December 22, 1978, p. 2839 and Table 8, p. 2840; for 1978: "Medical Education in the United States, 1978–79," *Journal of the American Medical Association*, Vol. 243, No. 9, March 7, 1980, Table 15, p. 880; for licentiates, 1950–1978: American Medical Association, *Physician Distribution and Medical Licensure in the U.S., 1978*, Center for Health Services Research and Development, Department of Statistical Analysis, 1979, Table 4, p. 357 and Table 5, p. 358.

Health Personnel

Chart E-21

Percent Distribution of M.D. Physicians in Private Practice, by Specialization Status (U.S.A., Selected Years, 1949–1978).

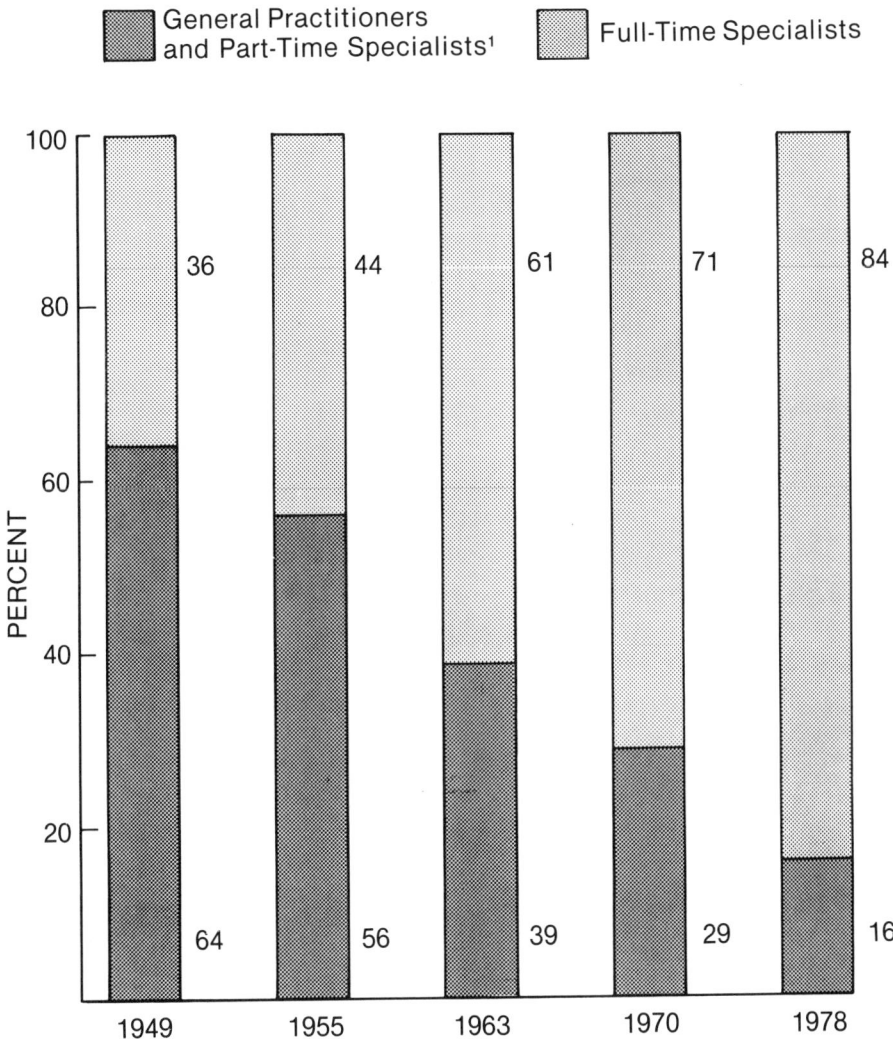

[1] Includes family practitioners.

SOURCES: For 1949 and 1955: Perrott, G. and M.Y. Pennell, *Health Manpower Chart Book,* Public Health Service, Washington, D.C., 1957, p. 30; for 1963: U.S. Public Health Service, Division of Public Health Methods, *Health Manpower Source Book, Section 18: Manpower in the 1960's,* Washington, D.C., 1964, Table 16, p. 28; for 1970: U.S. National Center for Health Statistics, *Health Resources Statistics, 1970,* DHEW, Public Health Service, Rockville, Maryland, 1971, Table 86, p. 155; for 1978: American Medical Association, *Physician Distribution and Medical Licensure in the U.S., 1978,* Center for Health Services Research and Development, Department of Statistical Analysis, 1979, Table A, p. 13.

Chart E-22

Number of Physicians Designated as Primary Care Physicians per 100,000 Persons, by Type of Practice (U.S.A., Selected Years, 1931-1978).

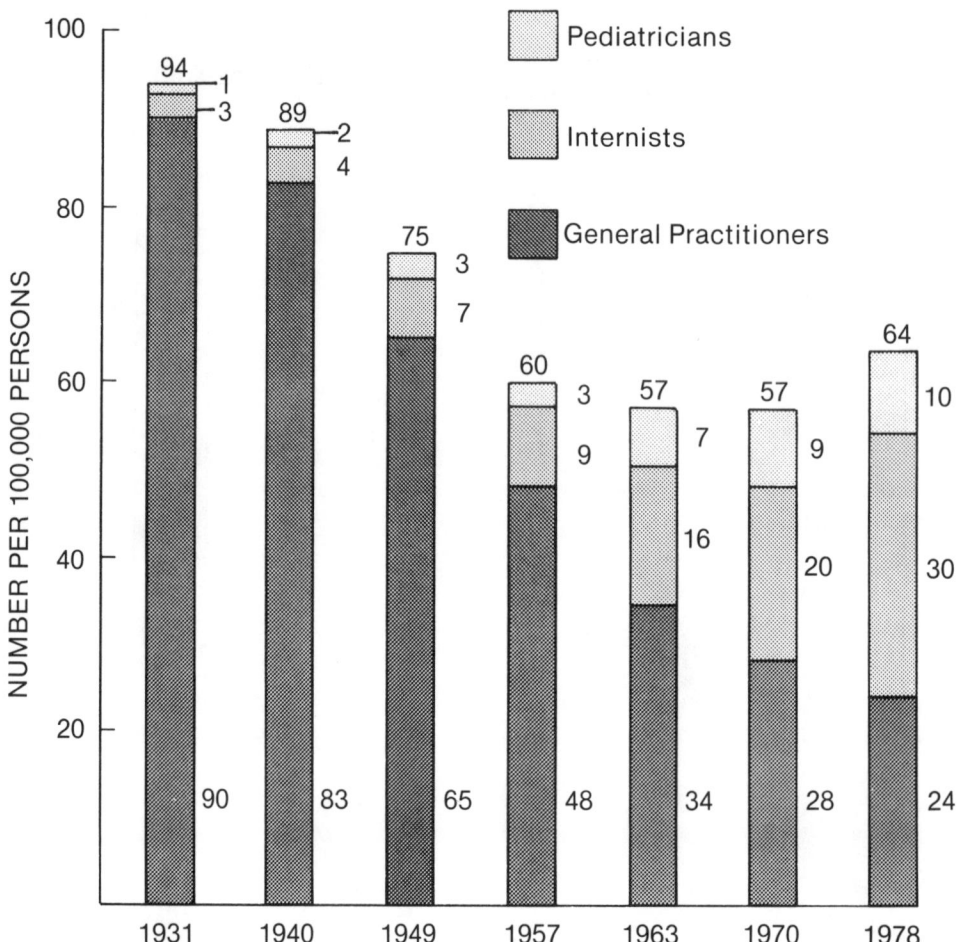

NOTE: For 1931-1957, primary care physicians include specialists who limit their practice to internal medicine and pediatrics, and physicians who are in general practice or part-time specialties. For 1963 and 1970, internal medicine includes allergy, nephrology, rheumatology, hematology, oncology, endocrinology, and infectious diseaes; pediatrics includes adolescent medicine, neonatal/perinatal medicine, pediatric endocrinology, pediatric hematology, and pediatric nephrology. For 1978, internal medicine includes allergy, cardiovascular disease, gastroenterology, and pulmonary disease; pediatrics includes pediatric allergy and pediatric cardiology. For 1970 and 1978, general practice includes family practice.

SOURCES: For 1931-1957: Overpeck, M.D., "Physicians in Family Practice, 1931-1967," *Public Health Reports,* Vol. 85, No. 6, June 1970, Table 2, p. 488; for 1963 and 1970: U.S. Department of Health, Education, and Welfare, *Interim Report of the Graduate Medical Education National Advisory Committee,* Public Health Service, Health Resources Administration, April 1979, Table 2, p. 29; for 1978: American Medical Association, *Physician Distribution and Medical Licensure in the U.S., 1978,* Center for Health Services Research and Development, Department of Statistical Analysis, 1979, Table G, p. 23 and Table 6, p. 74.

Chart E-23. Requirements for Certification, Licensure, and Training for Selected Non-physician Health Care Providers, and for Accreditation of Training Programs, by Type of Provider (U.S.A., 1980).

Type of Provider	Certification	Licensure	Length of Training	Minimal Education Requirements for Admission Into Training Program	Accreditation of Training Program
Nurse Practitioner (general)	American Nurses Association. License and 2 years of practice required; not required in most States.	No Mechanism for licensure. Registered nurse license obtained prior to nurse practitioner training. Some states require certification by state board of nursing and/or medicine.	8 to 12 months for certificate; 1 to 2 years for master's.	Registered nurse license for certificate; B.S. in nursing and RN license for master's	American Nurses Association responsible for accreditation at certificate level and the National League for Nursing at master's level.
Pediatric Nurse Practitioner	American Nurses Association. License and 2 years of practice required; not required in most states. The National Board of Pediatric Nurse Practitioners and Associates provides voluntary certification based on beginning competency exam.	No mechanism for licensure. Registered nurse license obtained prior to nurse practitioner training. Some states require certification by state board of nursing and/or medicine.	8 to 12 months for certificate; 1 to 2 years for master's.	Registered nurse license for certificate; B.S. in nursing and RN license for master's.	Accreditation not required. Programs can seek approval from the American Nurses Association (certificate level) or the National League for Nursing (master's degree).
Nurse-midwife	American College of Nurse-Midwives certification examination given after completion of accredited program.	No mechanism for licensure. Registered nurse licensure obtained prior to nurse-midwife training. American College of Nurse-Midwives certification is required in most states.	9 to 12 months for certificate; 1 to 2 years for master's.	Registered nurse license for certificate; B.S. in nursing and RN license for master's.	American College of Nurse-Midwives. Programs can seek National League for Nursing approval at master's level, but it is not required.
Physician's Assistant, MEDEX, Child Health Associate	National Board of Medical Examiners certification necessary to practice.	State licensing criteria vary, certification required by most states. Regulatory agencies also vary, the Board of Medical Examiners is most frequently designated.	18 to 24 months.	Usually 2 years of college-level courses in basic sciences, and 2 years of experience in the health field.	American Medical Association, Council on Medical Education responsible for program accreditation.

SOURCES: U.S. Department of Health, Education, and Welfare, Office of Health Research, Statistics, and Technology, Public Health Service, *Health United States, 1979*, Figure 1, p. 48; additional information provided by the Division of Nursing and the Division of Medicine, Bureau of Health Professions Education, and by the American College of Nurse Midwives.

Chart E-24 Percent Distribution of Selected Nonphysician Health Care Providers, by Type of Practice, Sex, and Color (U.S.A., 1979).

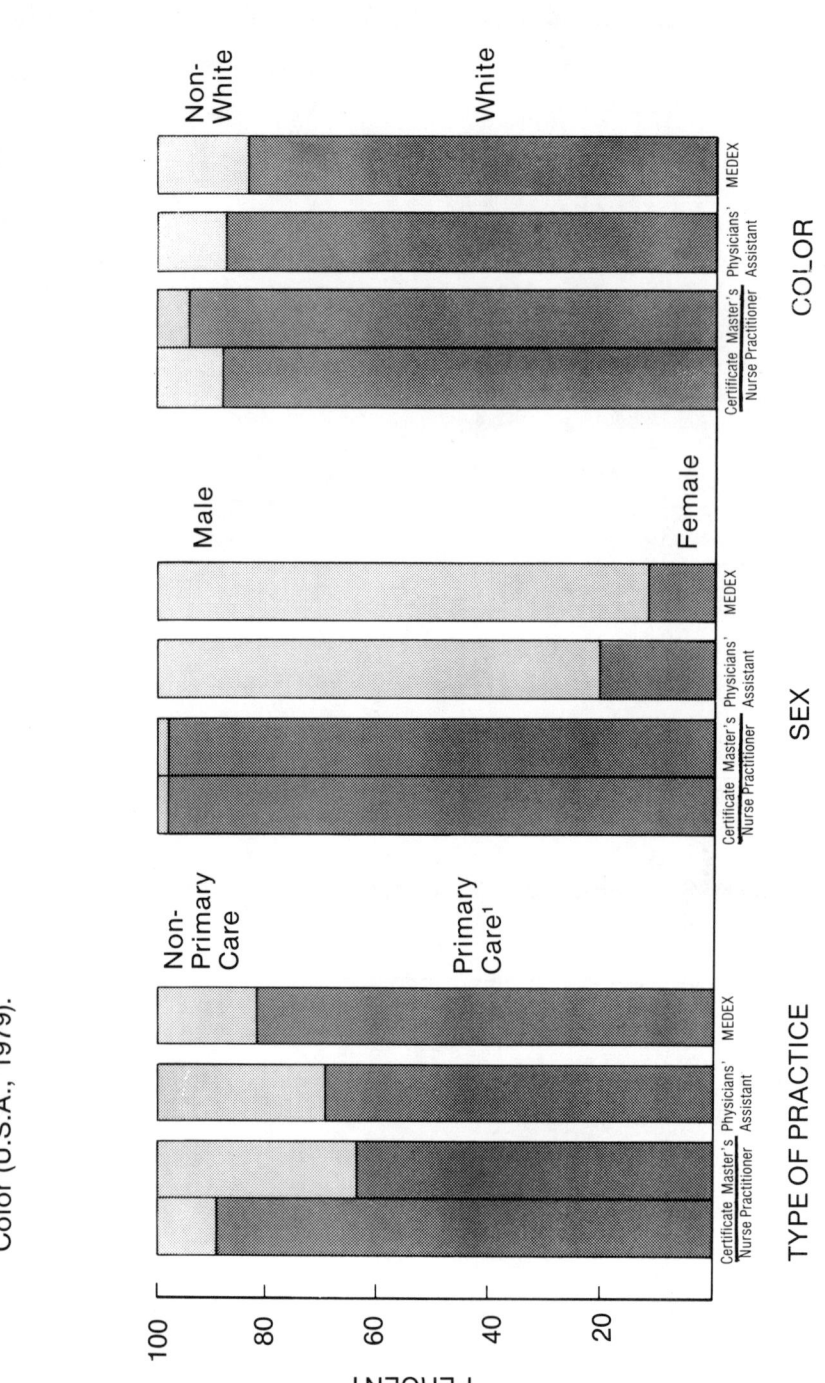

SOURCE: U.S. Department of Health, Education, and Welfare, *Health, United States, 1979*, Public Health Service, Office of Health Research, Statistics, and Technology, Hyattsville, Maryland, 1980, Table A, p. 46.

[1]Includes practice in pediatrics, family and general practice, and internal medicine.

Chart E-25

Percent Distribution of Full-time and Part-time Medical Faculty, by Specified Opinions Concerning the Quality of Students Going into Specified Medical Careers (12 Medical Colleges in U.S.A., Not Dated).[1]

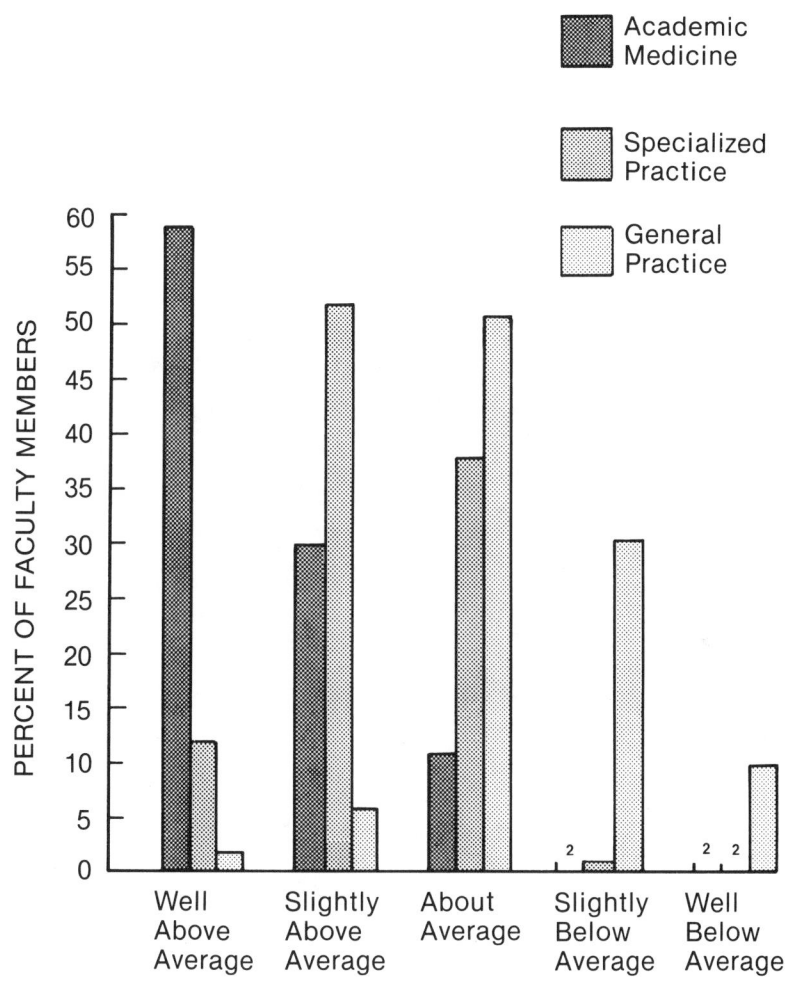

[1]Based on a survey of 694 full- and part-time faculty members with the rank of Instructor or higher at 12 medical colleges in the American Association of Medical Colleges. The response rate was 32%.

[2]None.

SOURCE: Guttentag, O., "The Teaching Physician, A Summary of Initial Findings," Unpublished Mimeograph, San Francisco Medical Center, August 1966, p. 3.

Chart E-26

Annual Number of Specialty Board Certificates Issued in Surgical and Non-Surgical Specialties (U.S.A., 1969–1978).

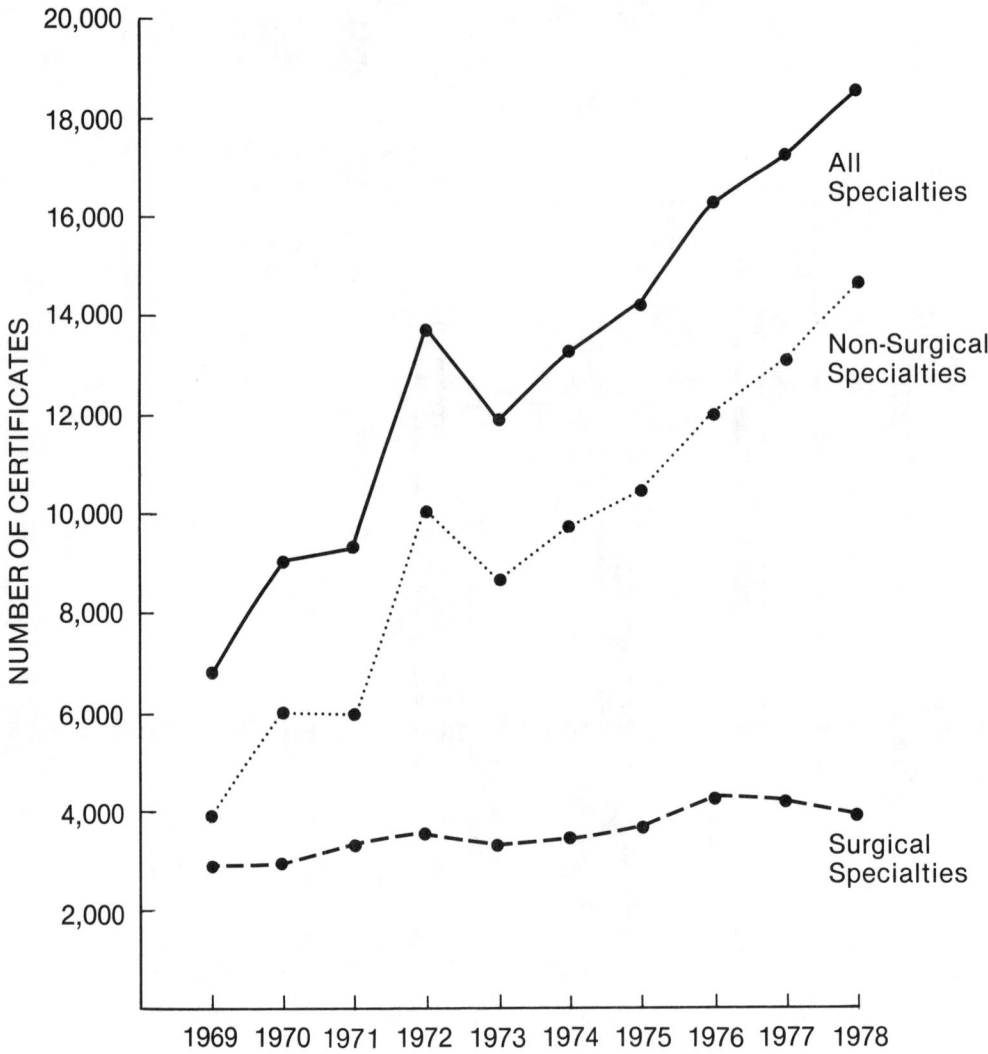

SOURCE: Haug, James N. and Kathleen Kuntzman, *Socio-Economic Factbook for Surgery, 1979,* American College of Surgeons, 1979, Table 10, p. 17 and Table 11, p. 18.

Chart E-27 Percent Distribution of Total Births, by Category of Personnel Performing Delivery, and Stillbirth Ratio Per 1000 Live Births, by Category of Personnel Performing Delivery (U.S.A., 1967).

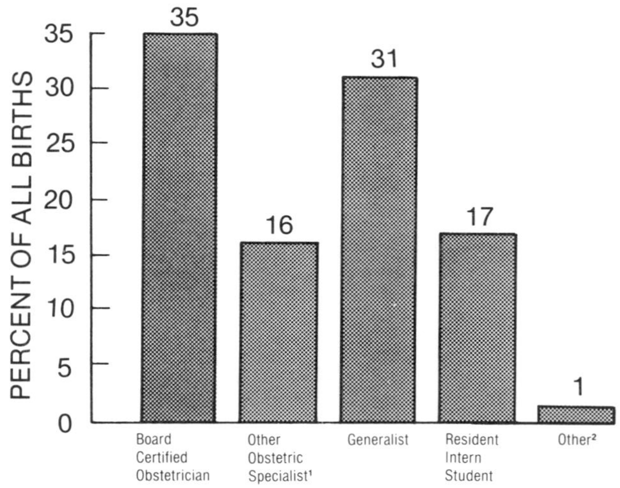

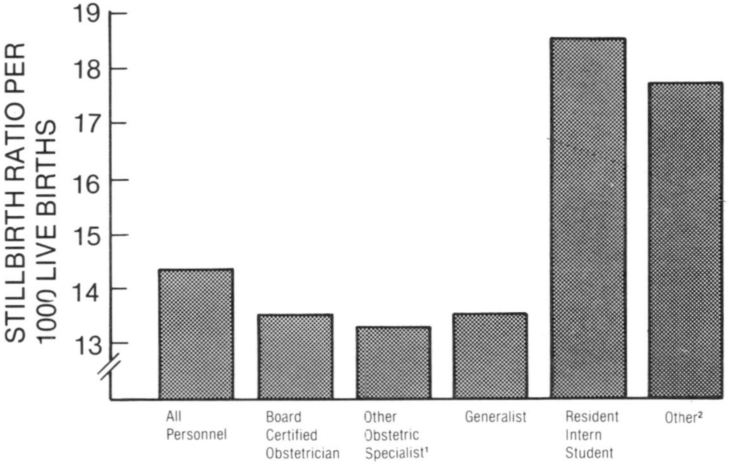

PERCENT OF ALL BIRTHS:
- Board Certified Obstetrician: 35
- Other Obstetric Specialist[1]: 16
- Generalist: 31
- Resident Intern Student: 17
- Other[2]: 1

STILLBIRTH RATIO PER 1000 LIVE BIRTHS:
- All Personnel: ~14
- Board Certified Obstetrician: ~15
- Other Obstetric Specialist[1]: ~15
- Generalist: ~15
- Resident Intern Student: ~18.5
- Other[2]: ~18

[1] Not board certified, but limiting practice to obstetrics and gynecology.
[2] Includes full-time, salaried hospital physicians (not trainees) and nurse-midwives.

SOURCE: *National Study of Maternity Care: Survey of Obstetric Practice and Associated Services in Hospitals in the United States*, A Report of the Committee on Maternal Health, American College of Obstetricians and Gynecologists, Chicago, 1970, Table III-1, p. 9 and Table IV-1, p. 11.

Health Personnel

Chart E-28

Percent of Active, Non-federal Physicians in Group Practice
(U.S.A., Selected Years, 1932–1975).[1]

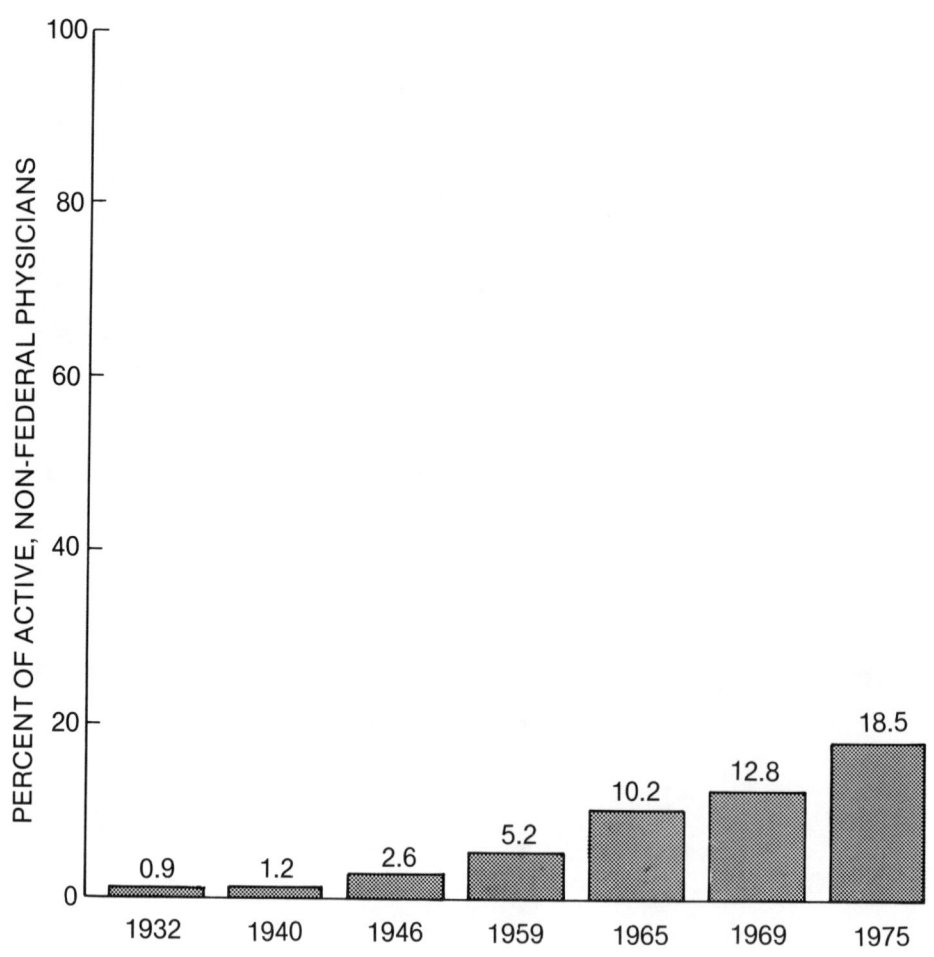

[1]Based on a definition of group practice as a formal association of three or more full-time physicians with income from medical practice pooled and redistributed to the members according to some prearranged plan.

SOURCE: Bureau of Health Manpower, *A Report to the President and Congress on the Status of Health Professions Personnel in the United States,* DHEW, Public Health Service, August 1978, Table IV-3, p. IV-47.

Chart E-29

Non-federal Physicians in Full-time and Part-time Group Practice as a Percent of all Physicians Delivering Patient Care, by Census Division (U.S.A., 1975).[1]

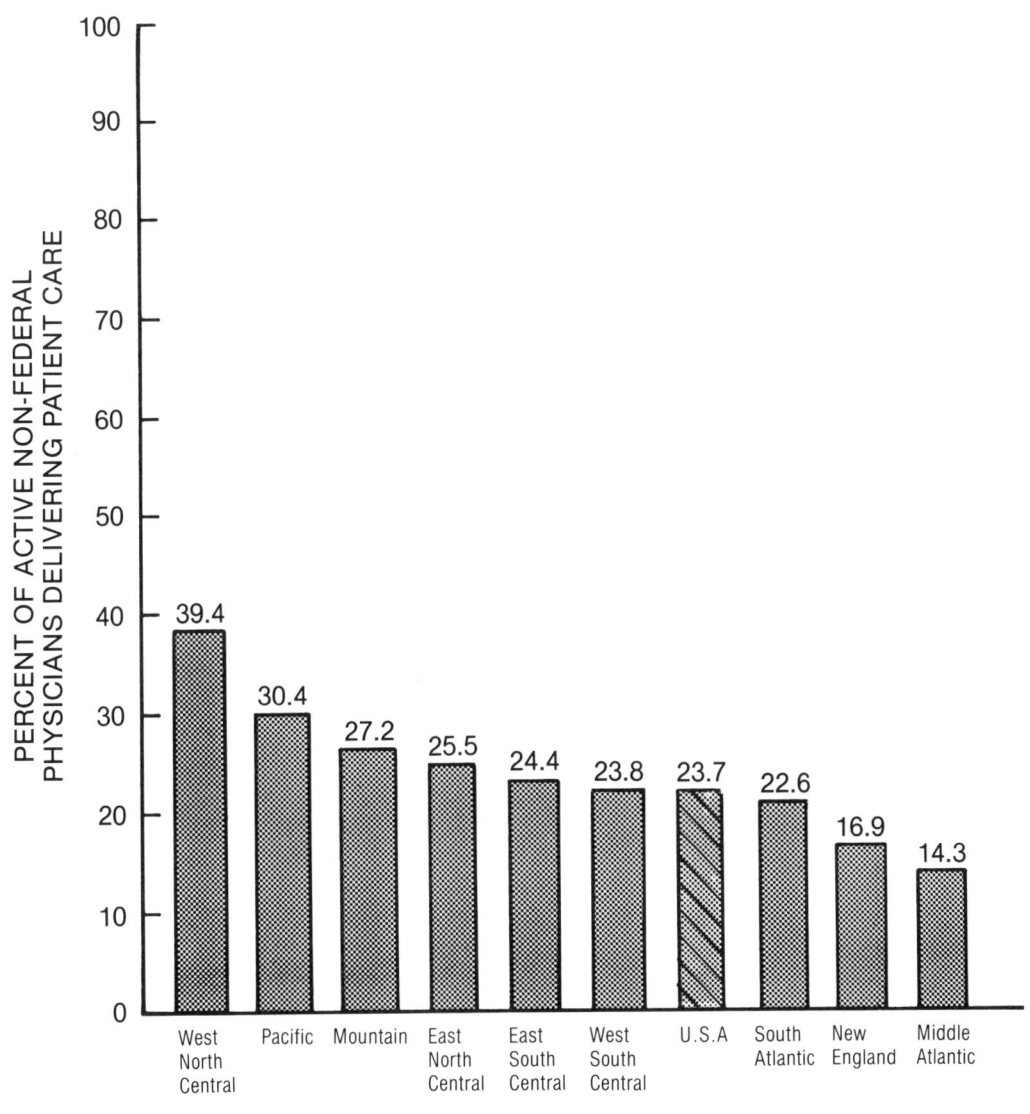

[1]Excludes interns and residents.

NOTE: Group practice is defined as three or more physicians formally organized to provide medical care, consultation, diagnosis, or treatment through the joint use of equipment and personnel, with income from medical practice distributed in accordance with methods previously determined by members of the group.

SOURCE: U.S. National Center for Health Statistics, *Health, United States, 1978*, DHEW, Public Health Service, Health Resources Administration, Hyattsville, Maryland, Table 128, p. 343.

Chart E-30 Percent Distribution of Medical Groups, and Percent of Group Physicians in General and Family Practice, by Size of Group (U.S.A., 1975).

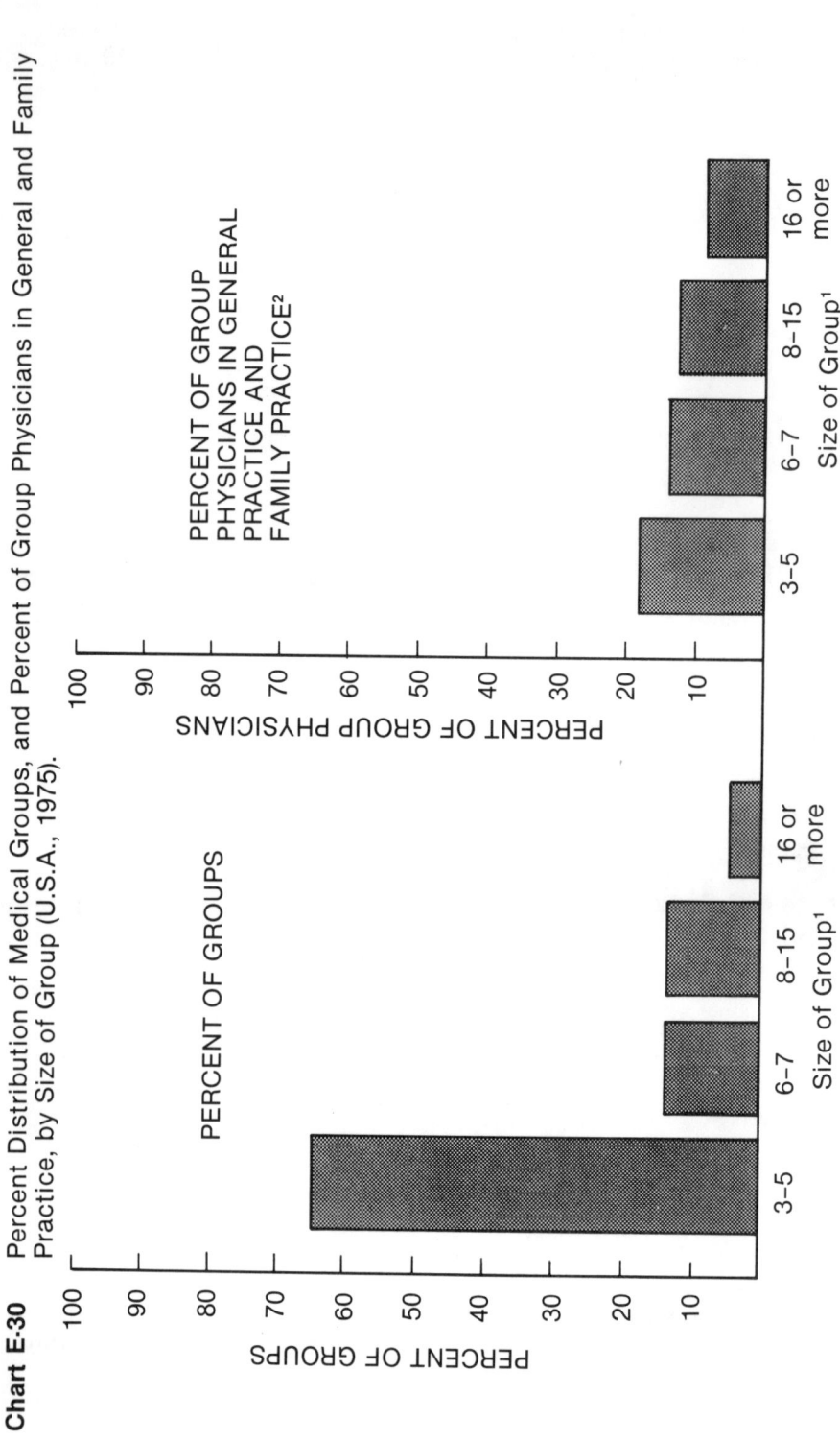

[1]Includes full-time and part-time physicians. Groups are both single-specialty and multi-specialty.

[2]Does not include physicians whose primary specialty is internal medicine.

SOURCE: Goodman, Louis J., Edward H. Bennett, and Richard J. Oden, *Group Medical Practice in the U.S., 1975*, American Medical Association, Center for Health Services Research and Development, Chicago, 1976, Table 5-3, p. 25 and Appendix Table 6, p. 105.

Chart E-31

Percent Distribution of Group Practices and Group Practice Physicians, by Type of Group (U.S.A., 1975).

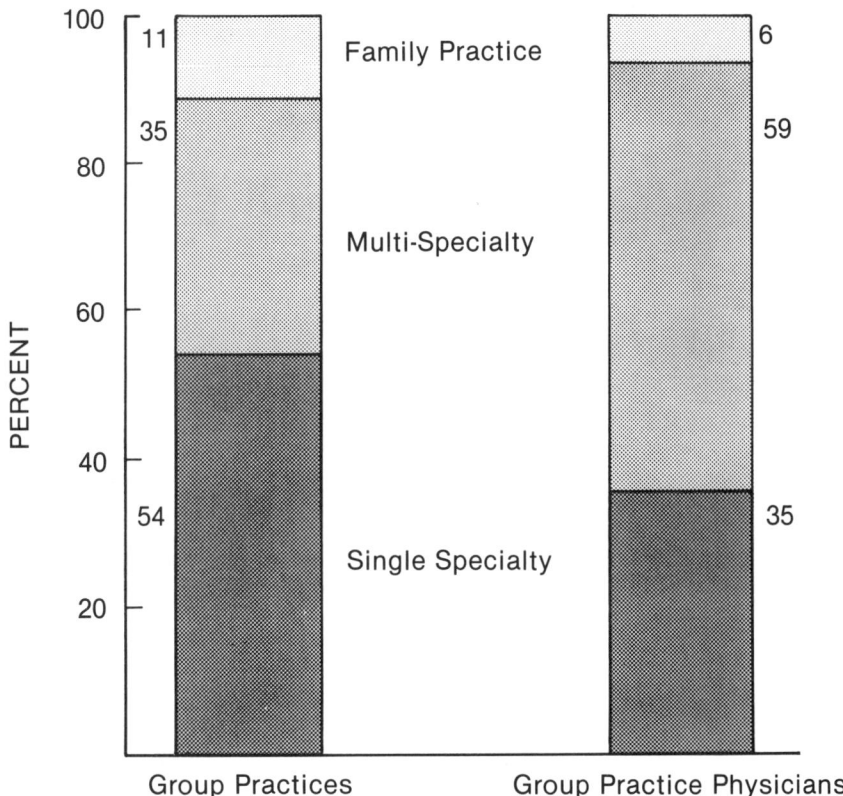

SOURCE: Goodman, L.J., Edward H. Bennett, and Richard J. Oden, *Group Medical Practice in the U.S., 1975,* American Medical Association, Table 3-1, p. 10.

Chart E-32 Numbers and Percent Distribution of Group Practices by Form of Organization, 1969 and 1975 (U.S.A.)

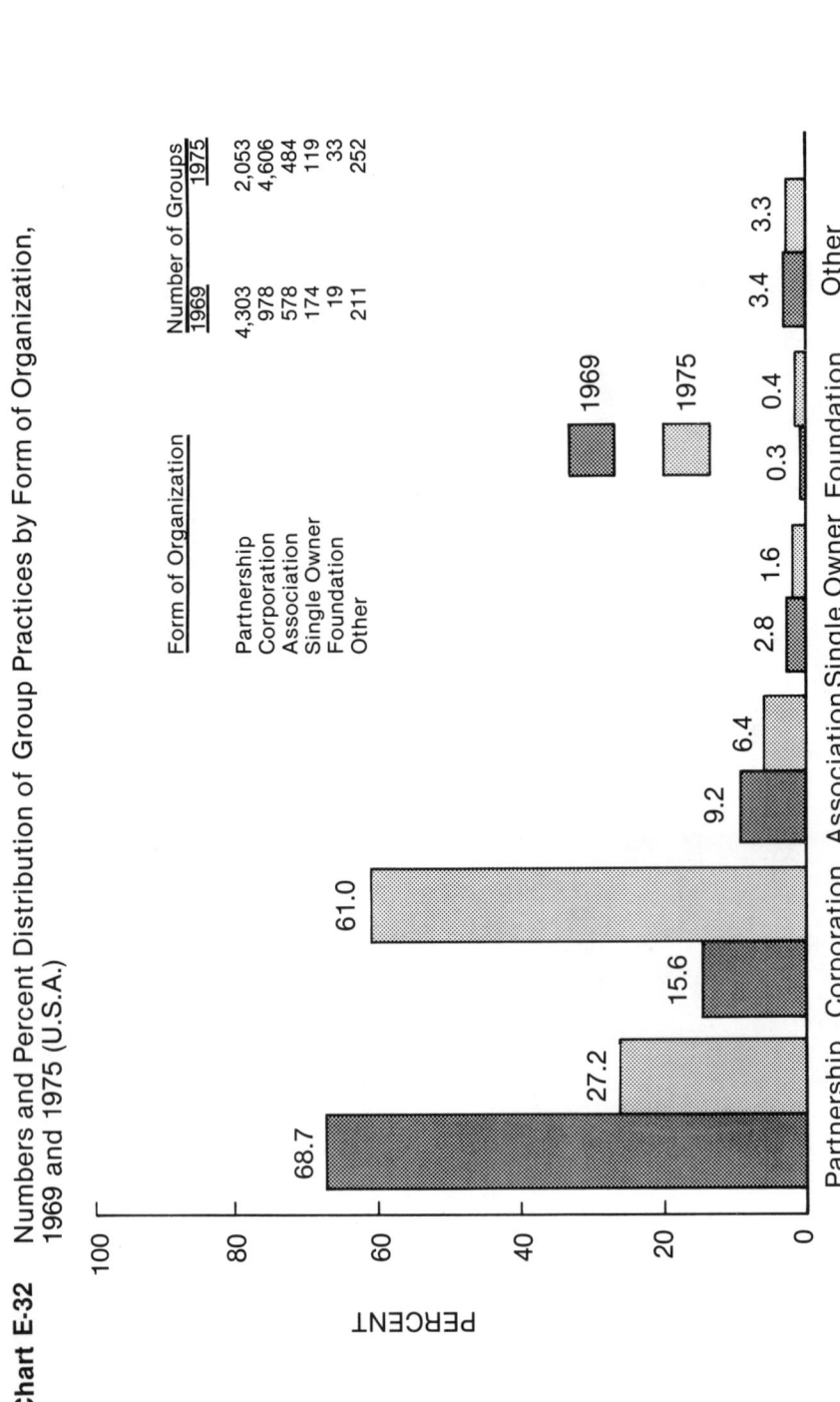

SOURCES: For 1969: Todd C. and M.E. McNamara, *Medical Groups in the United States, 1969*, American Medical Association, Chicago, 1971, Chart 2, p. 49; for 1975: Goodman, L.J., Edward H. Bennett, and Richard J. Oden, *Group Medical Practice in the United States, 1975*, American Medical Association, Chicago, Chart 8-1, p. 49.

Chart E-33

Attitudes of Physicians Toward Selected Aspects of Practice by Type of Practice[1] (U.S.A., 1970–1971).

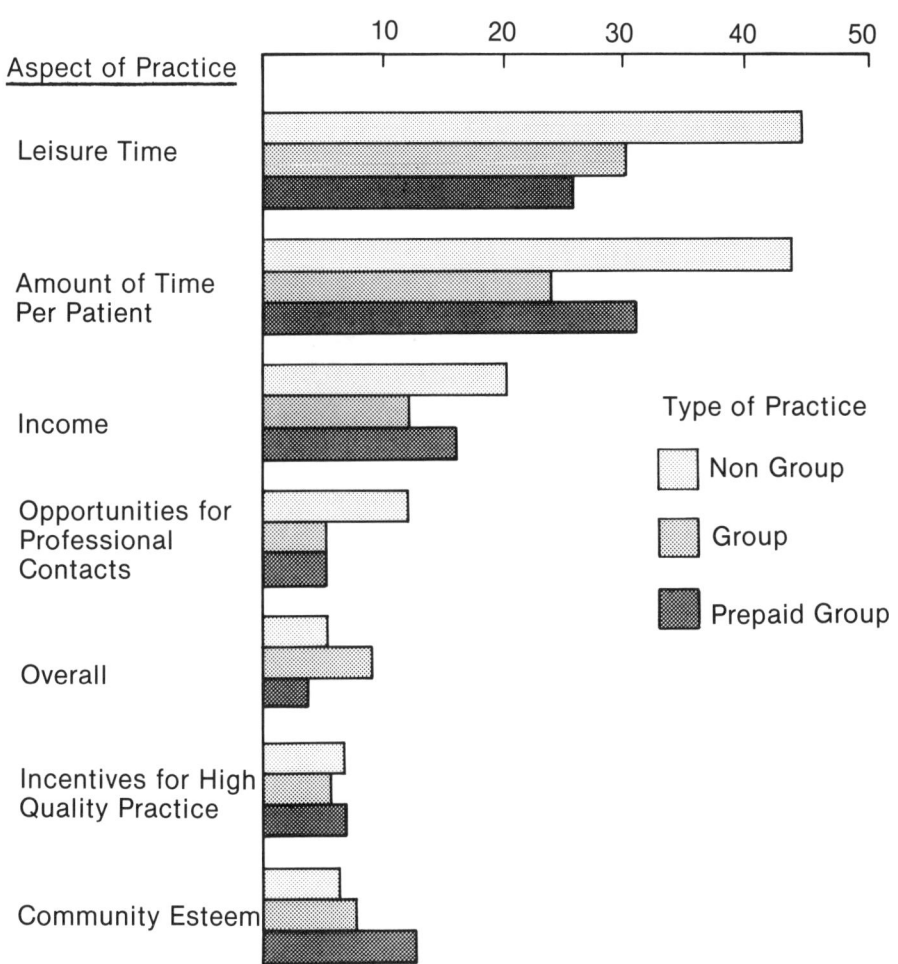

[1] Based on a national sample of pediatricians of whom 136 were in non-group, 43 in group, and 154 in prepaid group practice.

SOURCE: Mechanic, D., "The Organization of Medical Practice and Practice Orientations Among Physicians in Prepaid and Nonprepaid Primary Care Settings," *Medical Care*, Vol. 13, No. 3, March 1975, Table 7, p. 199.

Chart E-34

Percent of Physicians Remaining in Employment during the First Four Years Following Hire, Selected OEO Neighborhood Health Centers, and Kaiser-Permanente Group (1966–1970).

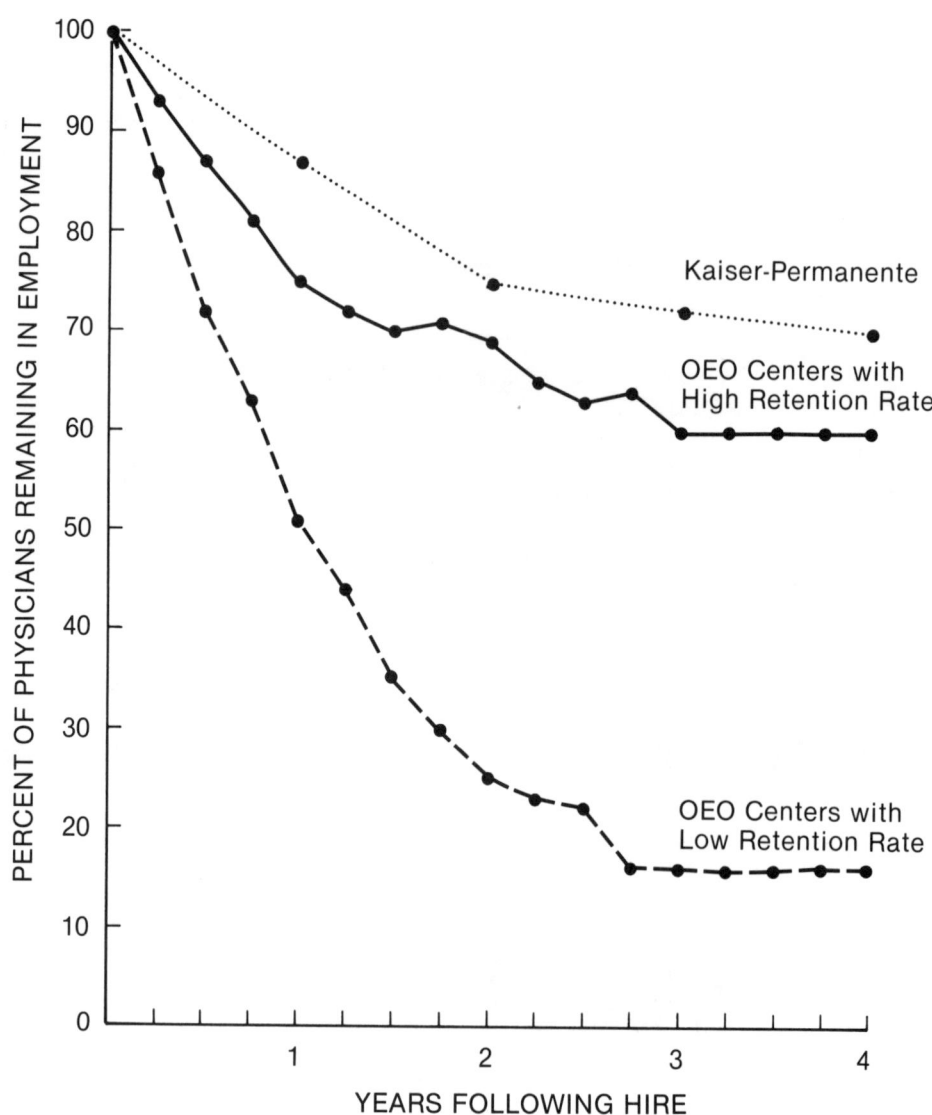

SOURCE: Tilson, Hugh H., "Stability of Physician Employment in Neighborhood Health Centers," *Medical Care,* Vol. XI, No. 5, September–October 1973, Figure 4, p. 390.

Chart E-35

Average Hours Practiced per Week, by Age of Physician and Selected Specialties (U.S.A., 1978).

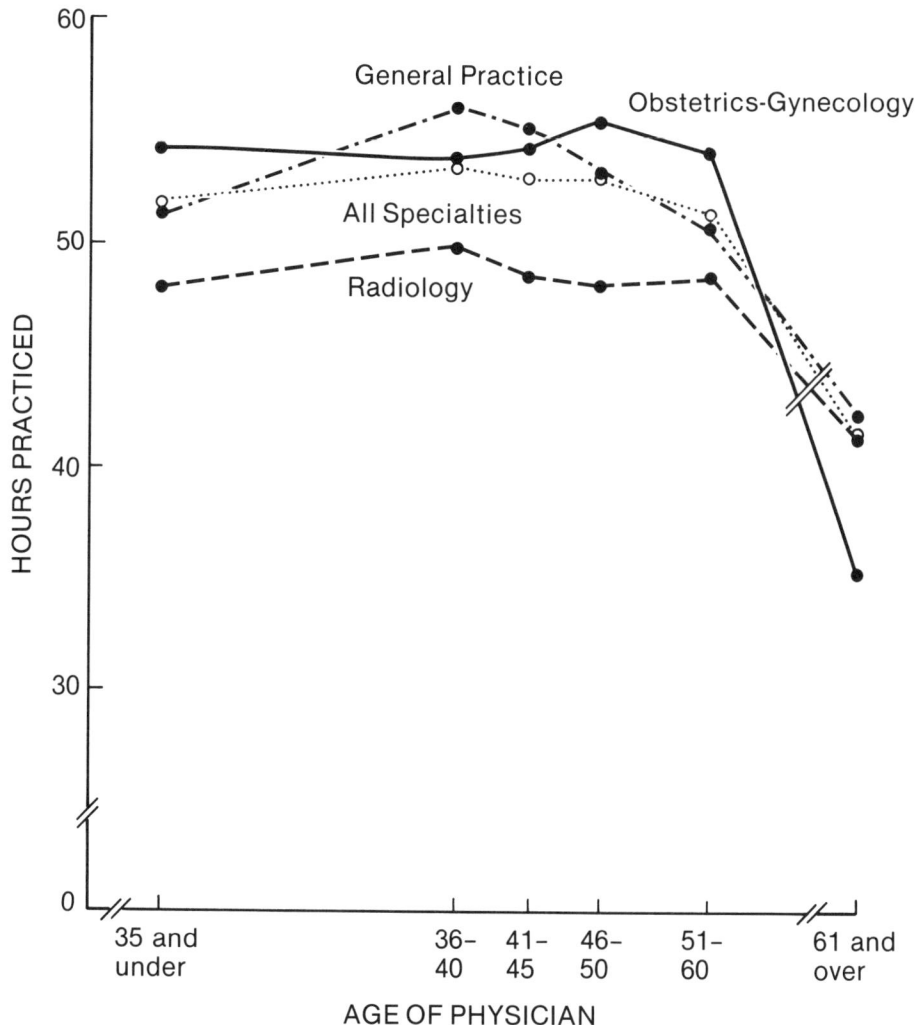

SOURCE: Gaffney, John C. and Gerald L. Glandon, editors, *Profile of Medical Practice, 1979*, Chicago, American Medical Association, 1979, Table 20, p. 207.

Chart E-36

Average Number of Office Visits and Hospital Visits per Physician per Week, by Specialty (U.S.A., 1978).[1]

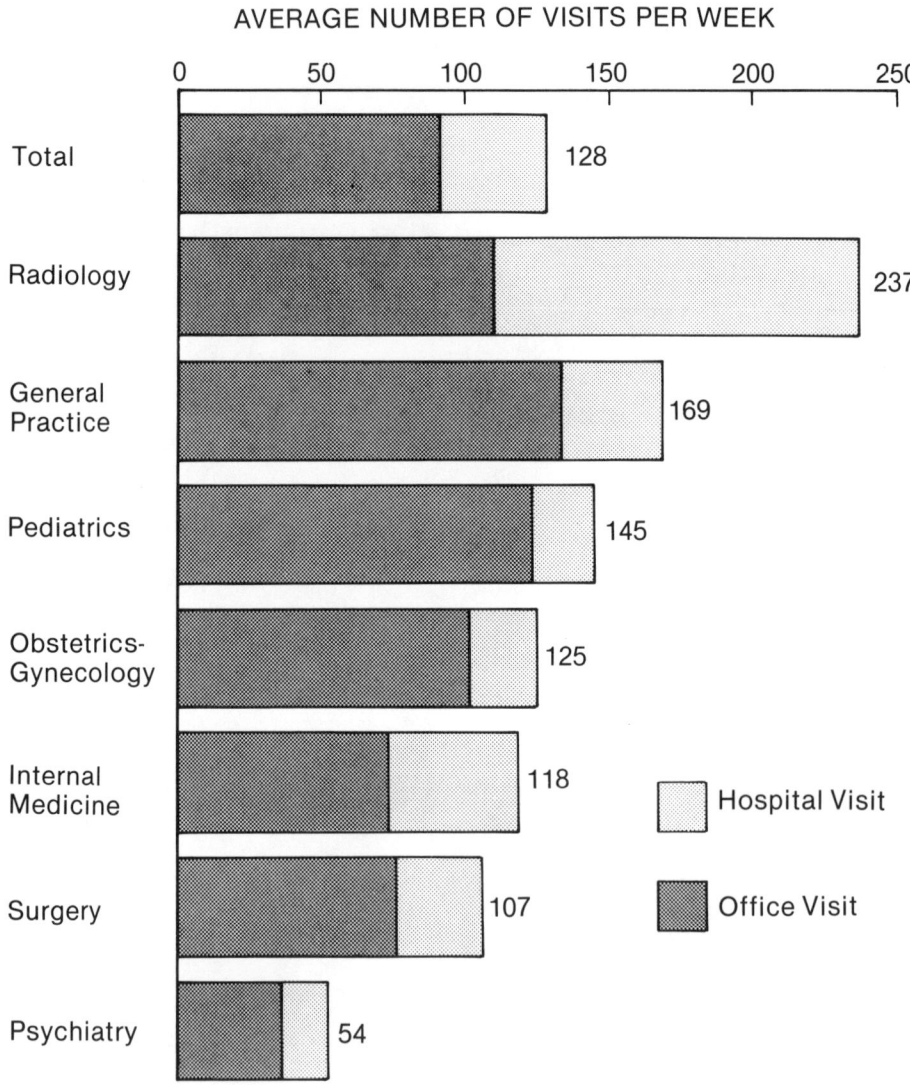

[1]Based on a survey of non-federal, office-based physicians in the United States.

SOURCE: Gaffney, John C. and Gerald L. Glandon, editors, *Profile of Medical Practice, 1979,* American Medical Association, 1979, Table 35, p. 222 and Table 37, p. 224.

Chart E-37

Average Net Income from Medical Practice of Physicians, by Age Group (U.S.A., 1977).

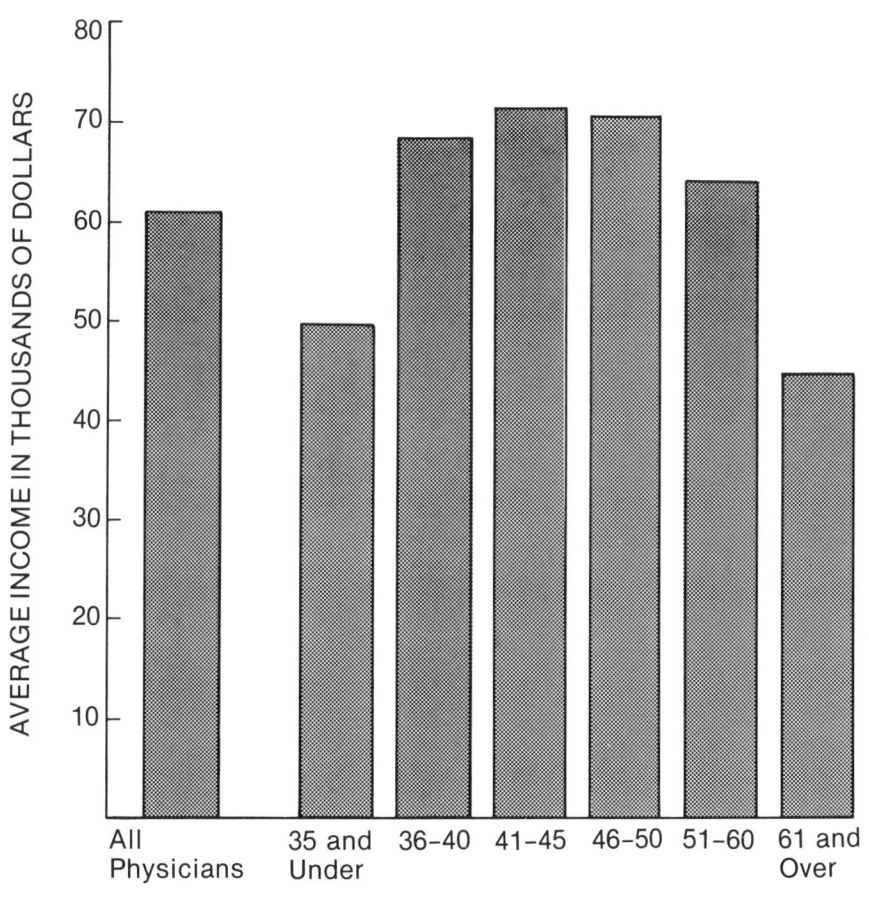

SOURCE: Gaffney, John C. and Gerald L. Olandon, editors, *Profile of Medical Practice, 1979*, American Medical Association, 1979, Table 77, p. 275.

Chart E-38

Relative and Actual Average Net Income, Number of Hours Practiced per Week, Number of Patient Visits per Week and Number of Patient Visits per Hour of Direct Care, for Physicians, by Type of Practice (U.S.A., 1977–1978).

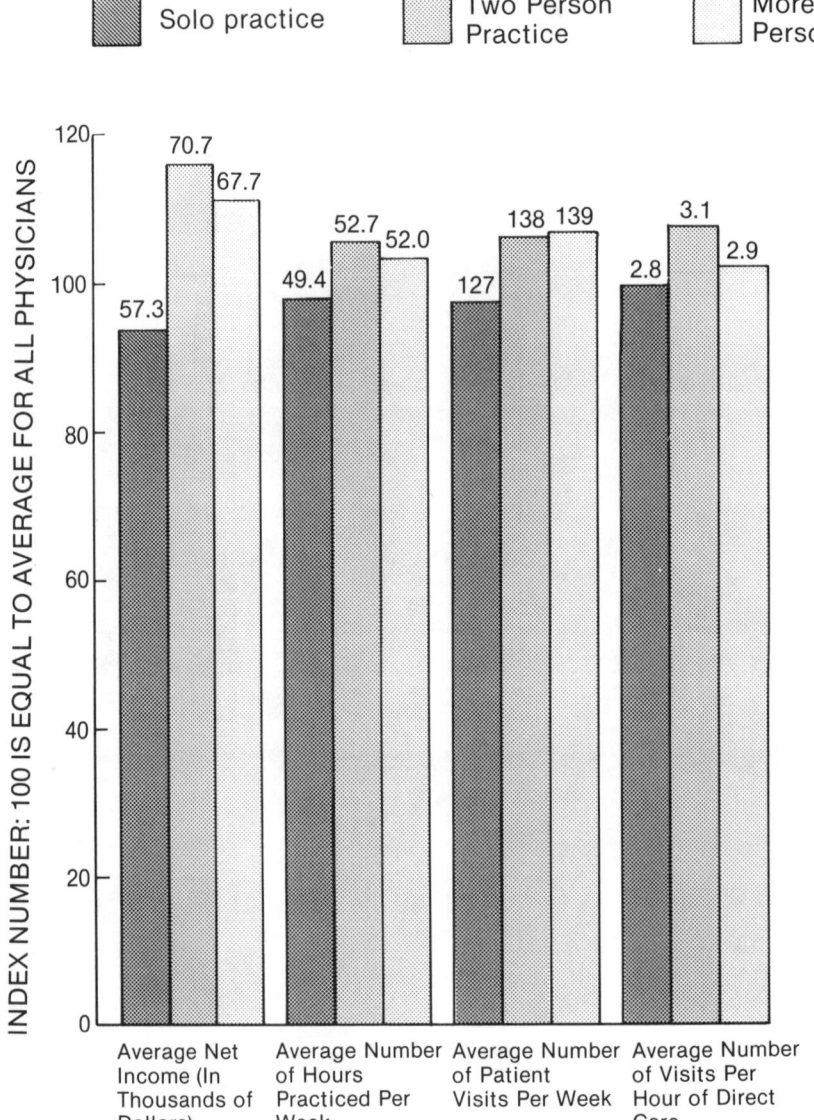

NOTE: Numbers above the bars are the actual values.

SOURCE: Gaffney, John C. and Gerald L. Glandon, editors, *Profile of Medical Practice, 1979,* Monroe, Wisconsin, American Medical Association, 1979, Table 17, p. 204, Table 22, p. 209, Table 31, p. 218, and Table 69, p. 261.

Medical Care Chartbook

Chart E-39 Average Net Income of Physicians, by Specialty (U.S.A., 1970 and 1978).

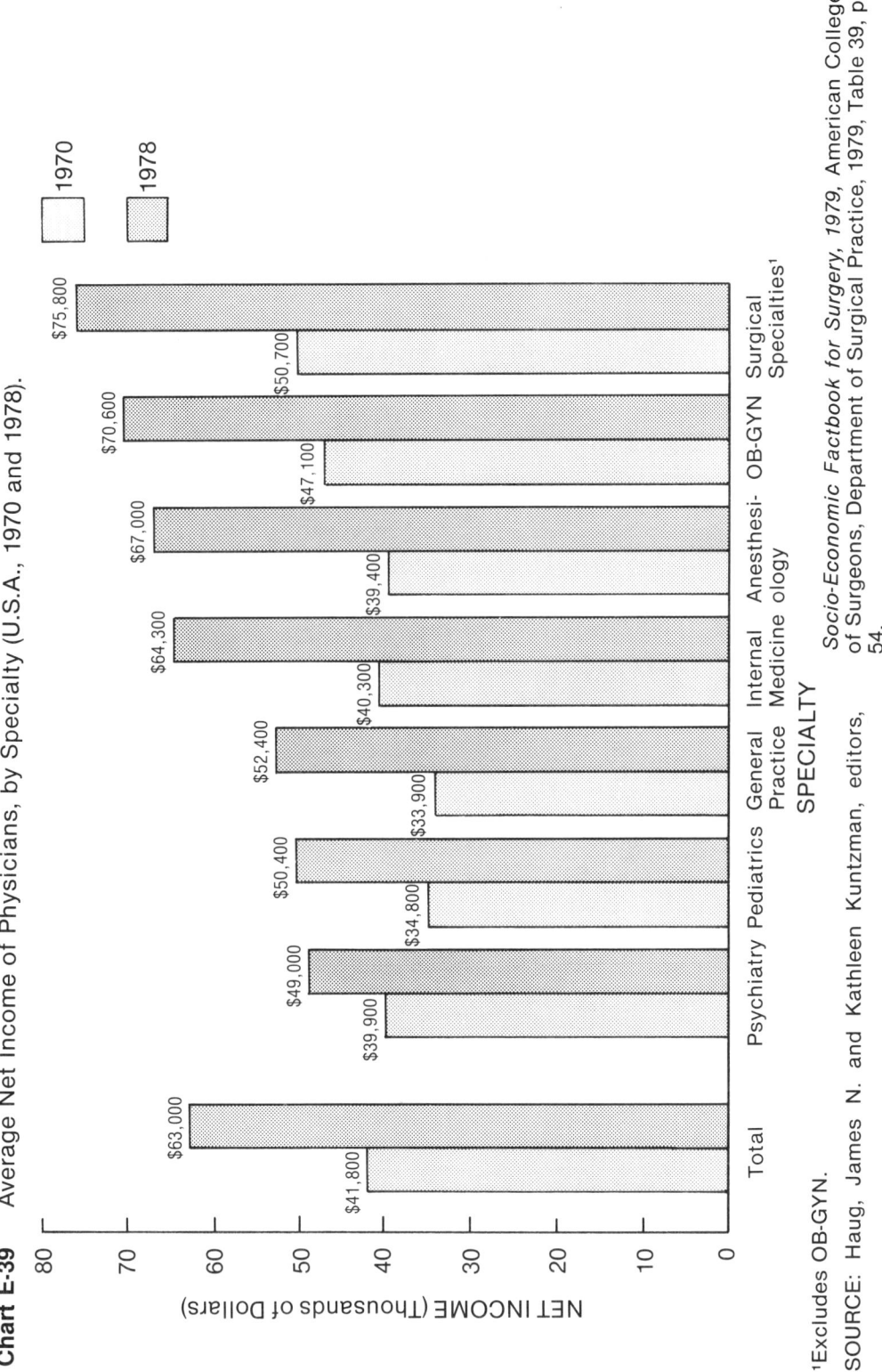

[1] Excludes OB-GYN.

SOURCE: Haug, James N. and Kathleen Kuntzman, editors, *Socio-Economic Factbook for Surgery, 1979*, American College of Surgeons, Department of Surgical Practice, 1979, Table 39, p. 54.

Health Personnel

Chart E-40 Average Physician Fees, by Specialty (U.S.A., 1978).

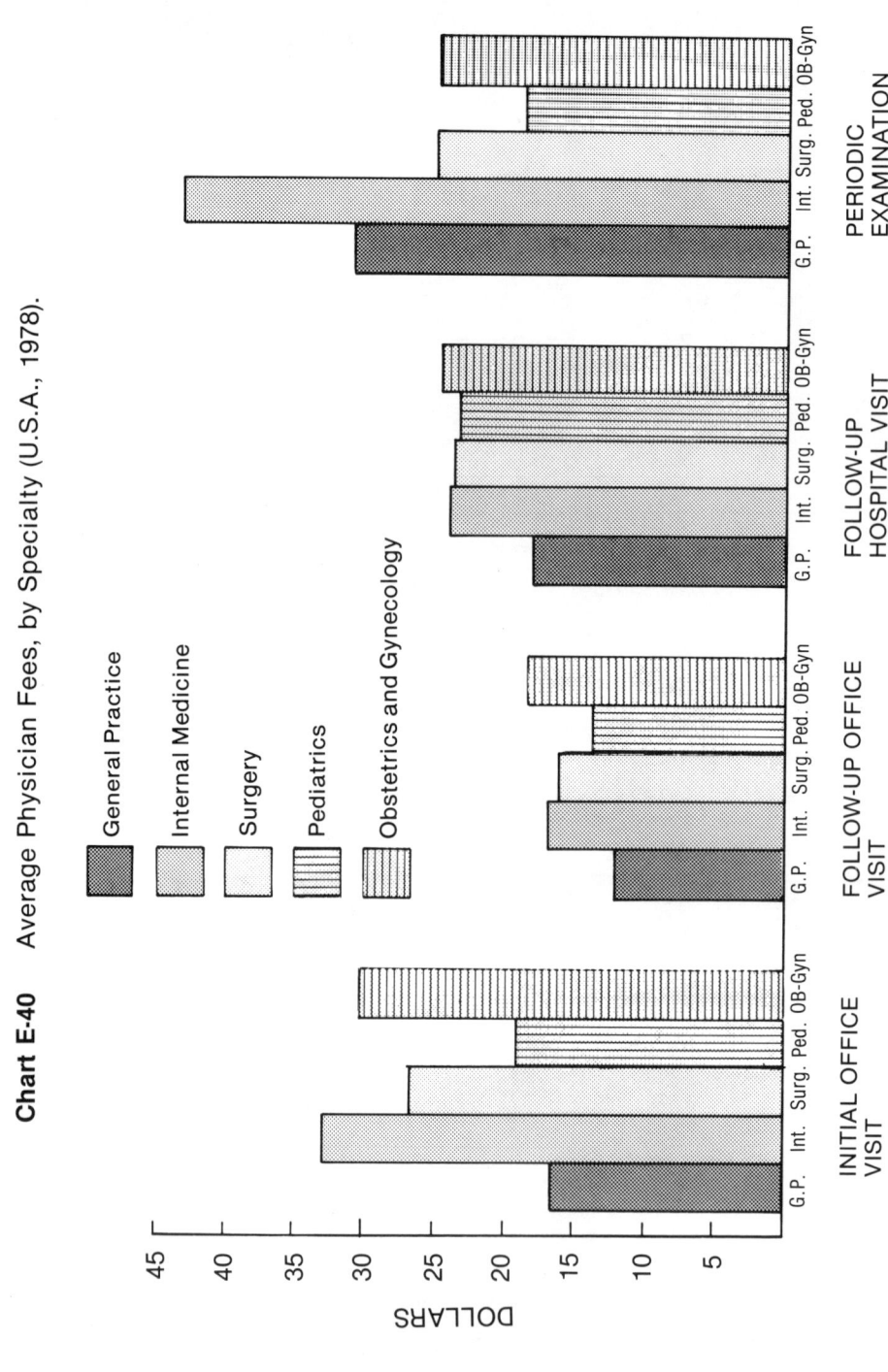

SOURCE: Haug, James N. and Kathleen Kuntzman, *Socio-Economic Factbook for Surgery, 1979*, American College of Surgeons, 1979, Table 40, p. 55.

Chart E-41

Percent Distribution of Methods of Paying Pathologists and Radiologists in Community Hospitals (U.S.A., 1965, 1969 and 1974).[1]

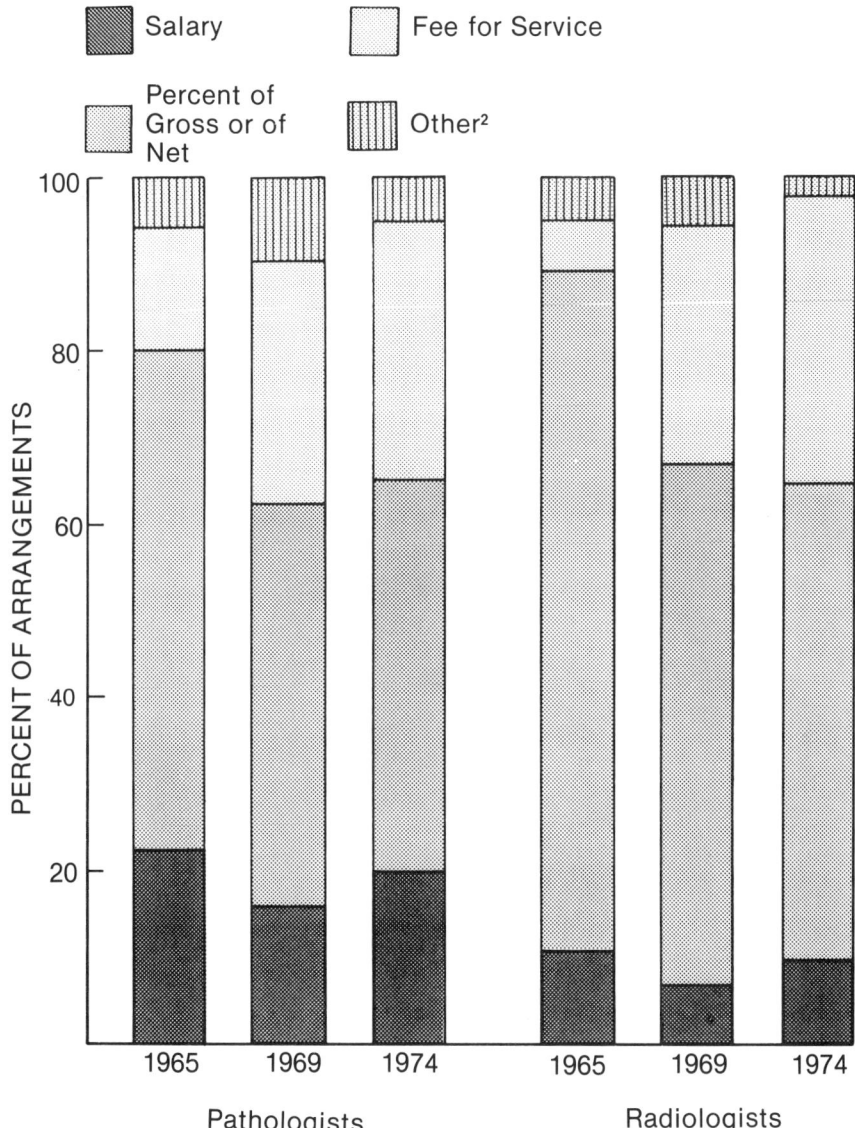

[1]For 1974, data refer to highest ranking radiologist and pathologist in the institution.

[2]The "other" category includes: the arrangement whereby the specialist leases space from the hospital, operating as an independent entrepreneur; and various combinations of methods of payment such as when the specialist receives a salary as well as a percentage of net departmental income.

SOURCES: For 1965 and 1969; Begole, C.M., P.J. Philip, and M. Williams, "Hospital Specialist Compensation Plans," *Hospitals*, Vol. 46, April 16, 1972, Table 1, p. 83; for 1974: *Modern Health Care*, Vol. 2, No. 4, October 1974, Table 2, p. 35.

Chart E-42

Number of Active Dentists, Hygienists, and Dental Assistants
(U.S.A., Selected Years, 1950–1977).

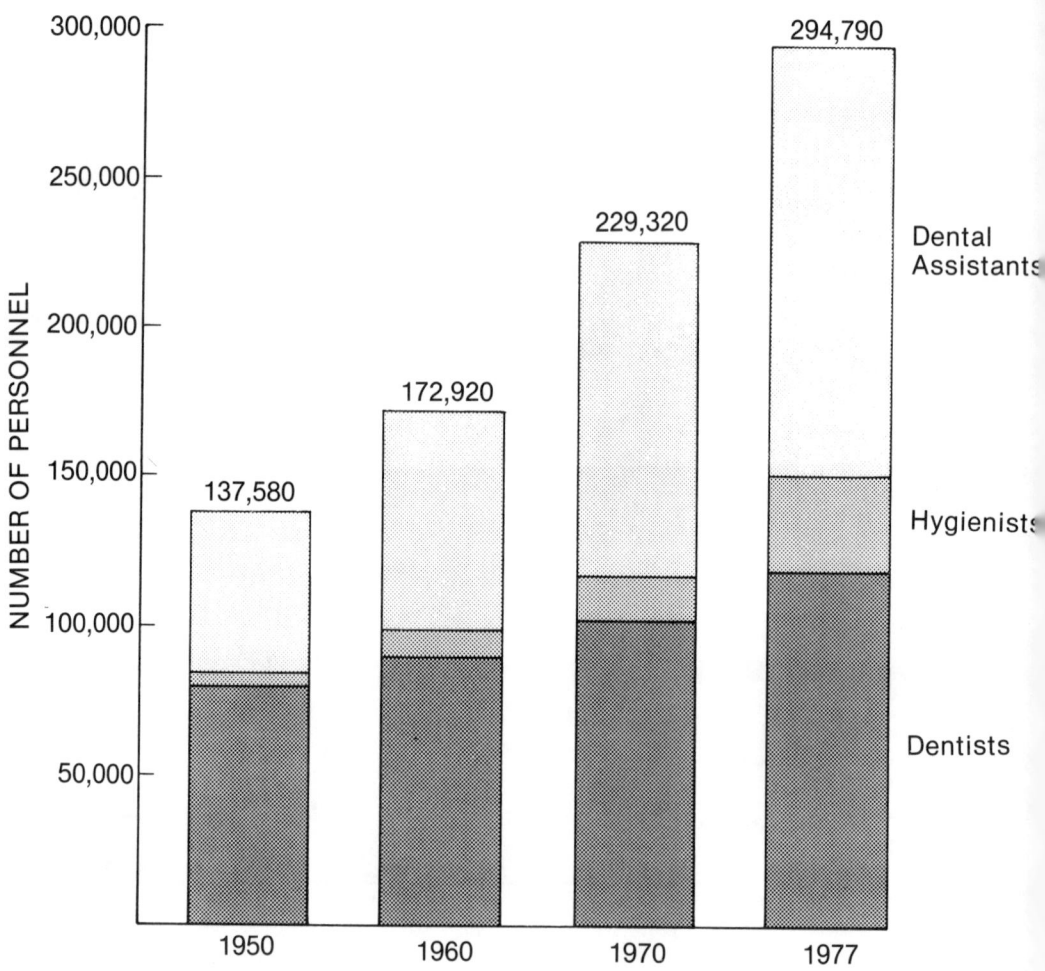

SOURCE: U.S. Department of Health, Education, and Welfare, *Dental Manpower Fact Book*, Public Health Service, Health Resources Administration, Bureau of Health Manpower—Division of Manpower Analysis, Hyattsville, Maryland, 1979, Table E-1, p. 65, Table E-4, p. 68 and Table A-1, p. 15.

Chart E-43

Dentists per 100,000 Persons by Geographic Area and Selected States (U.S.A., 1976).[1]

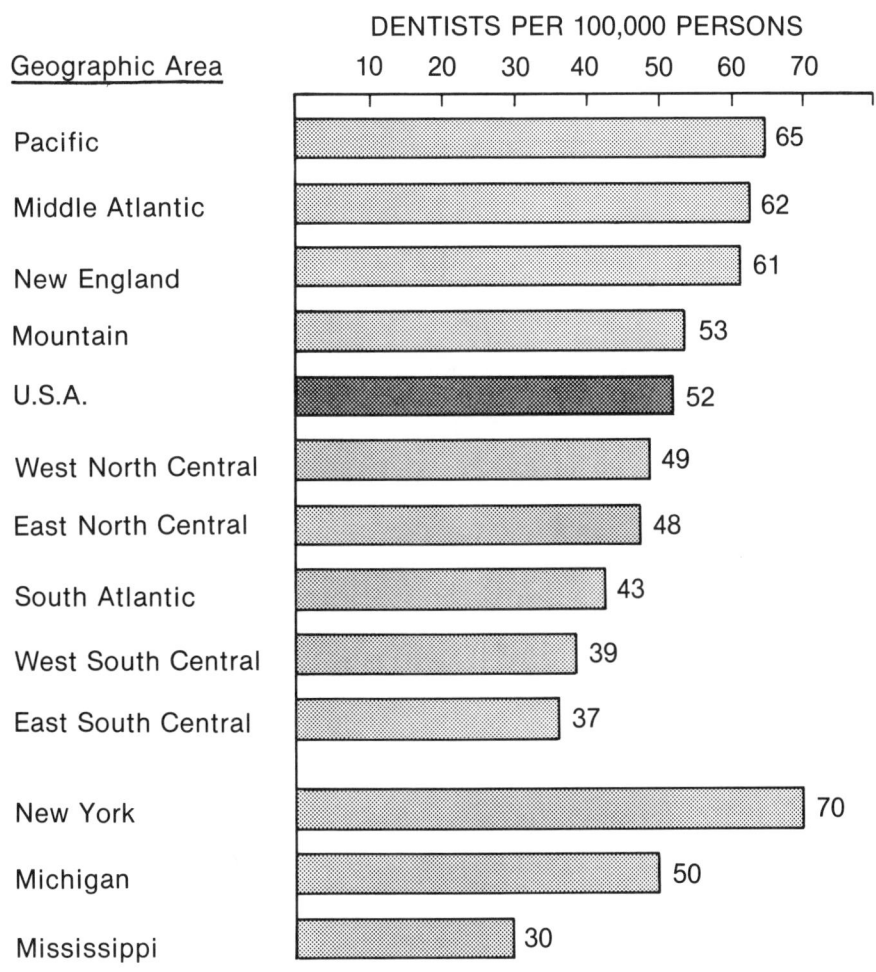

[1]Dentists in active practice only.
SOURCE: U.S. National Center for Health Statistics, *Health Resources Statistics, 1976-77*, DHEW, Public Health Service, Office of Health Research, Statistics, and Technology, Hyattsville, Maryland, 1976, Table 41, p. 70.

Chart E-44

States by Dentist-Population Ratios[1] and by per Capita Personal Income[2] (U.S.A., 1976).

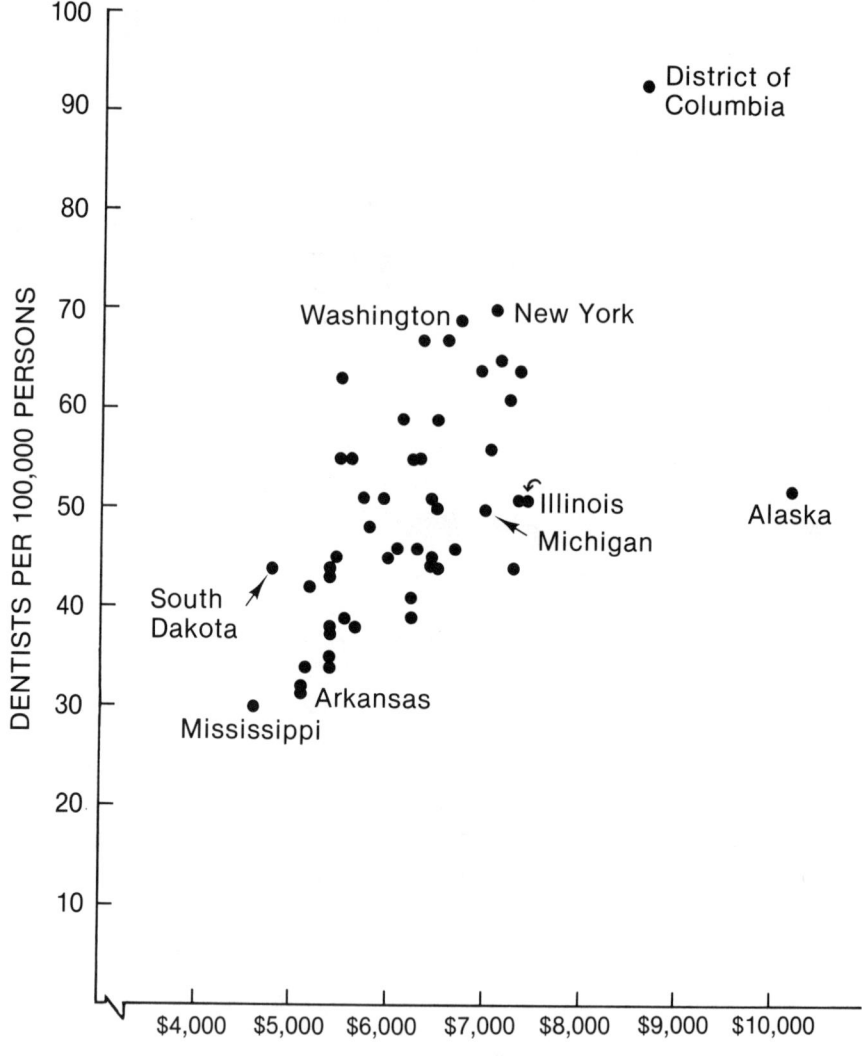

[1]Includes only active non-federal dentists.

[2]Personal income is the current income received by persons from all sources net of contributions for social insurance.

SOURCES: U.S. Department of Commerce, Bureau of the Census, *Statistical Abstract of the United States, 1977*, Washington, D.C., September 1977, Table 704, p. 437; U.S. National Center for Health Statistics, *Health Resources Statistics, 1976-77 Edition*, DHEW, Public Health Service, Office of Health Research, Statistics, and Technology, Hyattsville, Maryland, 1979, Table 41, p. 70.

Chart E-45

Percent of Active Physicians and Dentists, Including those in Federal Service, by Type of Practice (U.S.A., 1949–1976).

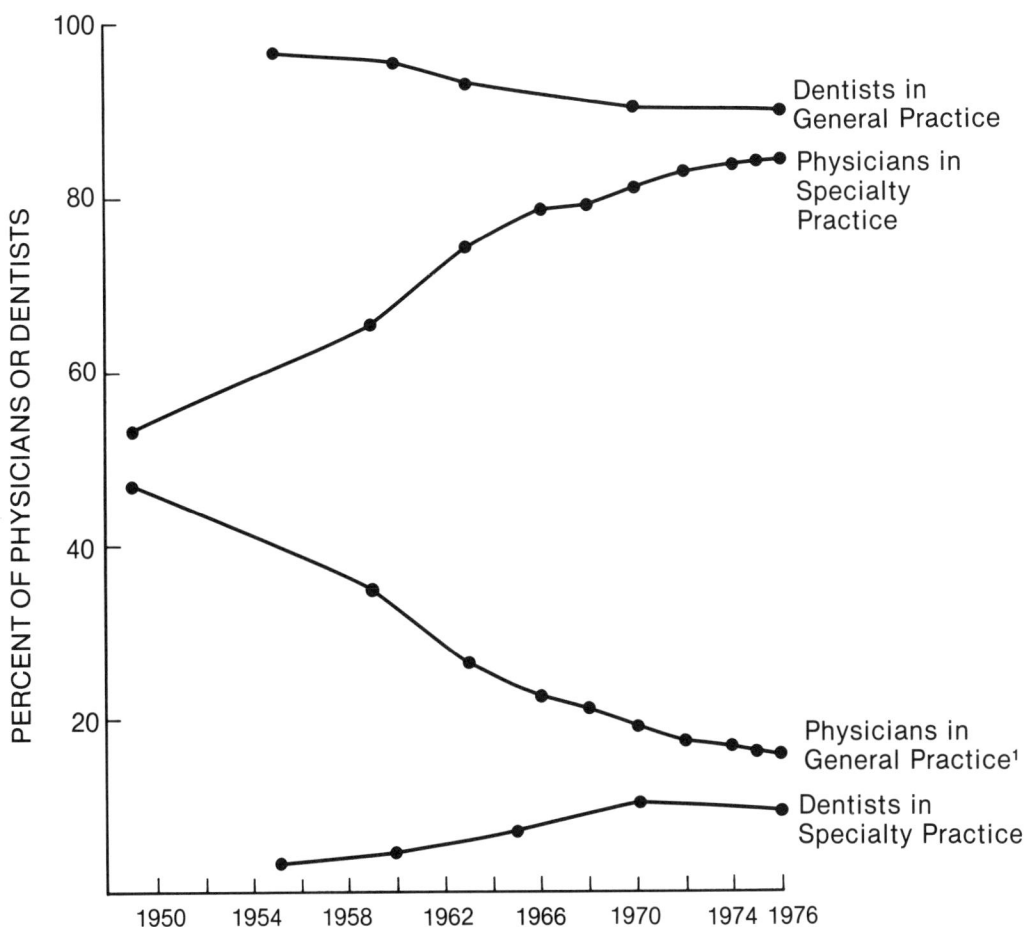

[1] Includes general and family practice.

SOURCES: U.S. National Center for Health Statistics, *Health, United States, 1978*, DHEW, Public Health Service, Hyattsville, Maryland, 1978, Table 125, p. 340; Division on Public Health Methods, *Chart Book on Health Status and Health Manpower*, DHEW, Public Health Service, Washington, D.C., September 1961, Table 20, p. 40; U.S. Bureau of Health Manpower, *A Report to the President and Congress on the Status of Health Professionals in the United States*, DHEW, Public Health Service, Health Resources Administration, Manpower Analysis Branch, August 1978, Table IV-2, p. IV-46 and Table V-1, p. V-19; U.S. National Center for Health Statistics, *Health Resources Statistics, 1976–77*, DHEW, Public Health Service, Office of Health Research, Statistics, and Technology, Hyattsville, Maryland, 1979, Table 40, p. 69 and Table 42, p. 71.

Chart E-46

Percent of Dentists, by Practice Organization or Employment (U.S.A., Selected Years, 1952–1976).

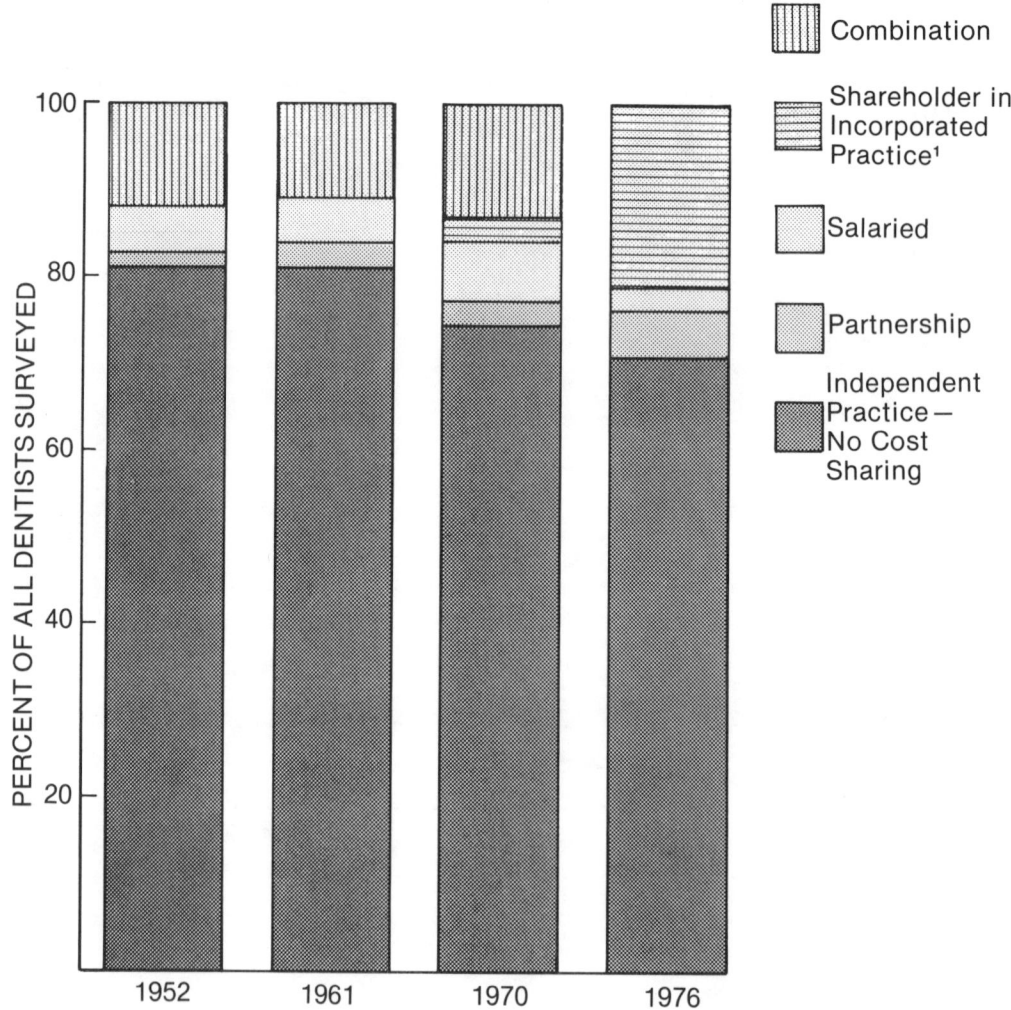

[1]Data not available for this category for the period prior to 1970.

SOURCE: Council on Dental Practice and Bureau of Economic and Behavioral Research, "An Analysis of Dental Practice from 1952 to 1976," *Journal of the American Dental Association,* Vol. 100, January 1980, Table 1, p. 91.

Chart E-47 Median Net Income of Dentists, by Type of Practice (U.S.A., 1952–1976).

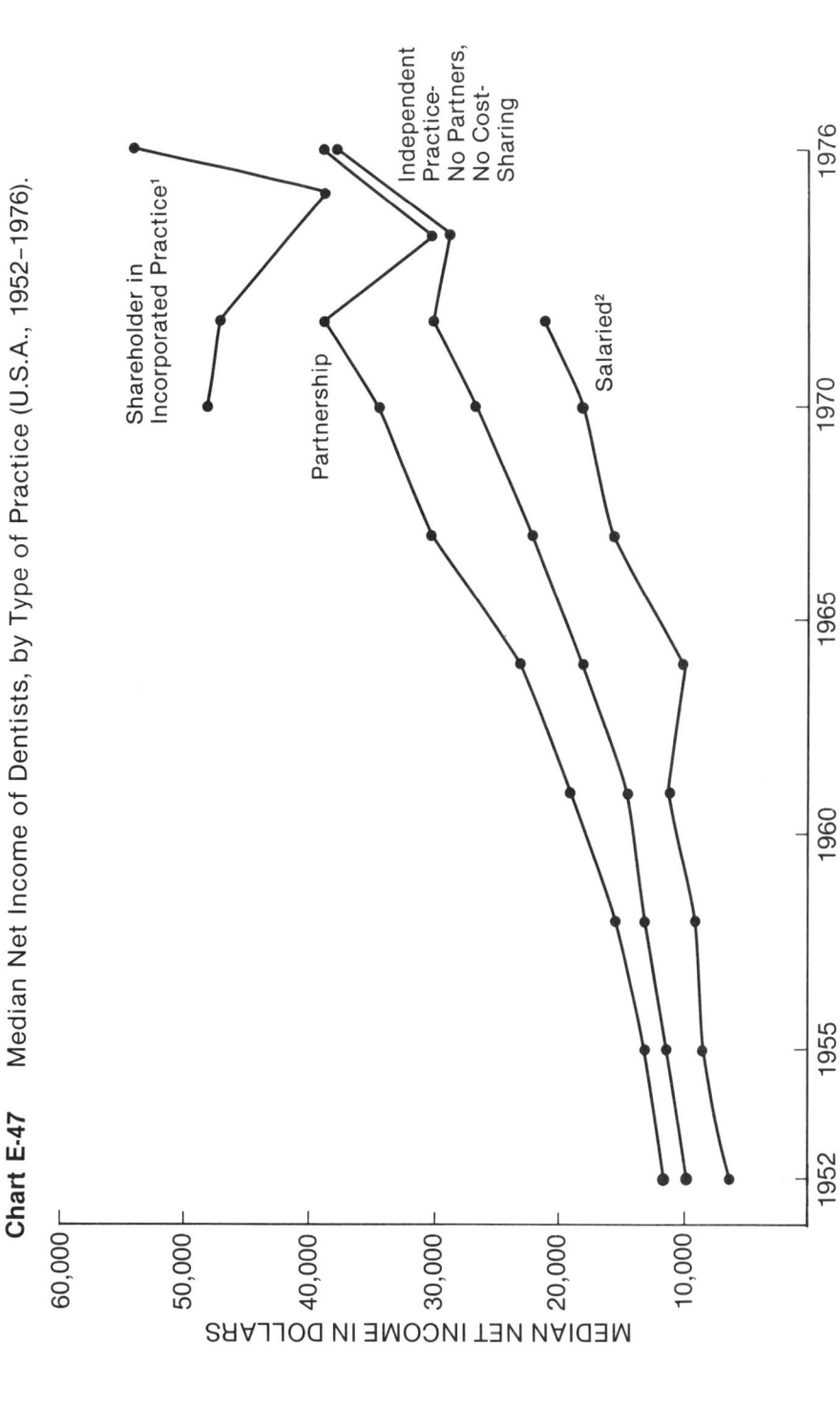

[1] Data not available for the period prior to 1970.
[2] Excludes those employed by another dentist or on staff at a dental school.

SOURCE: Council on Dental Practice and Bureau of Economic and Behavioral Research, "An Analysis of Dental Practice from 1952 to 1976," *Journal of the American Dental Association*, Vol. 100, January 1980, Table 5, p. 96.

Chart E-48

Mean Number of Patients per Year Seen by Independent or Nonsalaried Dentists, by Selected Ages of Dentist (U.S.A., Selected Years, 1952–1972).

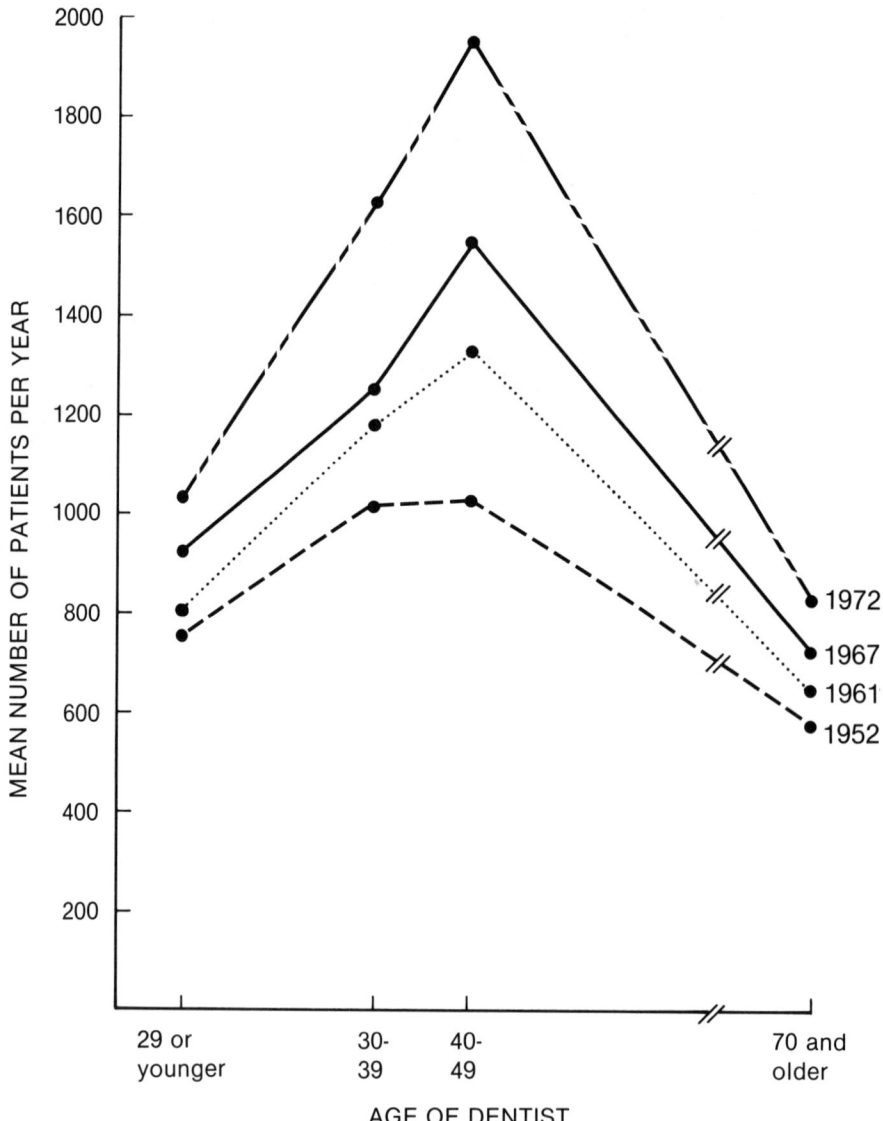

SOURCE: Council on Dental Practice and Bureau of Economic and Behavioral Research, "An Analysis of Dental Practice from 1952 to 1976," *Journal of the American Dental Association,* Vol. 100, January 1980, Figure 2, p. 90.

Chart E-49 Percent Increase in Mean Gross Income of Independent Dentists Related to the Facilities and Full time Staff Employed by the Dentist (U.S.A., 1970).

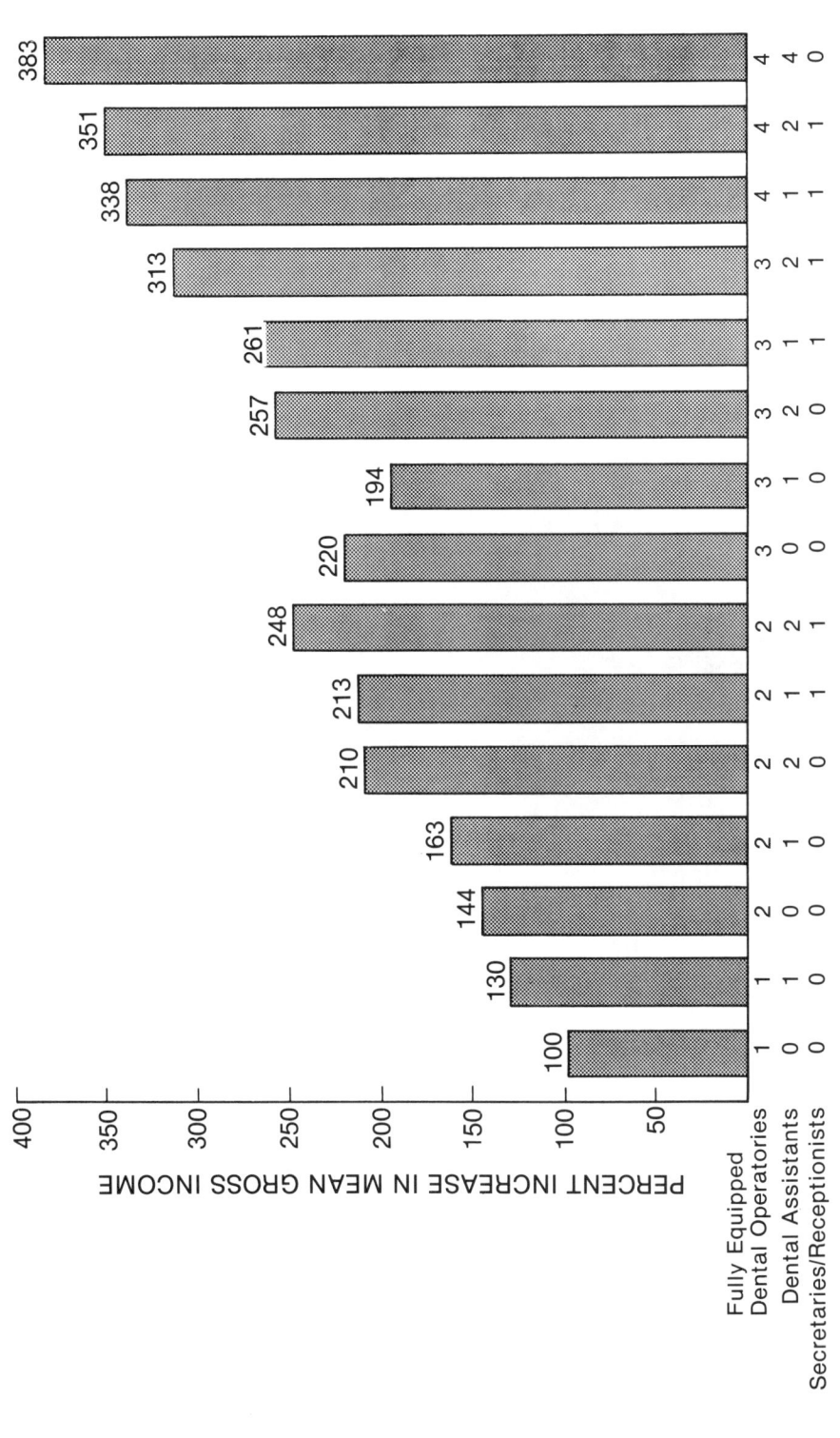

SOURCE: Reports of Councils and Bureaus, "1971 Survey of Dental Practice, III, Income of Dentists by Type of Practice, Personnel Employed, and Other Factors," *Journal of the American Dental Association*, Vol. 84, March 1972, Table 12, p. 637.

Chart E-50

Number and Percent Distribution of Active Nursing Personnel, by Type of Training (U.S.A., Selected Years, 1950–1976).

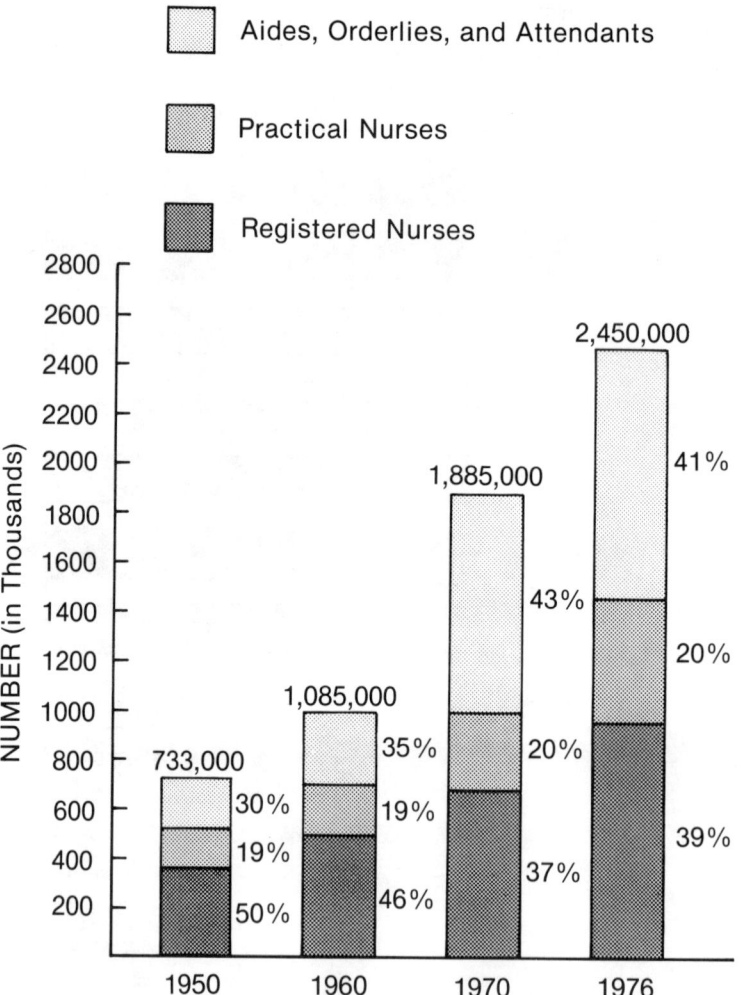

SOURCES: For 1950 and 1960; Division of Public Health Methods, *Health Manpower Source Book: Manpower in the 1960's*, DHEW, Public Health Service, Washington, D.C., Section 18, No. 263, 1964, Table 8, p. 14; for 1970: U.S. National Center for Health Statistics, *Health Resources Statistics, 1971*, DHEW, Public Health Service, Office of Health Research, Statistics and Technology, Rockville, Maryland, 1972, p. 173; for 1976: U.S. National Center for Health Statistics, *Health Resources Statistics, 1976-77*, DHEW, Public Health Service, Office of Health Research, Statistics, and Technology, Hyattsville, Maryland, 1976, Table 1, p. 11.

Health Personnel

Chart E-51

Nurse-Population Ratio, by Geographic Areas and Selected States (U.S.A., 1972).[1]

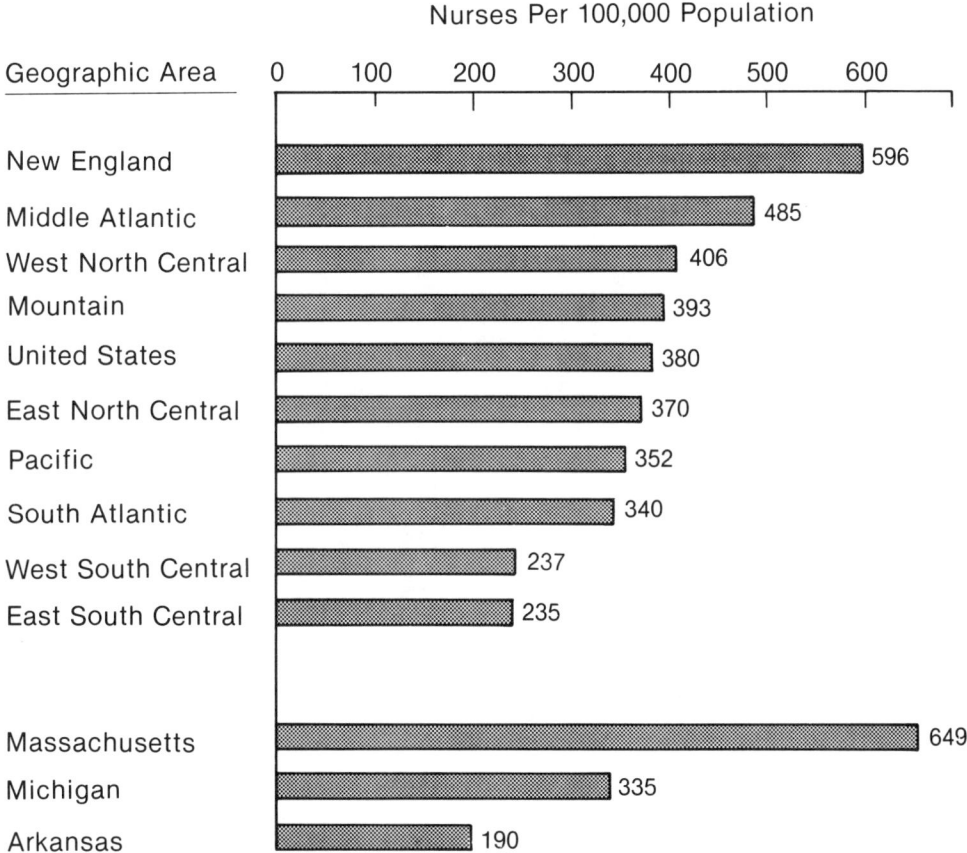

[1]Employed, registered nurses per 100,000 population.
SOURCE: American Nurses Association, *Facts About Nursing 1972-73*, Kansas City, American Nursing Association, Chart 1, p. 11.

Chart E-52 Educational Programs in Nursing and Related Career Opportunities (U.S.A., 1980).

Programs in Nursing	Usual Length of Study	Minimum Educational Requirements	Site of Training	Degree Awarded and License Eligibility	Type of Position Occupied Upon Graduation
Practical Nurse	1 year	High school diploma or graduate equivalent degree (GED)	Vocational high school, hospital, or community college	Certificate; eligible to take exam for licensure as L.P.N.	Bedside nursing (with supervision); primary care (with supervision)
Diploma (Hospital-Based)	2-3 years	High school or GED	Hospital and sometimes community college for liberal arts courses	Diploma; eligible to take exam for licensure as R.N.	Staff nurse; bedside nursing; Primary care, self-employed or in physician's office
Associate Degree	2 years	High school or GED	Community college or 4 year college, and clinical training in area hospitals	Associate Degree in Nursing; eligible to take exam for licensure as R.N.	Staff nurse; bedside nursing; Primary care, self-employed or in physician's office
Basic or Generic Baccalaureate	4 years	High school or GED	University or 4 year college, and clinical experience in area hospitals	Bachelor of Science (Nursing major) or Bachelor of Sciences; eligible for Nursing licensure as R.N.	Bedside nursing; PH nursing; Primary care, self-employed or in physician's office
Baccalaureate for R.N.	1½-2 years beyond Diploma or Associate Degree	R.N. Associate Degree or Diploma in Nursing	University or 4 year college, and clinical experience in area hospitals	Bachelor of Science (Nursing major) or Bachelor of Science in Nursing	Bedside nursing; PH nursing; Primary care, self-employed or in physician's office; Administration
Master's	2 years beyond Baccalaureate	B.S. in Nursing and R.N. licensure	University, and clinical experience in area hospitals	Master of Science or Master of Science in Nursing	Bedside nursing; PH nursing; primary care, self-employed or in physician's office; Administrator; Educator; Supervisor; clinical specialist
Doctoral	3 years or more beyond Baccalaureate, depending on choice of major	Baccalaureate Degree in Nursing	University and area hospitals if program requires	Ph.D.	All of the above for Master's and Researcher; Higher Education Administrator

SOURCE: Office of the Assistant Dean for Academic Affairs, School of Nursing, The University of Michigan, May 1980.

Chart E-53

Annual Number of Persons Graduating from Professional Nursing Programs, by Program (U.S.A., 1960-1961 through 1975-1976).

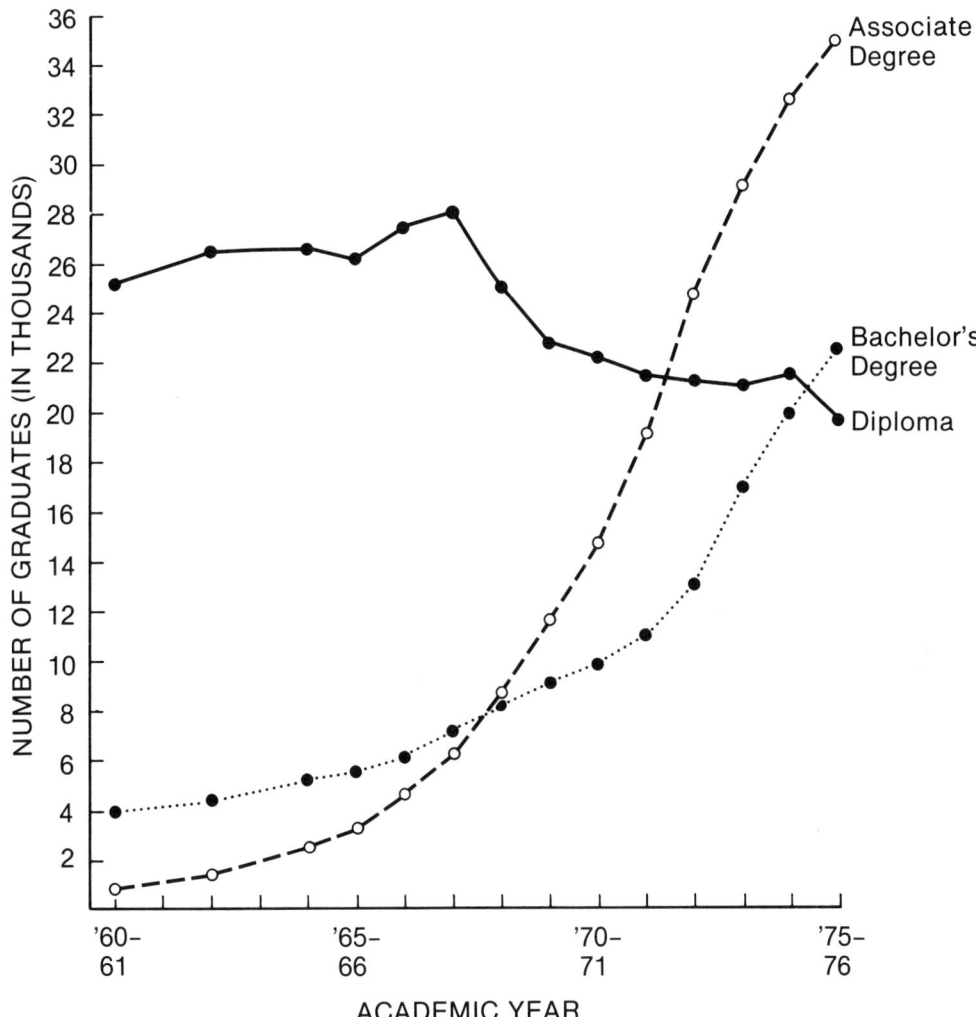

SOURCE: U.S. National Center for Health Statistics, *Health Resources Statistics, 1976-77,* DHEW, Public Health Service, Office of Health Research, Statistics, and Technology, Hyattsville, Maryland, Table 109, p. 175.

Health Personnel

Chart E-54

Percent Distribution of Registered Nurses, by Type of Practice or Field of Employment (U.S.A., 1977[1]).

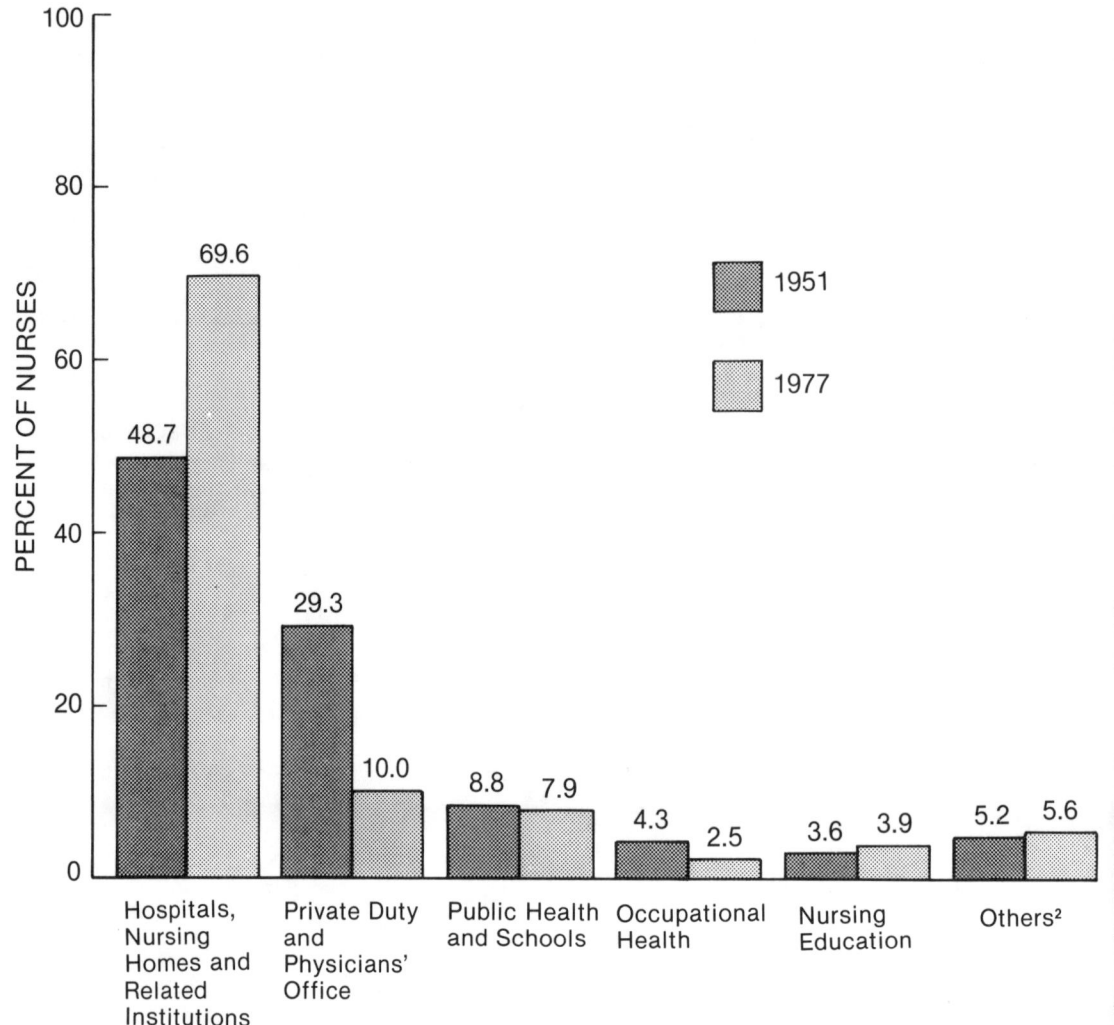

[1] Estimates from survey data.

[2] Other includes: State Boards of Nursing, Nursing and Health Associations, Central or Regional Offices of Federal Agencies, Health Planning Agencies, Placement (Referral) Services, Self Employed, Student Health, Miscellaneous, and not reported.

SOURCES: For 1951: *Facts About Nursing,* 1954 edition, The American Nurses' Association, New York, Table 2, p. 11; for 1977: Moses, E. and A. Roth, "Nursepower: What do Statistics Reveal About the Nation's Nurses?," *American Journal of Nursing,* October 1979, pp. 1750-1751.

Chart E-55

Numbers per 100,000 Persons of Specified Active Health Personnel (U.S.A., 1960 and 1976).

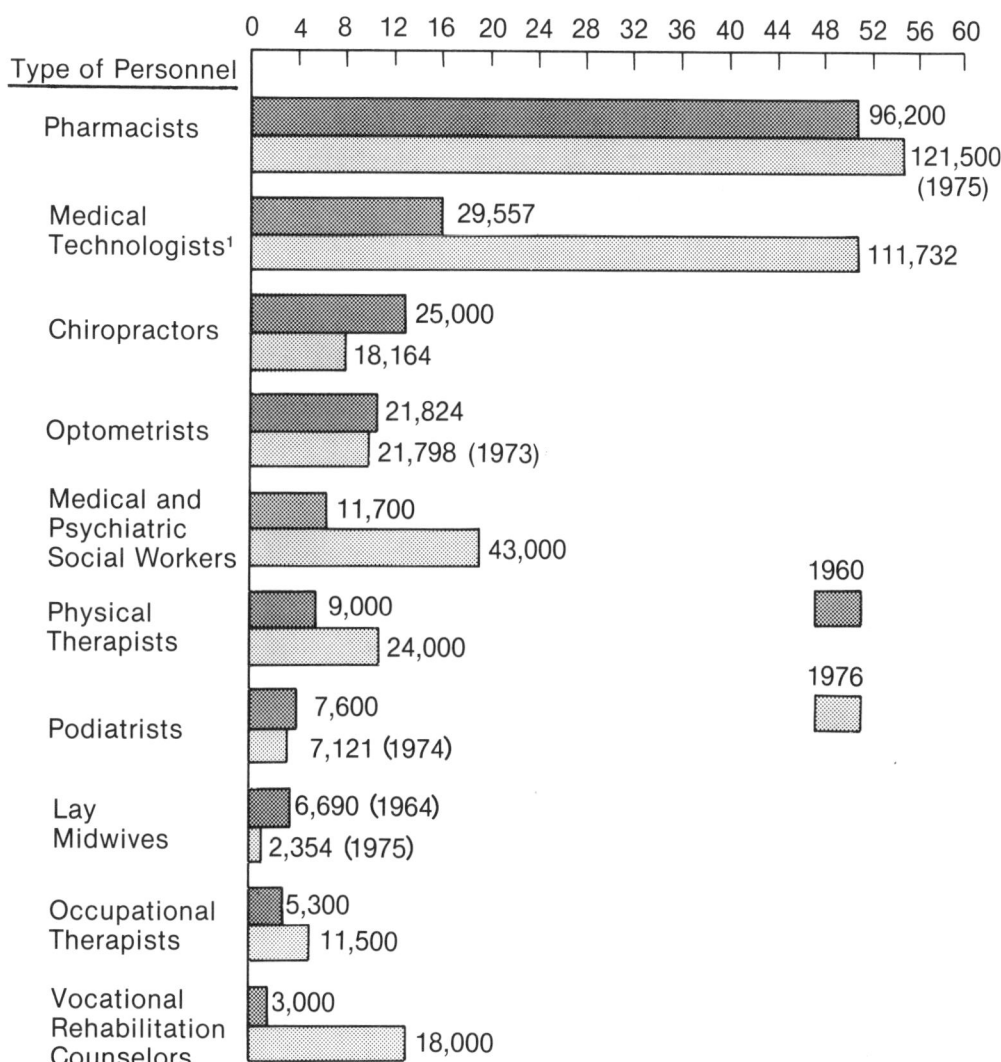

[1] Registered Medical Technologist certified by the American Society of Clinical Pathologists. Person does not necessarily have to be presently employed as a medical technologist.

NOTE: Total numbers for each personnel category are shown to the right of the bars.

SOURCE: U.S. National Center for Health Statistics, *Health Resources Statistics, 1976-1977 Edition,* DHEW, Public Health Service, Office of Health and Research, Statistics, and Technology, Hyattsville, Maryland, 1979, Table 23, p. 46, Table 28, p. 55, Table 89, p. 141, Table 100, p. 162, Table 120, p. 186, Table 130, p. 197, Table 137, p. 204, Table 142, p. 214, Table 152, p.230, Table 167, p. 249, and Table 190, p. 280.

Chart E-56

Percent of Persons in Selected Professions Who are Black (U.S.A., 1970).

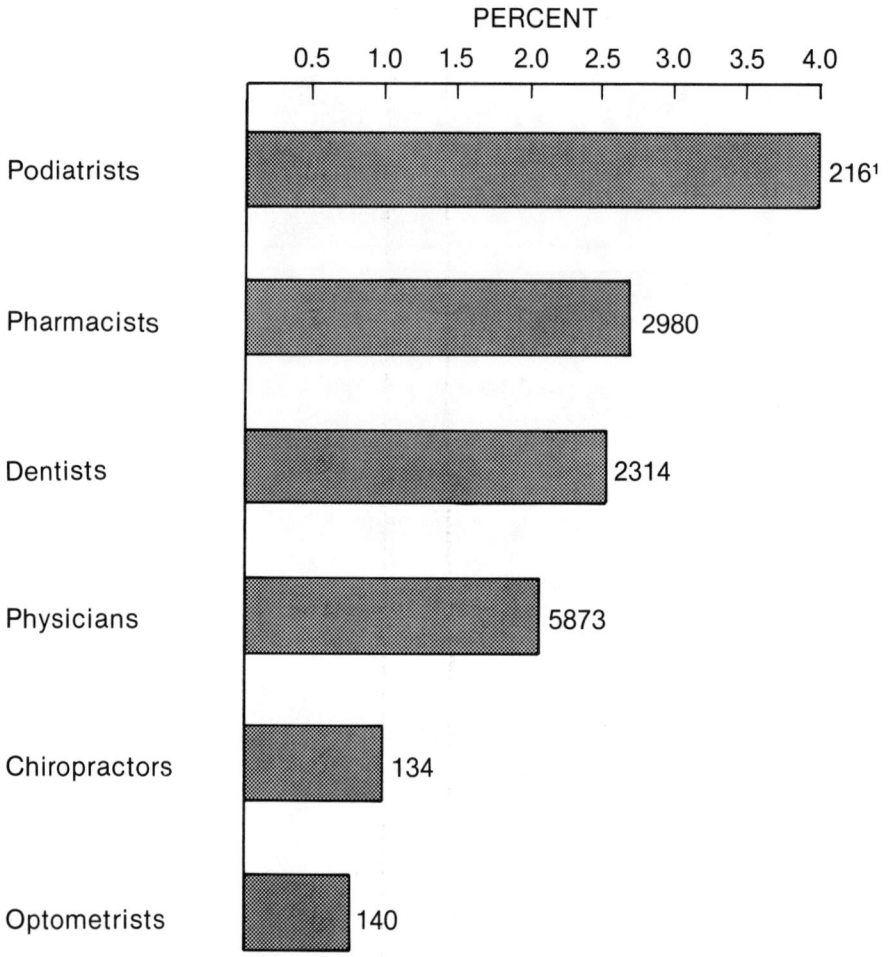

[1] Actual number in designated profession.
SOURCE: American Public Health Association, *Minority Health Chart Book*, 1974, p. 88.

SECTION F
Facilities

Chart F-1

Relative Increases in All Hospitals, Hospital Beds, and Ratio of Beds to Persons (U.S.A., 1909-1978).[1]

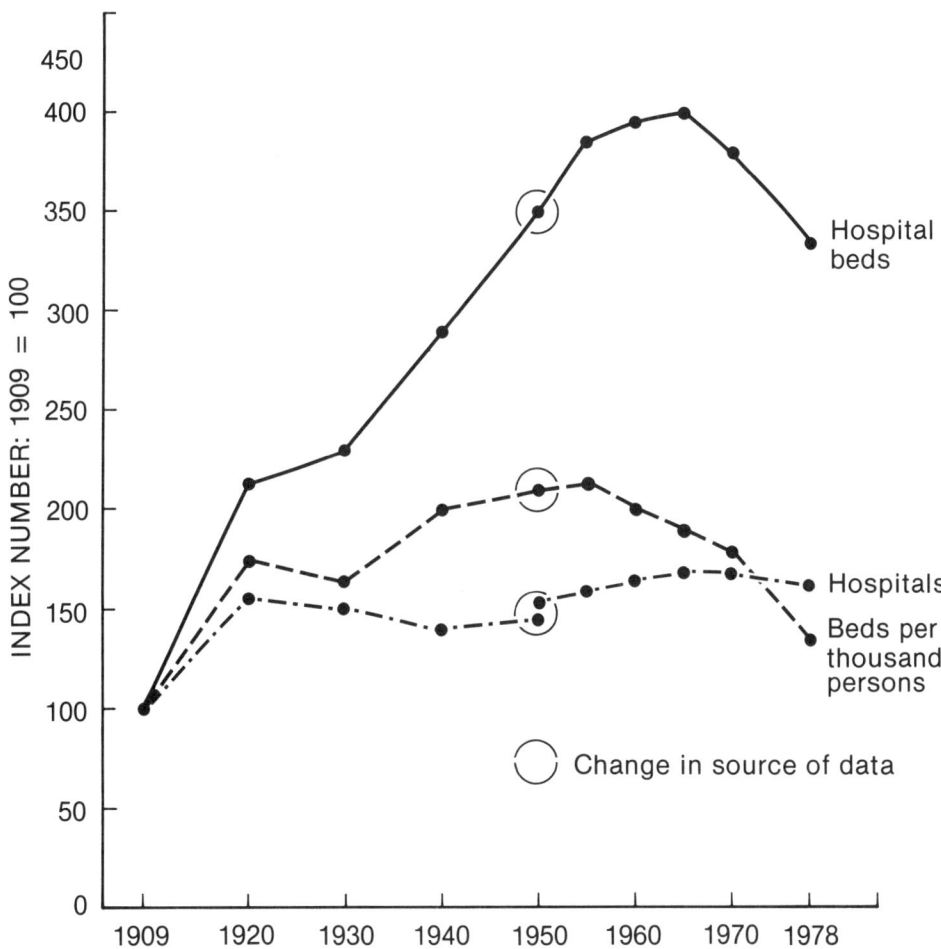

[1] The hospital data, compiled through 1950 by the American Medical Association do not correspond precisely to those compiled since 1950 by the American Hospital Association. From 1960, data include Alaska and Hawaii.

SOURCES: For 1909-1940: Arestad, F.H. and M.A. McGovern, "Hospital Services in the United States," *Journal of the American Medical Association,* Vol.149, May 10, 1952, p.149; for 1950-1978: American Hospital Association, "The Nations Hospitals: A Statistical Profile," *Hospital Statistics, 1979 Edition,* Chicago, Table 1, p.4; for population: U.S. Department of Commerce, Bureau of the Census, *Statistical Abstract of the United States-1978,* Table 2, p.6.

Chart F-2 Selected Statistics on Short-term and Long-term Hospitals Listed by the American Hospital Association, by Type of Control (U.S.A., 1978).

Selected Hospital Statistics	All Hospitals	Type of Control				
		Governmental			Non-Governmental	
		Federal	State	Local	Voluntary	Proprietary
Number of Hospitals	7,015 (100%)	370 (5%)	483 (7%)	1,749 (25%)	3,532 (50%)	881 (13%)
Number of Beds	1,380,645 (100%)	121,859 (9%)	259,114 (19%)	203,073 (15%)	704,202 (51%)	92,397 (6%)
Number of Admissions	37,243,182 (100%)	1,997,176 (5%)	1,309,753 (4%)	6,402,547 (17%)	24,545,959 (66%)	2,987,747 (8%)
Average Daily Census	1,041,936 (100%)	95,585 (9%)	205,821 (20%)	142,225 (13%)	538,428 (52%)	59,877 (6%)

SOURCE: American Hospital Association, *Hospital Statistics, 1979 Edition*, Chicago, Table 2A, pp. 8-9 and Table 2B, pp. 10-11.

Facilities

Chart F-3

Non-federal Short-term General and Other Special Hospital Beds per 1000 Persons by Geographic Area and Selected States (U.S.A., 1970 and 1978).[1]

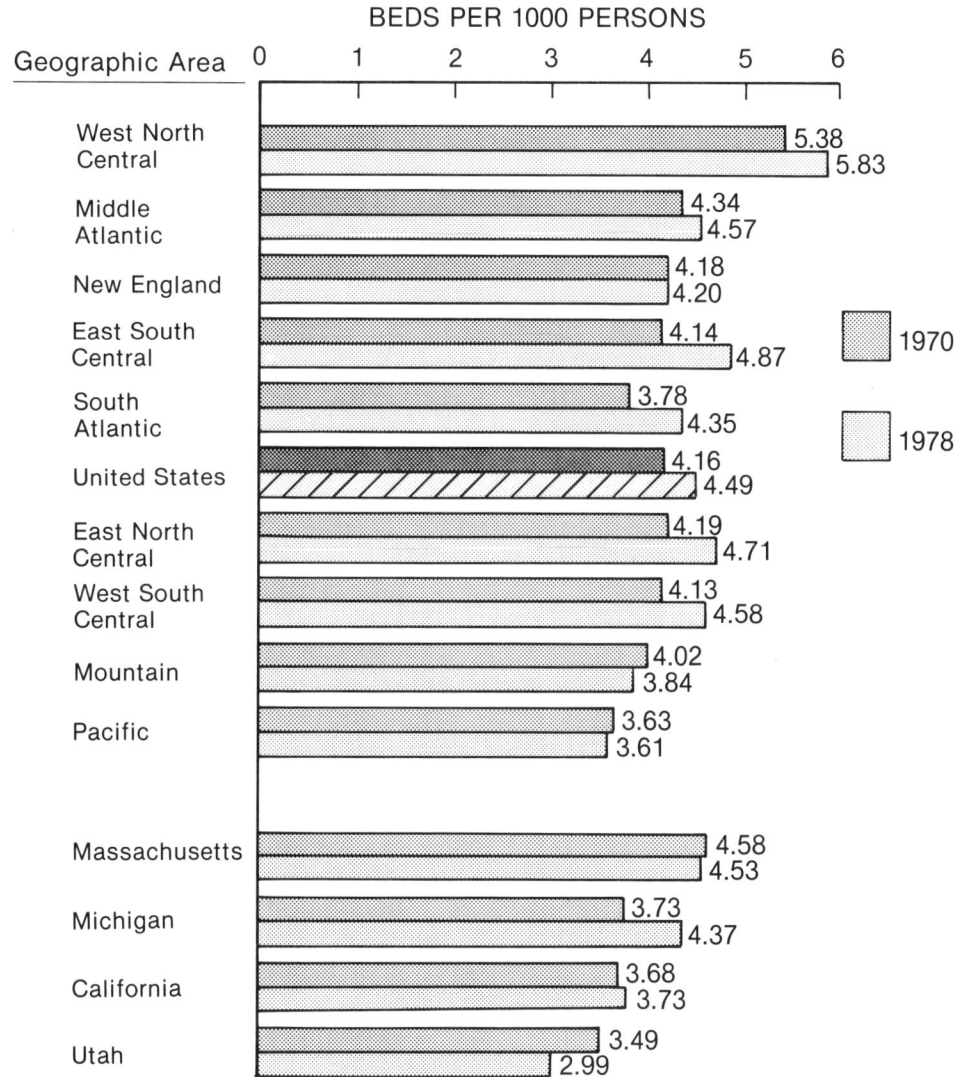

[1]Hospitals listed by the American Hospital Association.
SOURCES: For Population, 1970 and 1978: U.S. Department of Commerce, Bureau of the Census, *Statistical Abstract of the United States, 1979 Edition,* Table II, p. 14; for 1970: American Hospital Association, *Hospitals,* Guide Issue, August 1, 1971, Part II, Table 3, pp. 468–479; for 1978: American Hospital Association, *Hospital Statistics, 1979 Edition,* Chicago, 1979, Table 5A, p. 20, Table 5B, pp. 22–38, and Table 5C, pp. 48, 82, 84, 128.

Chart F-4

Percent Distribution of Short-term and Long-term Hospitals and Hospital Beds Listed by the American Hospital Association, by Governmental and Non-governmental Control (U.S.A., 1960, 1970, and 1978).

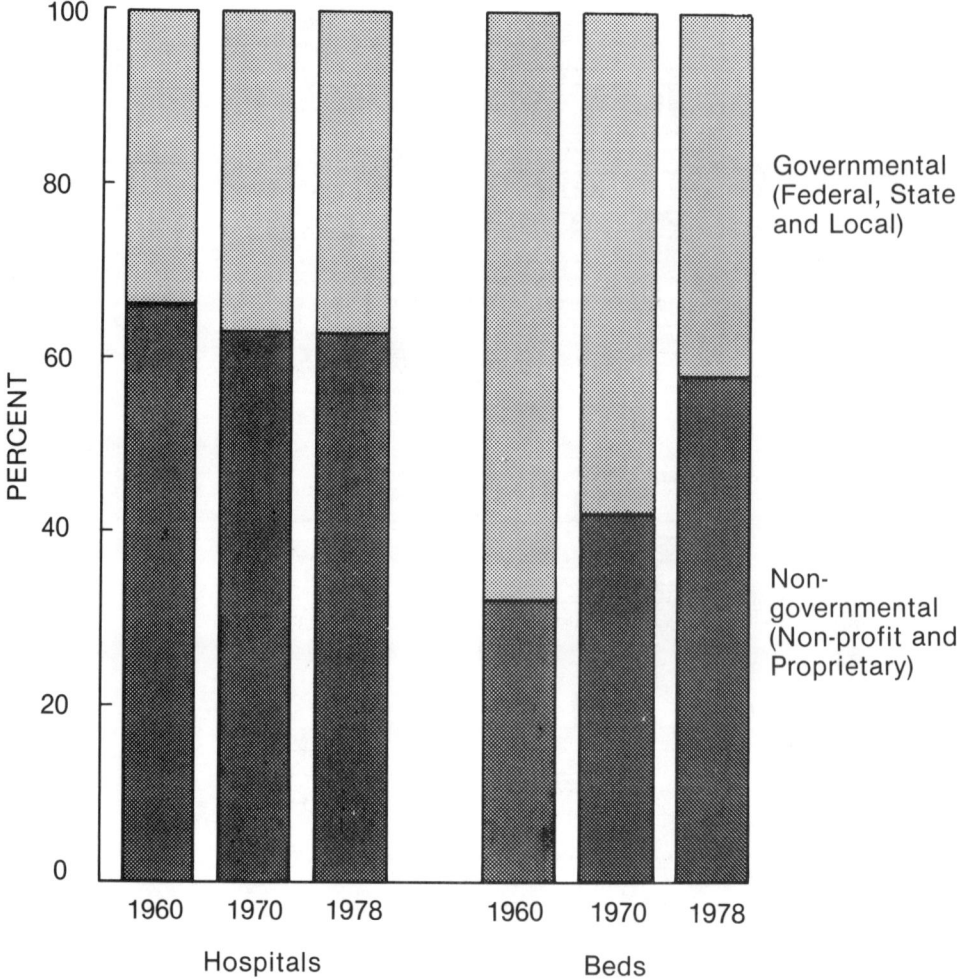

SOURCES: For 1960: *Hospitals,* Guide Issue, Vol.35, Part 2, August 1, 1961, Table 2, pp. 396–401; for 1970: *"Hospital Statistics," Hospitals,* Guide Issue, Vol.45, Part 2, August 1, 1971, Table 2B, pp.464–467; for 1978: American Hospital Association, *Hospital Statistics,* 1979 Edition, Chicago, Table 2A, pp.8–9 and Table 2B, pp.10–11.

Facilities

Chart F-5

Percent Distribution of Non-federal Short-term General and Other Special Hospitals and of Hospital Beds Listed by the American Hospital Association, by Type of Ownership (U.S.A., Selected Years, 1946–1978).

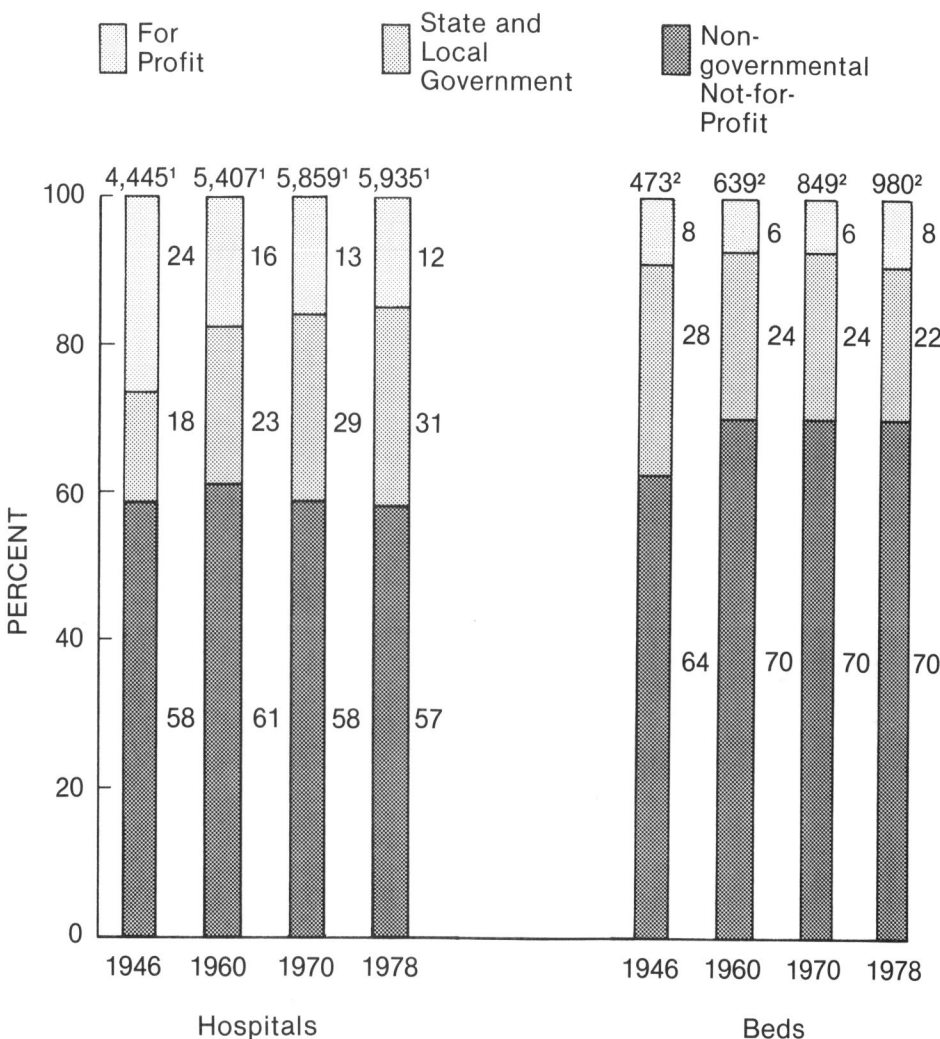

[1] Total number of hospitals.
[2] Total number of beds, in thousands.
SOURCE: American Hospital Association, *Hospital Statistics, 1979 Edition,* Chicago, Table 1, p. 6.

Facilities

Chart F-6

Percent Distribution of Hospital Beds by Ownership, and by Type of Hospital (U.S.A., 1978).

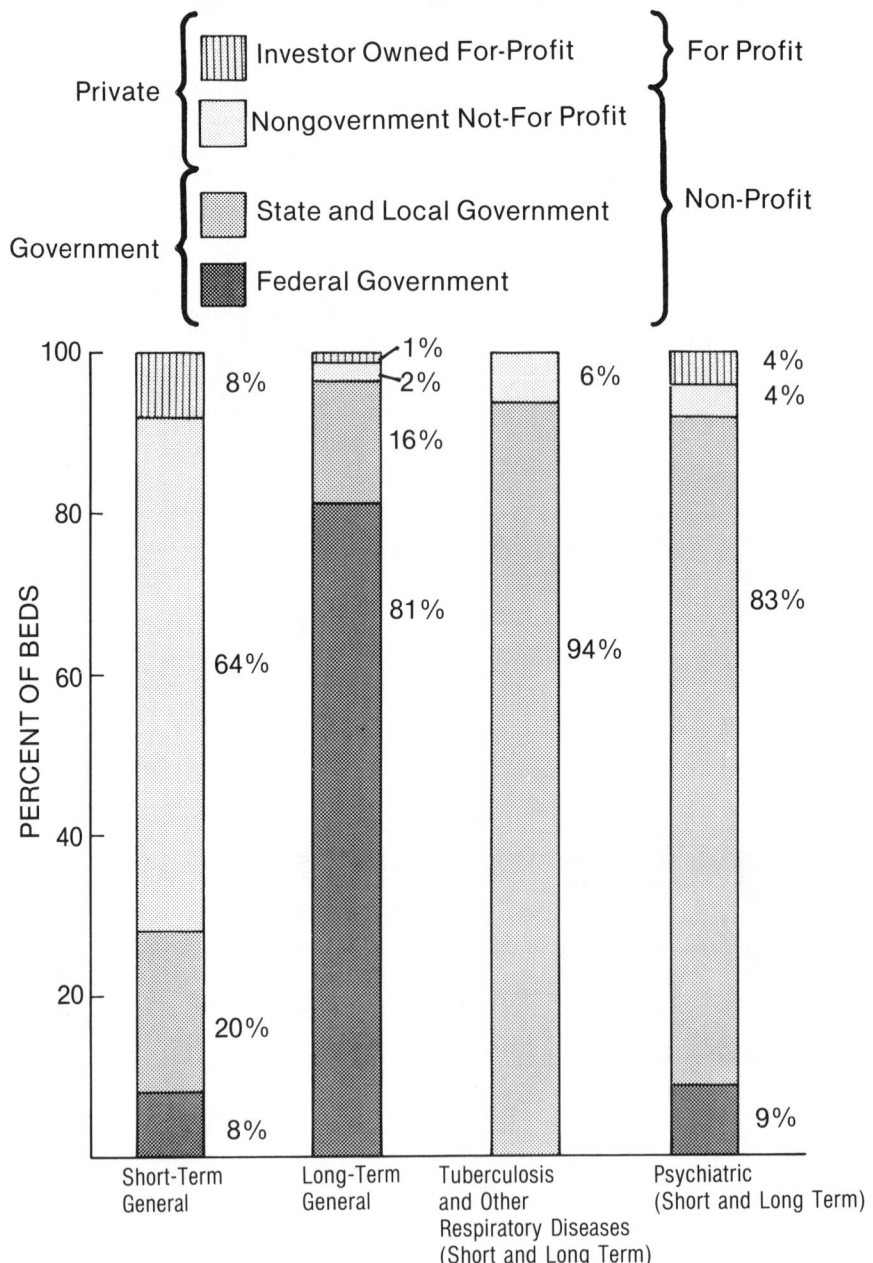

NOTE: Where there are no hospital beds for a given category, that category does not appear.

SOURCE: American Hospital Association, *Hospital Statistics, 1979 Edition,* Table 2A, pp. 8–9 and Table 2B, pp.10–11.

Facilities

Chart F-7

Percent Change in Admissions to Hospitals, by Type of Stay and by Type of Control (U.S.A., 1950–1978).

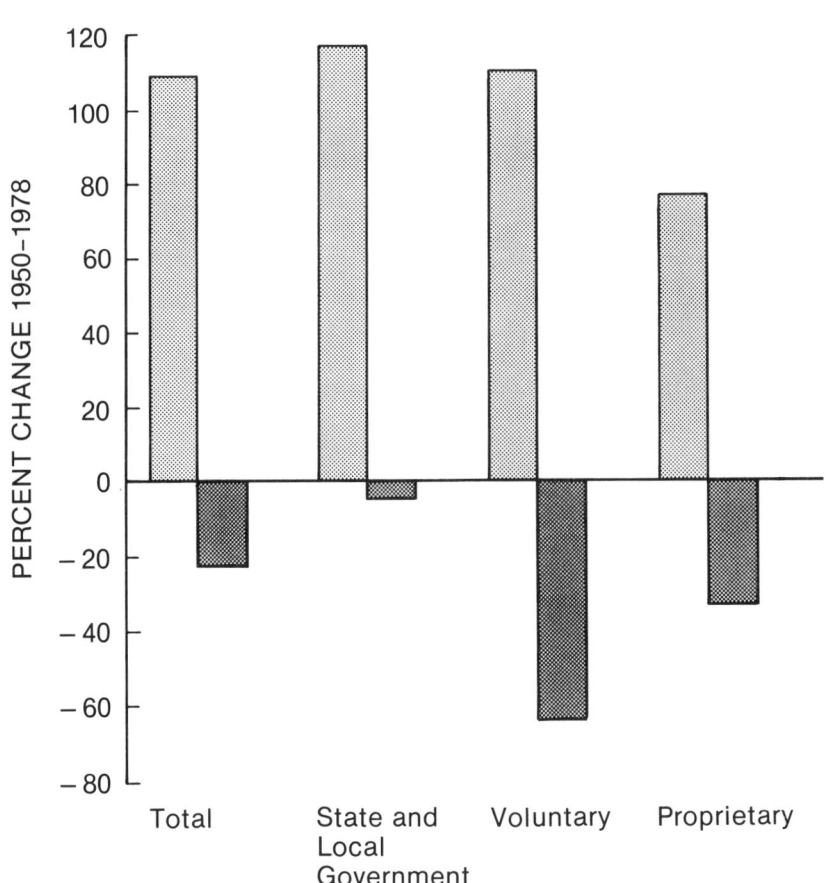

SOURCES: For 1950: "Statistical Guides," *Hospitals*, American Hospital Association, Guide Issue 25, June 1951, Part 2, Table 3, p. 10; for 1978: American Hospital Association, *Hospital Statistics, 1979 Edition*, Chicago, Table 2A, pp. 8–9, and Table 2B, pp. 10–11.

Facilities

Chart F-8

Percent Distribution of Hospitals and Beds, by Type of Hospital (U.S.A., 1978).[1]

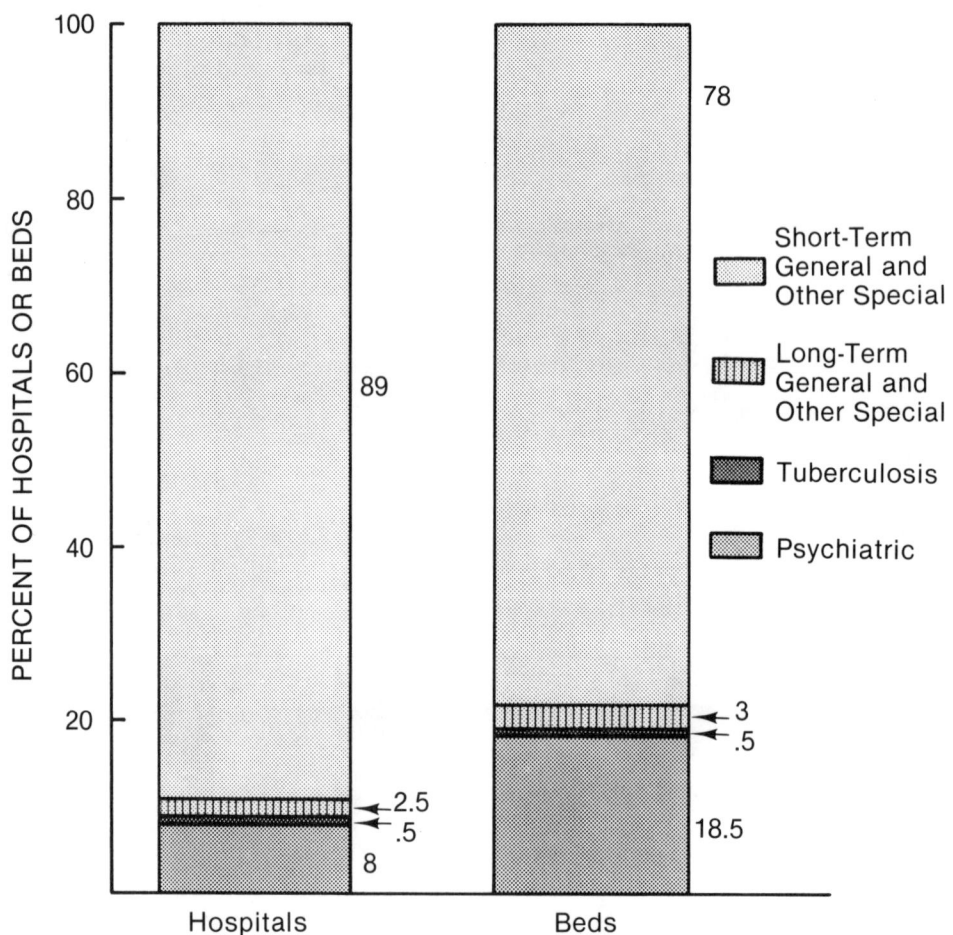

[1]Hospitals listed by the American Hospital Association. Excludes federal hospitals.
SOURCE: American Hospital Association, *Hospital Statistics, 1979 Edition*, Chicago, 1979, Table 2A, pp. 8–9 and Table 2B, pp. 10–11.

Facilities

Chart F-9

Mean Hospital Size and Beds per 1,000 Persons, by Type of Hospital (U.S.A., 1970 and 1978).[1]

TYPE OF HOSPITAL	MEAN HOSPITAL SIZE, IN BEDS		BEDS PER 1000 POPULATION	
	1970	1978	1970	1978[2]
All non-Federal Hospitals	217	189	7.1	5.8
Short-Term General and Other Special Hospitals	145	165	4.2	4.5
Long-Term General and Other Special Hospitals	254	245	0.3	0.2
Tuberculosis Hospitals	195	186	0.1	0.01
Psychiatric Hospitals	1,015	447	2.6	1.1

[1]Hospitals listed by the American Hospital Association. Excludes federal hospitals.

[2]Based on the estimated total resident population in 1978 of 218,059,000.

SOURCES: American Hospital Association, *Hospital Statistics, 1979 Edition*, Chicago, 1979, Table 2A, pp. 8–9 and Table 2B, pp. 10–11; for population: U.S. Department of Commerce, Bureau of the Census, *Statistical Abstract of the United States, 1979 Edition*, Washington, D.C., Table 11, p. 14.

Facilities

Chart F-10

Percent Distribution of Non-federal Short-term General and Other Special Hospitals and Hospital Beds, by Size of Hospital (U.S.A., 1978).[1]

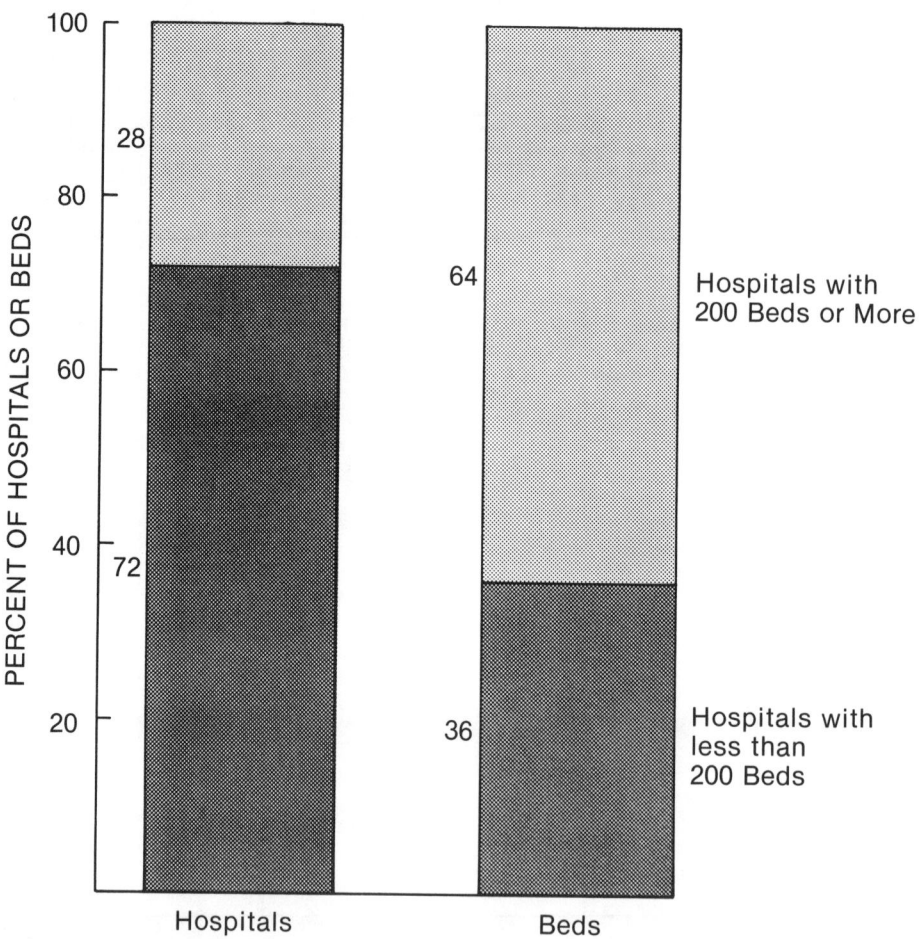

[1]Hospitals listed by the American Hospital Association

SOURCE: American Hospital Association, *Hospital Statistics, 1979 Edition*, Chicago, 1979, Table 2A, pp. 8-9.

Facilities

Chart F-11 Percent Distribution of Hospitals and Hospital Beds, by Size, Non-federal Short-term General and Other Special Hospitals (U.S.A., 1978).[1]

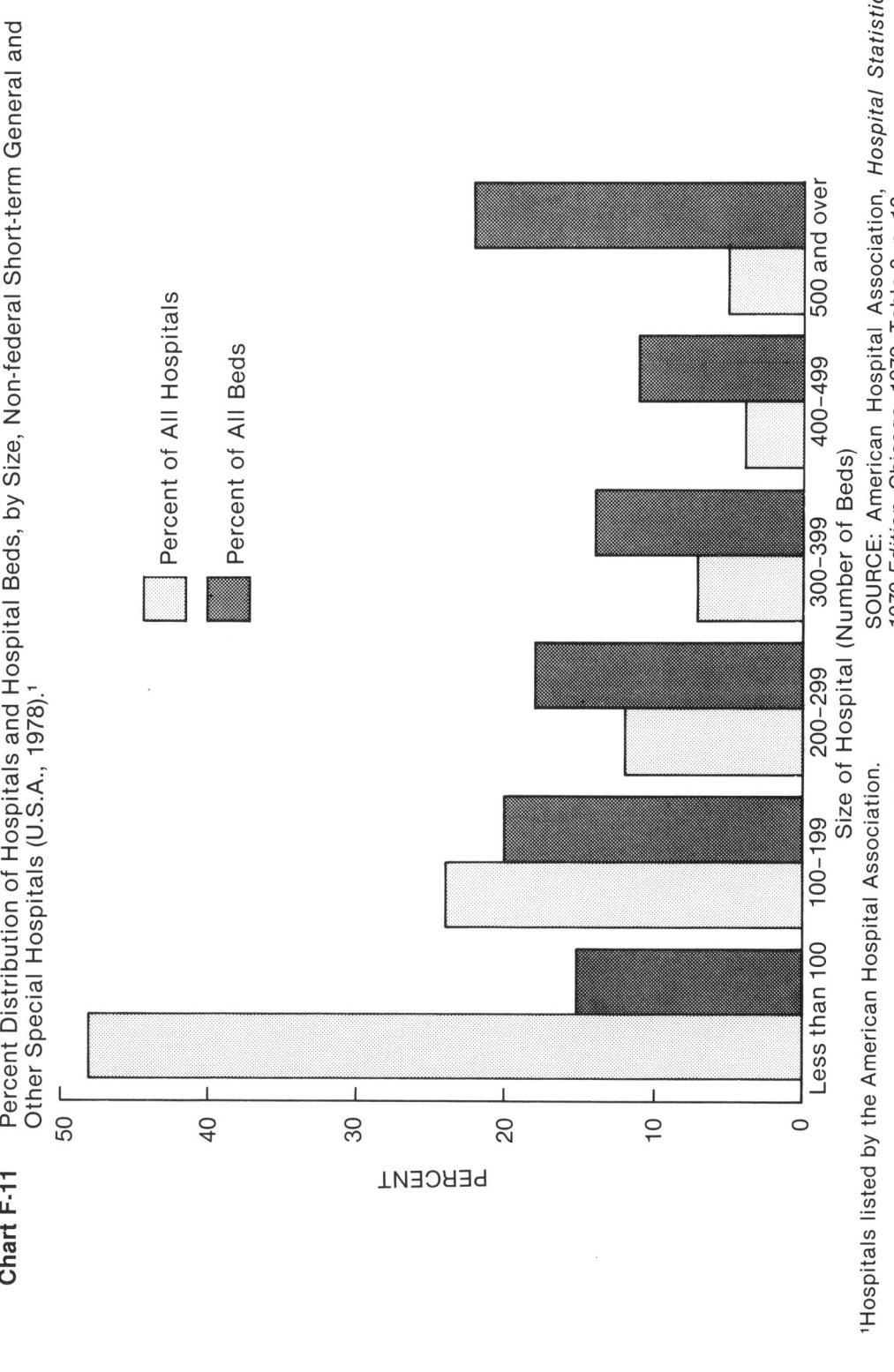

[1]Hospitals listed by the American Hospital Association.

SOURCE: American Hospital Association, *Hospital Statistics, 1979 Edition*, Chicago, 1979, Table 3, p. 12.

Facilities

Chart F-12 Occupancy Rate and Length of Stay, by Size of Hospital, Non-federal, Short-term General and Other Special Hospitals (U.S.A., 1978).[1]

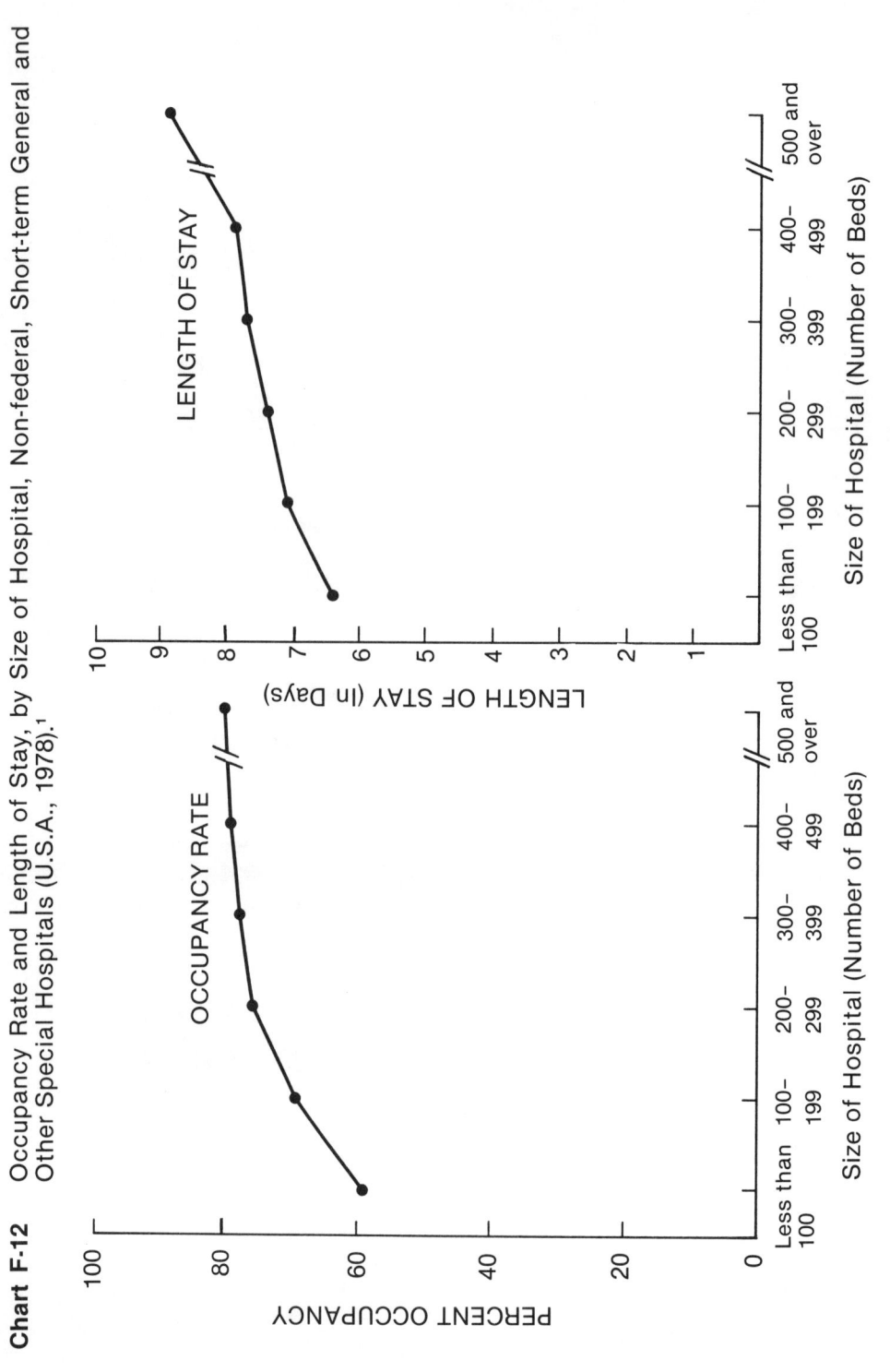

[1]Hospitals listed by the American Hospital Association.

SOURCE: American Hospital Association, *Hospital Statistics, 1979 Edition*, Chicago, 1979, Table 3, p. 12.

Chart F-13

Average Length of Hospital Stay, by Age of Patient and Size of Hospital (U.S.A., 1977).[1]

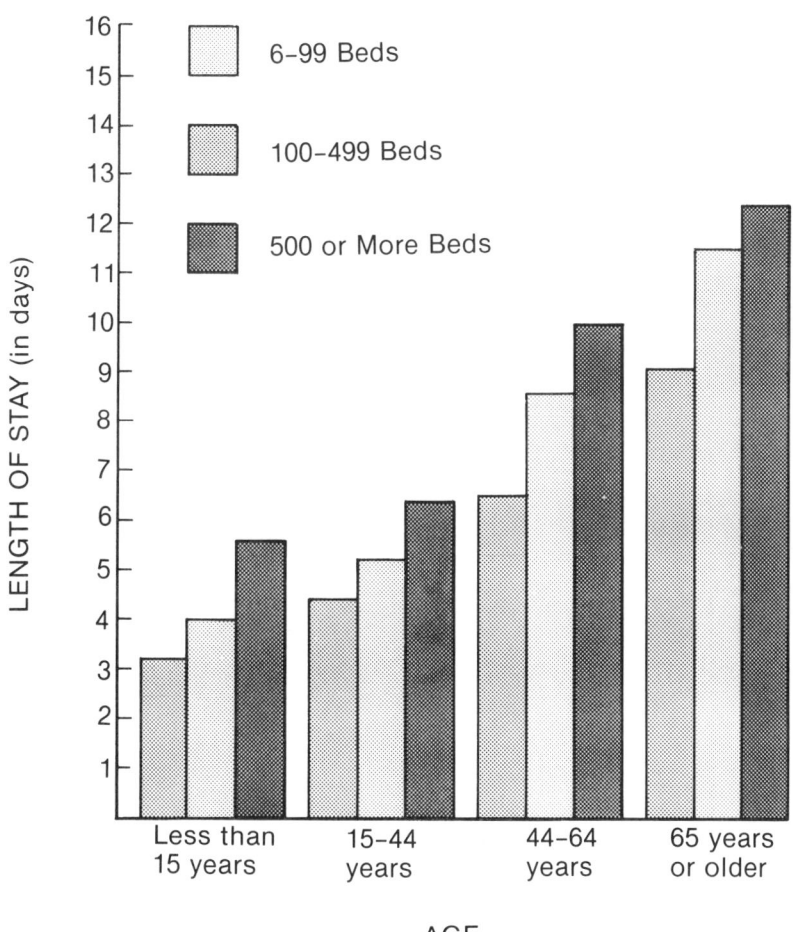

[1]Data are for non-federal short-stay hospitals and exclude newborn infants.
SOURCE: U.S. National Center for Health Statistics, *Utilization of Short-Term Hospitals: Annual Summary for the United States, 1977*, DHEW, Public Health Service, Office of Health Research, Statistics, and Technology, Hyattsville, Maryland, Series 13, No. 41, March 1979, Table 7, p. 28.

Facilities

Chart F-14

Percent of Hospitals with JCAH Accreditation and Percent with Medicare Participation, by Size of Hospital, Non-federal, Short-term General and Other Special Hospitals (U.S.A., 1978).[1]

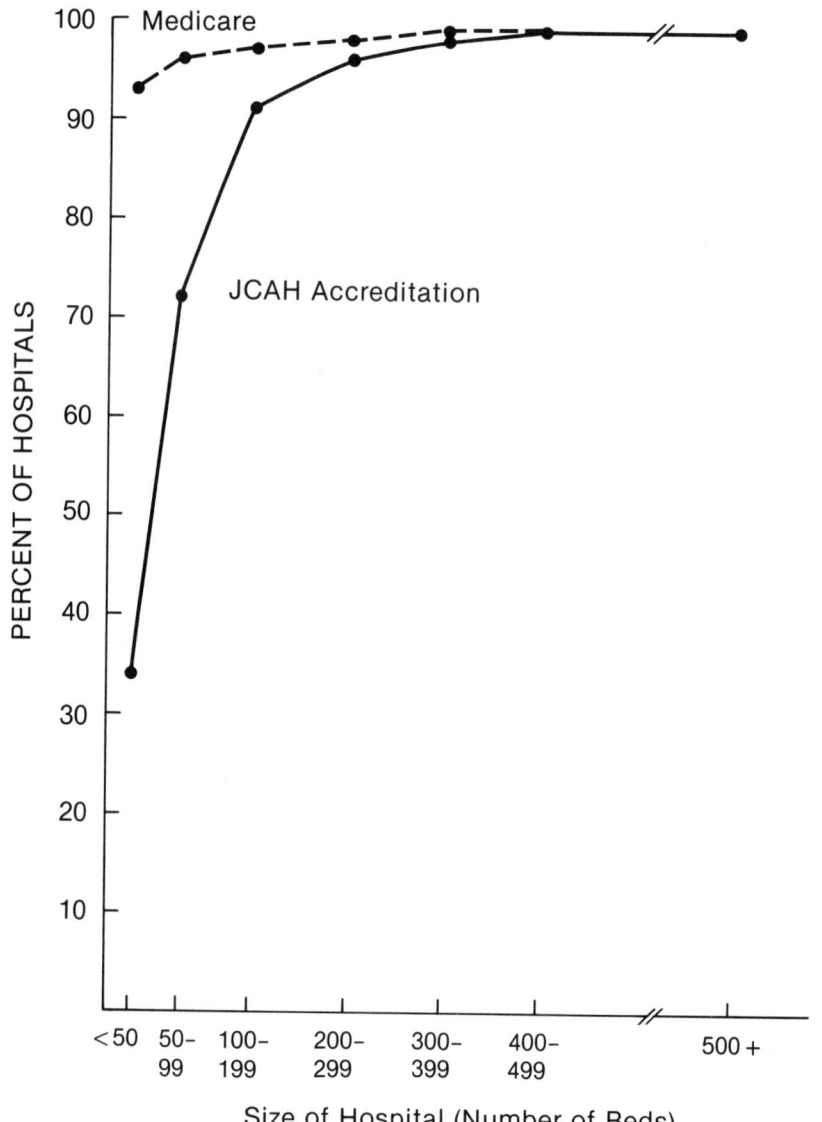

[1]Listed by the American Hospital Association.

SOURCE: American Hospital Association, *Hospital Statistics, 1979 Edition*, Chicago, 1979, Table 10A, p. 186.

Chart F-15

Percent of Non-federal Short-term Hospitals, by Size, Type of Control, and Accreditation by the Joint Commission on Accreditation of Hospitals (U.S.A., 1978).[1]

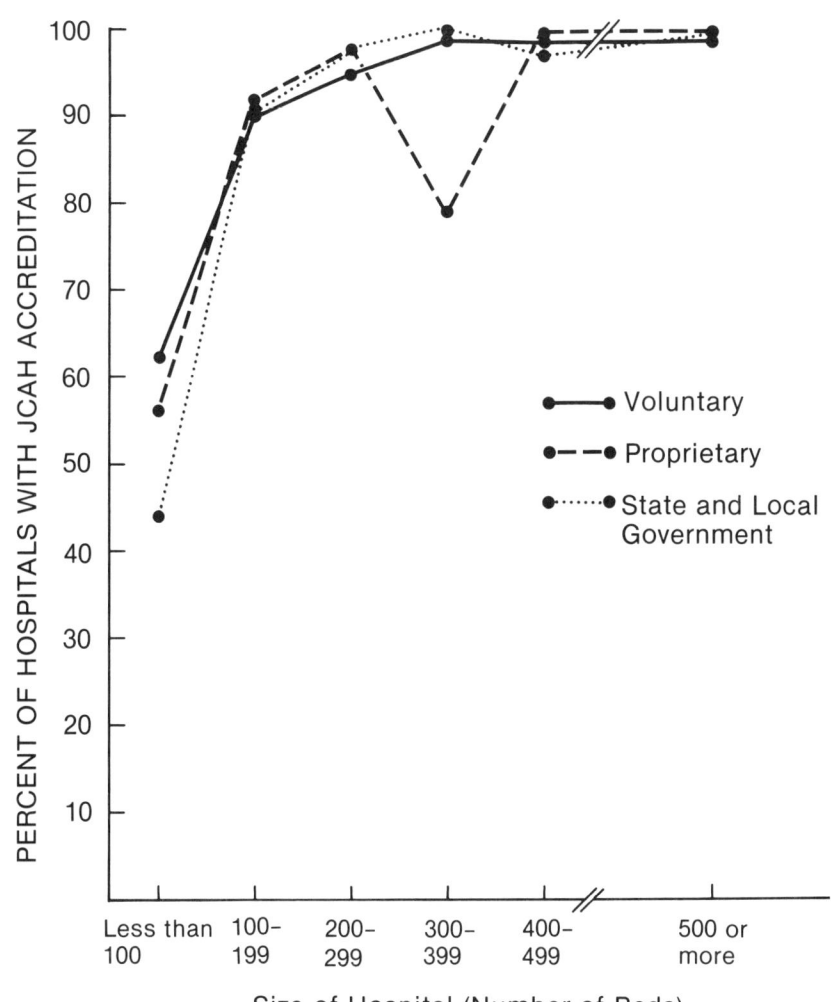

[1] Hospitals listed by the American Hospital Association.

SOURCE: American Hospital Association, *Hospital Statistics, 1979 Edition*, Chicago, 1979, Table 10A, p. 186.

Facilities

Chart F-16

Relative Magnitudes of Specified Indicators of the Operations of Hospital Maternity Services, by Hospital Size (U.S.A., 1967).

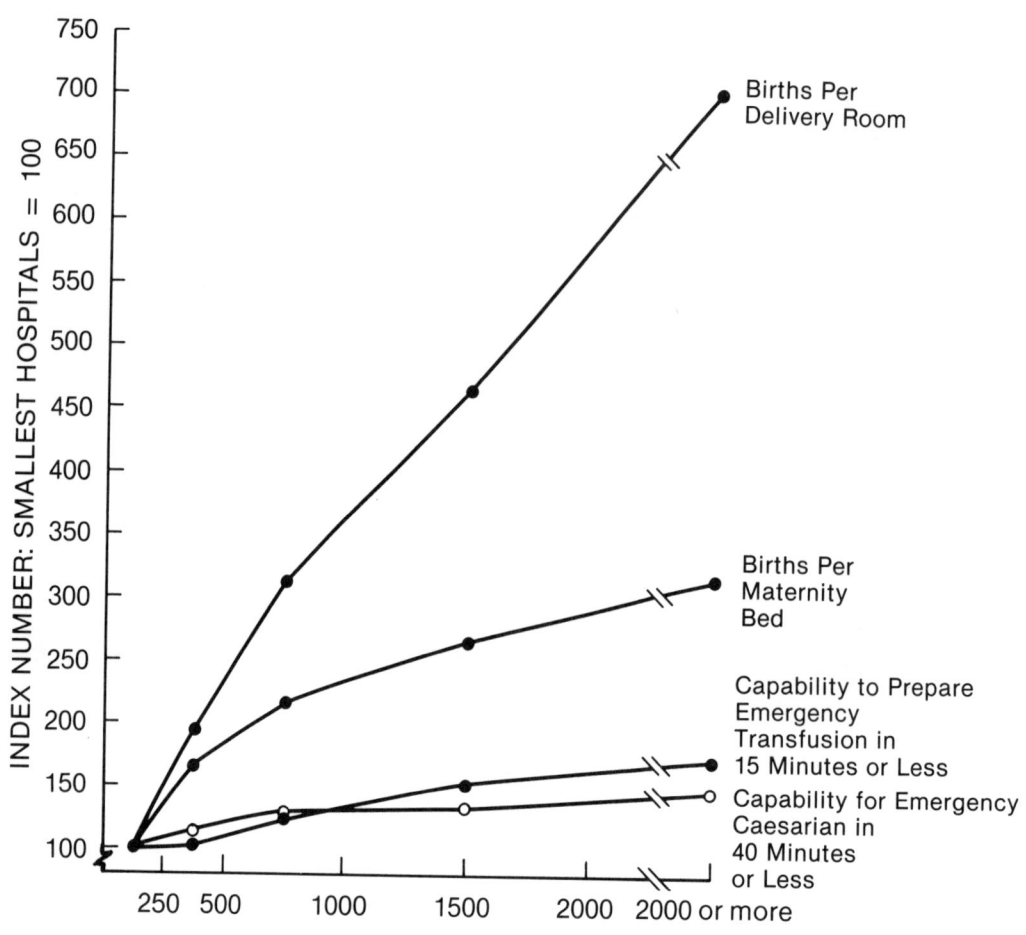

SOURCE: Committee on Maternal Health, The American College of Obstetricians and Gynecologists, *National Study of Maternal Care*, Chicago, 1970, Table 2-bl, pp. 80–81, Table 2-b3, pp. 84–85, Table 6-e, p. 120, and Table 7-d, pp. 132–133.

Facilities

Chart F-17

Percent of Patients Discharged per Day for Short-stay, Non-federal Hospitals, by Specified Lengths of Stay, All Persons and Persons 65 Years and Older (U.S.A., 1977).[1]

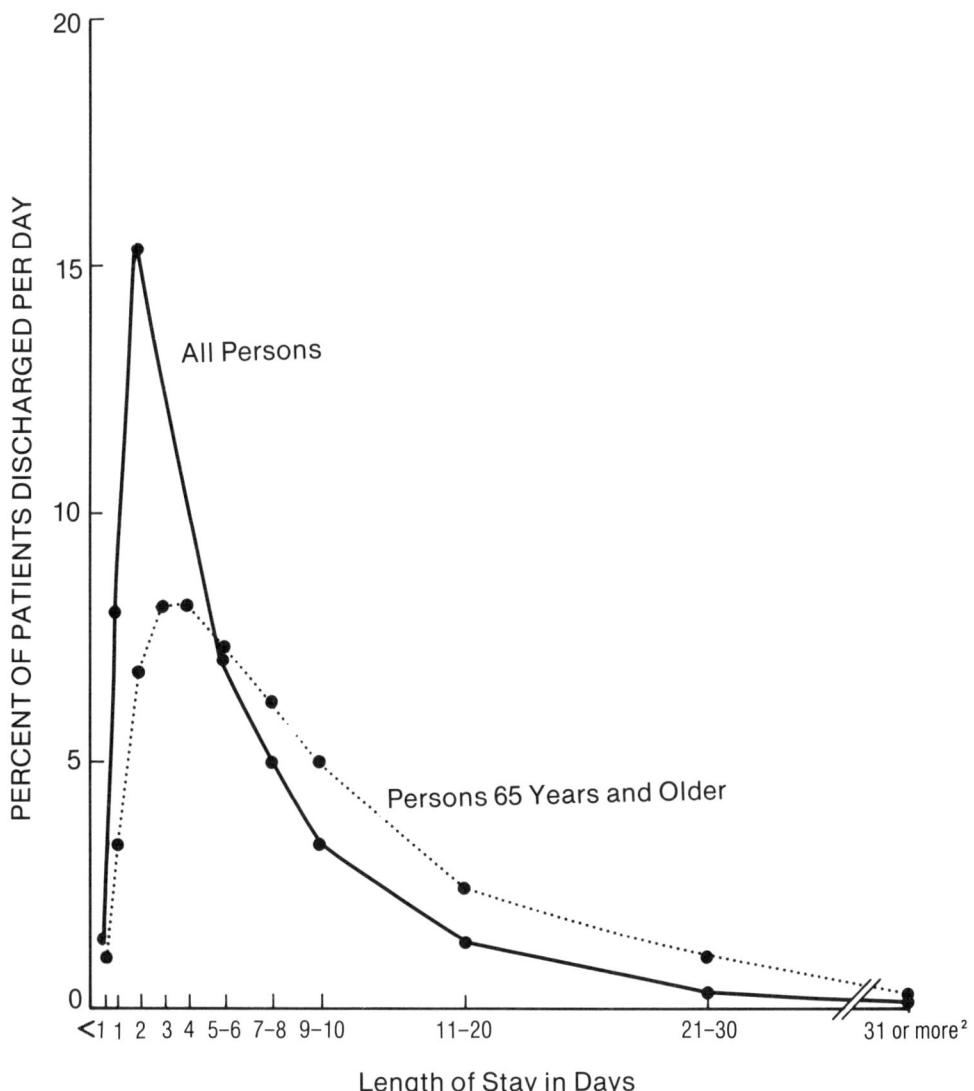

[1]Excludes newborn infants.
[2]The interval for 31 days or more is assumed to terminate on day 59.
SOURCE: U.S. National Center for Health Statistics, *Utilization of Short-stay Hospitals: Annual Summary for the United States, 1977*, DHEW, Public Health Service, Office of Health Research, Statistics, and Technology, Hyattsville, Maryland, Series 13, No. 41, March 1979, Table 3, pp. 23-24.

Facilities

Chart F-18

Cumulative Distribution of Discharges from Short-stay Non-federal Hospitals, by Length of Stay for All Persons and Those 65 Years and Older (U.S.A.,1977).[1]

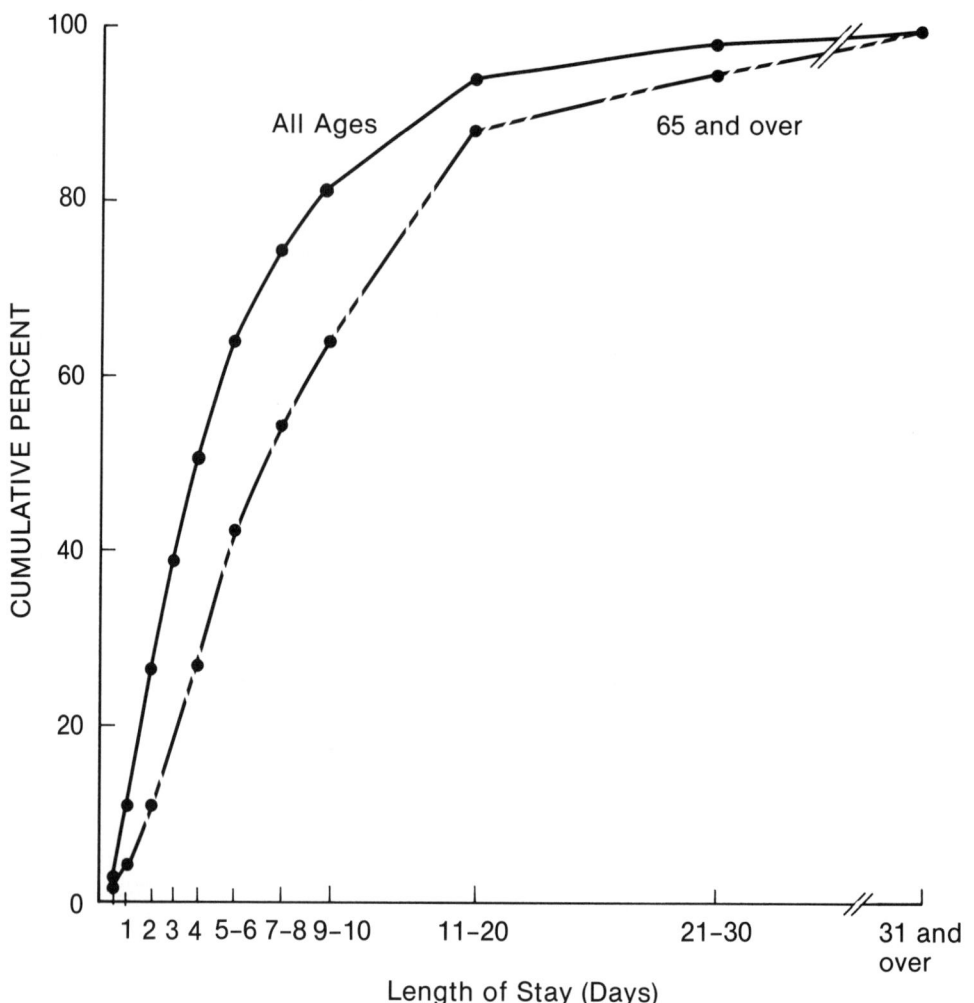

[1] Excludes newborn infants.

SOURCE: U.S. National Center for Health Statistics, *Utilization of Short-stay Hospitals: Annual Summary for the United States, 1977*, DHEW, Public Health Service, Office of Health Research, Statistics, and Technology, Hyattsville, Maryland, Series 13, No. 41, March 1979, Table 3, pp. 23-24.

Facilities

Chart F-19

Percent Distribution of Patients Discharged From, and Days Stayed in, Non-federal, Short-stay Hospitals, by Length of Stay (U.S.A., 1977).[1]

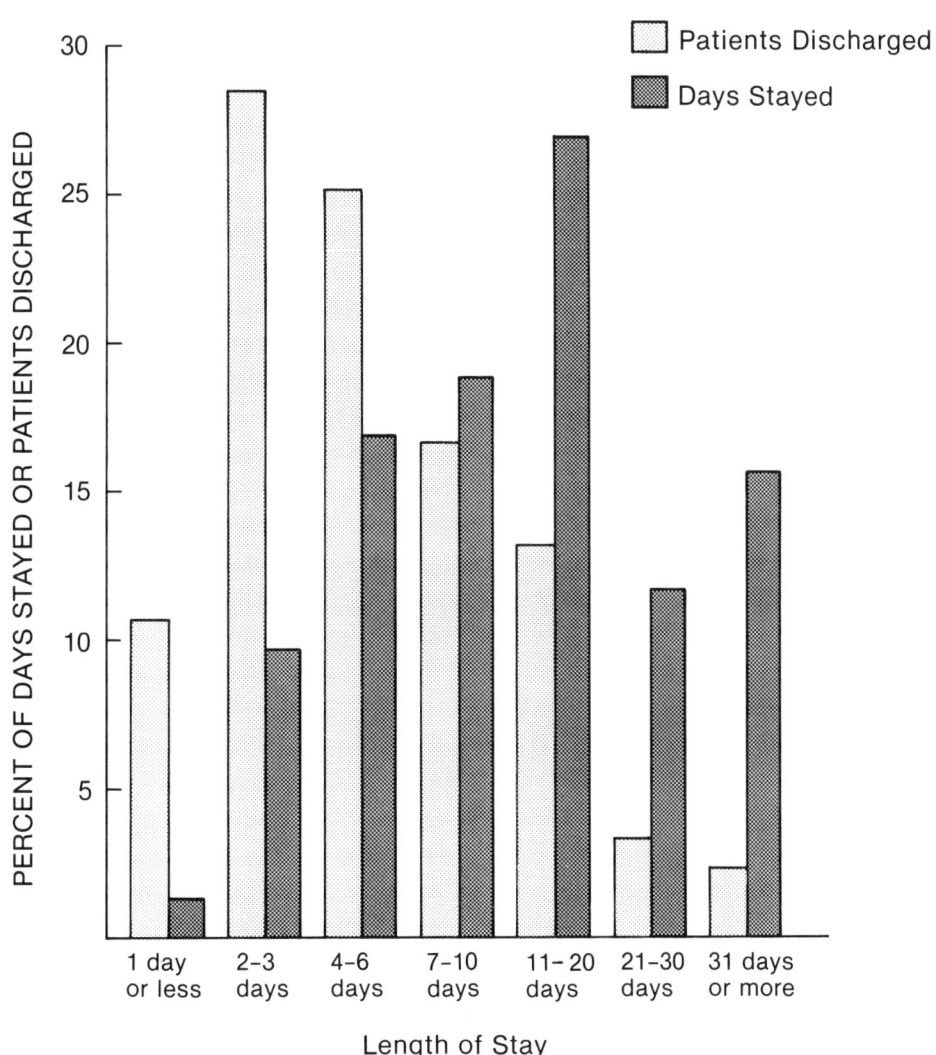

[1] Excludes newborn infants.

SOURCE: U.S. National Center for Health Statistics, *Utilization of Short-stay Hospitals: Annual Summary for the United States, 1977*, DHEW, Public Health Service, Office of Health Research, Statistics and Technology, Hyattsville, Maryland, Series 13, No. 41, March 1979, Table 3, p. 24.

Facilities

Medical Care Chartbook

Chart F-20 Relative Average Length of Stay, Number of Discharges per 1,000 Persons per Year, and Number of Days of Care per 1,000 Persons per Year, by Region (U.S.A., 1977).[1]

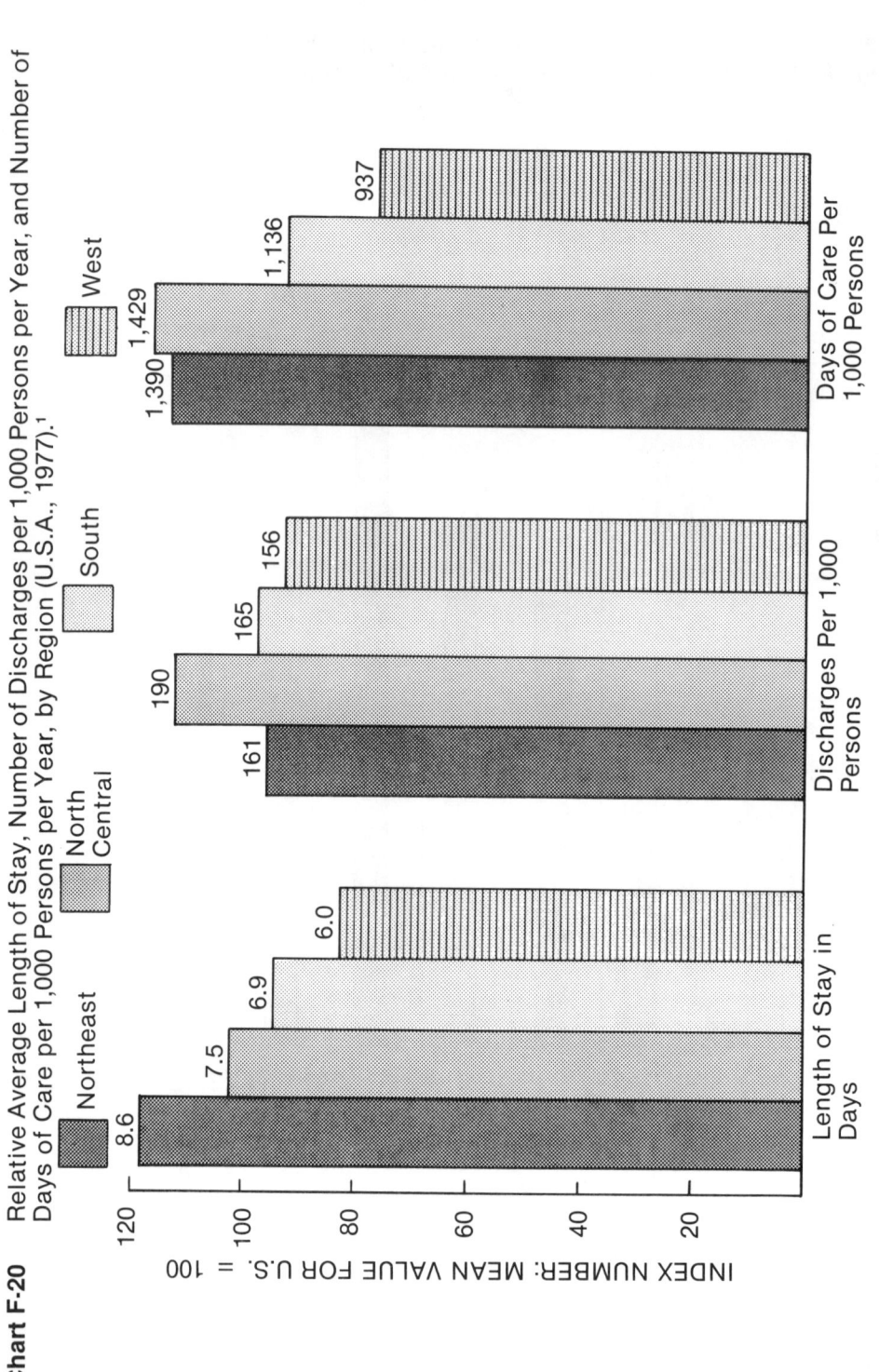

[1] All non-federal short-stay hospitals. Excludes newborn infants.

NOTE: Numbers above bars are actual values.

SOURCE: U.S. National Center for Health Statistics, *Utilization of Short-Stay Hospitals: Annual Summary for the United States, 1977*, DHEW, Public Health Service, Office of Health Research, Statistics, and Technology, Hyattsville, Maryland, Series 13, No. 41, March 1979, Table 8, p. 31 and Table 9, p. 32.

Facilities

Medical Care Chartbook

Chart F-21 Average Length of Stay for Selected Diagnoses, by Region (U.S.A., 1977).[1]

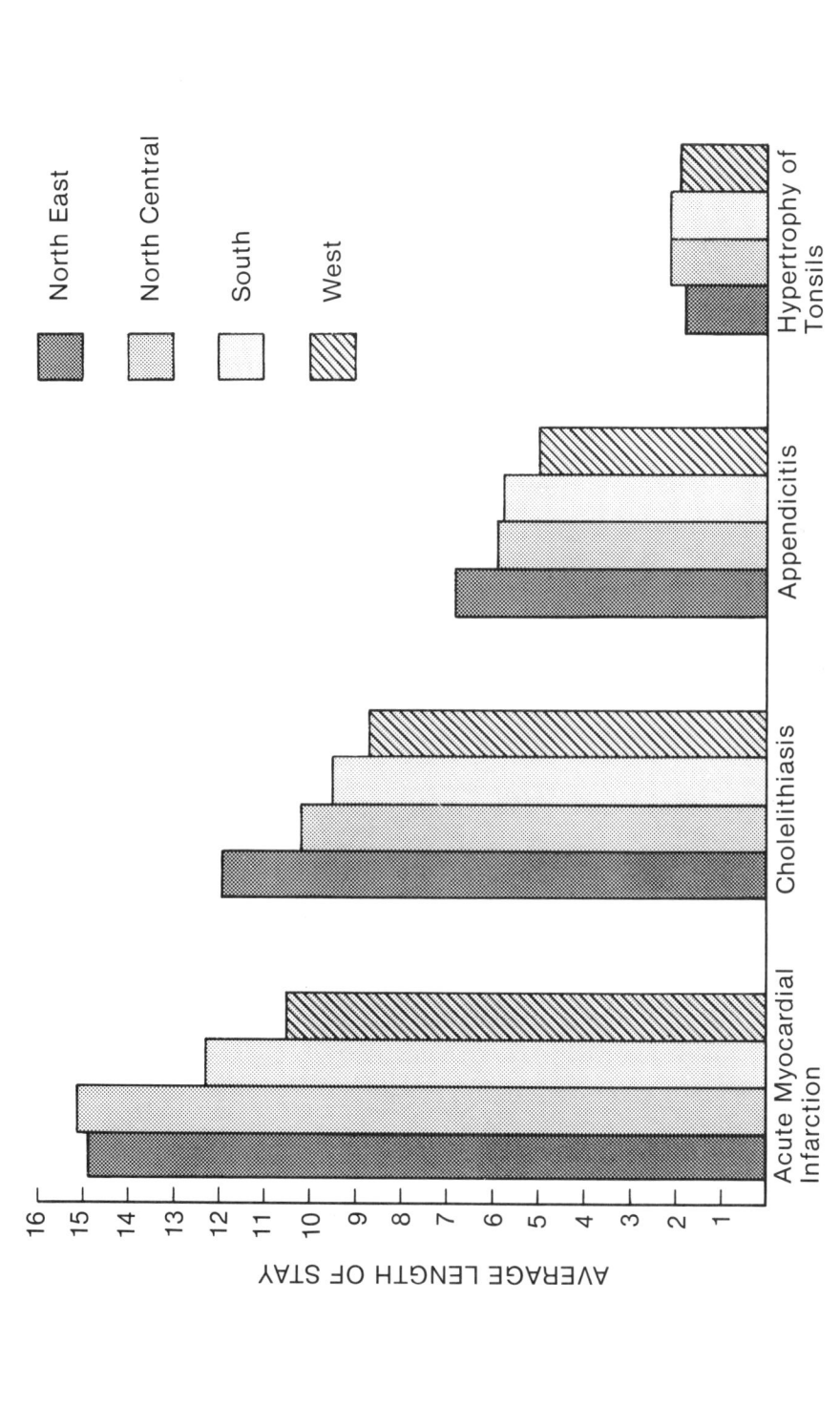

[1] Data are for non-federal short-stay hospitals.
SOURCE: U.S. National Center for Health Statistics, *Utilization of Short-Stay Hospitals: Annual Summary of the United States, 1977*, Public Health Service, Office of Health Research, Statistics, and Technology, Hyattsville, Maryland, Series 13, No. 41, March 1979, Table 15, p. 41.

Chart F-22 Percent of All Hospitals with Specified Characteristics (U.S.A., 1960 and 1978).[1]

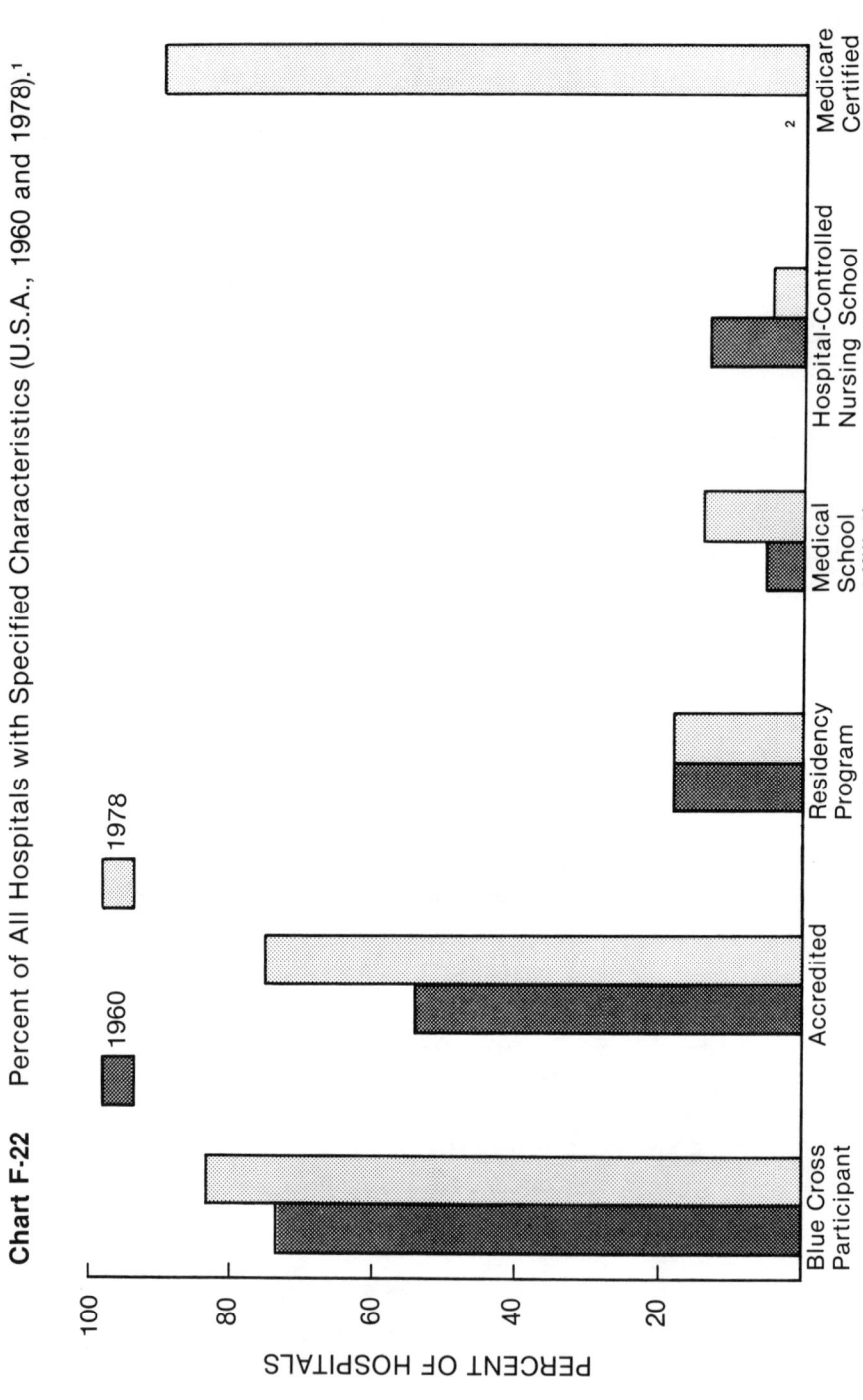

SOURCES: For 1960: "Hospitals," *Journal of the American Hospital Association*, Guide Issue, Vol. 35, Part 2, August 1961, Table 7, p. 430; for 1978: American Hospital Association, *Hospital Statistics, 1979*, Chicago, 1979, Table 10A, p. 186.

[1]Hospitals listed by the American Hospital Association.
[2]Not applicable.

Facilities

Medical Care Chartbook

Chart F-23 Percent of Hospitals that Have Specified Facilities and Services (U.S.A., 1950 and 1978).[1]

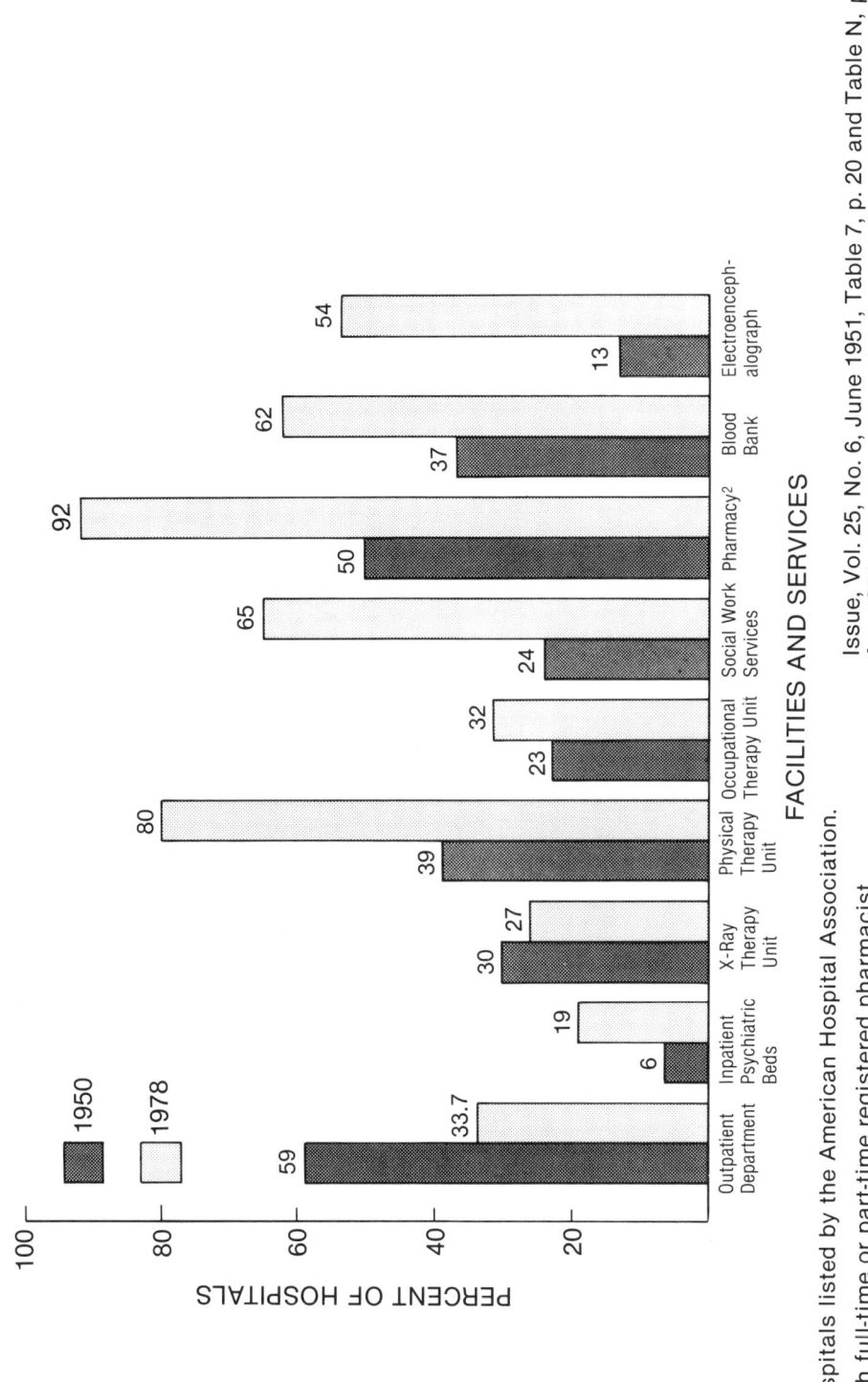

[1] Hospitals listed by the American Hospital Association.
[2] With full-time or part-time registered pharmacist.

SOURCES: For 1950: "Statistical Guide," *Hospitals*, Guide Issue, Vol. 25, No. 6, June 1951, Table 7, p. 20 and Table N, p. 32; for 1978: American Hospital Association, *Hospital Statistics, 1979*, Chicago, 1979, Table 12A, pp. 192-199.

Facilities

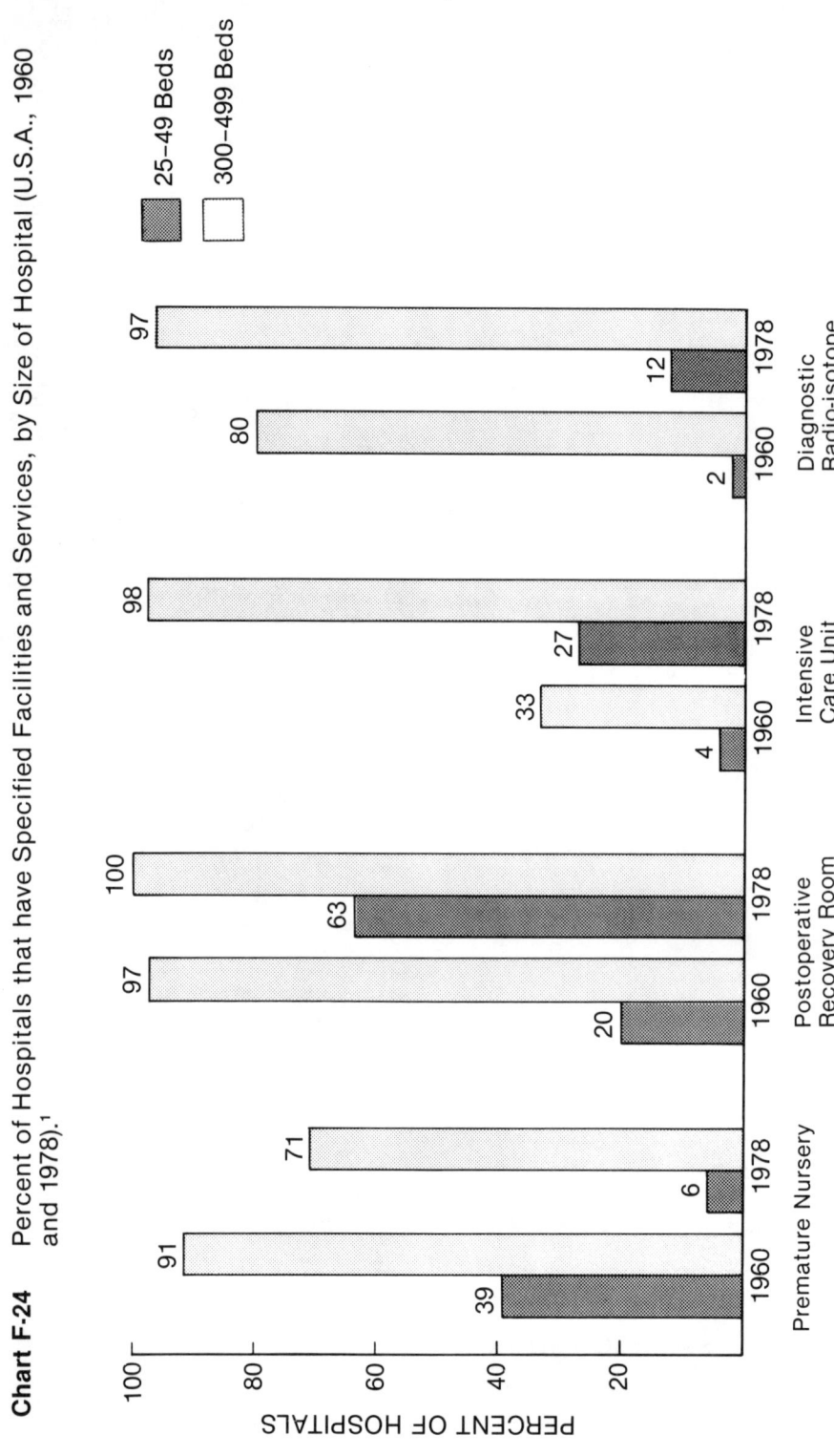

Chart F-24 Percent of Hospitals that have Specified Facilities and Services, by Size of Hospital (U.S.A., 1960 and 1978).[1]

[1]Includes non-federal short-term general and other special hospitals listed by the American Hospital Association.

SOURCES: For 1960: "Hospitals," *Journal of the American Hospital Association*, Guide Issue, Vol. 35, Part 2, August 1961, Table 5, pp. 424–427; for 1978: American Hospital Association, *Hospital Statistics, 1979*, Chicago, 1979, Table 12A, pp. 192–199.

Facilities

Chart F-25 Percent of All Hospitals and of All Non-federal Short-term General and Other Special Hospitals with Specified Facilities and Services (U.S.A., 1960 and 1978).[1]

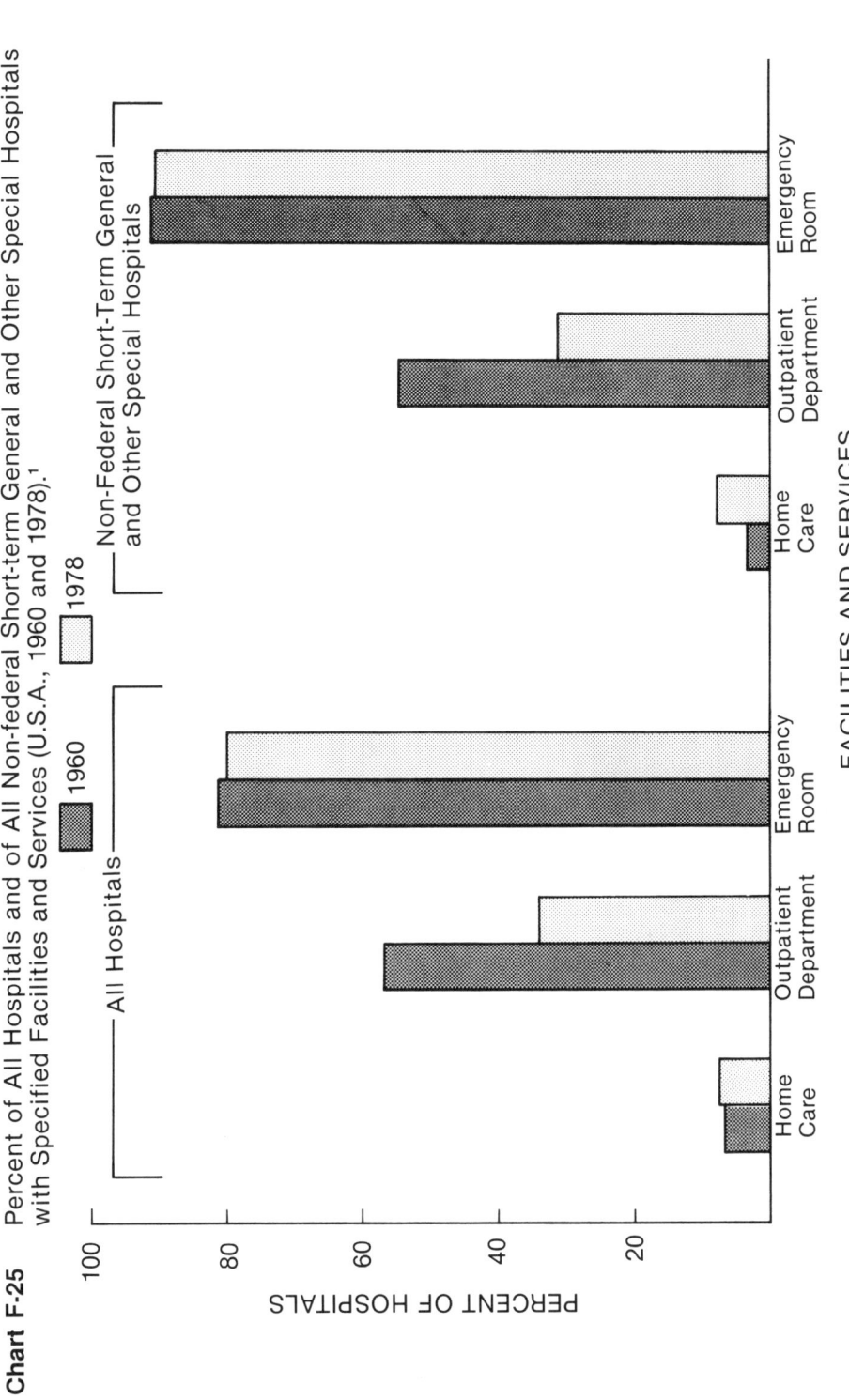

[1]Hospitals listed by the American Hospital Association.

SOURCES: For 1960: "Hospitals," *Journal of the American Hospital Association*, Guide Issue, Vol. 35, Part 2, August 1961, Table 5, pp. 424–427; for 1978: American Hospital Association, *Hospital Statistics, 1979*, Chicago, 1979, Table 12A, pp. 192–199.

Facilities

Chart F-26

Percent Increase in Use of Selected Hospital Services per Patient per Day[1] (U.S.A., 1946–1961).

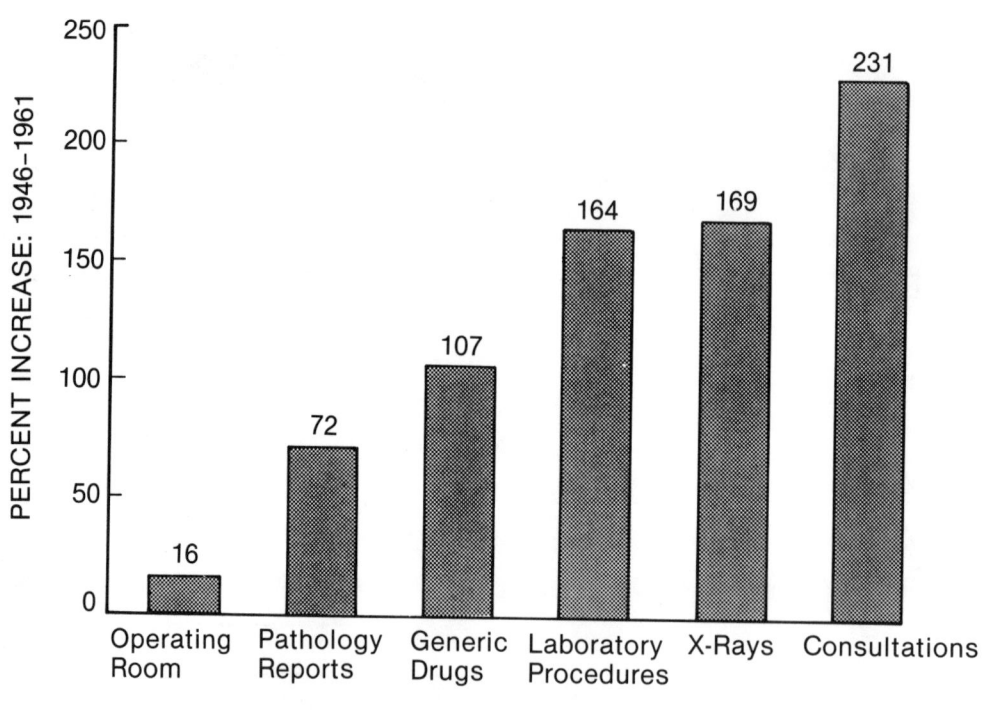

[1] Adjusted for length of stay using ratio of mean length of stay 1961/1946.

NOTE: Based on a nationwide sample of non-federal general, short-term hospitals.

SOURCE: Commission on the Cost of Medical Care, *The Cost of Medical Care, Vol. IV, Changing Patterns of Hospital Care,* American Medical Association, Chicago, 1964, Tables 21, 22, 23, 24, 25, 26, 27.

Facilities

Medical Care Chartbook

Chart F-27 Number of Selected Services Provided to Patients Hospitalized with Myocardial Infarction (U.S.A., 1939 and 1969).

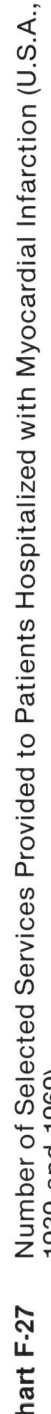

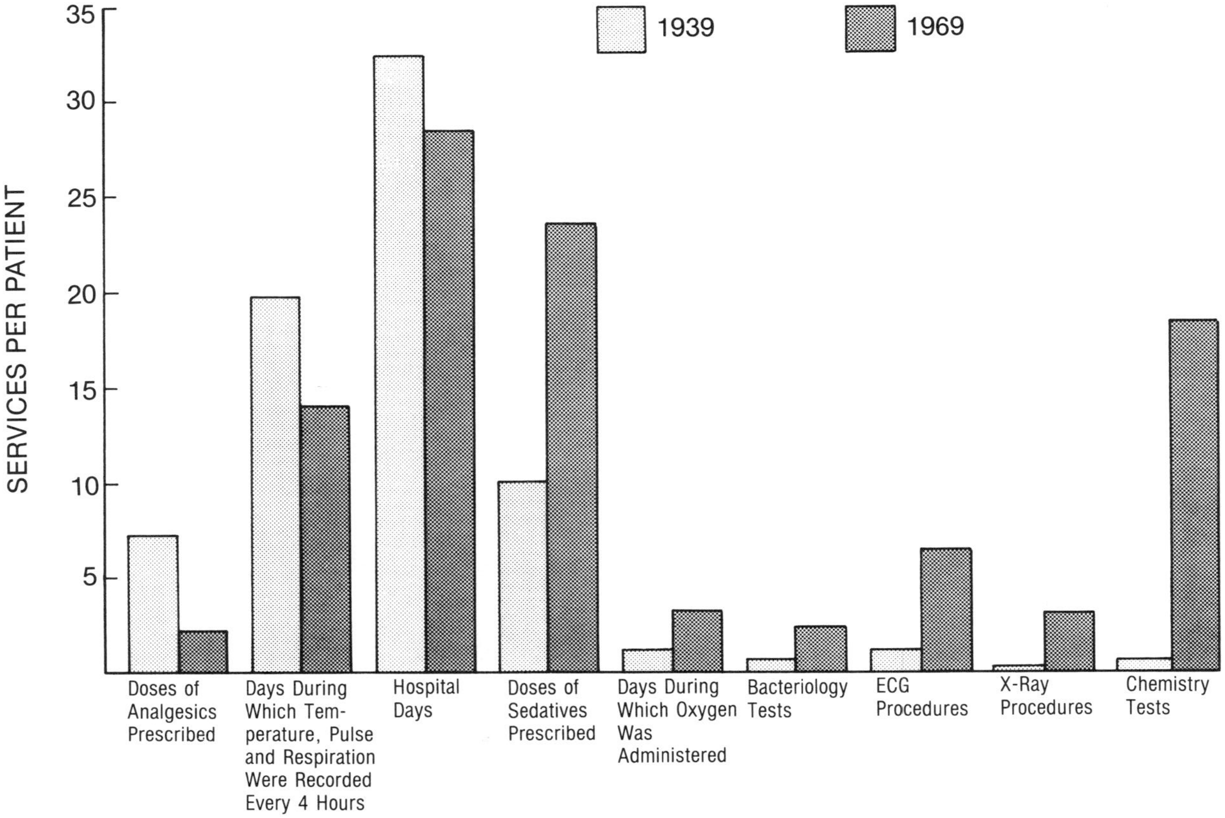

SOURCE: Martin, S.P., et al., "Inputs into Coronary Care During 30 Years," *Annals of Internal Medicine,* Vol. 81, No. 3, September 1974, Table 5, p. 292.

Facilities

Chart F-28 Charges per Patient Day by Type of Charge and Length of Stay, Medicare Patients[1] (U.S.A., and Outlying Areas, July 1, 1966–June 30, 1967).

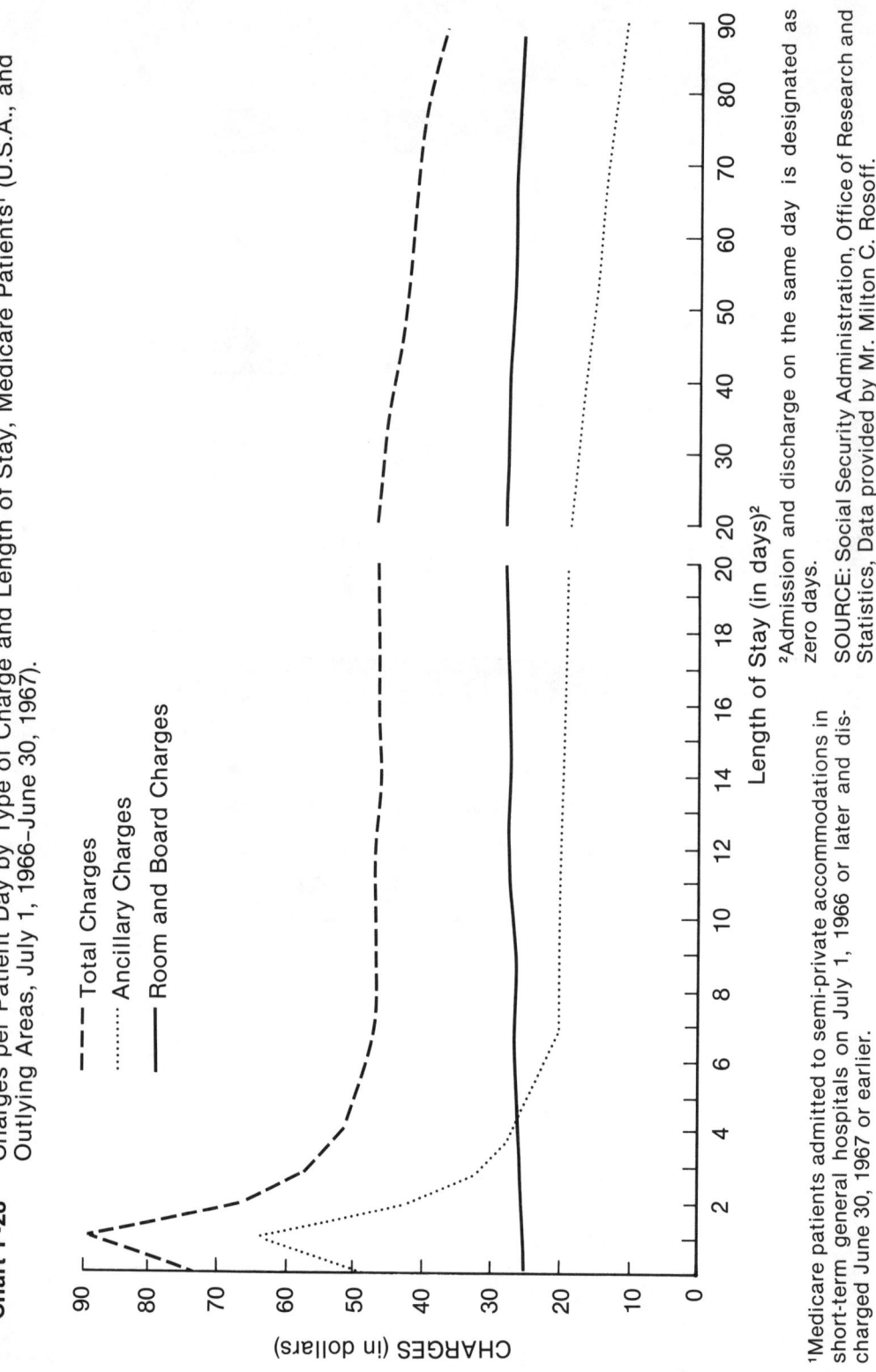

[1] Medicare patients admitted to semi-private accommodations in short-term general hospitals on July 1, 1966 or later and discharged June 30, 1967 or earlier.

[2] Admission and discharge on the same day is designated as zero days.

SOURCE: Social Security Administration, Office of Research and Statistics, Data provided by Mr. Milton C. Rosoff.

Facilities

Chart F-29

Hospital Personnel per 100 Patients, and Payroll Expenses per Patient Day, by Type of Hospital (U.S.A., 1946–1978).[1]

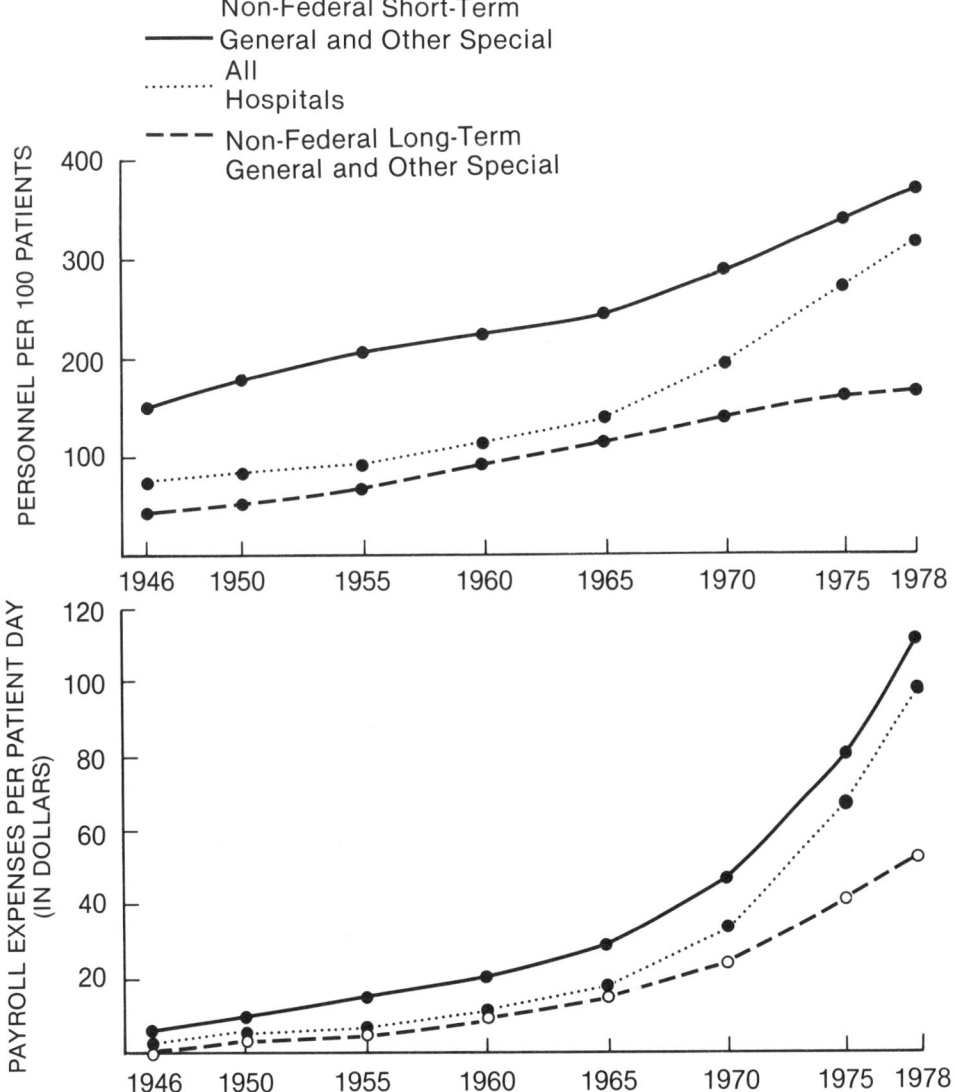

[1]Personnel data exclude residents, interns, and students from 1952 on. They include not only full-time personnel, but also, for 1954 and thereafter, full-time equivalents of part-time personnel. The hospitals included are those listed by the American Hospital Association.

SOURCES: For 1946–1970: "Hospitals," *Journal of the American Hospital Association*, Guide Issue, Vol. 45, No. 15, Part 2, August 1, 1971, Table 1, pp. 460–462; for 1975–1978: American Hospital Association, *Hospital Statistics, 1979*, Chicago, 1979, Table 1, pp. 4–7.

Facilities

Chart F-30

Percent Distribution of Judgments[1] Concerning Level of Care Required by Patients in Seven Hospitals (Monroe County, New York, March 13–April 30, 1961).

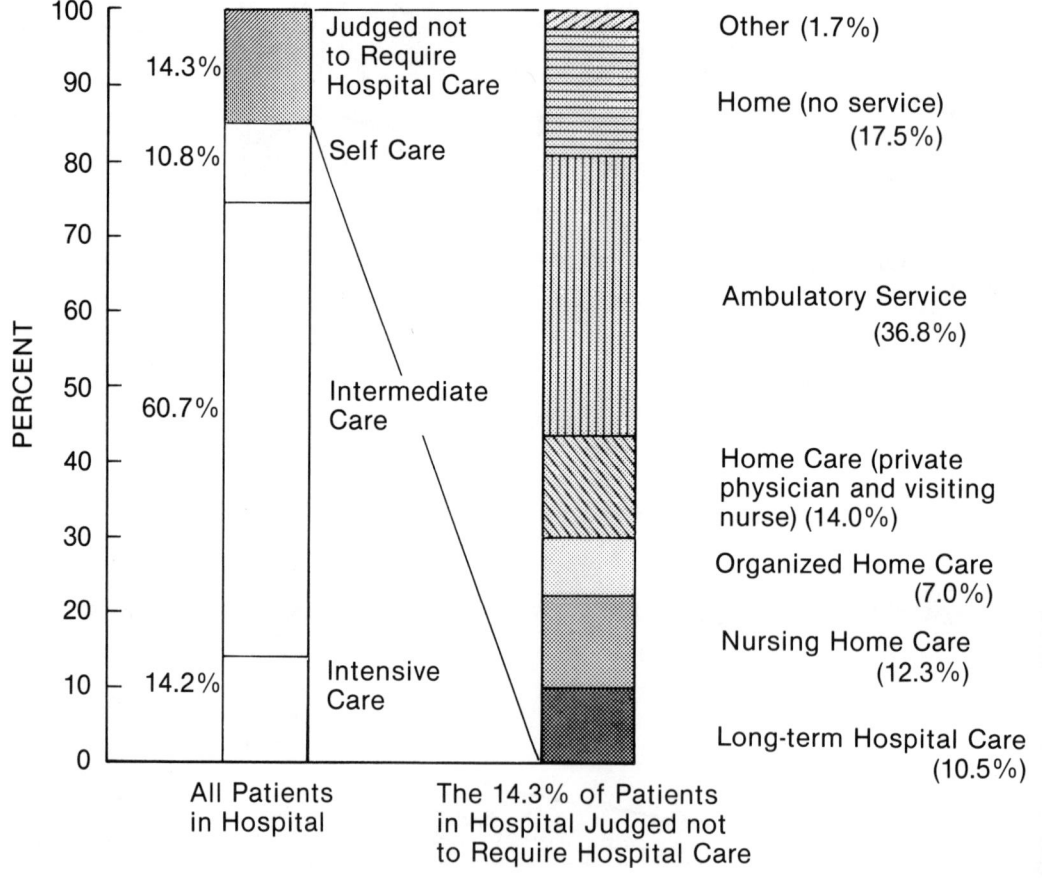

[1]Made by a team of local physicians.

SOURCE: Berg, R.L., et. al, "Bed Utilization Studies for Community Planning," *Journal of the American Medical Association,* Vol. 207, March 31, 1969, Tables 1, 2 and 3, pp. 2411–2413.

Facilities

Chart F-31 Percent Distribution of Patients Hospitalized in Medical-Surgical Beds, by Appropriateness of Hospitalization and Distribution of Suggested Alternative Levels of Care for Those Inappropriately Hospitalized (Onondaga County, New York, 1967).

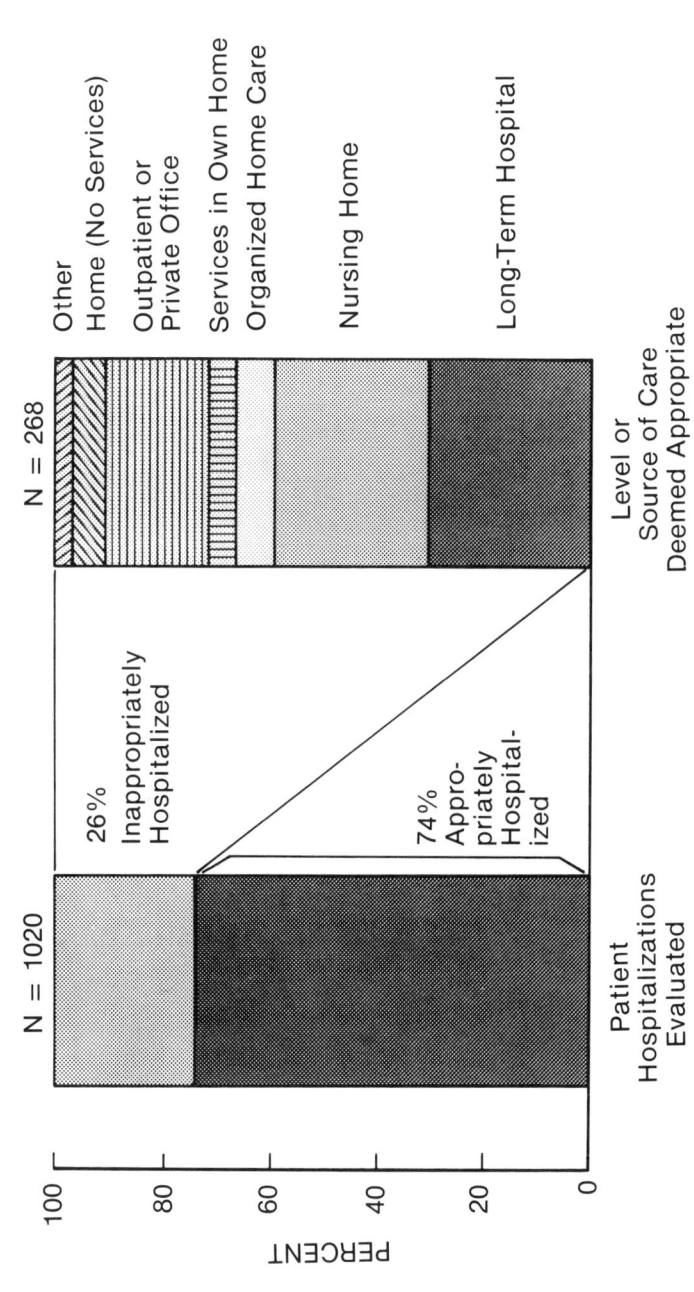

SOURCE: Shelton, D.S., R.H. Schlesinger, H.W. Fibiger, "Bed Utilization—A Community Study," *Hospital Management*, Vol. 105, June 1968, Table 1, p. 47.

Chart F-32

Emergency Visits, Outpatient Visits, and Hospital Admissions for Non-federal Short-term General and Other Special Hospitals per 100 Persons (U.S.A., 1955 and 1978).[1]

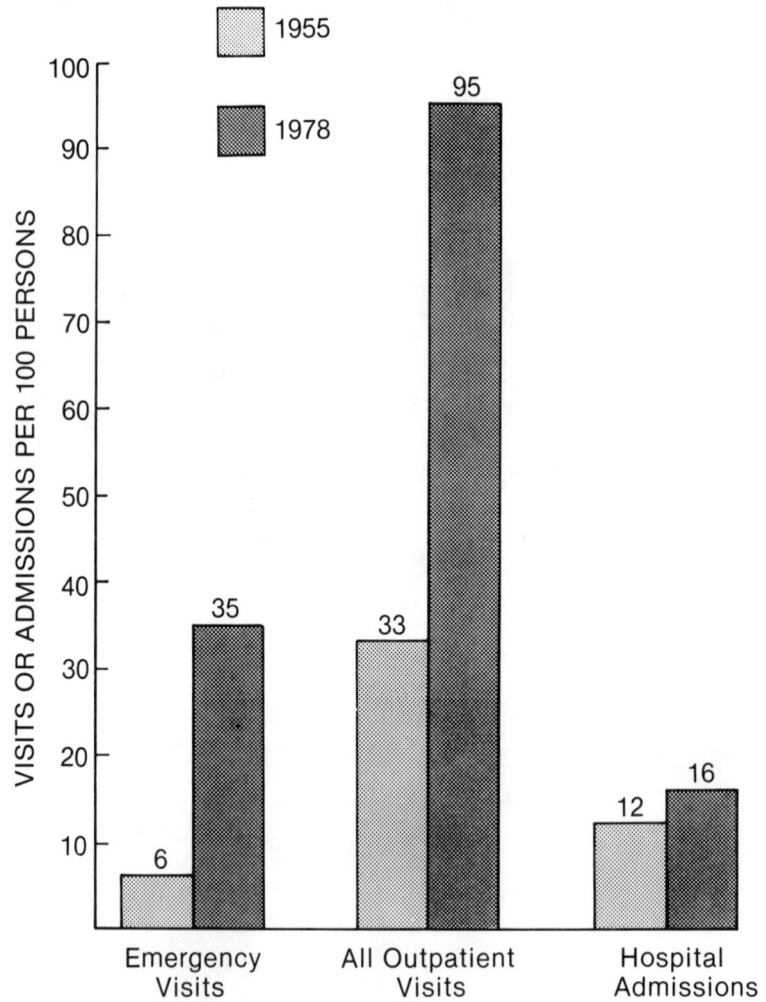

[1] "All outpatient visits" include emergency visits. Data are for hospitals listed by the American Hospital Association.

SOURCES: For 1955: "Hospitals," *Journal of the American Hospital Association*, Guide Issue, Part 2, August 1, 1956, Table 1, p. 14 and Table 17, p. 62; for 1978: American Hospital Association, *Hospital Statistics, 1979*, Chicago, 1979, Table 5A, p. 20.

Facilities

Chart F-33

Percent Distribution of Patients' Primary Reason for Visit to Hospital Emergency Service (Michigan, 1965).[1]

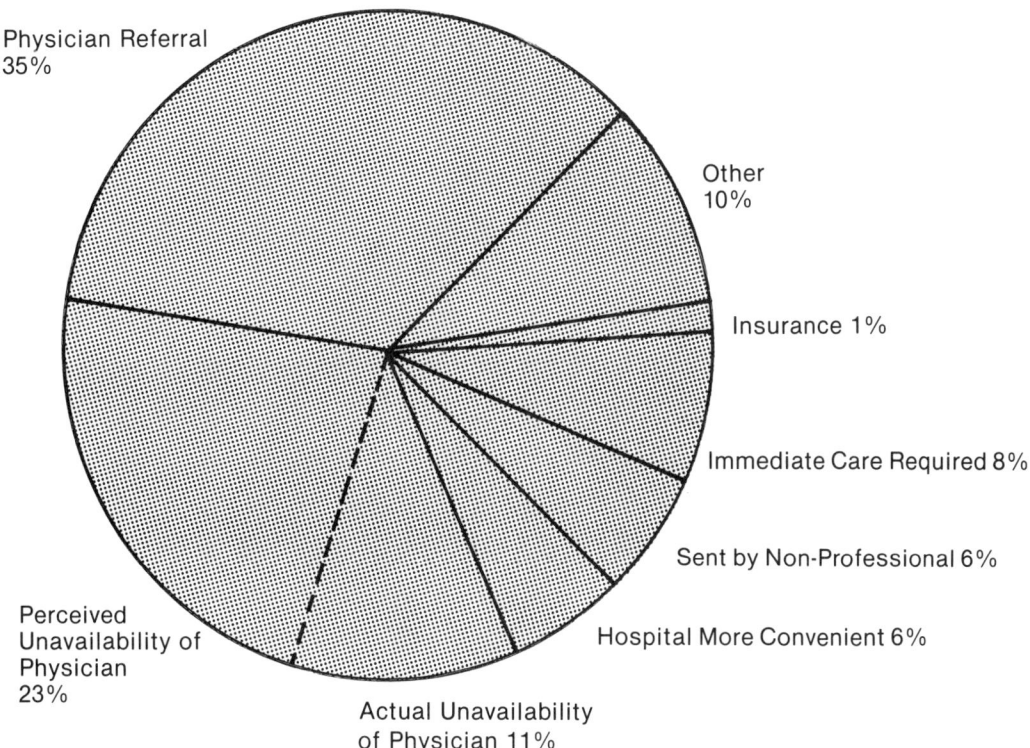

[1] Based on a sample of emergency room care in 22 hospitals during a seven day period in January, 1965.

SOURCE: Vaughan, H. and C. Gamester, "Hospital Emergency Room Utilization in Michigan," *Inquiry,* Vol. 3, May 1966, Table 5, p. 45.

Chart F-34

Emergency Visits, by Type of Visit and Source of Payment (Boston, 1972).

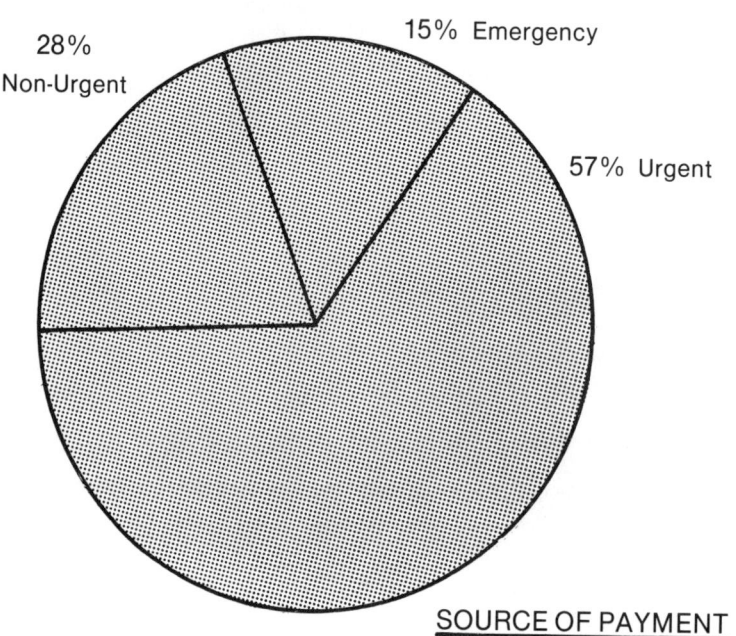

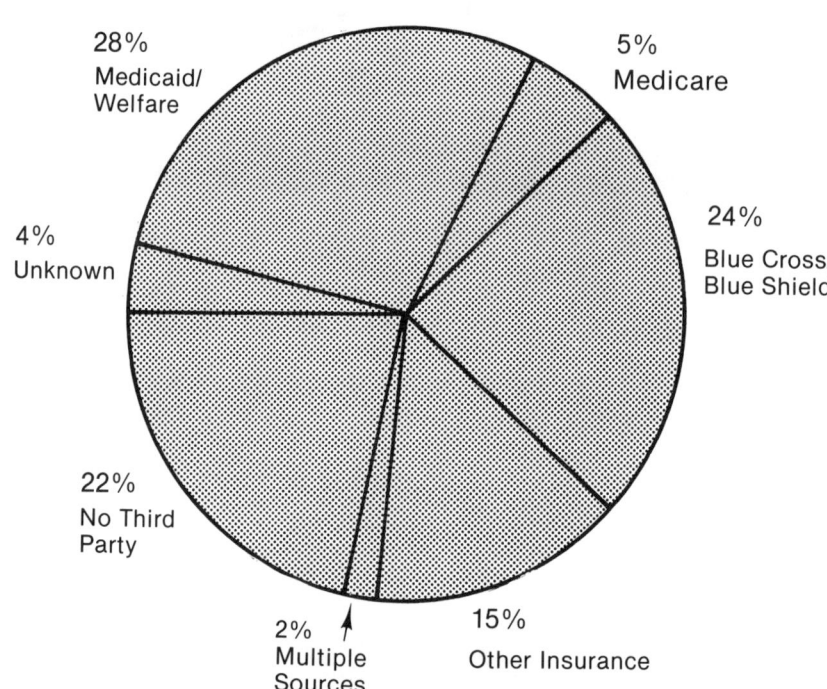

SOURCE: Kleinman, J.C., et al., "Planning for Emergency Medical Services in Boston," *Public Health Reports,* Vol. 90, No. 5, September–October 1975, Tables 1 and 2, p. 463.

Chart F-35 Number and Percent Distribution of Patients Admitted to Emergency Service and Seen in Triage, and Disposition of Patients Seen in Triage (Yale-New Haven Medical Center, 1963).

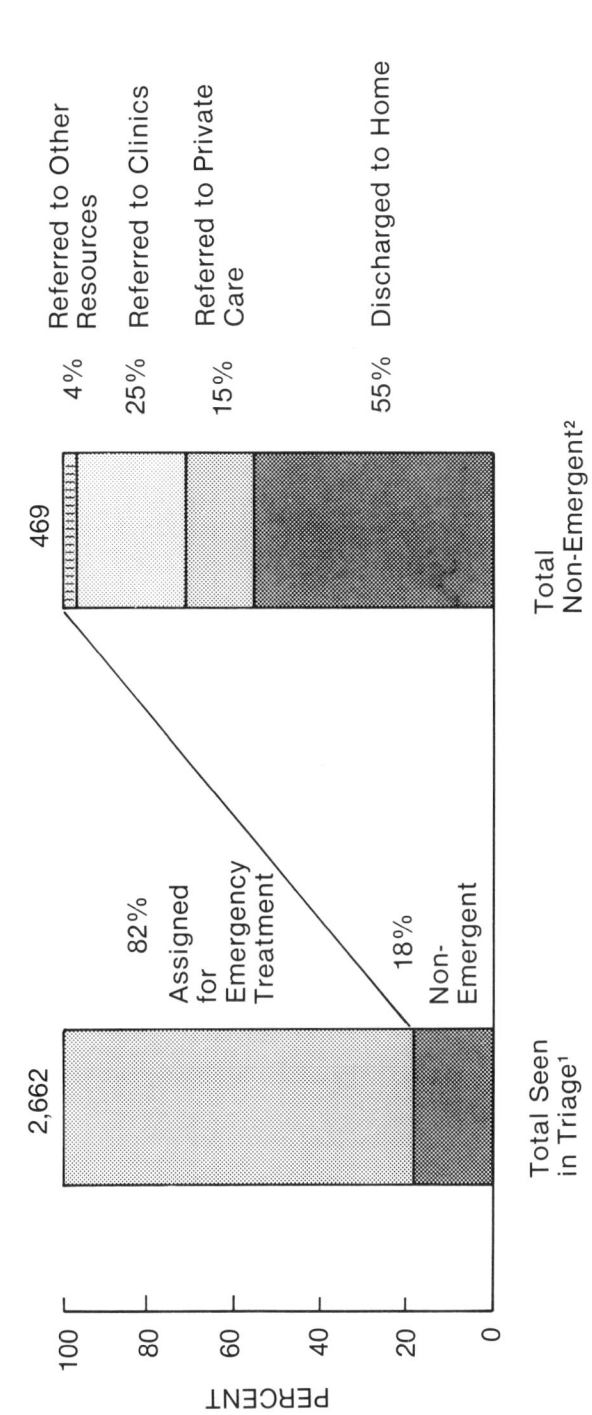

[1] The triage program operated only from 10 a.m. to 10 p.m. The total admissions to emergency service were 3,743, of which 1,081 were not seen in triage.

[2] The categories of non-emergent admissions represented the following percents of the total seen in triage: discharged to home—10%; referred to private care—3%; referred to clinics—4%; referred to other resources—1%.

SOURCE: Weinerman, E.R., S.R. Rutzen, and D.A. Pearson, "Effects of Medical 'Triage' in Hospital Emergency Service," *Public Health Reports*, Vol. 80, May 1965, Table 5, p. 393.

Chart F-36 Percent of Emergency Department Patients Not Needing Emergency Treatment by Selected Patient and Visit Characteristics (Buffalo, New York, 1972).

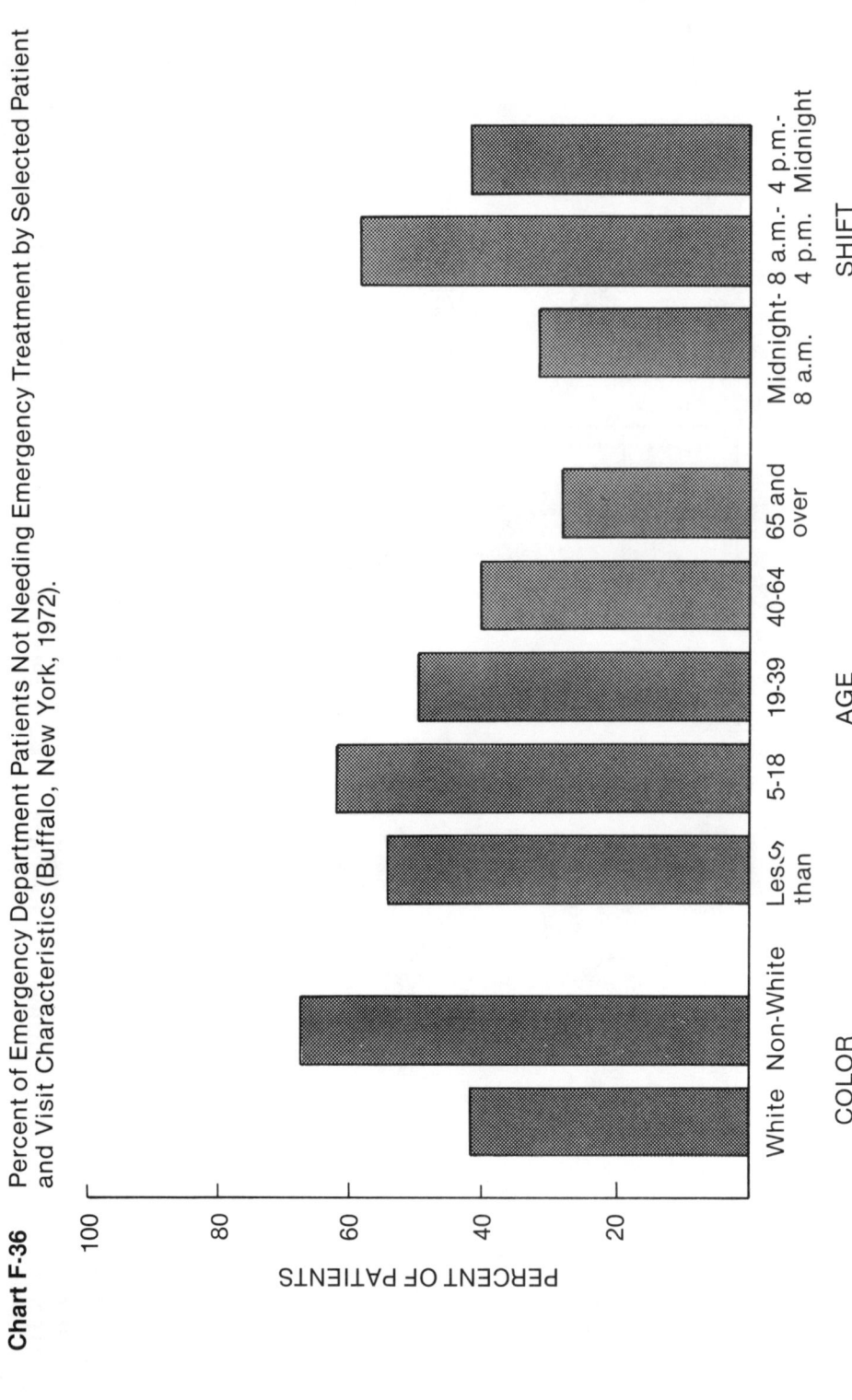

SOURCE: Gibson, Geoffrey, "Categorization of Hospital Emergency Capabilities—Some Empirical Methods to Evaluate Appropriateness of Emergency Department Utilization," *The Journal of Trauma*, Vol. 18, No. 2, February 1978, Table IX, p. 99.

Chart F-37 Percent Hospital Emergency Facilities that Meet Specified Criteria, by Hospital Size (New Jersey, 1973).

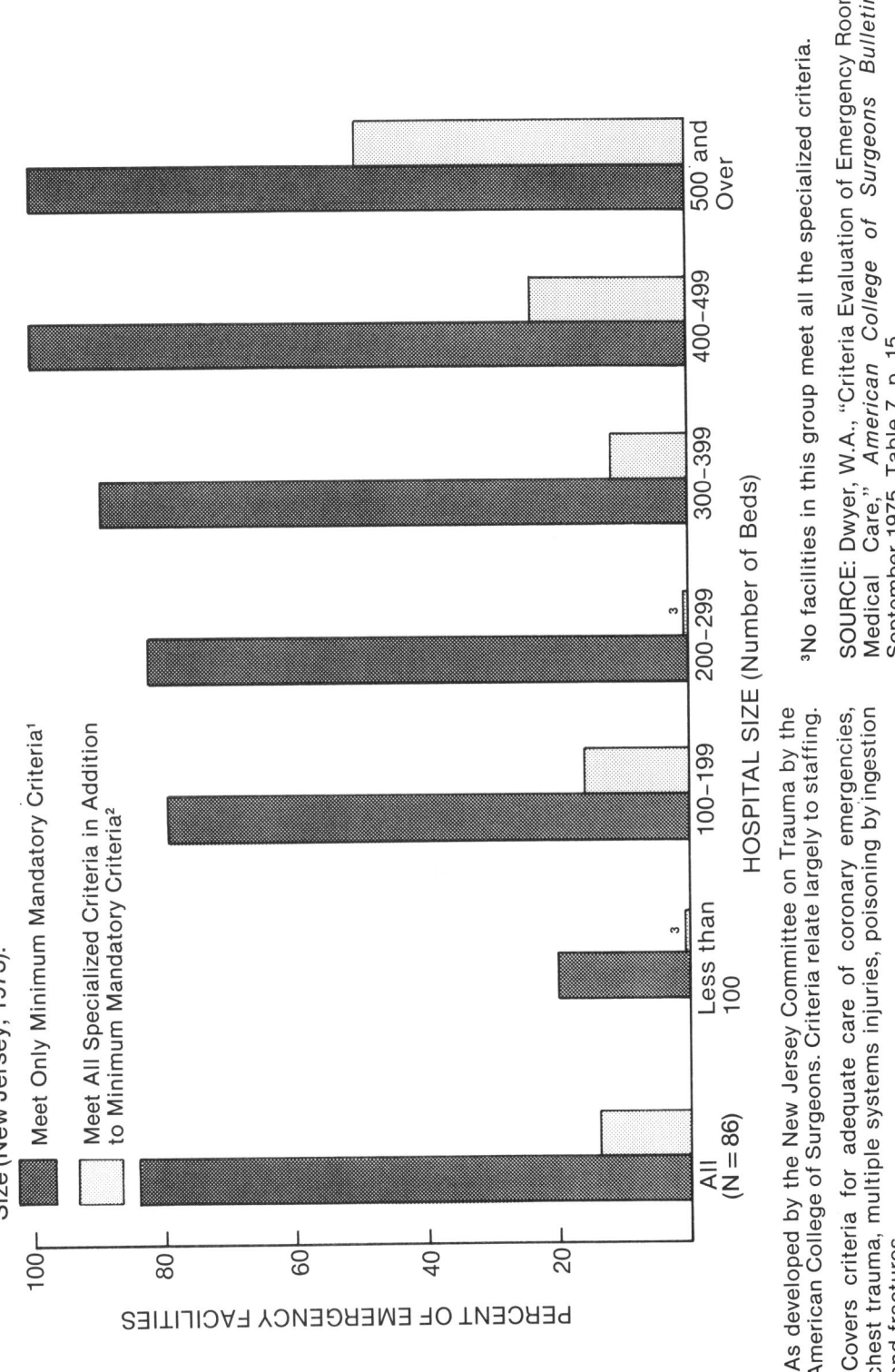

[1] As developed by the New Jersey Committee on Trauma by the American College of Surgeons. Criteria relate largely to staffing.

[2] Covers criteria for adequate care of coronary emergencies, chest trauma, multiple systems injuries, poisoning by ingestion and fractures.

[3] No facilities in this group meet all the specialized criteria.

SOURCE: Dwyer, W.A., "Criteria Evaluation of Emergency Room Medical Care," *American College of Surgeons Bulletin*, September 1975, Table 7, p. 15.

Chart F-38

Percent of Patients of Emergency Departments by the Appropriateness of Match Between the Clinical Need of the Patient and the Type of Facility (Buffalo, New York, 1972).

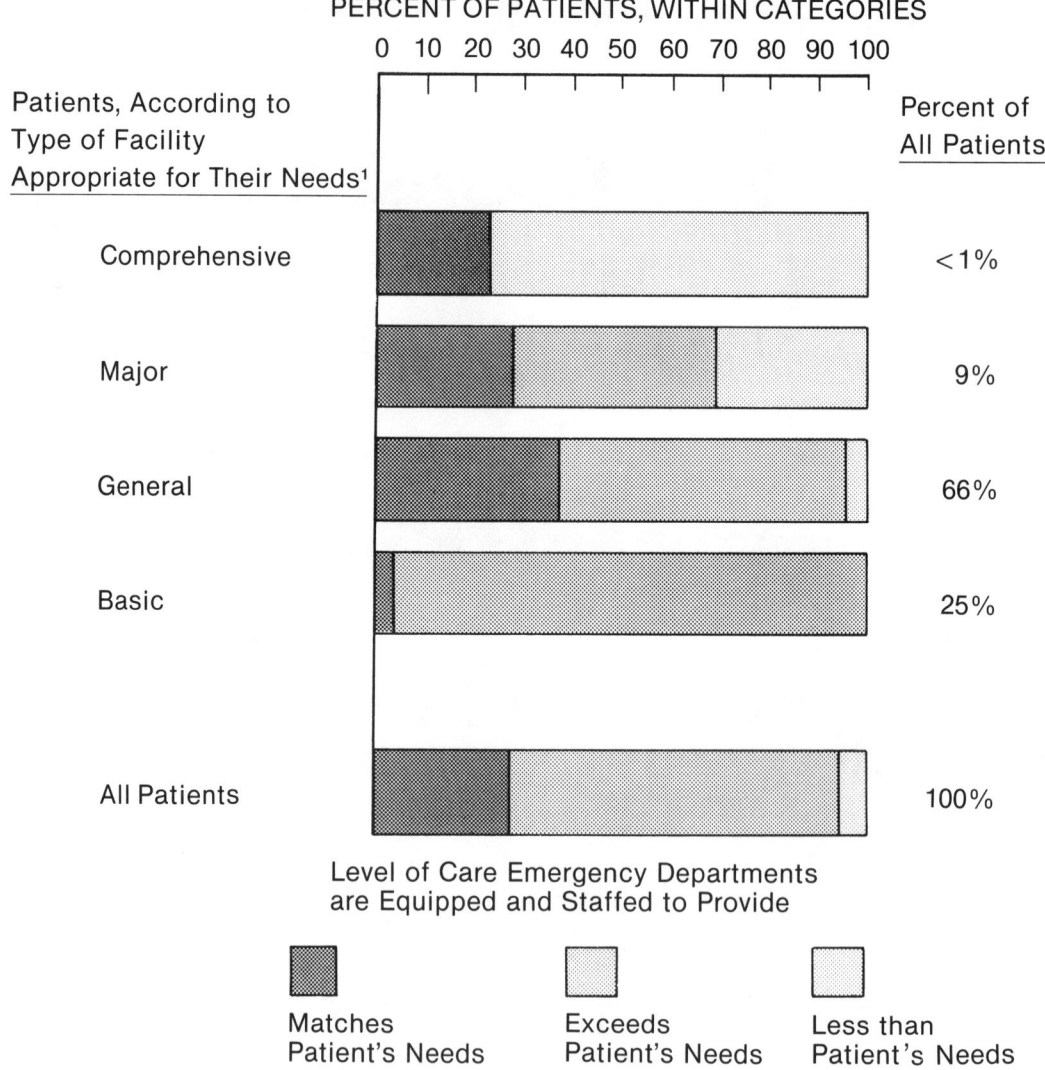

[1] Based on 24,212 emergency patients whose clinical needs were determined by an experienced trauma nurse on the basis of the medical record. Facility requirements are in terms of the four-stage A.M.A. categorization of emergency departments.

SOURCE: Gibson, G., *Measures of Appropriateness of Hospital Emergency Department Utilization,* Paper presented at A.P.H.A. meeting, San Francisco, November 1973, Tables 3 and 5, p. 10.

Facilities

Chart F-39

Percent Distribution of Patients of Emergency Departments, By the Appropriateness of Match Between the Clinical Need of the Patient and the Type of Facility, and by the Patient's Insurance Coverage
(Buffalo, New York, 1972).

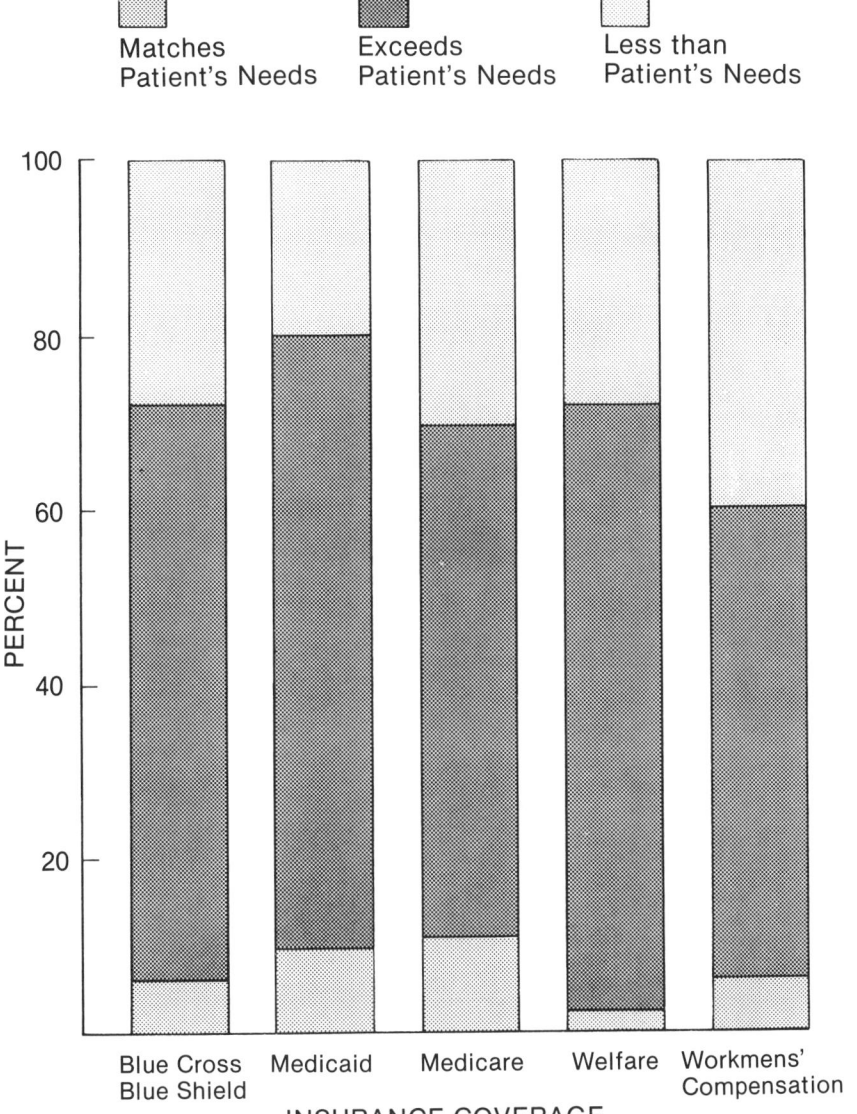

SOURCE: Gibson, Geoffrey, "Categorization of Hospital Emergency Capabilities — Some Empirical Methods to Evaluate Appropriateness of Emergency Department Utilization," *The Journal of Trauma*, Vol. 18, No. 2, February 1978, Table VI, p. 98.

Chart F-40

Percent Distribution of Emergency Departments, by Types of Physician Staffing Patterns (Connecticut, 1966 and 1971).

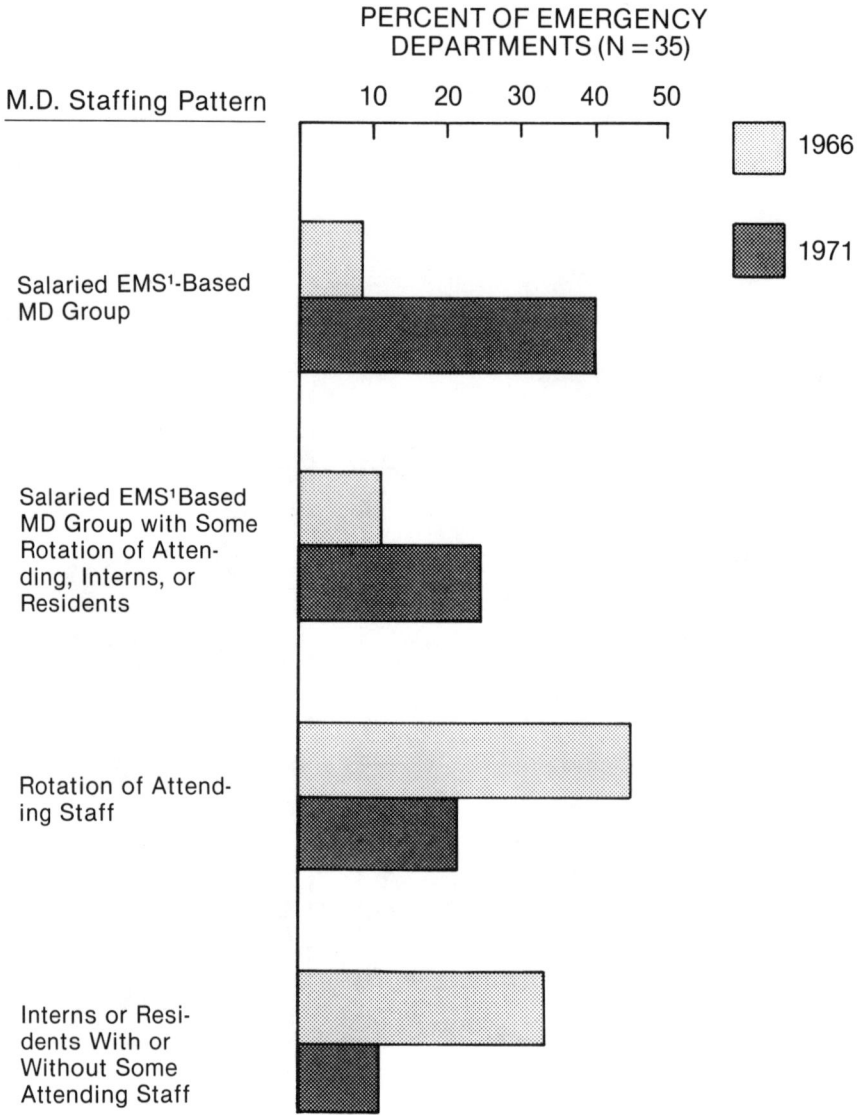

[1] Emergency Medical Service.
SOURCE: Fenhagen, H.P., et al., "Emergency Medical Services and the Hospital: A State-wide Analysis, Part III: Physician Staffing of Hospital Emergency Departments," *Hospital Administration,* Vol. 18, No. 4, Fall 1973, Table 1, p. 95.

Facilities

Medical Care Chartbook 237

Chart F-41 Relative and Actual Number of Nursing Care Homes[1] and Beds (U.S.A., Selected Years, 1963–1976).

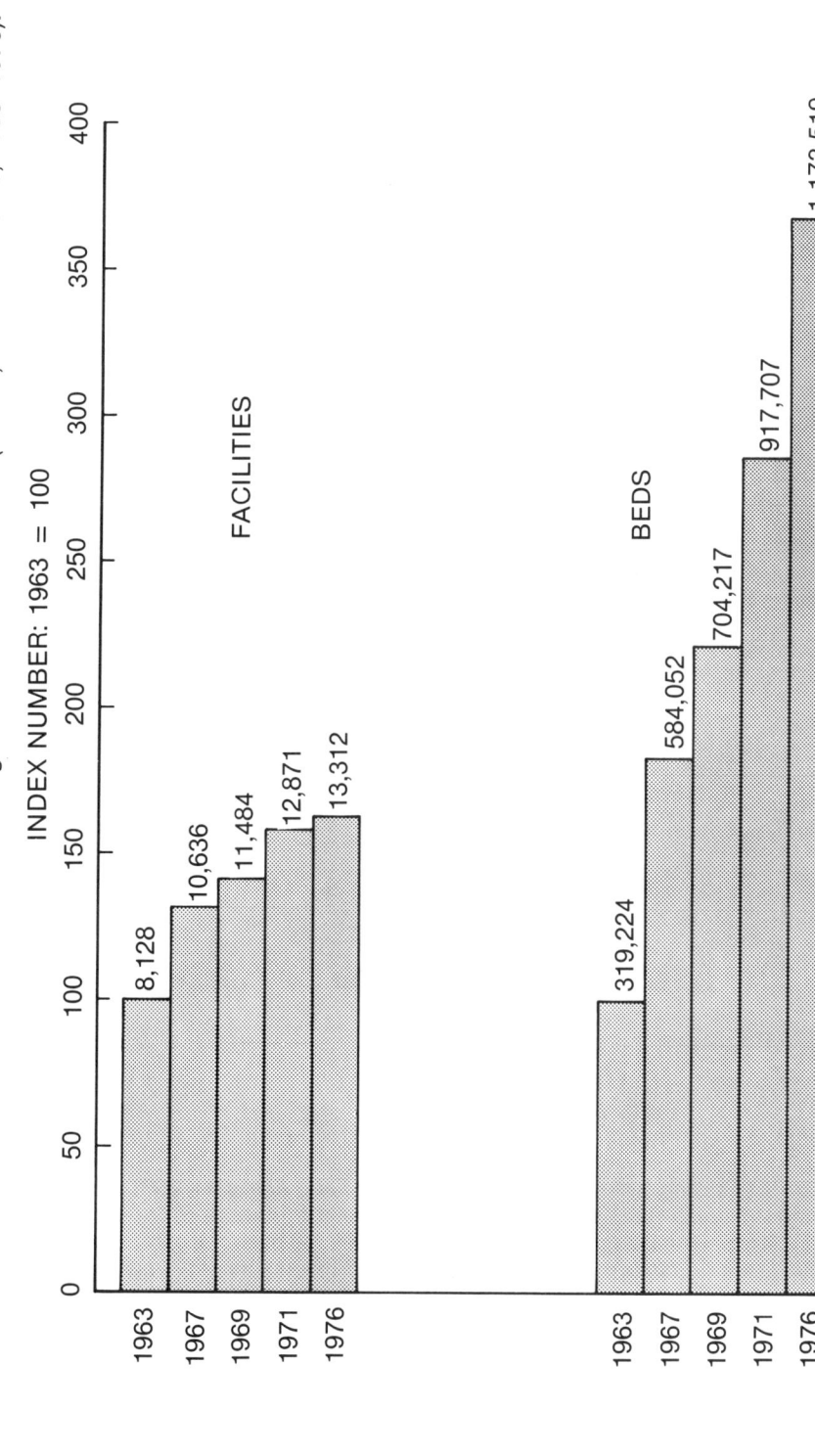

[1] Homes in which at least 50 percent of the residents received one or more nursing services, and where at least one registered nurse or licensed practical nurse was employed 35 hours or more per week.

SOURCES: For 1963, 1969, and 1971: U.S. National Center for Health Statistics, *Health Resources Statistics, 1974*, DHEW, Public Health Service, Rockville, Maryland, 1974, Table 217, p. 383; for 1967 and 1976: U.S. National Center for Health Statistics, *Health Resources Statistics, 1976–1977*, DHEW, Public Health Service, Hyattsville, Maryland, 1979, Table 226, p. 329.

Chart F-42

Percent Distribution of Nursing Care and Related Homes and Beds, by Type of Care (U.S.A., 1976).

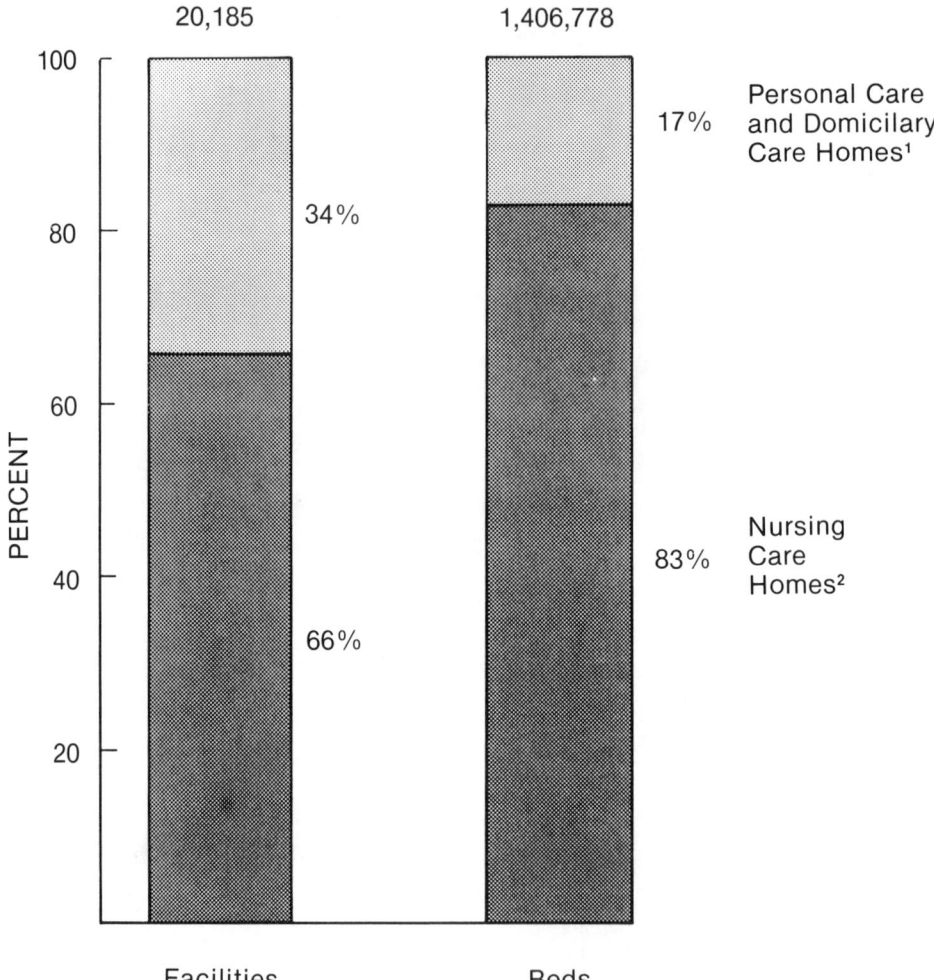

[1]Includes (1) personal care homes *with* nursing, in which either (a) some of the residents but less than 50 percent receive nursing care or (b) more than 50 percent of the residents receive nursing care, but no RNs or LPNs are employed full-time on the staff; (2) personal care homes *without* nursing, in which the facility routinely provides three or more personal services but no nursing service; and (3) domiciliary care homes in which the facility has as its primary function to provide room and board, while also having responsibility for providing some personal care services.

[2]In nursing care homes at least 50 percent of the residents receive one or more nursing services, and at least one registered nurse or licenses practical nurse is employed 35 hours or more per week.

SOURCE: U.S. National Center for Health Statistics, *Health Resources Statistics, 1976-77*, DHEW, Public Health Service, Office of Health Research, Statistics, and Technology, Hyattsville, Maryland, 1979, Table 226, p. 329.

Facilities

Chart F-43

Number of Nursing Care Home Beds[1] per 1000 Civilian Population Age 65 and Over, by Geographic Regions and Selected States (U.S.A., 1976).

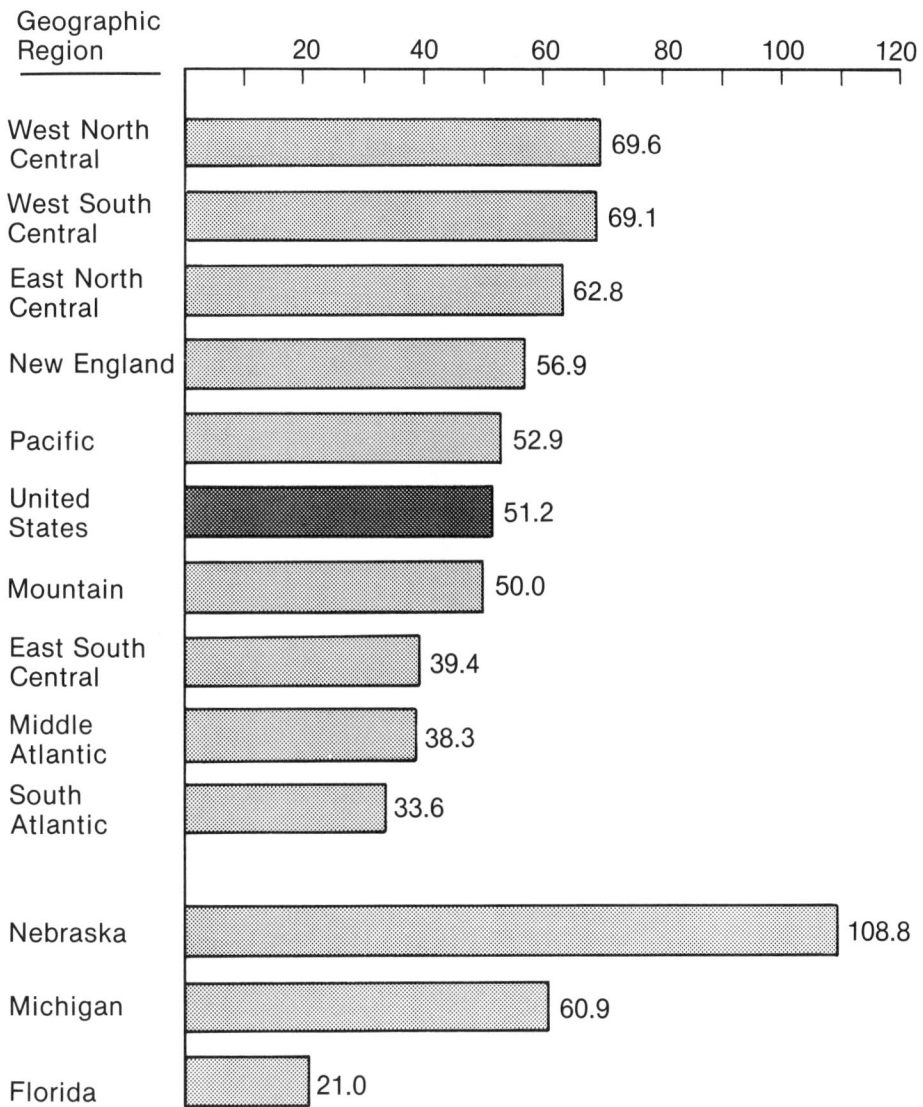

[1]Homes in which at least 50 percent of the residents received one or more nursing services, and where at least one registered nurse or licensed practical nurse was employed 35 hours or more per week.

SOURCE: U.S. National Center for Health Statistics, *Health Resources Statistics*, 1976-77, DHEW, Public Health Service, Office of Health Research, Statistics, and Technology, Hyattsville, Maryland, 1979, Table 231, p. 333 and Table 232, p. 334.

Facilities

Chart F-44

Percent Distribution of Facilities and Beds for Nursing Homes[1] and Hospitals,[2] by Type of Control (U.S.A., 1977).

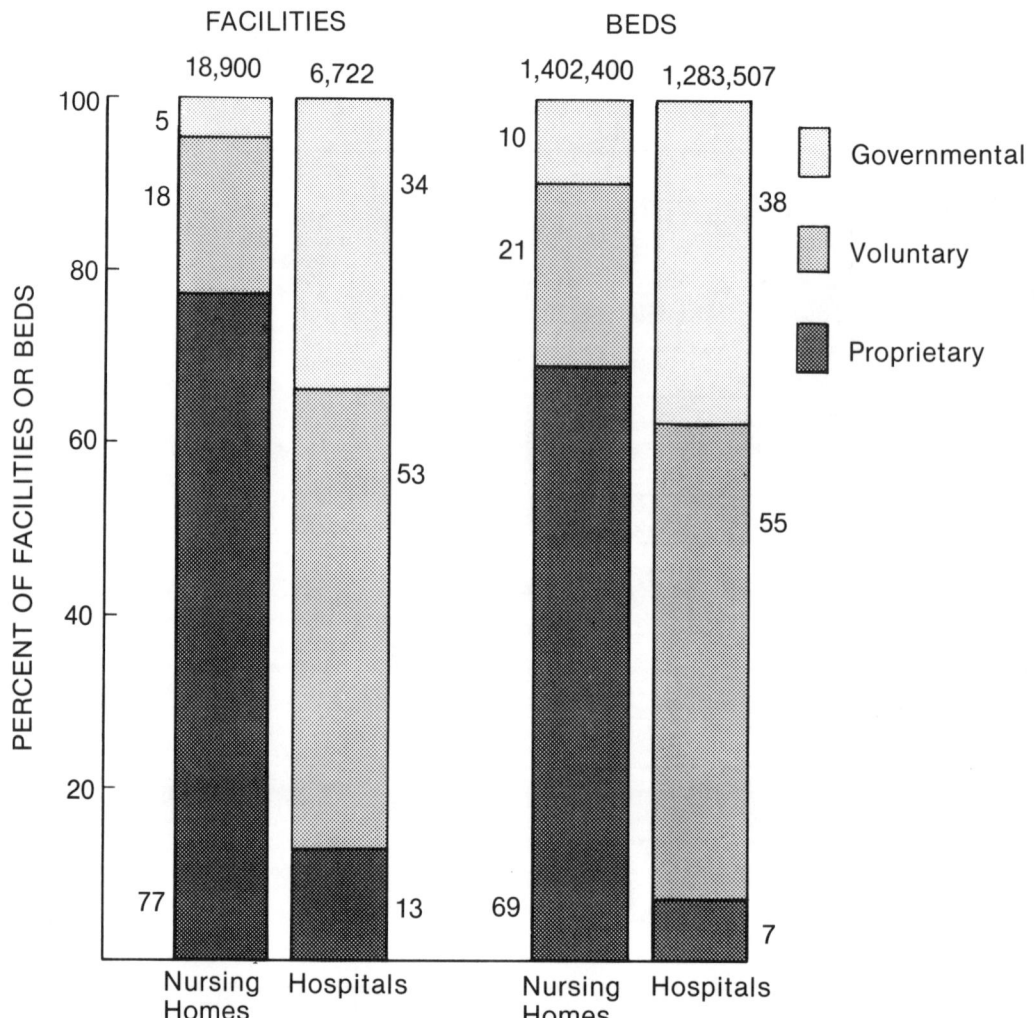

[1] A nursing care home is one in which at least 50 percent of the residents receive one or more nursing services, and where at least one registered nurse or licensed practical nurse is employed 35 hours or more per week.

[2] Listed by the American Hospital Association.

SOURCES: For nursing homes: U.S. National Center for Health Statistics, *The National Nursing Home Survey: 1977 Summary for the United States*, DHEW, Public Health Service, Office of Health Research, Statistics, and Technology, Hyattsville, Maryland, Series 13, No. 43, July 1979, Table 1, p. 8; for hospitals: American Hospital Association, *Hospital Statistics, 1978 Edition*, Chicago, 1978, Table 3, p. 12.

Facilities

Chart F-45

Percent Distribution of Nursing Homes and Beds, by Size of Nursing Home (U.S.A., 1977).

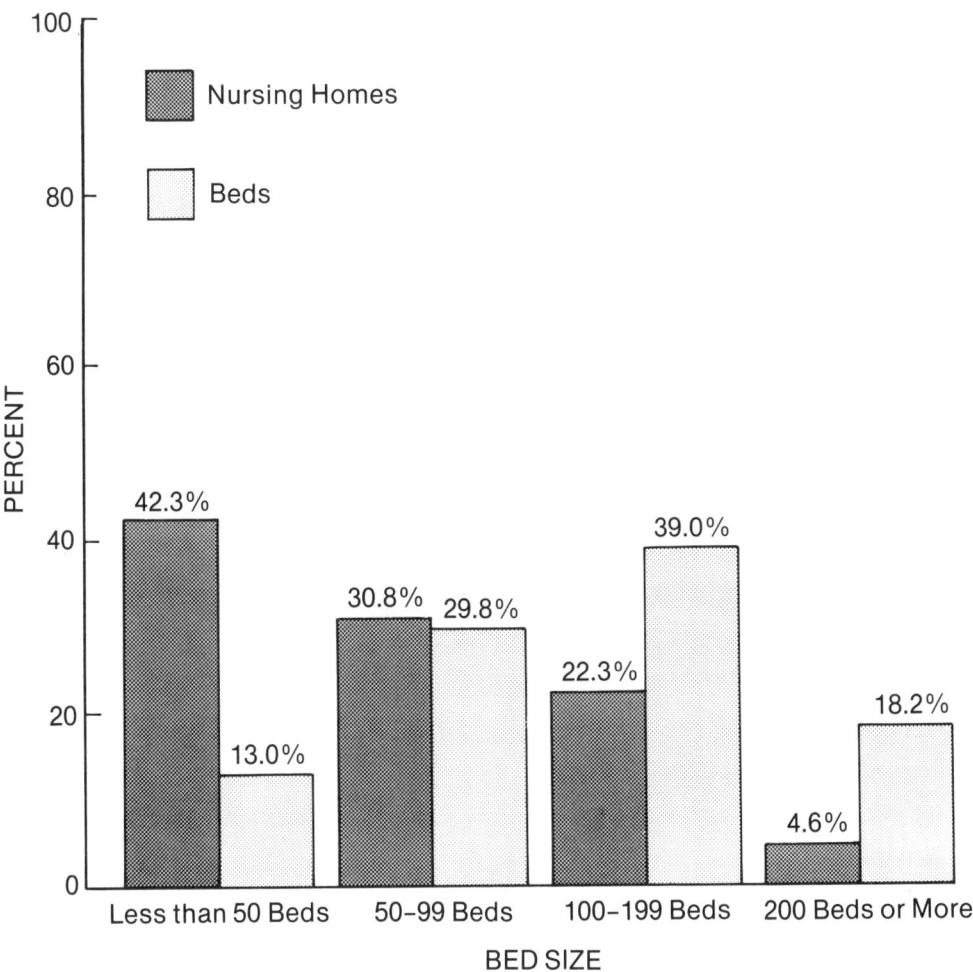

SOURCE: U.S. National Center for Health Statistics, *The National Nursing Home Survey: 1977 Summary for the United States,* DHEW, Public Health Service, Office of Health Research, Statistics, and Technology, Hyattsville, Maryland, Series 13, No. 43, July 1979, Table 1, p. 8.

Facilities

Chart F-46 Percent Distribution of Nursing Home Residents and Discharges, by Primary Source of Payment (U.S.A., 1976 and 1977).[1]

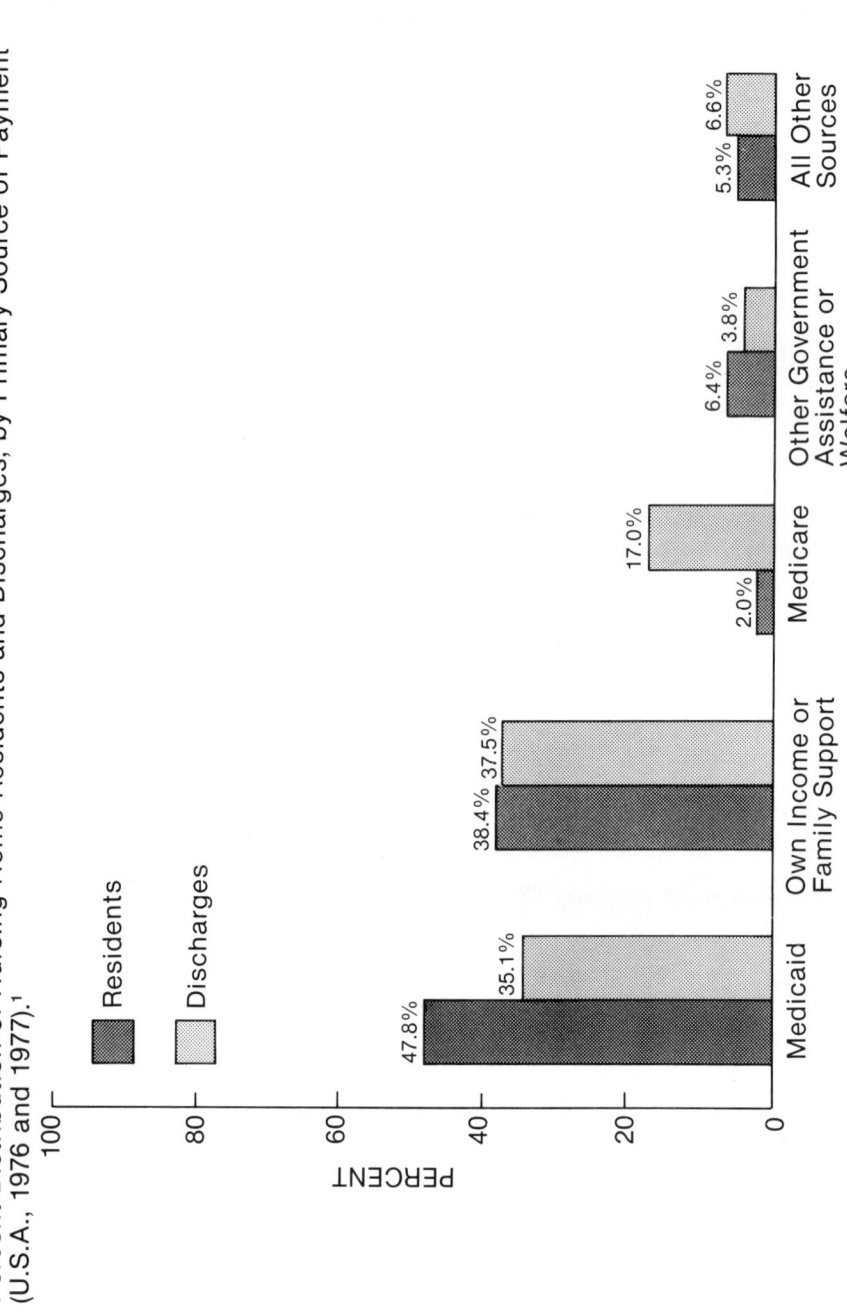

[1] Data on discharges are for 1976; data on residents are for 1977.
[2] All other sources includes religious organizations, foundations, volunteer agencies, Veterans Administration contract, initial payment life care funds and other sources or no charge.

SOURCE: U.S. National Center for Health Statistics, *The National Nursing Home Survey: 1977 Summary for the United States*, DHEW, Public Health Service, Office of Health Research Statistics, and Technology, Hyattsville, Maryland, Series 13, No.43, July 1979, Table 43, pp. 111-112.

Chart F-47

Percent Distribution of Full-Time Employees of Skilled Nursing Care Homes, Excluding Administrators, by Type of Employee (U.S.A., August 1973–April 1974).

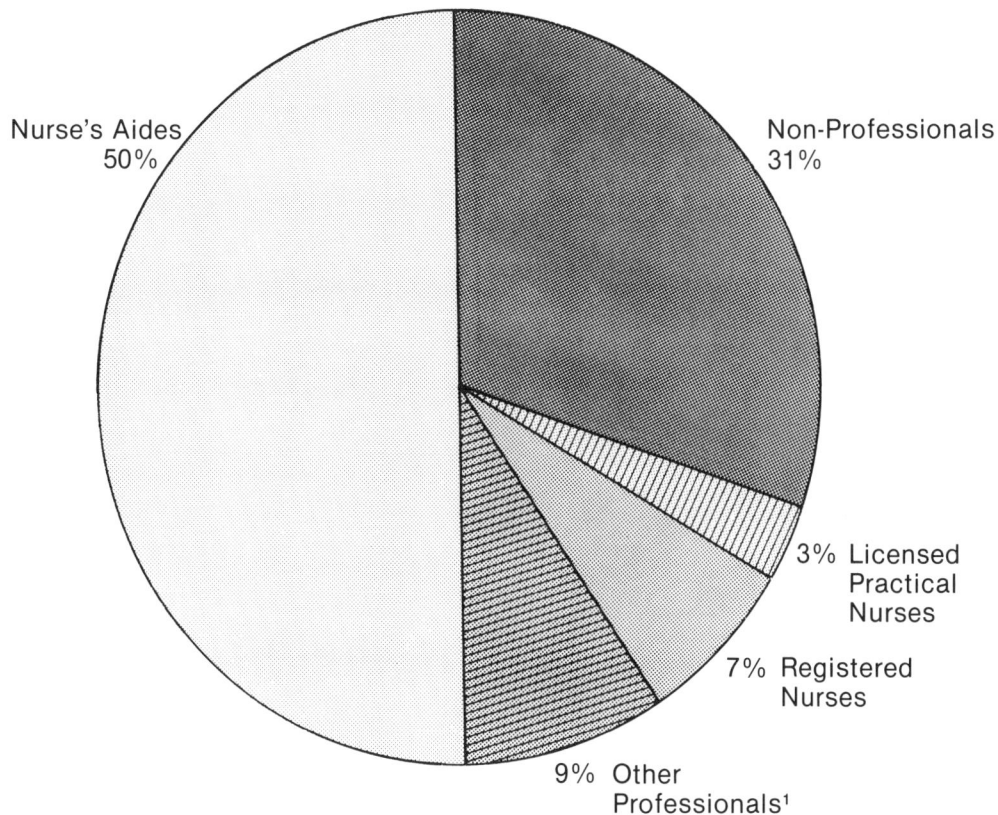

[1] Other professionals include dentists, dietitians, pharmacists, physicians, and therapeutic recreators. Administrators and medical record administrators are not included in this category.

NOTE: Skilled nursing care homes are homes in which fifty percent or more of the residents received services normally performed by a registered or licensed practical nurse and which had a registered nurse or licensed practical nurse employed fifteen or more hours per week.

SOURCE: U.S. National Center for Health Statistics, *Employees in Nursing Homes in the United States: 1973-74 National Nursing Home Survey*, DHEW, Public Health Service, Office of the Assistant Secretary for Health, Hyattsville, Maryland, Series 14, No. 20, February 1979, Table 1, p. 12.

Facilities

Chart F-48

Percent Distribution of Patients Receiving Skilled Nursing Care in Long-term Care Facilities, by Appropriateness of Care Received (Rhode Island, 1973–1974.

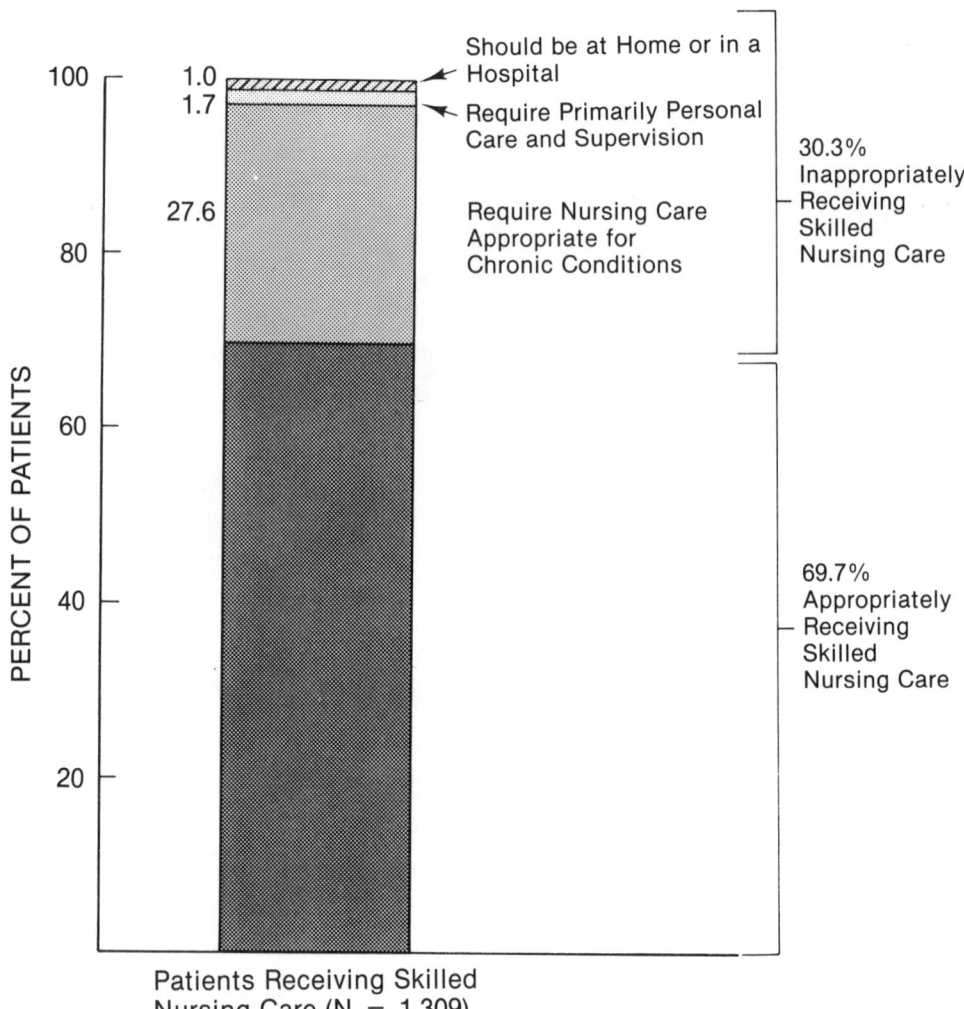

SOURCE: Allison-Cooke, S. and H. Thornberry, "Factors Affecting Nursing Home Medical Review, Implications for Program and Facility Planning," *Medical Care*, Vol. 15, No. 6, June 1977, Table 4, p. 498.

Facilities

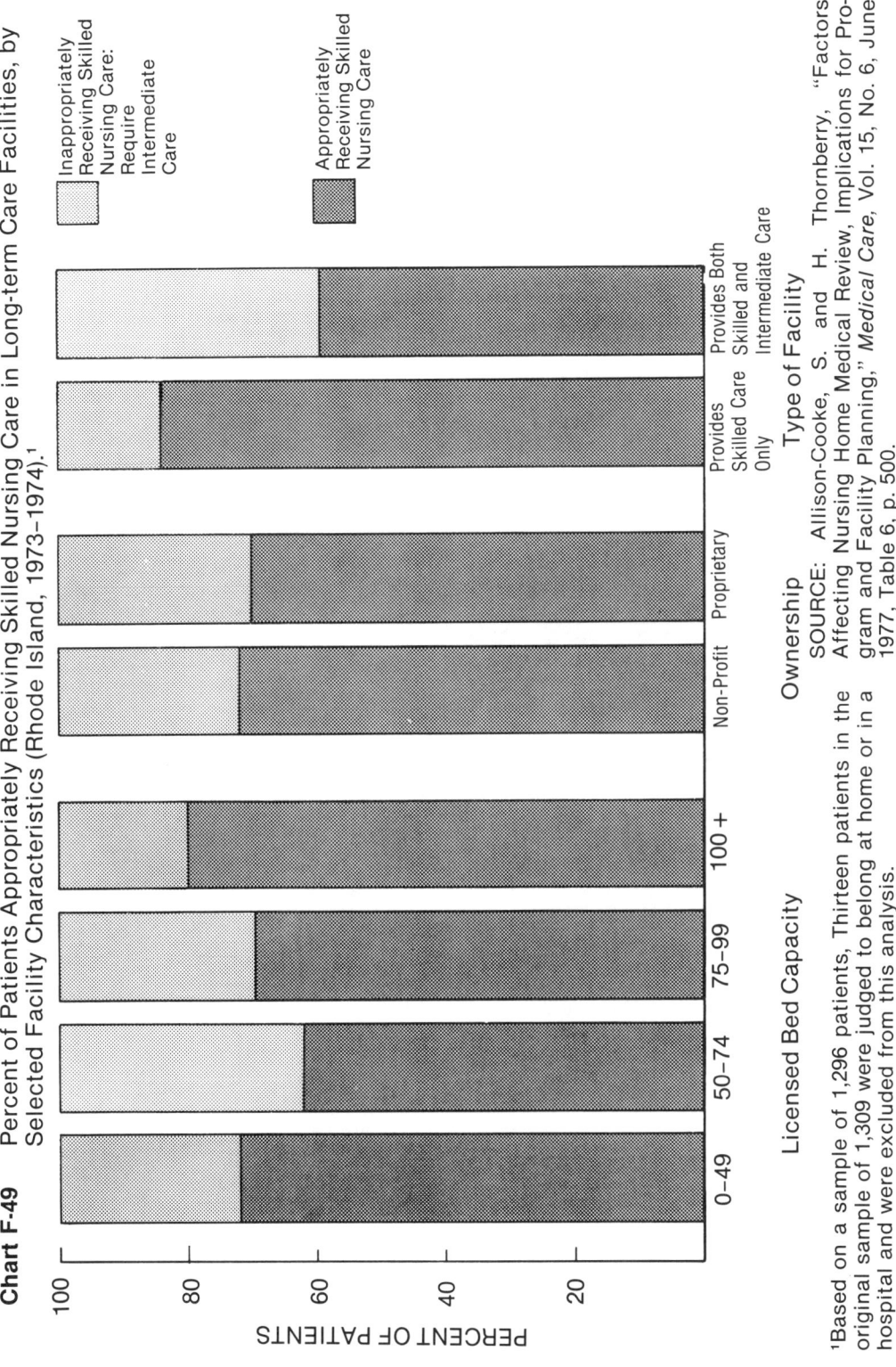

Chart F-49 Percent of Patients Appropriately Receiving Skilled Nursing Care in Long-term Care Facilities, by Selected Facility Characteristics (Rhode Island, 1973–1974).[1]

[1] Based on a sample of 1,296 patients. Thirteen patients in the original sample of 1,309 were judged to belong at home or in a hospital and were excluded from this analysis.

SOURCE: Allison-Cooke, S. and H. Thornberry, "Factors Affecting Nursing Home Medical Review, Implications for Program and Facility Planning," *Medical Care*, Vol. 15, No. 6, June 1977, Table 6, p. 500.

Chart F-50

Percent Change in Number of Home Health Agencies
and Skilled Nursing Facilities Participating in Medicare (U.S.A., 1967–1976).

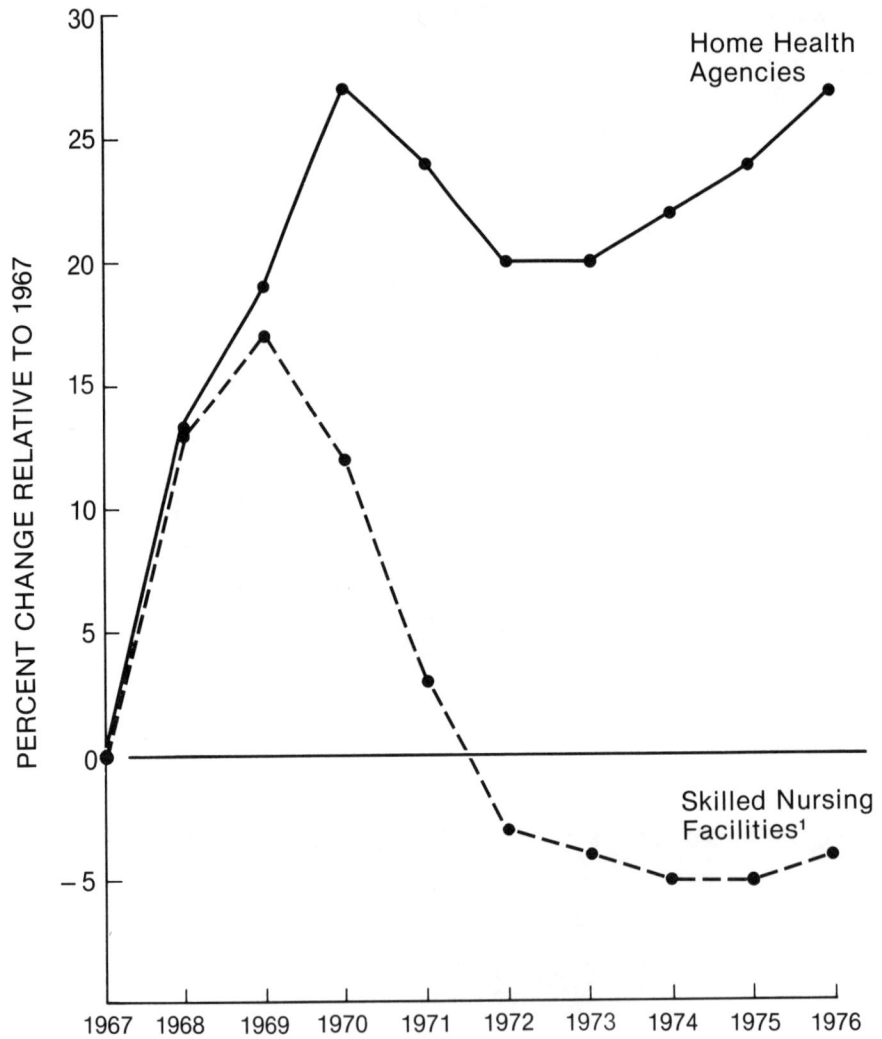

[1]Prior to 1972, Skilled Nursing Facilities were designated as Extended Care Facilities.

SOURCES: For 1967–1974: U.S. Department of Health, Education, and Welfare, Social Security Administration, *Health Insurance Statistics,* No. NI-6, April 8, 1968, Table 2, p. 6, No. N1-14, June 20, 1969, Table 2, p. 20, No. NI-18, May 5, 1970, Table 2, p. 17, No. N1-23, January 15, 1971, Table 2, p. 18, No. N1-34, February 17, 1972, Tables G and J, p. 8, No. N1-48, July 20, 1973, Table G and J, p. 10; for 1975: U.S. Department of Health, Education, and Welfare, Social Security Administration, *Social Security Bulletin — Annual Statistical Supplement 1975,* Office of Research and Statistics, 1977, Table 153, p. 173; for 1976: U.S. Department of Health, Education, and Welfare, Social Security Administration, *Social Security Bulletin — Annual Statistical Supplement, 1976,* Office of Research and Statistics, 1980, Table 146, p. 186.

Facilities

Chart F-51

Number and Percent Distribution of Home Health Agencies, by Type of Agency (U.S.A., Selected Years, 1945-1977).

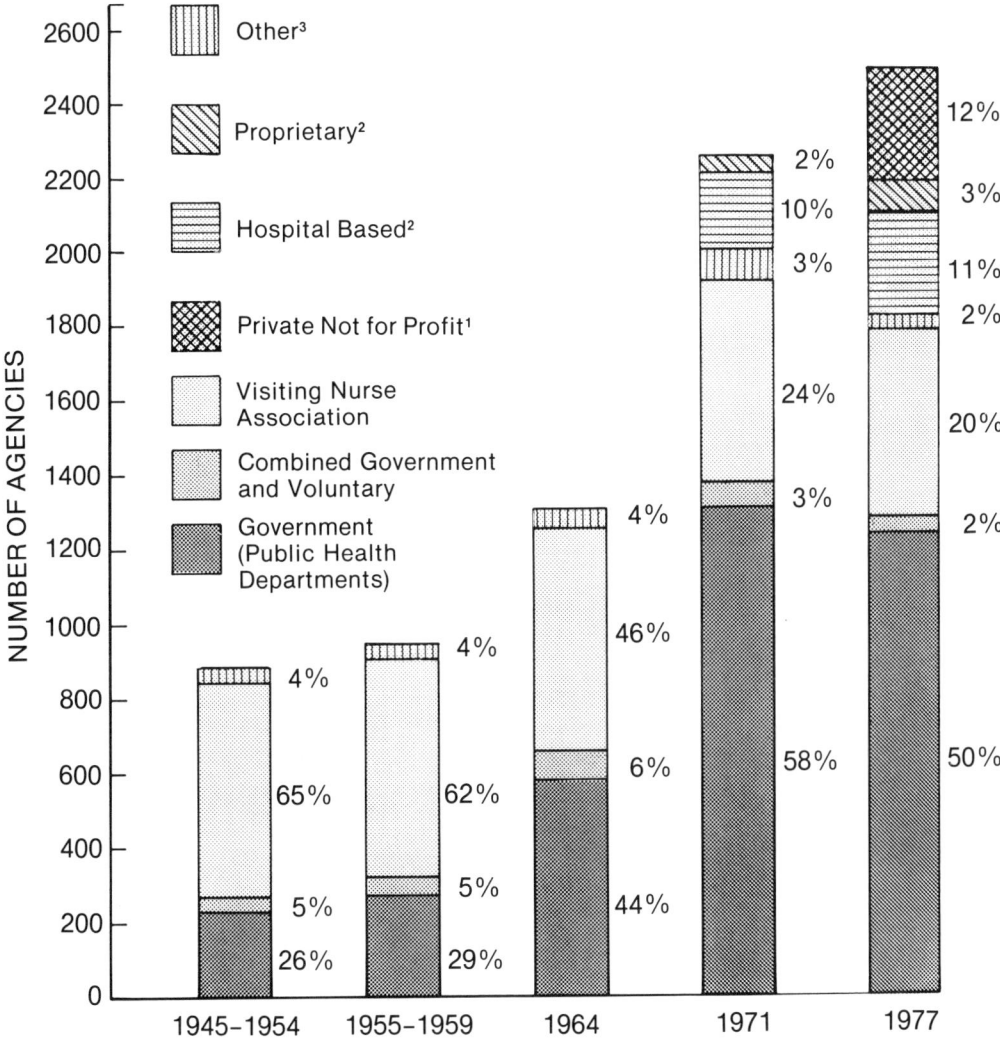

[1] No data available before 1977 for this category.

[2] No data available before 1971 for this category.

[3] For 1971 only, includes: extended care facility based (0.4%); rehabilitation facility based (0.5%); and miscellaneous (2.6%).

SOURCES: For 1945-1964: Ryder, C.F., P.G. Stitt, and W.F. Elkin, "Home Health Services, Past, Present, and Future," *American Journal of Public Health,* Vol. 59, No. 9, September 1969, Table 1, p. 1721; for 1971: *Home Health Services in the United States, A Report to the Special Committee on Aging,* U.S. Senate, U.S. Government Printing Office, Washington, D.C., 1972, Table C-2, p. 18; for 1977: U.S. Department of Health, Education, and Welfare, *Research and Statistics Note No. 2, Medicare: Utilization of Home Health Services,* Health Care Financing Administration, Office of Policy, Planning, and Research, June 1978, Table 6.

Facilities

Chart F-52 Number of Home Health Visits and Reimbursement for Home Health Services Under the Medicare Program (U.S.A., 1969–1976).

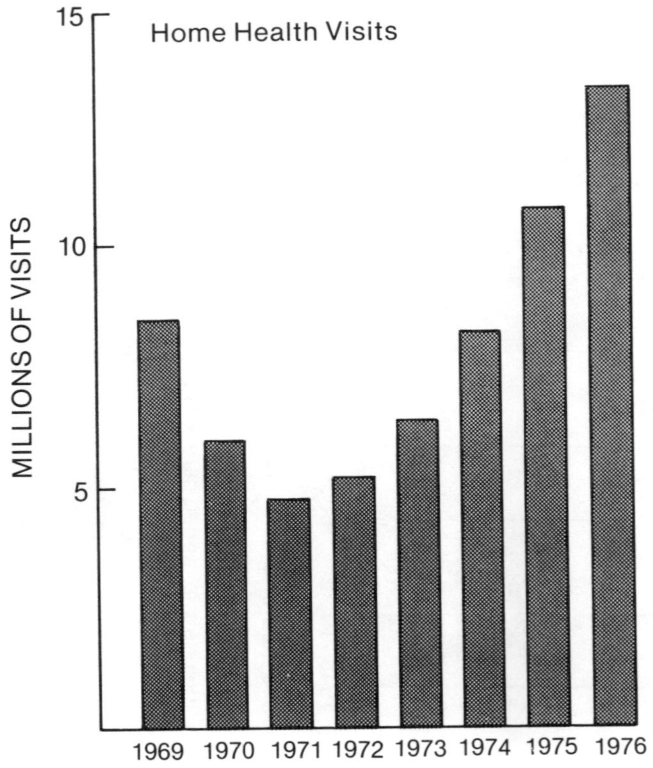

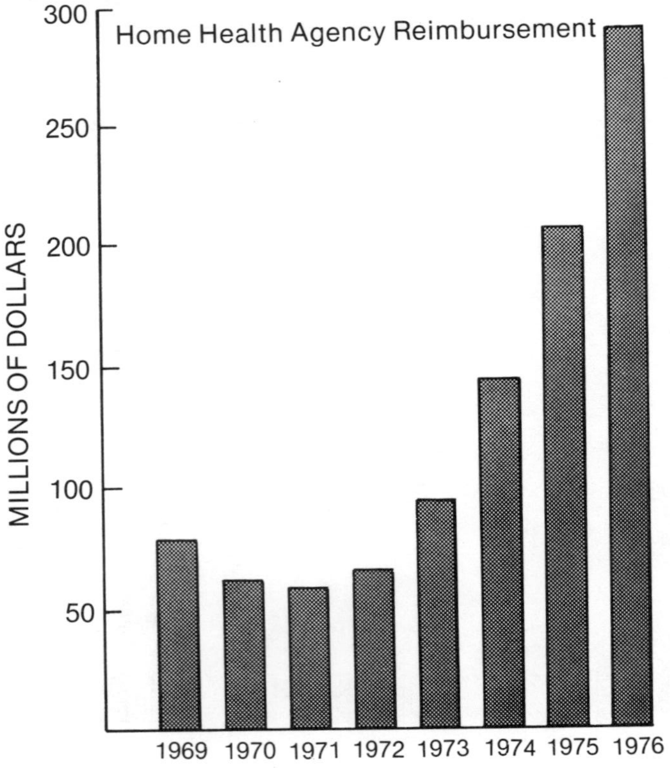

SOURCE: Health Care Financing Administration, *Health Care Financing Program Statistics, Medicare: Use of Home Health Services, 1976*, Office of Research, Demonstrations, and Statistics, May 1980, Table 1, p. 3.

Facilities

Chart F-53

Number and Percent of Home Health Agencies Certified to Participate in Medicare that Provide Specified Services (U.S.A., 1980).

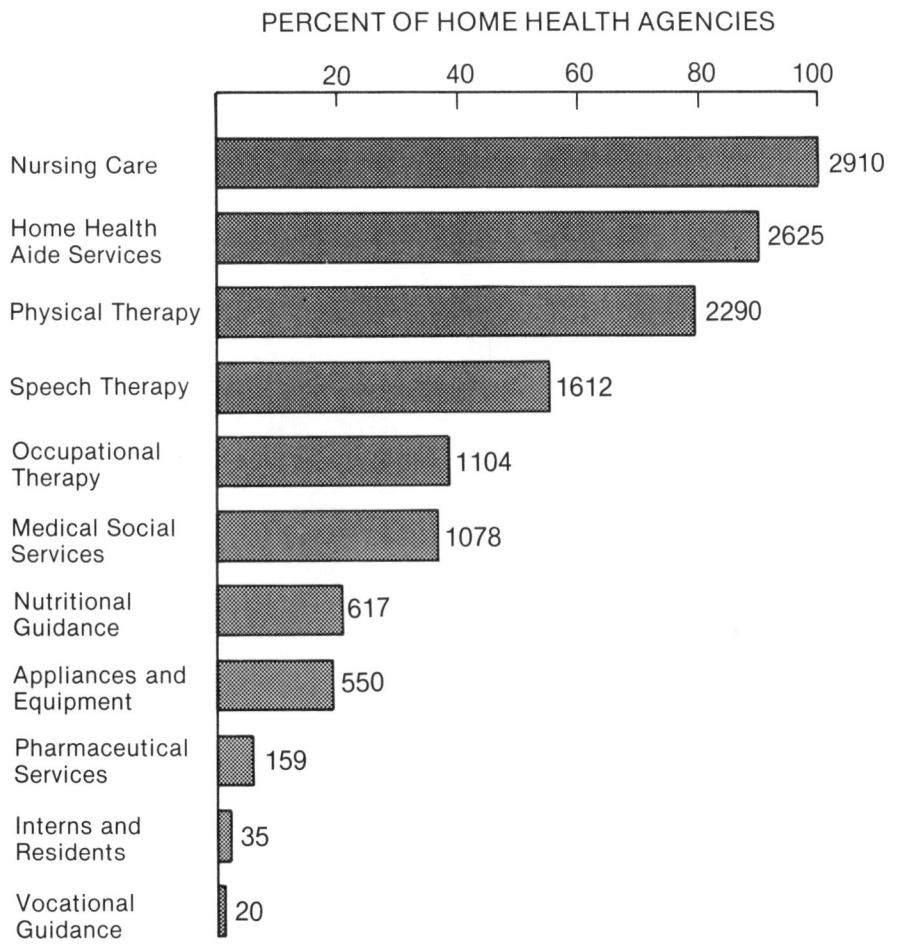

SOURCE: Data from the Medical Care Provider Service file, supplied by Charles Helbing, Health Care Financing Administration, June 1980.

Chart F-54

Percent Change in Utilization of Health Services in a Study Group of Cardiac Patients Provided with Home Care Services Relative to a Control Group that did not Receive Such Services (Boston, 1954).

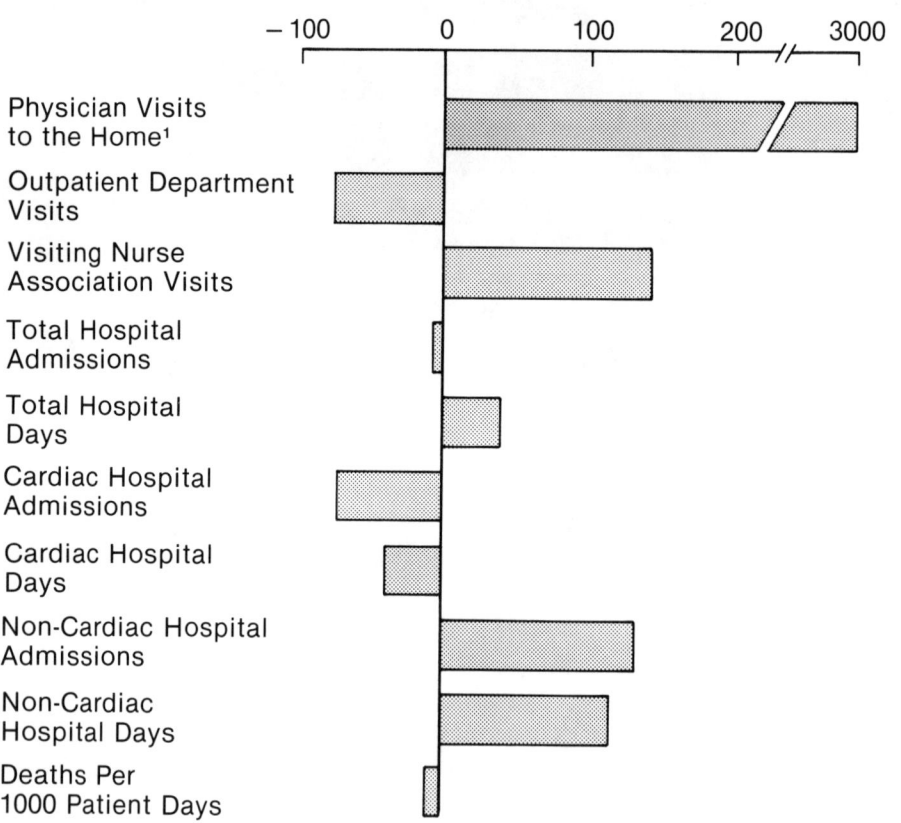

[1] Approximate number.
SOURCE: Bakst, J. N. and E. F. Marra, "Experience with Home Care for Cardiac Patients," *American Journal of Public Health*, Vol. 45, April 1955, Table 1, p. 446 and Table 2, p. 447.

Facilities

Chart F-55

Percent Change in Use of Hospital Service in a Study Group of Cardiac Patients That Received Public Health Home Nursing Services Relative to a Control Group That Did Not Receive Such Services[1] (St. Lukes Hospital Center, New York City, January 1964–September 1966).

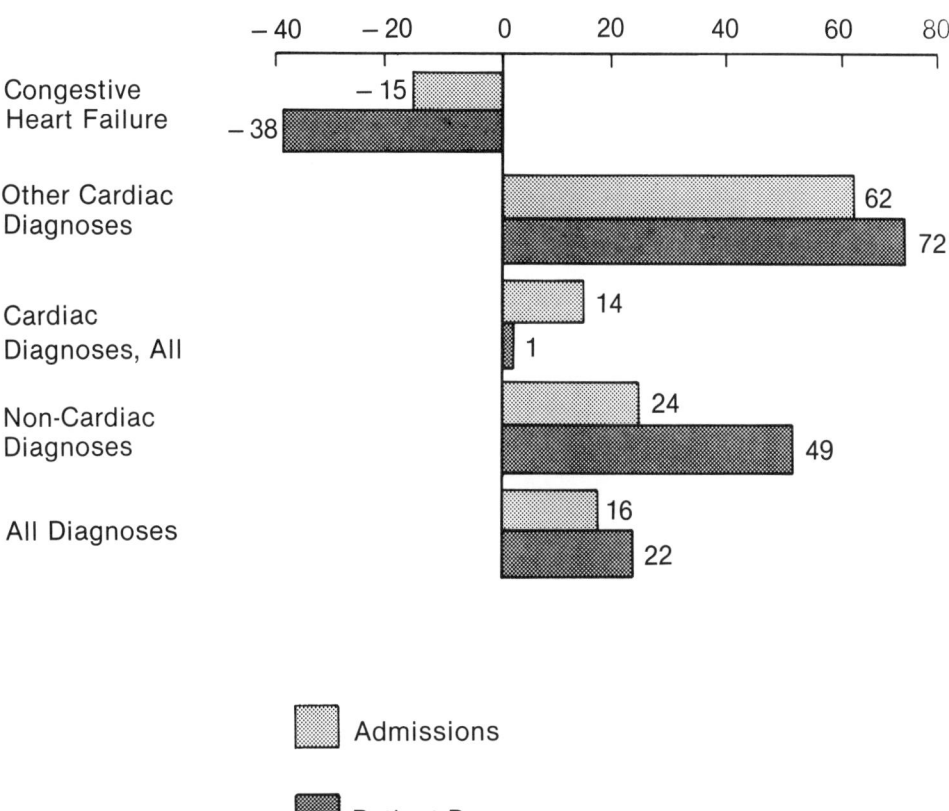

1 Both groups of patients continued to receive supervision from the outpatient clinics. The study group patients also received public health nursing follow-up from two public health nurses working full time in the hospital based program. Hospital utilization rates were computed per 100 months of follow-up.

SOURCE: Hanchett, E. and P.R. Torrens, "A Public Health Home Nursing Program for Outpatients with Heart Disease," *Public Health Reports,* Vol. 82, August 1967, pp. 683–688.

Facilities

Chart F-56 Percent Distribution of Home Health Visits under the Medicare Program, by Type of Agency Providing Care, and Percent Distribution of Visits Provided by each Type of Agency, by Type of Service Provided (U.S.A., 1976).

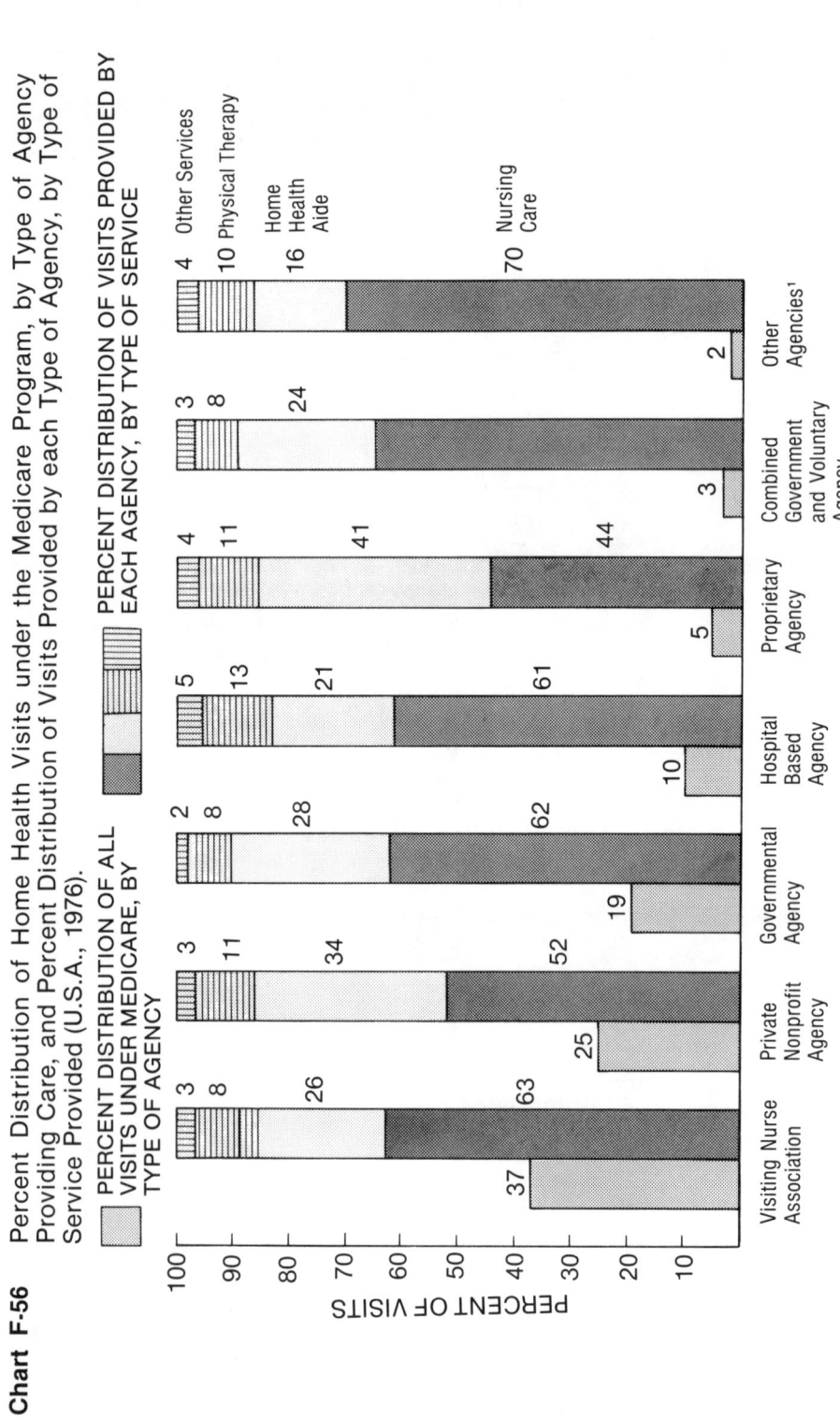

[1] "Other Agencies" include rehabilitation and skilled nursing facility-based organizations.

SOURCE: Health Care Financing Administration, *Health Care Financing Program Statistics, Medicare: Use of Home Health Services, 1976,* Office of Research, Demonstrations, and Statistics, May 1980, Table 6, p. 9.

Facilities

Chart F-57 Total Medicare Payments per Person for Persons Allocated Randomly to a Control Group and to Experimental Groups Which Were Eligible for Specified Additional Services for One Year (Six U.S. Cities, 1975–1977).[1]

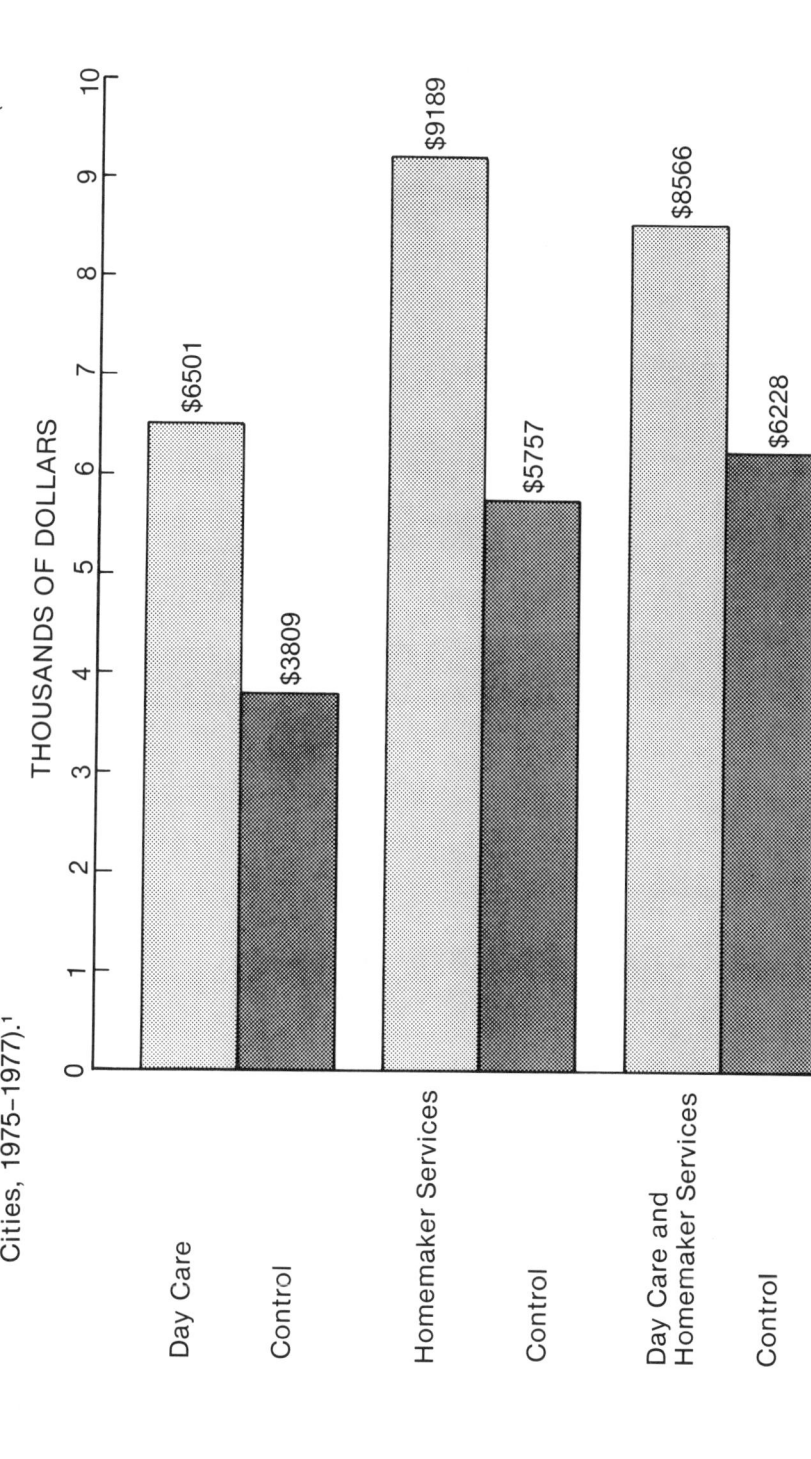

[1] Medicare payments are for all covered services, including nursing home and hospital care utilized by the experimental and control groups. Outcomes measured in terms of physical function, death rates, contentment, mental functioning, and social activity, were generally more favorable for the groups receiving additional services than for the control groups.

SOURCE: National Center for Health Services Research, *Effects and Costs of Day Care and Homemaker Services for the Chronically Ill: A Randomized Experiment*, DHEW, Public Health Service, Office of Health Research, Statistics, and Technology, August 1979, Table 2, p. 16, Table 3, p. 22, and Table 4, p. 25.

Chart F-58 Percent Distribution of Aged Population, by Type of Care Received and Needed (Monroe County, New York, 1964).

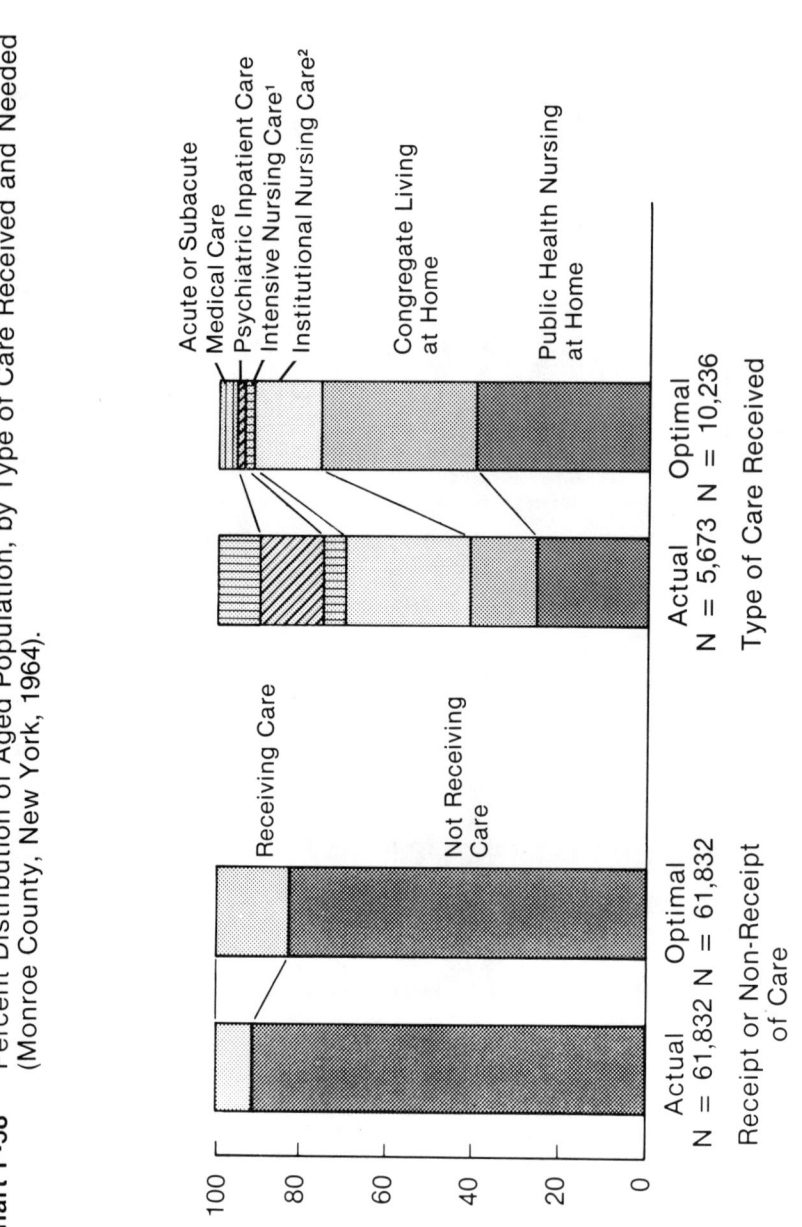

[1] Includes convalescent and rehabilitation services for persons who might otherwise develop into long-term domiciliary patients.
[2] Provided in proprietary nursing homes, nursing units of homes for the aged, infirmaries or hospitals.

SOURCE: Berg, Robert L., et. al., "Assessing the Health Care Needs of the Aged," *Health Services Research*, Spring 1970, Table 6, p. 49.

Facilities

SECTION G
Quality of Care

Chart G-1

Percent Distribution of Patient Opinion of Hospital Care Received, by Clinical Experts' Judgment of Care (New York City Area, Late 1960).

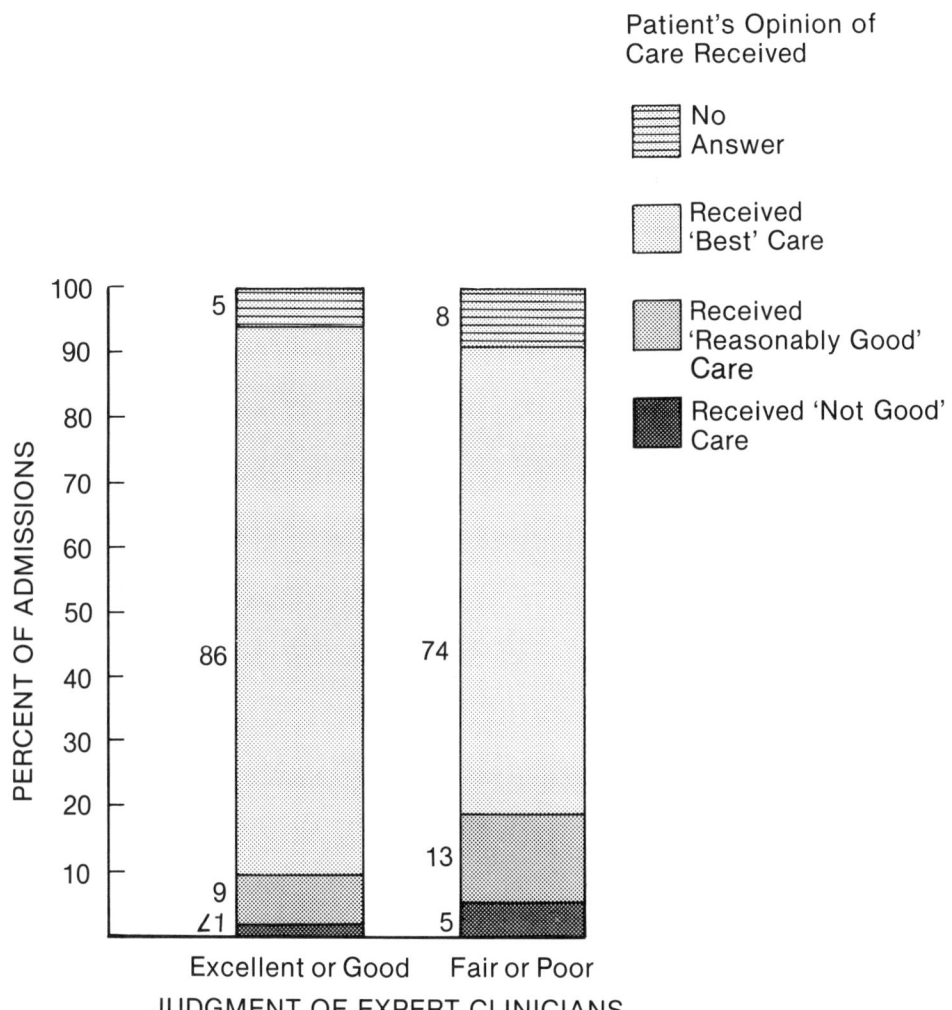

SOURCE: Columbia University School of Public Health and Administrative Medicine, *The Quantity, Quality and Costs of Medical and Hospital Care Secured by a Sample of Teamster Families in the New York Area*, New York, p. 79.

Chart G-2

Percent of Cases of Cancer of the Cervix Which Survived for Five Years, By Year in Which the Cases Were Recorded in the Cancer Registry and by Categories of Hospitals
(New York State, Excluding New York City, 1949, 1959-62).

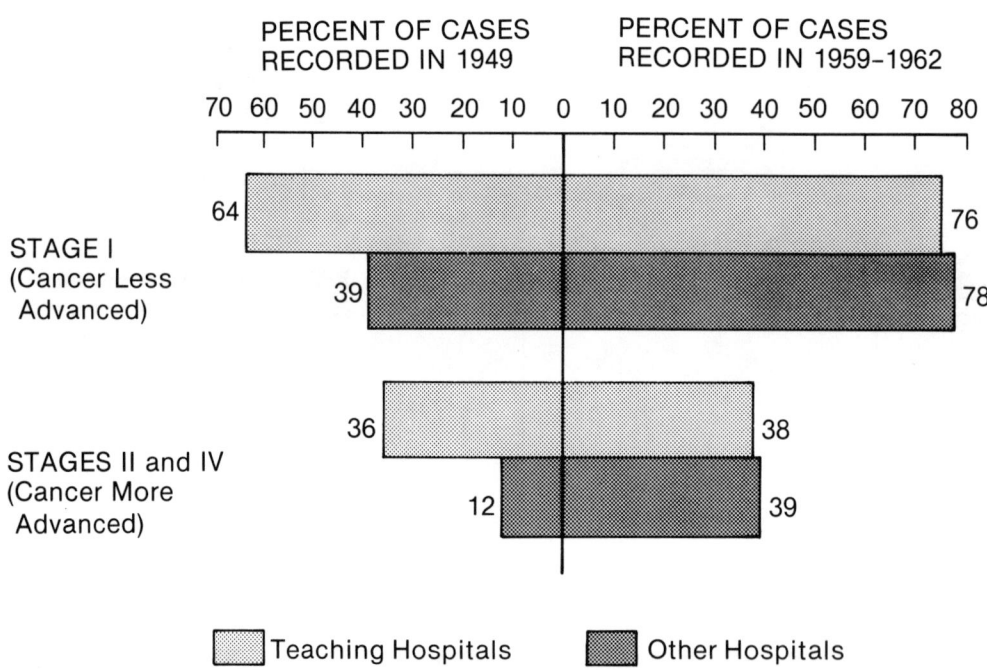

SOURCE: Graham, J. B. and F. P. Paloucek, "Where Should Cancer of the Cervix be Treated?" *American Journal of Obstetrics and Gynecology*, Vol. 87, October 1, 1963, pp. 405-409, with additional data provided by Dr. Graham.

Quality of Care

Chart G-3

Percent of All Perinatal Deaths, and of All Perinatal Deaths in Mature Infants with Specified Responsibility Factors,[1] to Have Been Judged Preventable (New York City, 1950-51).

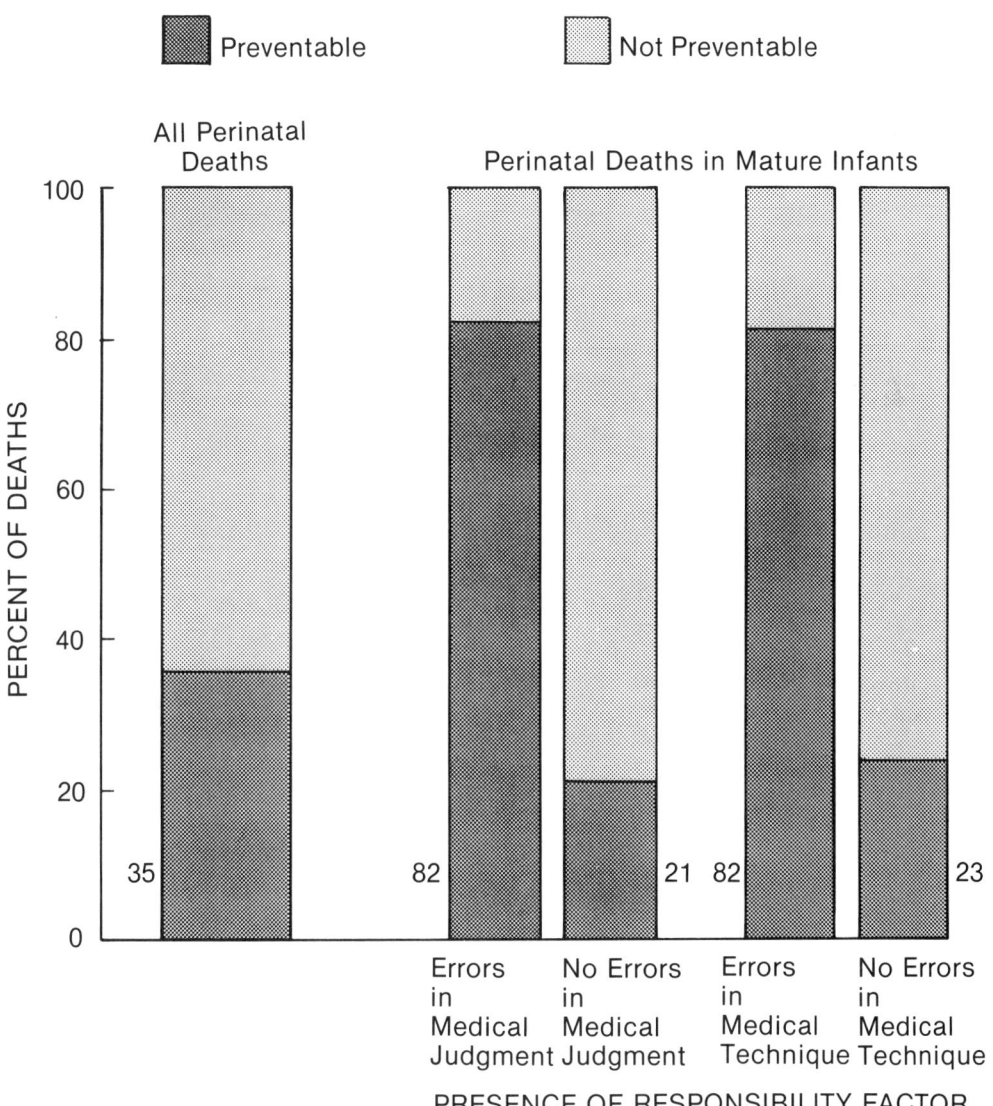

[1] Some deaths may have involved more than one responsibility factor.
SOURCE: Kohl, S.G., *Perinatal Mortality in New York City*, Harvard University Press, Cambridge, 1955, Table XIV, p. 18, Table XV, p. 24 and Table XVI, p. 26.

Quality of Care

Chart G-4

Percent of Perinatal Deaths Judged to Have Been Preventable, by Characteristics of Medical Care Received (New York, 1950–1951).

	Percent of Preventable Deaths	
	Mature Infants	Premature Infants
A. All Deaths	42	29
B. By Place of Birth		
Voluntary Teaching Hospital	24	18
Voluntary Non-Teaching Hospital	43	26
Municipal Teaching Hospital	43	35
Municipal Non-Teaching Hospital	62	36
Proprietary Hospital	34	28
Home Deliveries	79	56
C. By Service Status		
Private	38	26
Ward	47	33
D. By Type of Professional Service		
Obstetrician	32	29
House Staff	48	32
Other Physician	42	25
Unknown	30	30

SOURCE: Kohl, S. G., *Perinatal Mortality in New York City*, Harvard University Press, Cambridge, 1955.

Quality of Care

Chart G-5

Total Maternal Mortality and Maternal Mortality Judged To Be Preventable, by Size of Obstetrical Service (New York City, 1930-1932).

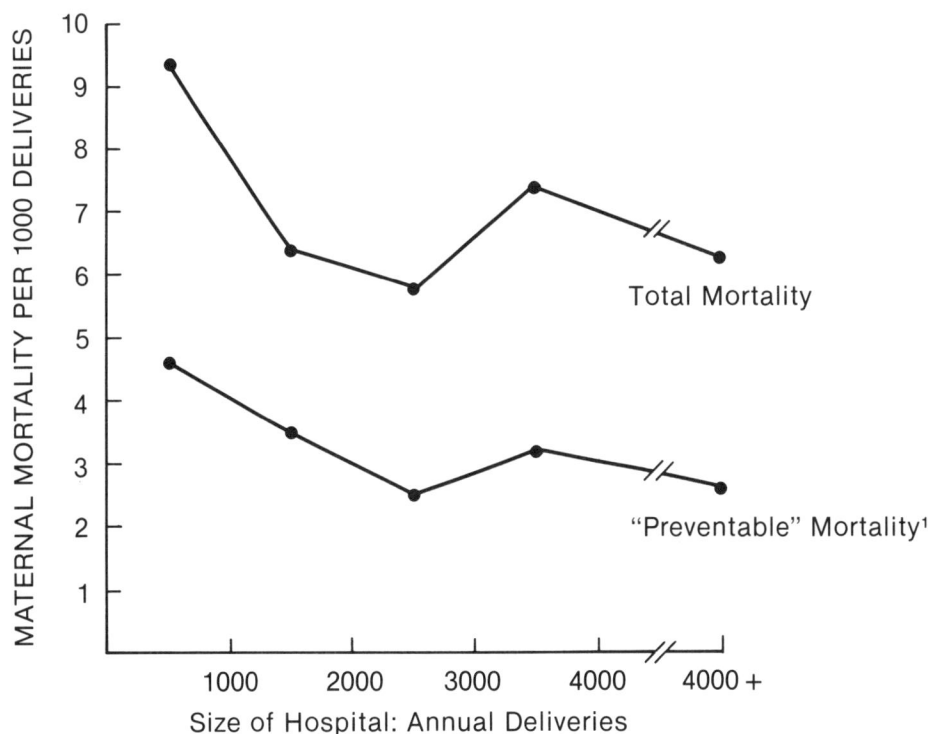

[1] Judgments of preventability are based on review by a committee of information from the hospital record and interview with the medical attendants of each case.

SOURCE: Committee on Public Health Relations, New York Academy of Medicine, *Maternal Mortality in New York City*, New York, Oxford University Press, Commonwealth Fund, 1933, pp. 250-255.

Chart G-6

Percent Distribution of Maternal Deaths[1] by Avoidability of, and Responsibility for, Death[2] (Women Under the Care of Osteopathic Physicians, Michigan, 1954–1963).

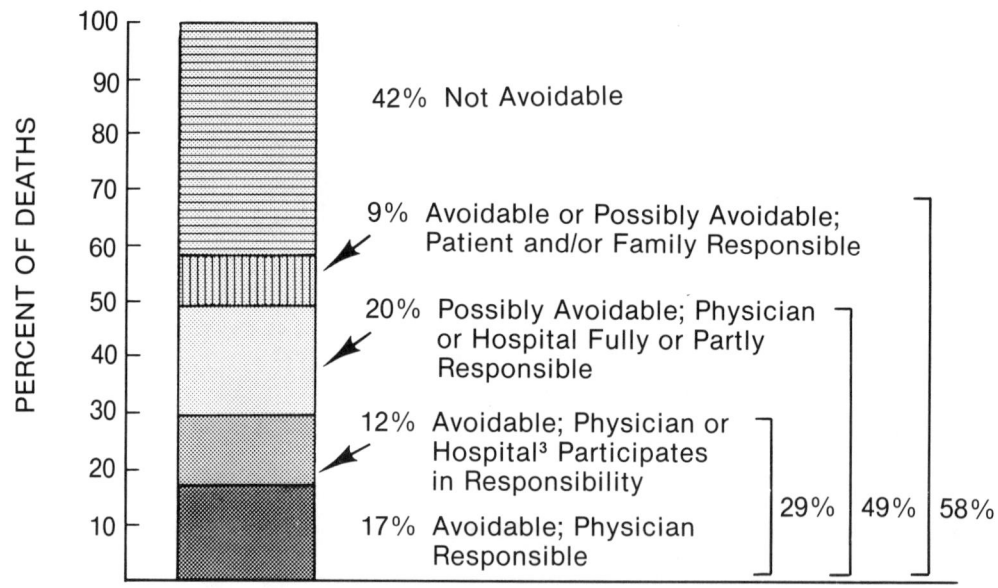

All Maternal Deaths (N = 104)

[1] A maternal death is defined as "the death of any woman dying from any cause whatsoever while pregnant or within 90 days of the termination of the pregnancy..."

[2] As judged by a committee of osteopathic physicians based on information abstracted from records supplemented with interviews with the attending physician in each case.

[3] Hospital exclusively responsible in one case and shares in eight cases.

SOURCES: Bubeck, Roy G. Jr., et. al., "Maternal Mortality: Report of Ten-Year Study of Patients Under Osteopathic Care," *Journal of the American Osteopathic Association*, Vol. 67, December 1967, Table 10, p. 391.

Chart G-7 Fatality Rates, by Type of Condition and Type of Hospital (England and Wales, 1956–59).[1]

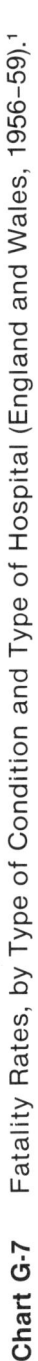

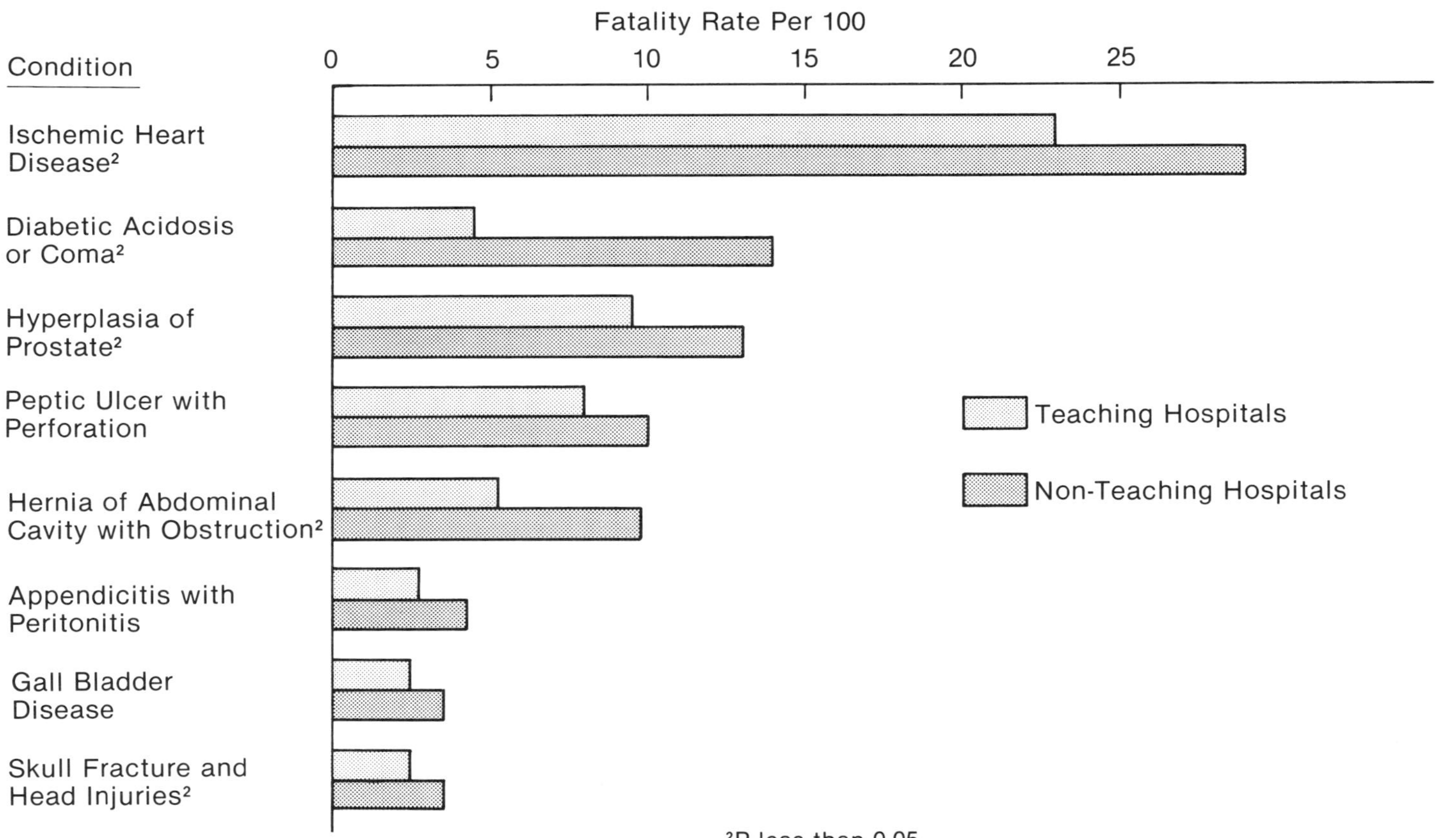

Condition	Teaching Hospitals	Non-Teaching Hospitals
Ischemic Heart Disease[2]	23	28
Diabetic Acidosis or Coma[2]	4.5	14
Hyperplasia of Prostate[2]	9.5	13
Peptic Ulcer with Perforation	8	10
Hernia of Abdominal Cavity with Obstruction[2]	5.2	9.8
Appendicitis with Peritonitis	2.7	4.2
Gall Bladder Disease	2.5	3.5
Skull Fracture and Head Injuries[2]	2.5	3.5

[1] The case fatality rate in non-teaching hospitals is standardized on the age and sex distribution of admissions to teaching hospitals.

[2] P less than 0.05.

SOURCE: Lipworth, L., J.A.H. Lee, and J.N. Morris, "Case-Fatality in Teaching and Non-Teaching Hospitals, 1956–59," *Medical Care*, Vol. 1, April–June 1963, Table 1, p. 71 and Table 3, p. 72.

Quality of Care

Chart G-8

Crude and Adjusted Death Rates[1] by Type of Hospital[2]
(Los Angeles County, California, 1964).

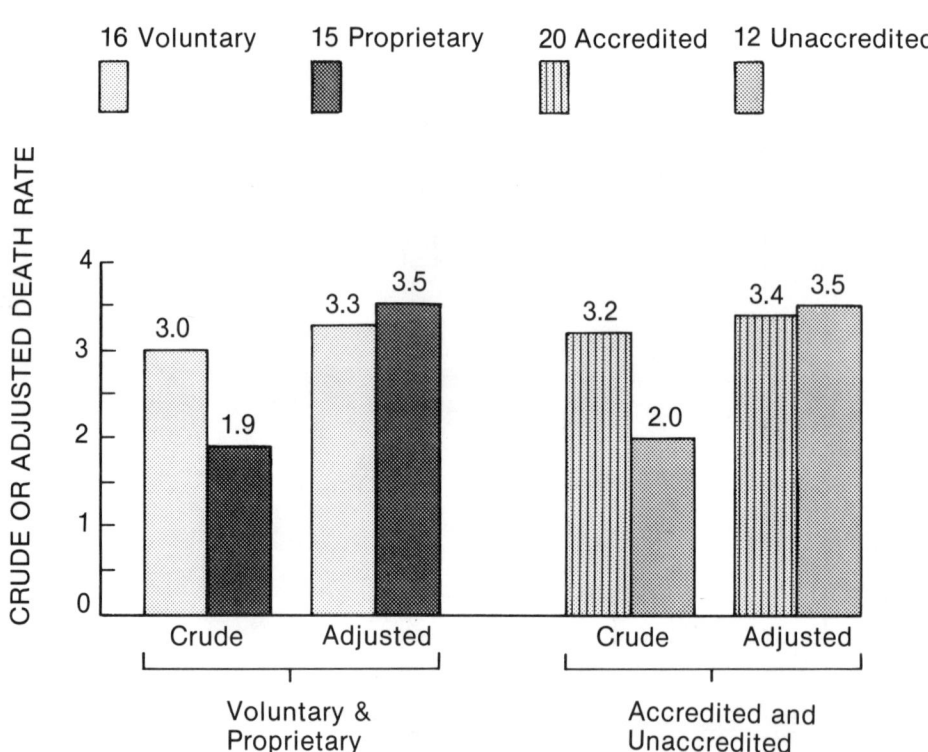

[1]Crude death rates are all deaths occurring in the hospital except the newborn as a percentage of all admissions, except maternity admissions. Adjustment for case severity is made indirectly by correcting for hospitals' average length of stay and occupancy rate.

[2]Sample of general hospitals stratified by size and type of control.

SOURCE: Roemer, M. I., A. T. Moustafa, and C. A. Hopkins, "A Proposed Quality Index: Hospital Death Rates Adjusted for Case Severity," *Health Services Research*, Vol. 3, Summer 1968, pp. 96–118.

Quality of Care

Chart G-9

Relative Post-Operative Mortality Ratios[1], Adjusted to Account for Variation Among Institutions in Specified Patient Characteristics, 34 Medical Centers in the Collaborative National Halothane Study (U.S.A., 1959-1962).

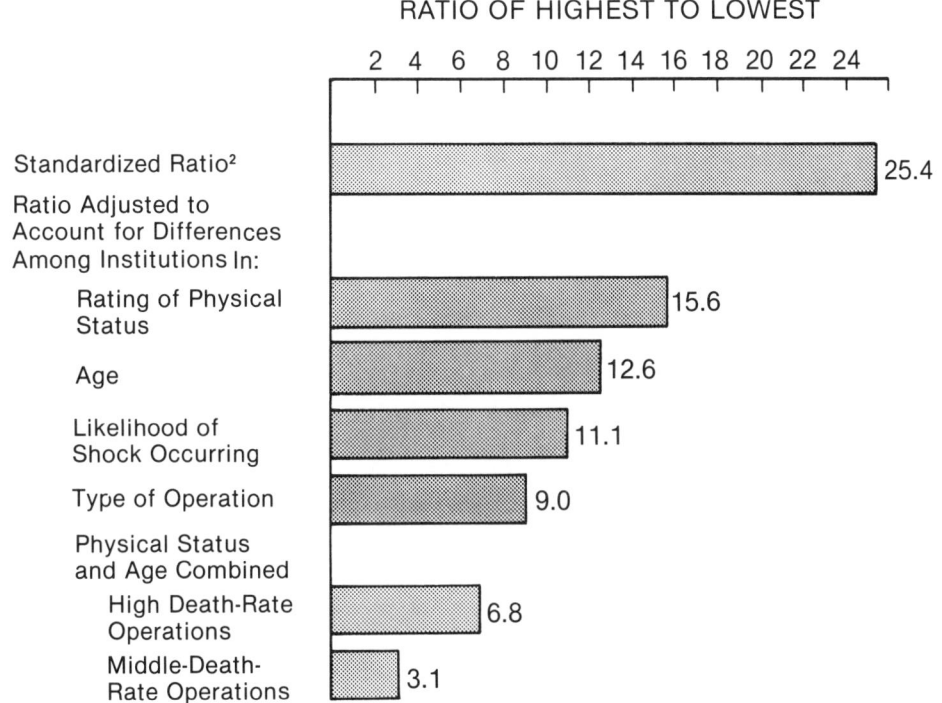

[1]Post-operative deaths are those that occurred in the hospital within 6 weeks of a general anesthetic. There were about a million operations and 17,000 deaths. The Death Ratio is Deaths/Deaths + Operations. The chart shows the quotient of The Highest Mortality Ratio/The Lowest Mortality Ratio among 34 institutions for each array. The sample of institutions was not random, since participation was voluntary. All hospitals had a "teaching connection." They ranged from 350 to 1500 beds with a median of 650.

[2]Mortality ratio for the entire sample equals 1. The unstandardized ratio ranged from 2.68 to 64.05 per 1000 operations.

SOURCE: Bunker, J. P., et. al., *National Halothane Study*, Report of the Subcommittee on the National Halothane Study, National Academy of Sciences — National Research Council, Washington, D.C., 1969, Tables 5 and 12, pp. 196, 334 and 341.

Chart G-10

Percent Distribution of Hospitals by Standardized Mortality Ratio for Two Diagnostic Categories (U.S.A., PAS Hospitals, 1972).[1]

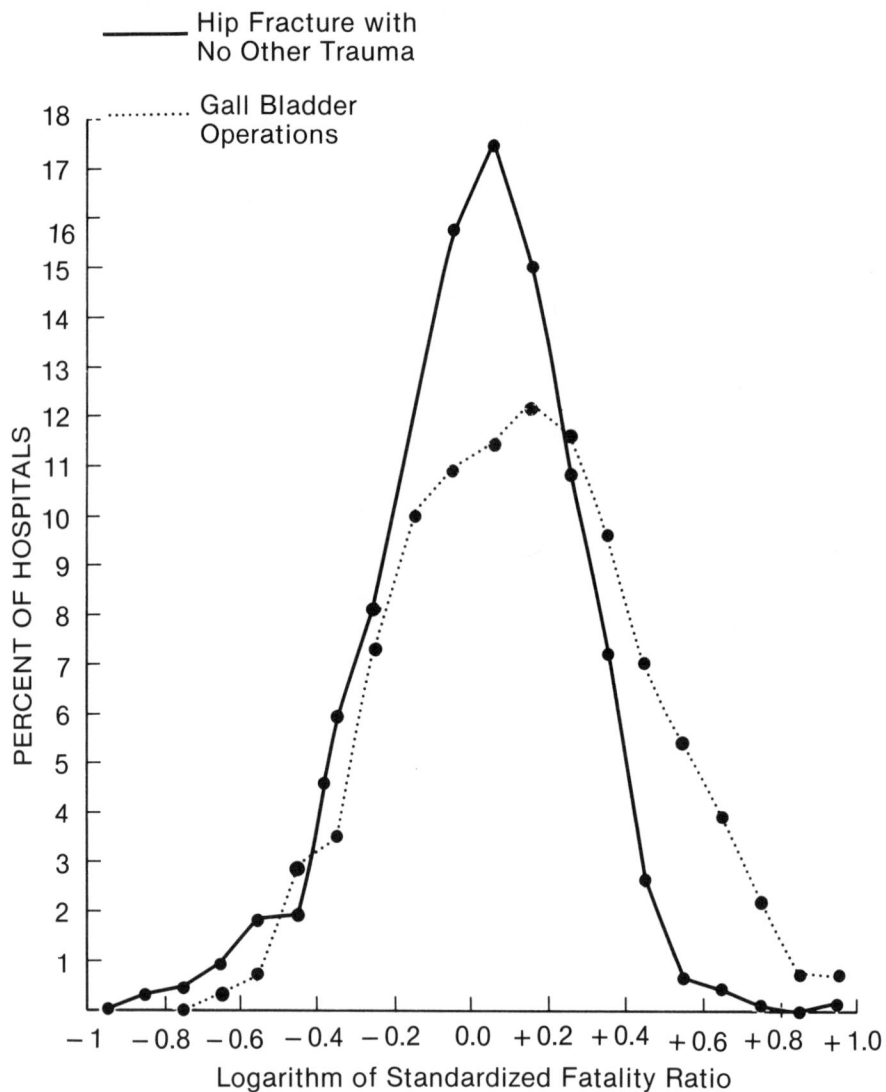

[1]Hospitals in the Professional Activities Study of the Commission on Professional and Hospital Activities, excluding those with no deaths and with fatality ratios of 10.0 or more. The fatality ratio is that of observed postoperative deaths to deaths expected after correcting for the effect of selected patient characteristics.

SOURCE: Center for the Institutional Differences Study, *Study of Institutional Differences in Postoperative Mortality*, Stanford, Calif., The Center, Dec. 15, 1974, Appendix II.B.13.

Quality of Care

Chart G-11

Hospital Service Areas[1] by Appendectomy Rate and by Death Rate from Appendicitis (11 Counties in Western New York State, Appendectomies in 1948 and Average of Deaths From Appendicitis 1944-1948).

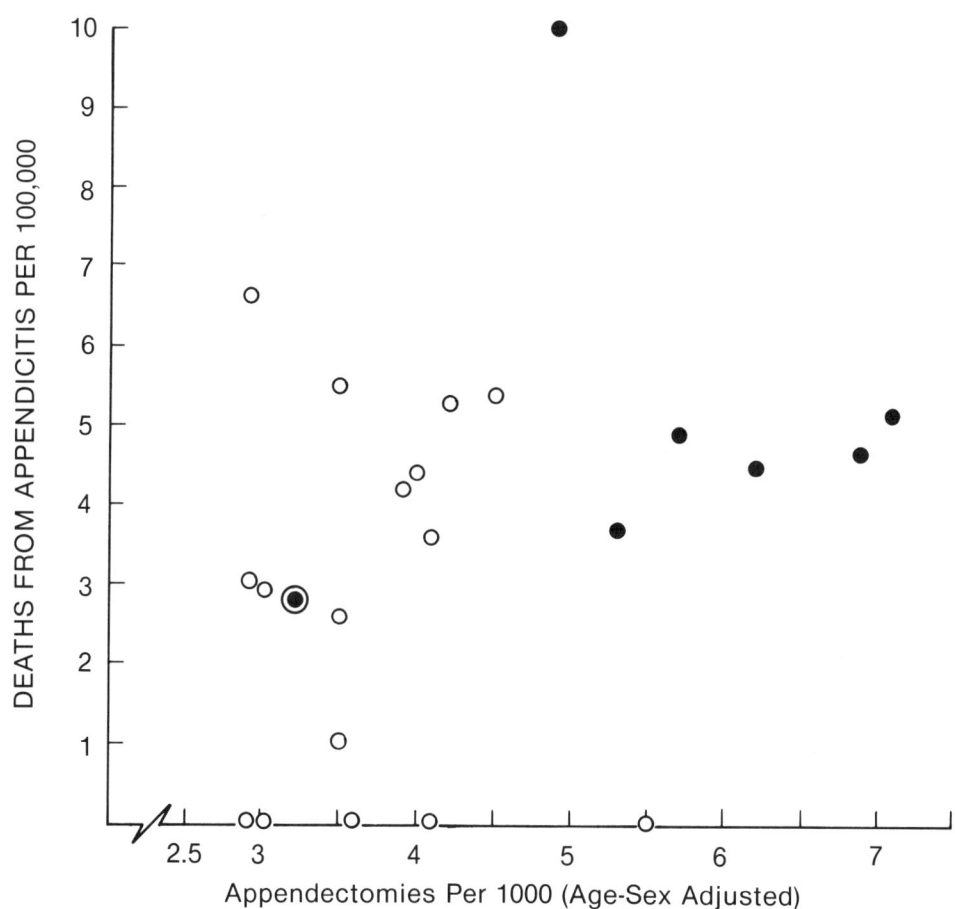

◉ Rochester Service Area: Considered to Serve As "Standard"

● Service Areas with Appendectomy Rates Significantly Higher ($p < 0.001$) Than the Rate for the Rochester Area.

[1] "Studies of the place of residence of all patients, except new-born infants, who were hospitalized in 1946, served to outline 23 distinct and mutually exclusive hospital service areas.... Each hospital service area accounted for 75 to 95 percent of all hospitalizations per person who resided therein."

SOURCE: Lembcke, Paul A., "Measuring the Quality of Medical Care Through Vital Statistics Based on Hospital Service Areas: 1. Comparative Study of Appendectomy Rates," *American Journal of Public Health*, Vol. 42, March 1952, pp. 276-286.

Quality of Care

Chart G-12 Tonsillectomies per 10,000 Children 14 Years of Age or Less in 13 Hospital Service Areas (Vermont, 1969 and 1973).

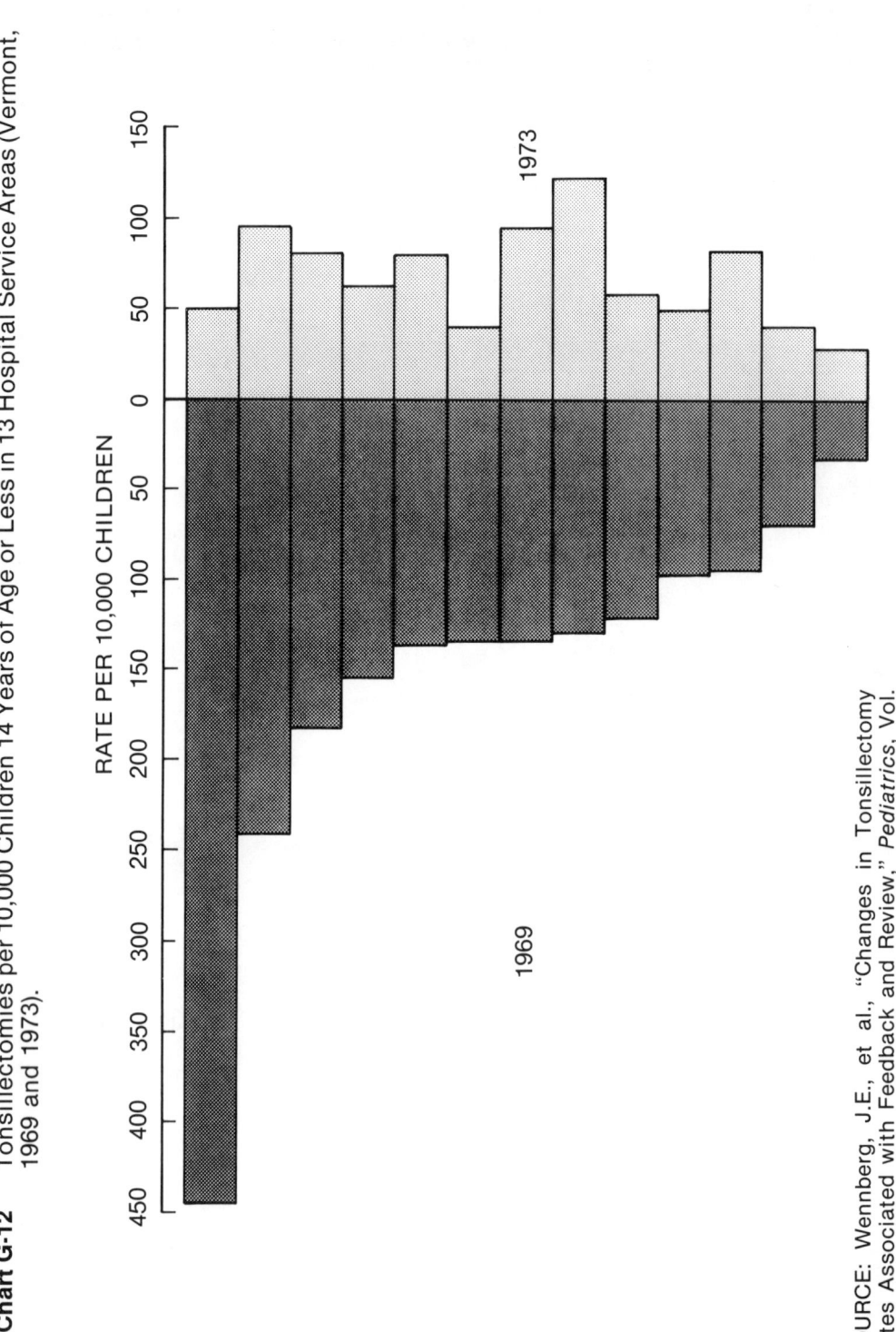

SOURCE: Wennberg, J.E., et al., "Changes in Tonsillectomy Rates Associated with Feedback and Review," *Pediatrics*, Vol. 59, June 1977, Table III, p. 824.

Chart G-13

Percent of 11-Year Old Children Who Were Either Found to Have Had a Tonsillectomy or for Whom Tonsillectomy was Recommended at Specified School Medical Examinations (New York City, 1933).

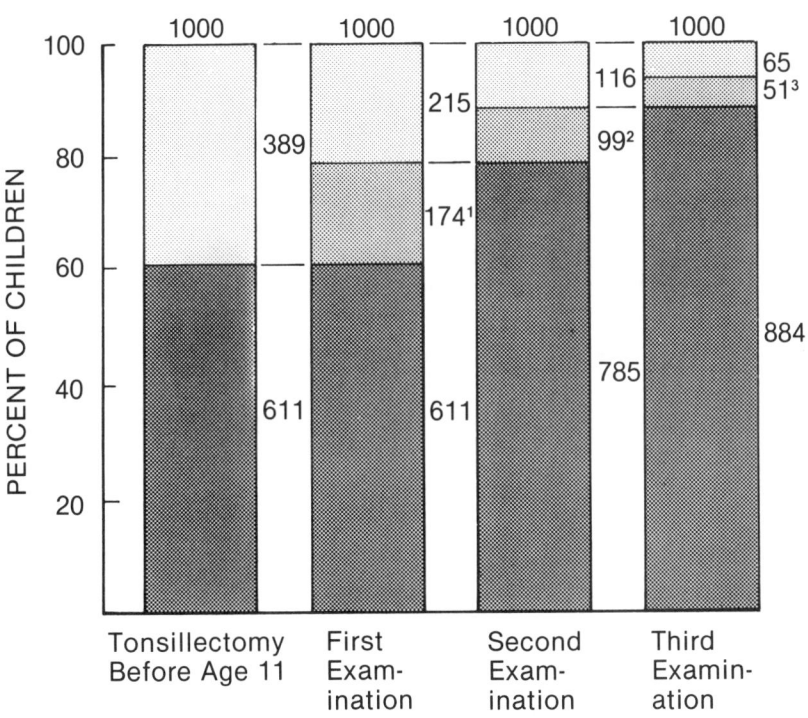

[1]Represents 45% of children without tonsillectomies at the previous stage.
[2]Represents 46% of children without tonsillectomies at the previous stage.
[3]Represents 44% of children without tonsillectomies at the previous stage.

SOURCE: American Child Health Association, Research Division, *Physical Defects, The Pathway to Correction*, American Child Health Association, New York, 1934, pp. 80–84.

Chart G-14

Percent of Primary Appendectomies in Which "No Disease" was Reported After Pathological Examination of the Removed Tissues
(19 Selected Hospitals, Southwest Michigan, 1956–1957).

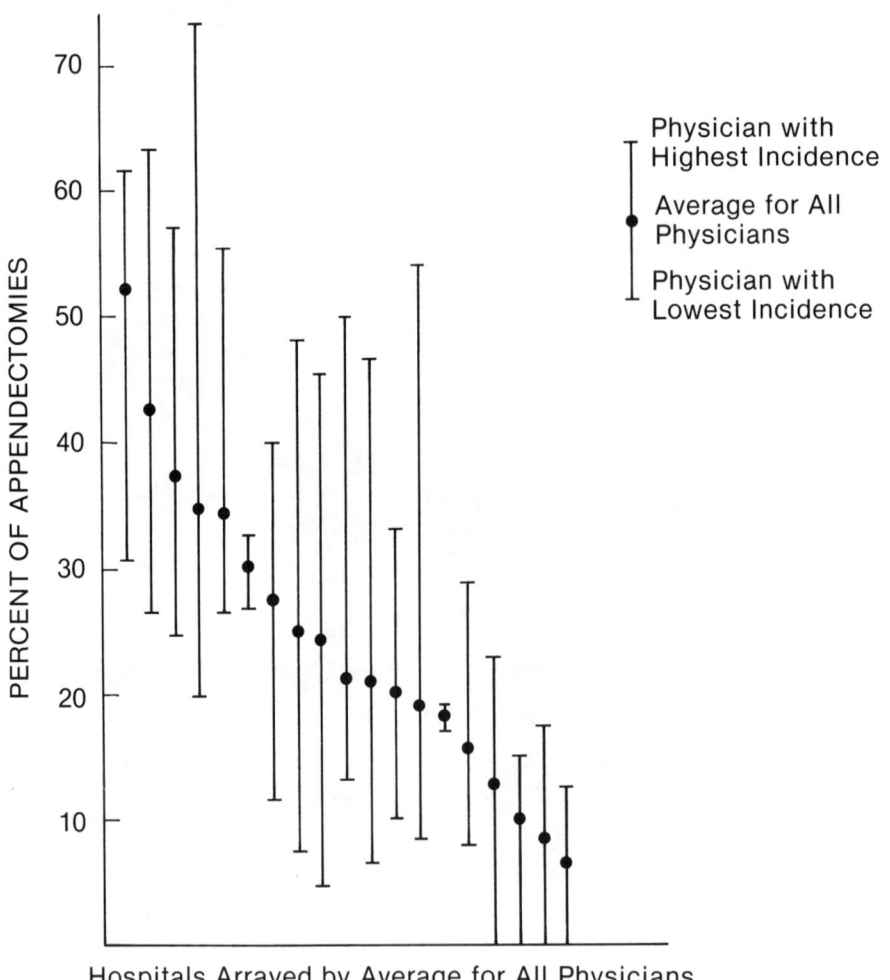

SOURCE: Weeks, H.A., "Tightness of Organization Related to Patterns of Patient Care," Bureau of Public Health Economics, School of Public Health, The University of Michigan, Ann Arbor, Michigan.

Quality of Care

Chart G-15

Percent Distribution of Hysterectomies Performed in 35 Non-governmental Hospitals, by Justification of Operation
(Los Angeles and Vicinity, California, 1948).

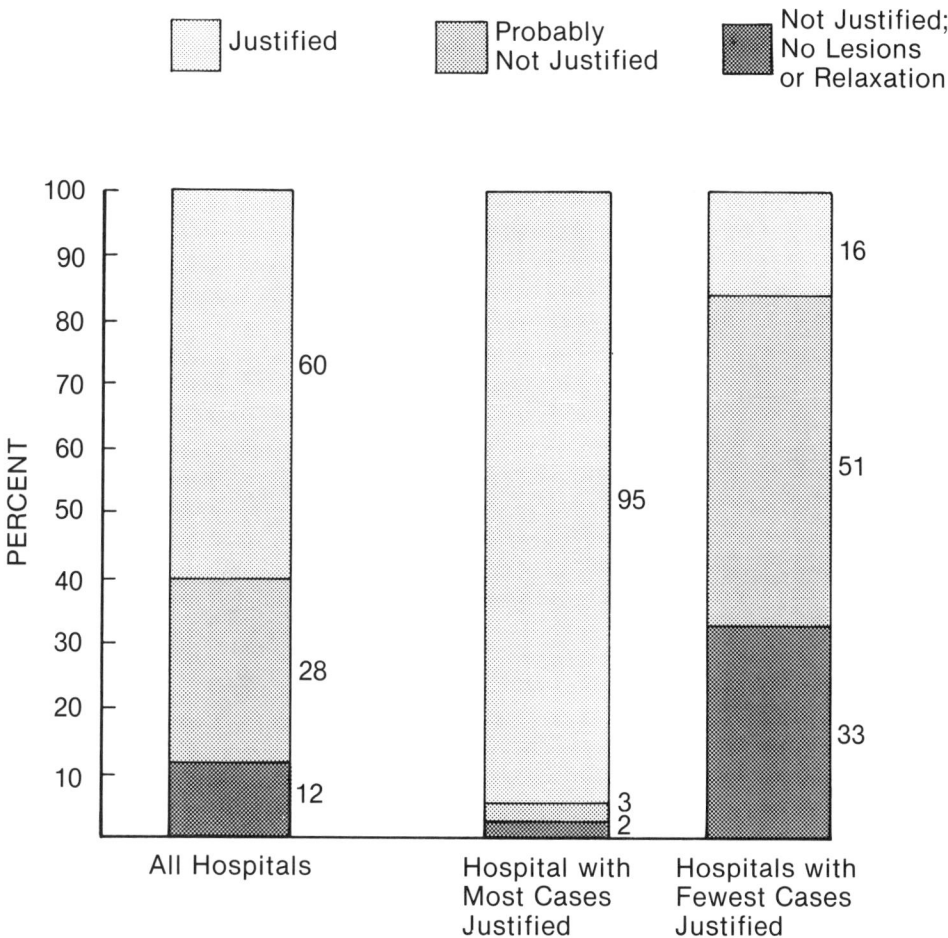

SOURCE: Doyle, J. C., "Unnecessary Hysterectomies: Study of 6248 Operations in Thirty-Five Hospitals During 1948," *Journal of the American Medical Association*, Vol. 151, January 31, 1953, pp. 360–365.

Chart G-16

Percent of Appendectomies Classified Pathologically as "Unnecessary" or "Doubtful" in Two Universities and Three Community Hospitals, by Type of Hospital and Patient Pay Status (Baltimore, 1957 and 1958).

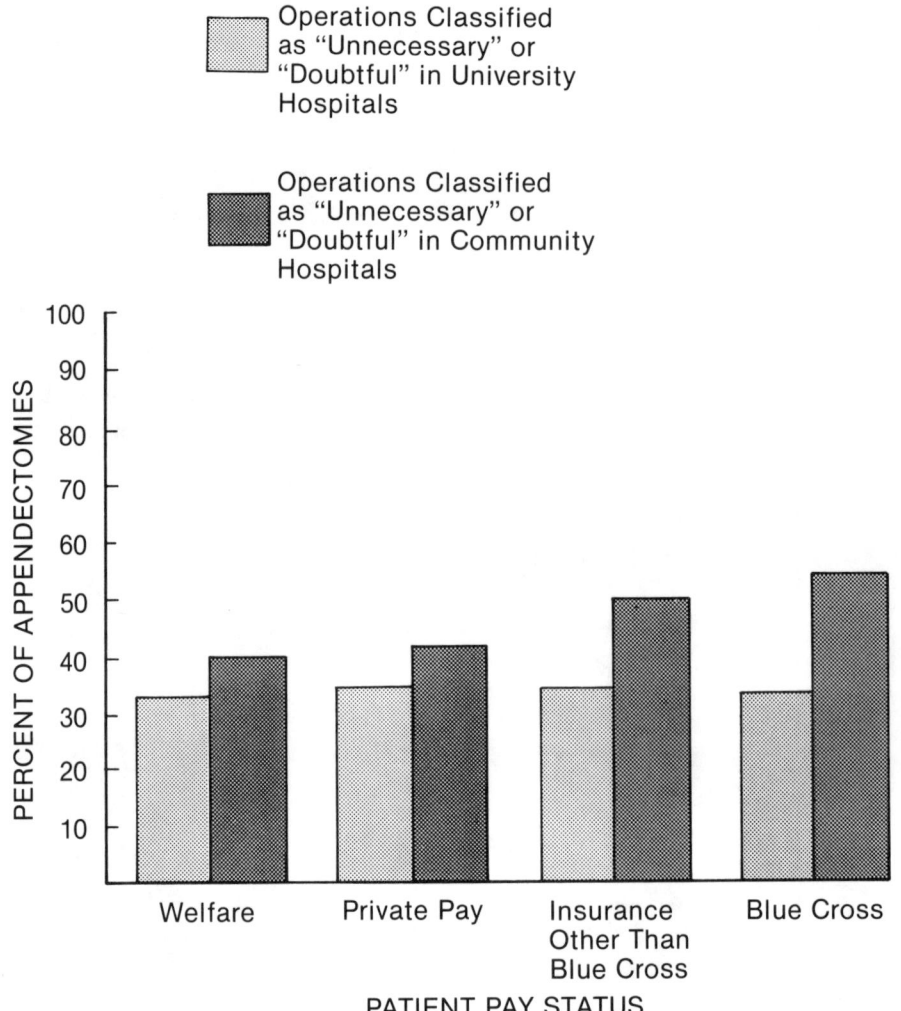

SOURCE: Sparling, J. F., "Measuring Medical Care Quality: A Comparative Study," *Hospitals*, Vol. 36, March 16, 1962, p. 67.

Chart G-17 Disposition of Patients Admitted with Appendicitis as Initial Diagnosis, by Correctness of Diagnosis (Glasgow, Scotland).

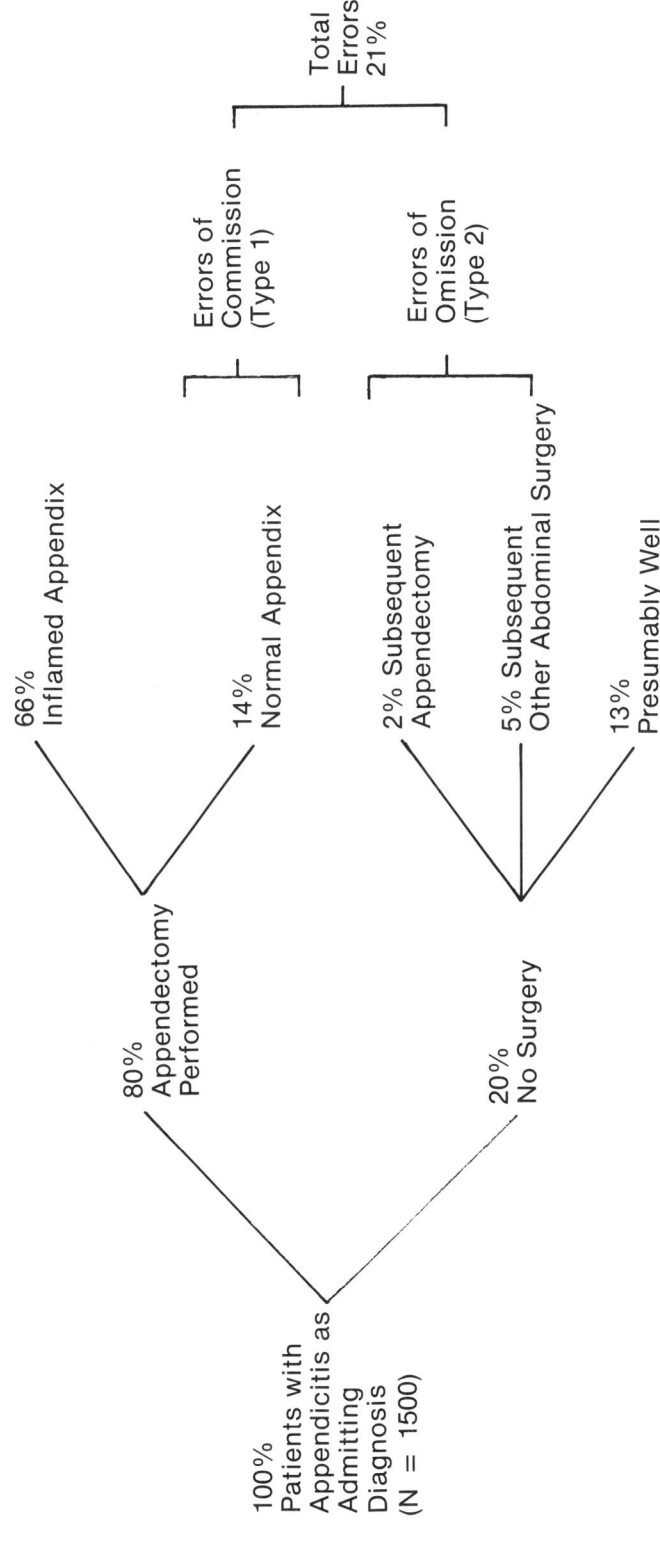

SOURCE: Study by J.G.R. Howie, as cited in: Thomas, E.J. and C. Barbara Mueller, "Appendectomy: Diagnostic Criteria and Hospital Performance," *Hospital Practice*, April 1969, p. 73.

Chart G-18

Percent Distribution of Persons (12–29 Years of Age) Admitted for Possible Appendicitis by Whether Operated, Nature of Tissue Removed and Subsequent Recurrence of Symptoms, and by Type of Approach to Surgery (Western Infirmary of Glasgow, Scotland, 1963).

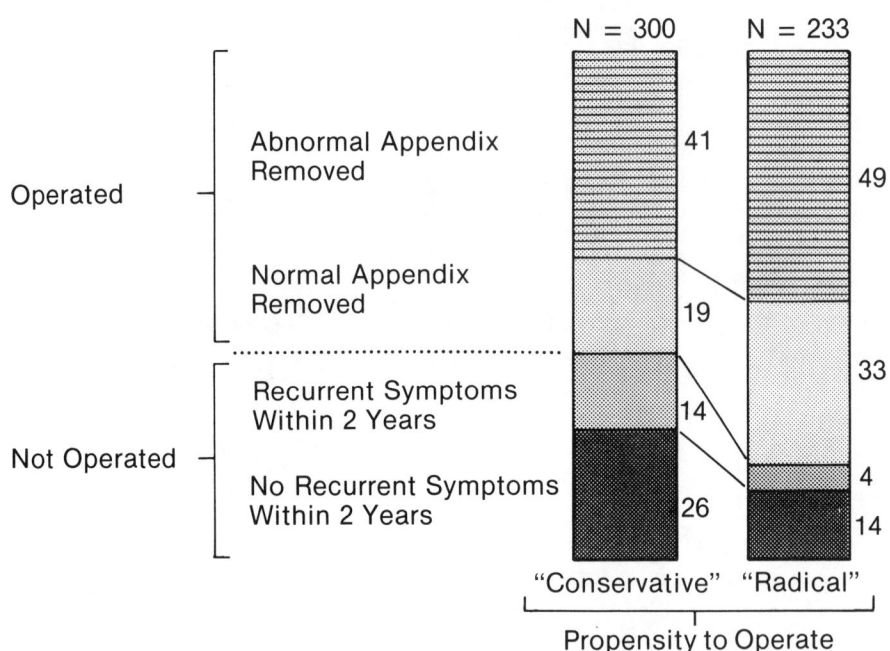

Computation of Expected Avoidable Mortality For Each Approach, Based on Estimates of Risk

State of Appendix	Percent by State	Mortality Risk	Expected Mortality[2]
	"Conservative Approach"		
Normal, Removed	19	0.02	0.0038%
Abnormal, Not Removed	8[1]	0.04	0.0032
Both	—	—	0.0070
	"Radical Approach"		
Normal, Removed	33	0.02	0.0066%
Abnormal, Not Removed	0	0.04	— —
Both	—	—	0.0066

[1]49% − 41% = 8%   [2]Product of Preceding Columns

SOURCE: Howie, J.G.R., "The Place of Appendectomy in the Treatment of Young Adult Patients With Possible Appendicitis," *Lancet*, Vol. 1, June 22, 1968, p. 1365–1367.

Chart G-19

Expected Deaths, Hospital Costs, and Convalescent Days Associated with Performing Appendectomies on Patients Who Present Themselves with Signs and Symptoms that Correspond to Increasing Probabilities of the Presence of True Appendicitis.

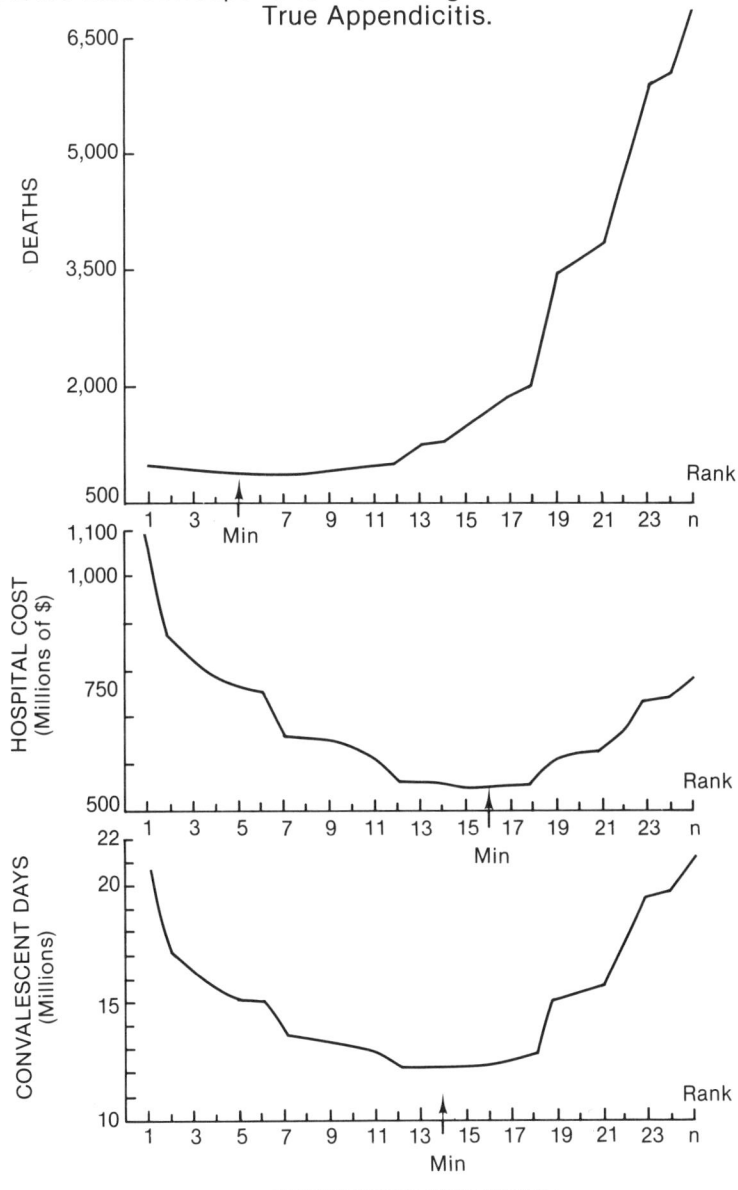

NOTE: The assumption was made that 100% of true appendicitis cases not operated on would result in perforation of the appendix. The appendicitis risk score corresponds to twenty-four possible symptom combinations ranked from least likely to most likely of being associated with appendicitis.

SOURCE: Neutra, Raymond, "Indications for the surgical treatment of suspected acute appendicitis: a cost-effectiveness approach," in *Costs, Risks, and Benefits of Surgery*, J.P. Bunker, B.A. Barnes and F. Mosteller, editors, New York, 1977, Figure 18-3, p. 289.

Chart G-20

Percent Distribution of Children under 14 Admitted to the Pediatric Service of the Johns Hopkins Hospital with a Possible Diagnosis of Appendicitis, by Whether Surgery Was Done, and by the Clinical-Pathological Findings after Surgery, During Two Periods that Differed in the Prevailing Strategy of Management (Baltimore, 1965-1974).

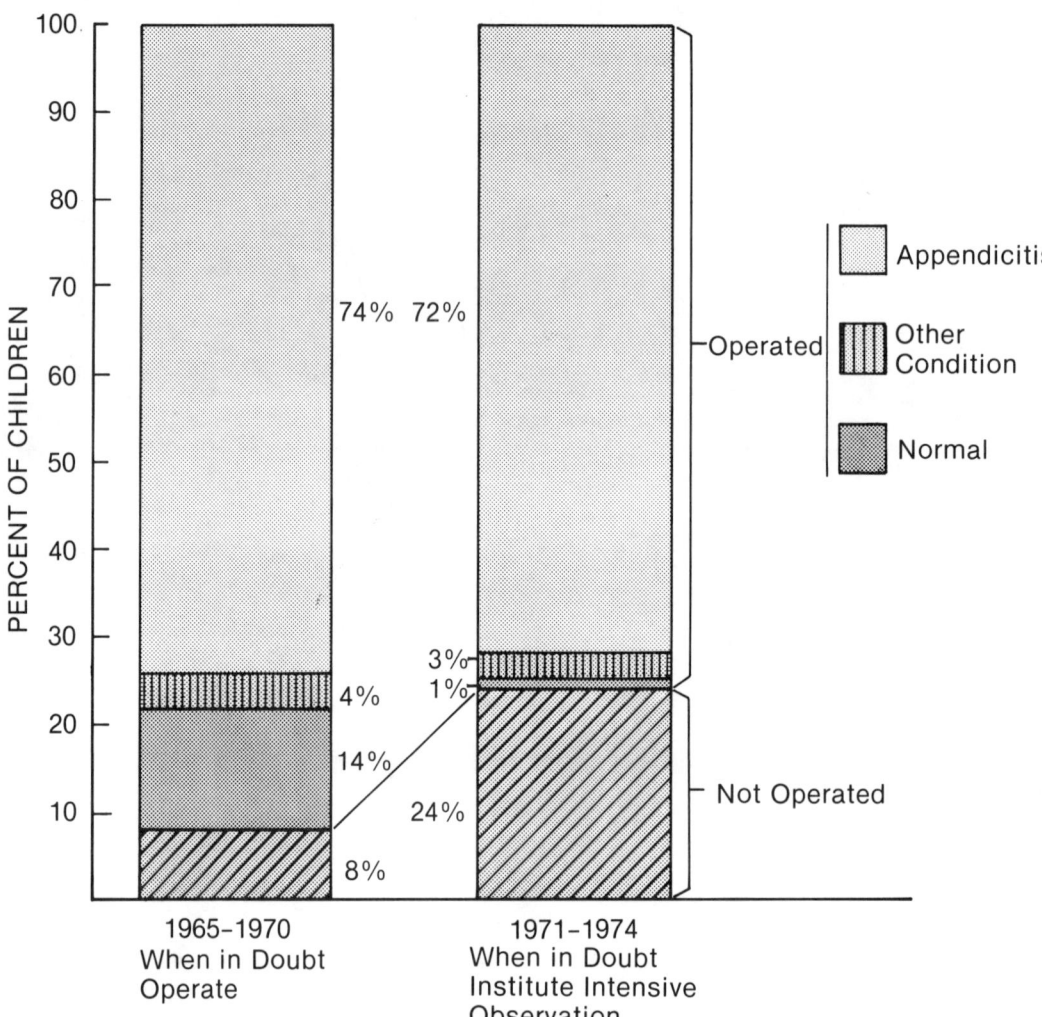

NOTE: During the two periods 27 and 28 percent of appendectomies were for a ruptured appendix, but no rupture occurred during the period of observation. The mortality rates were 0.75 and 0.96 percent of operations (0.96 and 0.73 percent of all cases). None of the cases discharged without an operation has returned with, or been treated elsewhere for, recurrent appendicitis. Seven out of 213 cases included in the category of "appendicitis" during 1965-1970 had "pinworm infestation."

SOURCE: White, J.J., M. Santillana, and J.A. Haller, "Intensive In-Hospital Observation: A Safe Way to Decrease Unnecessary Appendectomy," *American Surgeon,* Vol. 41, December 1975, Tables 1 and 2, p. 794.

Quality of Care

Chart G-21 Percent Distribution of Persons Participating in a Mandatory Second Opinion Program for Elective Surgery, by Specified Status, Reported One Year After Being Seen by the Consultant Surgeon (Cornell University Program, New York, February 1972 - February 1978).

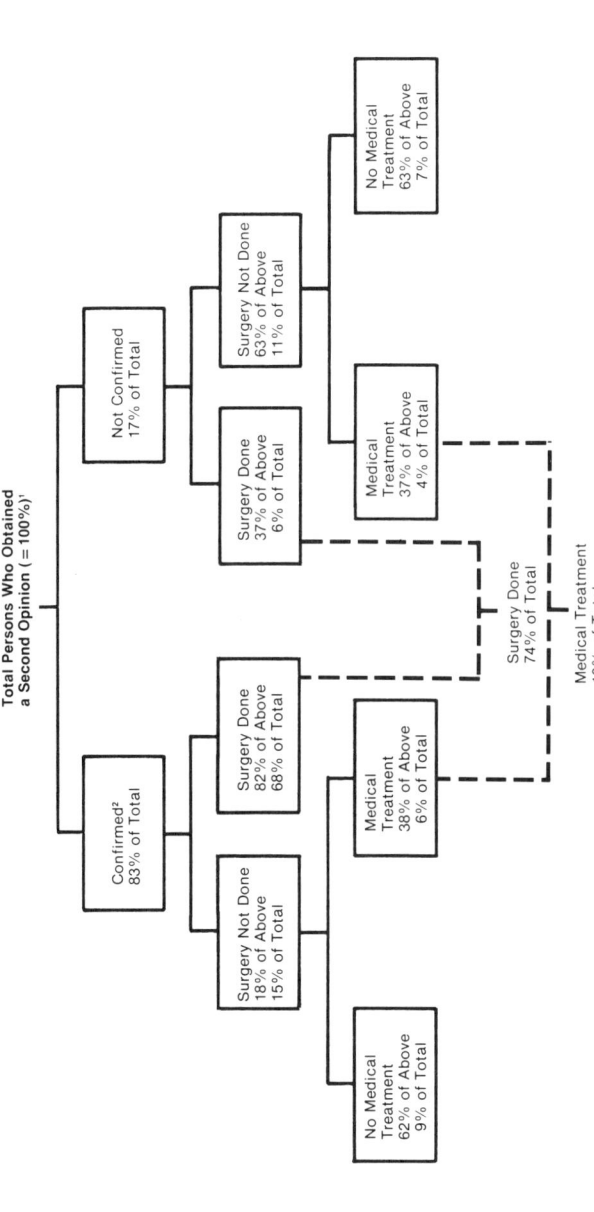

[1] Persons participating in an insurance program requiring that whenever elective surgery is recommended, a board-certified surgeon examine the patient and provide a second opinion on the need for the operation

[2] Cases in which the consultant surgeon confirmed that surgery is needed.

NOTE: The figure of 17% "not confirmed" is an estimate based on data for the period February 1972–October 1977 reported by E. G. McCarthy and M. C. Finkel in a paper presented at the HCFA Conference on Research Results from Physician Reimbursement Studies, Washington D.C., 1978. This figure was used to compute the total number of persons who obtained a second opinion under the assumption that a 70 percent response rate applies equally to confirmed and non-confirmed cases. Data reported for the sample of "confirmed" cases who were followed up were taken to apply to all confirmed cases.

SOURCE: McCarthy, E.G. and M.L. Finkel, "Second Opinion Elective Surgery Programs: Outcome Status over Time," *Medical Care*, Vol. 61, December 1978, Tables 1, 2, 5 and 6, pp. 988 and 990.

Chart G-22 Number of Total and Unjustified Abdominal Hysterectomies, and Percent of Total Abdominal Hysterectomies that were Judged to be Unjustified, Before and After the Institution of External Review (Five Hospitals, Saskatchewan, Canada, 1970 and 1974).

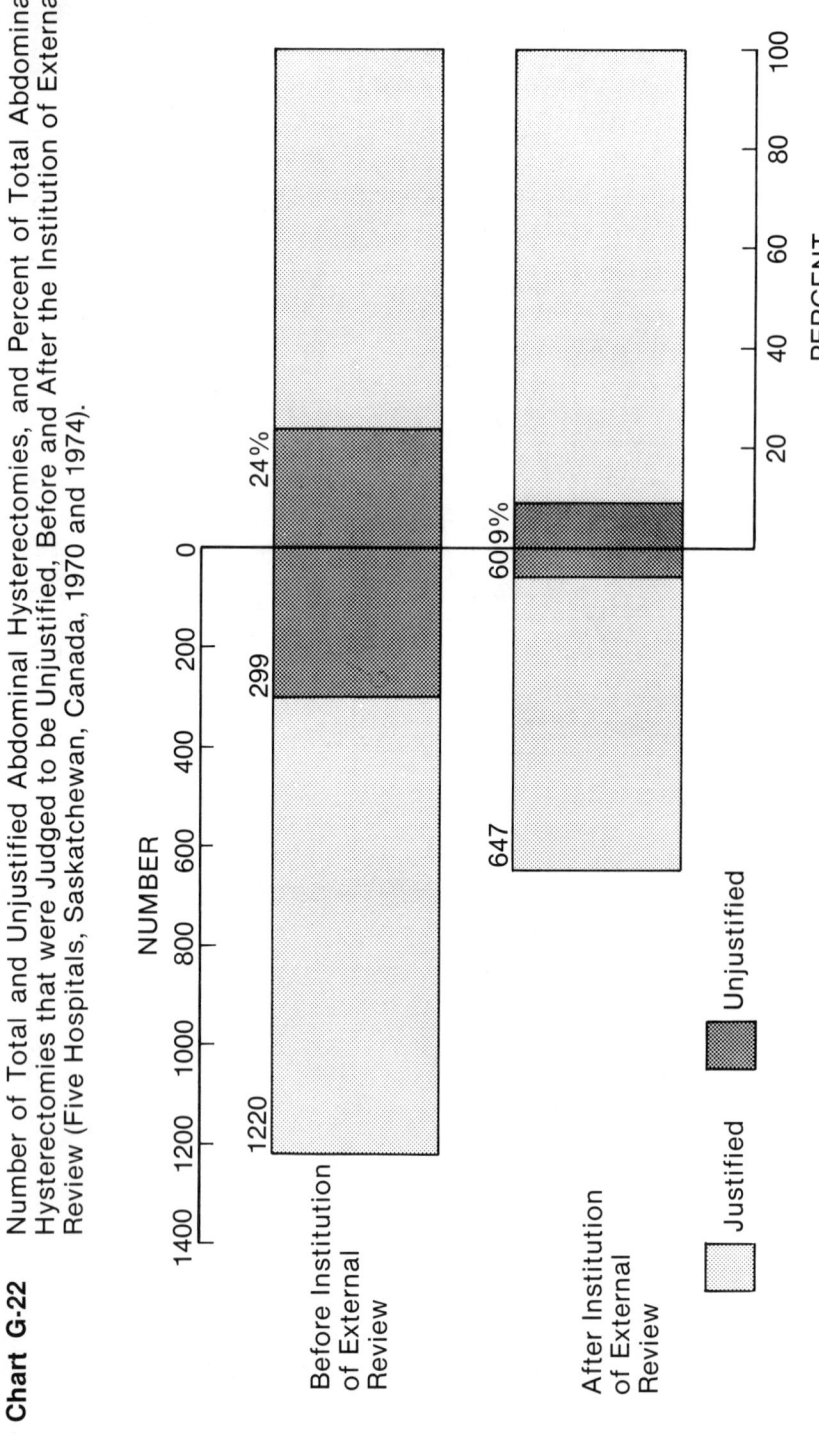

NOTE: A committee of the College of Physicians and Surgeons specified indications of abdominal hysterectomy, reviewed hospital records for compliance with indications, and discussed the findings with the medical staff, the administrative officers and the board of governors of each hospital.

SOURCE: Dyck, F. J., et al., "Effect of Surveillance on the Number of Hysterectomies in the Province of Saskatchewan," *New England Journal of Medicine*, Vol. 296, June 9, 1977, Table 1, p. 1327.

Chart G-23

Comparative Assessment of Clinic Patients[1] with Suspected Urinary Tract Infection (Medical School Outpatient Department, Spring 1965).

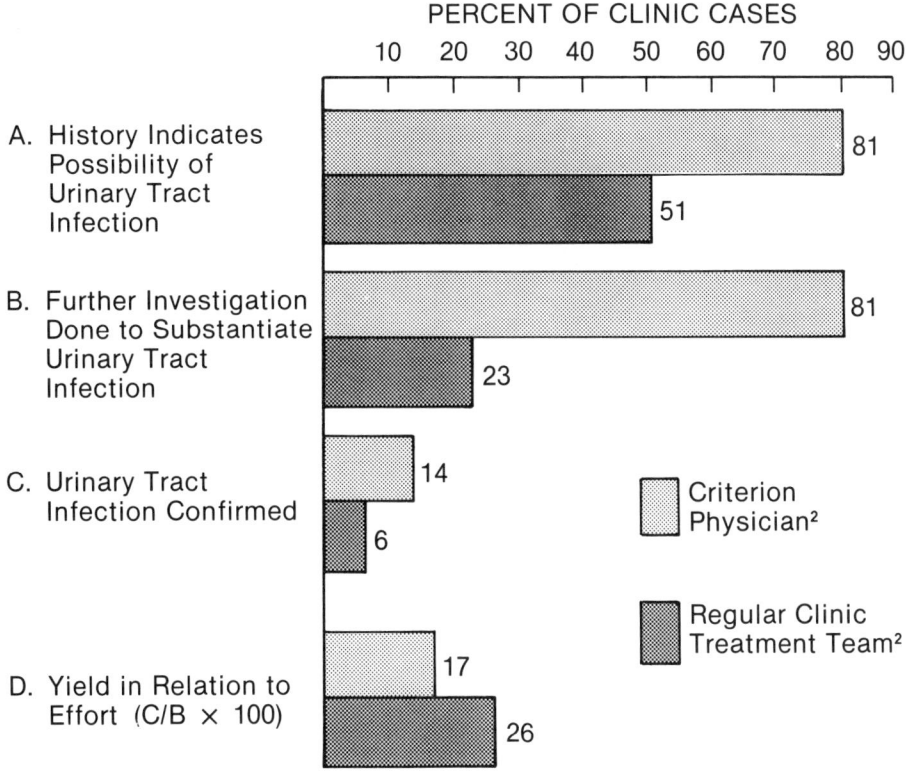

[1] All new patients (N = 133) accepted for the medical clinic during a three-month period.

[2] The criterion physician was the researcher who used standard criteria compiled from an extensive review of the literature. The regular clinic treatment team consisted of a senior medical student and an attending physician.

SOURCE: Gonnella, J.S., et al, "Evaluation of Patient Care: An Approach," *Journal of the American Medical Association*, Vol. 214, December 14, 1970, pp. 2040–2043.

Chart G-24

Hospitals by Percent of Deficiencies in Management[1] Which Were Considered to be "Presumptive" Evidence and Those Which Were Considered to be "Substantial" Evidence of Poor Management[2]
(Four Hospitals, Metropolitan Boston, 1956).

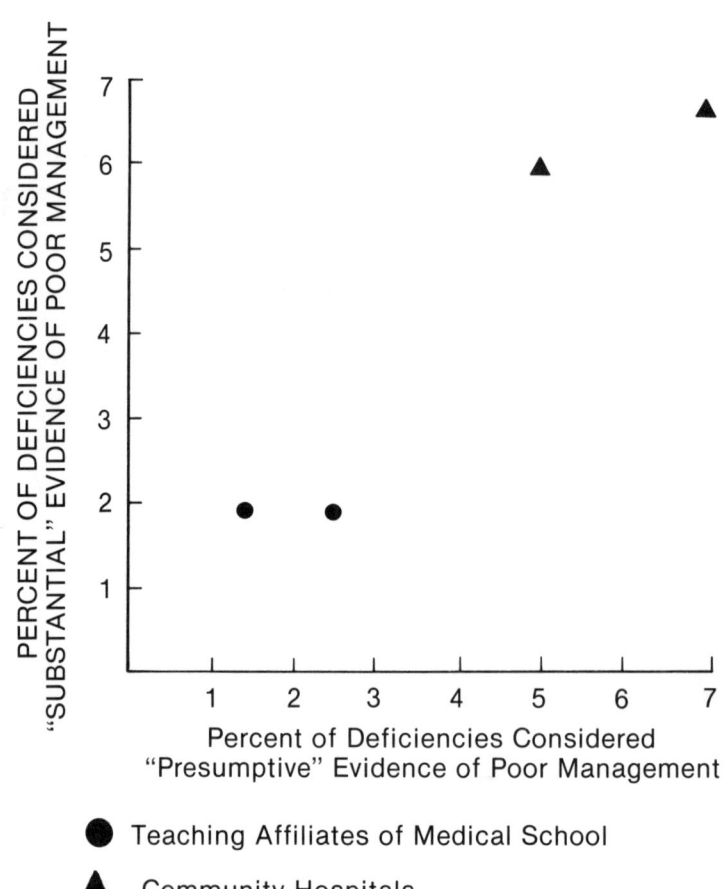

[1]Judgments of deficiencies made by review of charts in selected diagnoses from the departments of medicine, surgery and obstetrics-gynecology.

[2]The "presumptive" category was composed of those that might reflect inadequacy in recording alone and not necessarily important omissions or mistakes in diagnosis or treatment. The "substantial" category was composed of instances of omission of essential diagnostic or therapeutic procedures which would be recorded routinely if they had been done, or use of contraindicated therapy, or unacceptable surgical procedures.

SOURCE: Rosenfeld, Leonard S., "Quality of Medical Care in Hospitals," *American Journal of Public Health*, Vol. 47, July 1957, p. 862.

Quality of Care

Chart G-25

Percent of Hospitalized Cases Judged to Have Received "Less Than Optimal" Medical Care and Percent Admitted Unnecessarily to the Hospital, by Medical Specialty (Teamster Family Members, New York City, 1962).

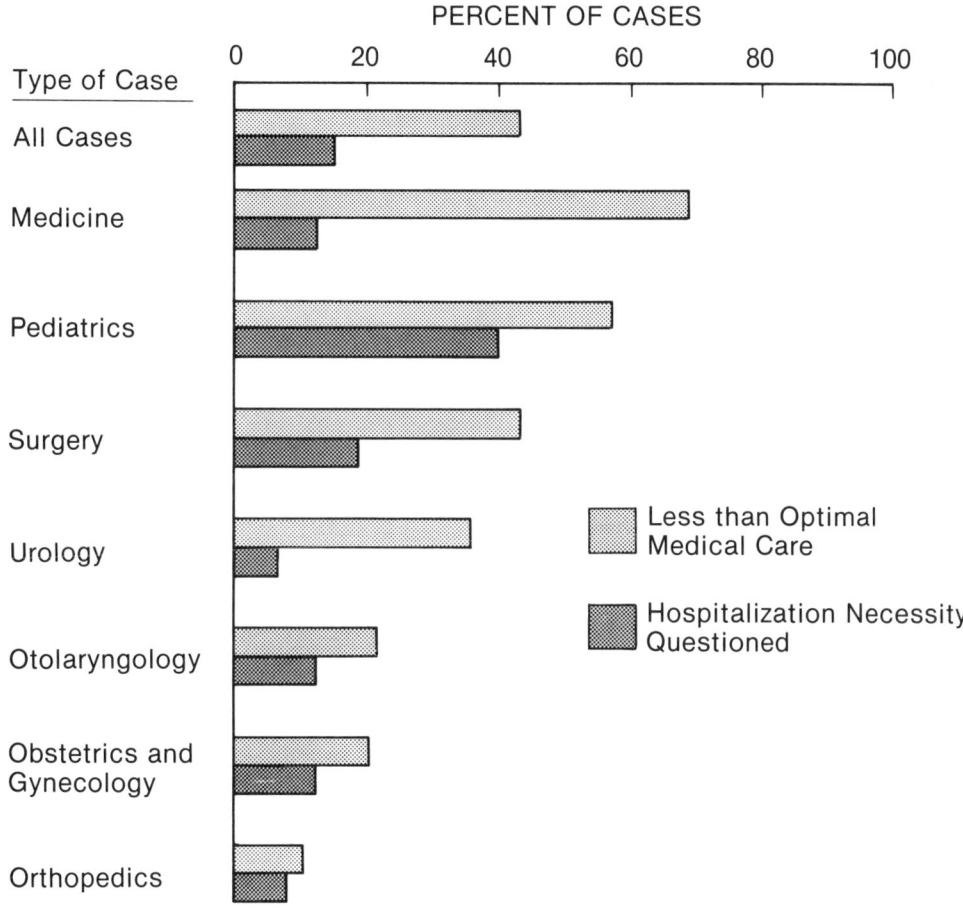

SOURCE: Morehead, M.A. and R.S. Donaldson, *A Study of the Quality of Hospital Care Secured by a Sample of Teamster Family Members in New York City*, Columbia University, School of Public Health and Administrative Medicine, New York, 1964, Table 3, p. 47 and Table 5, p. 52.

Quality of Care

Chart G-26

Percent of Hospital Admissions Judged to be Unnecessary, by Selected Diagnostic, Hospital, and Physician Characteristics (Teamster Family Members, New York City, 1962).

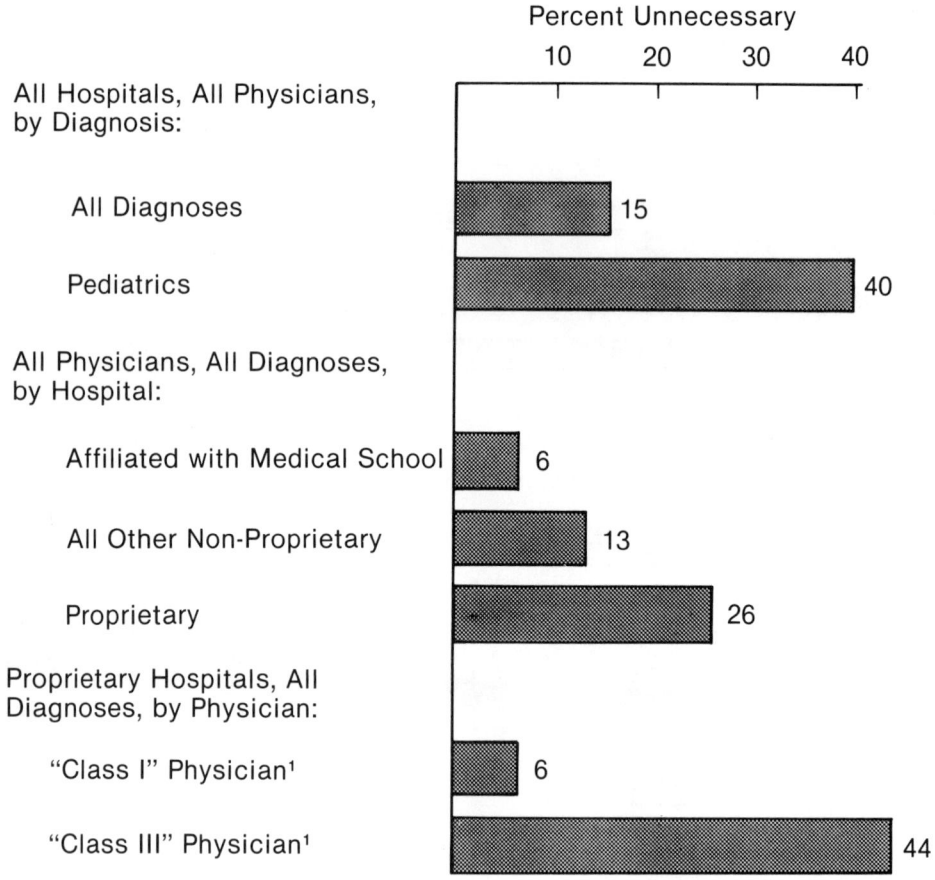

[1]Class I physicians are diplomates of an American Specialty Board or Fellows of an American College; Class III physicians are not Diplomates or Fellows and have no staff appointments in a voluntary or municipal hospital.

SOURCE: Morehead, M.A. and R.S. Donaldson, *A Study of the Quality of Hospital Care Secured by a Sample of Teamster Family Members in New York City*, Columbia University, School of Public Health and Administrative Medicine, New York, 1964, Table 8, p. 52, Table 9, p. 53, and Table 10, p. 54.

Quality of Care

Chart G-27

Percent of Hospital Admissions Judged to Have Received "Less Than Optimal" Care, by Type of Hospital
(Teamster Family Members, New York City, 1962).

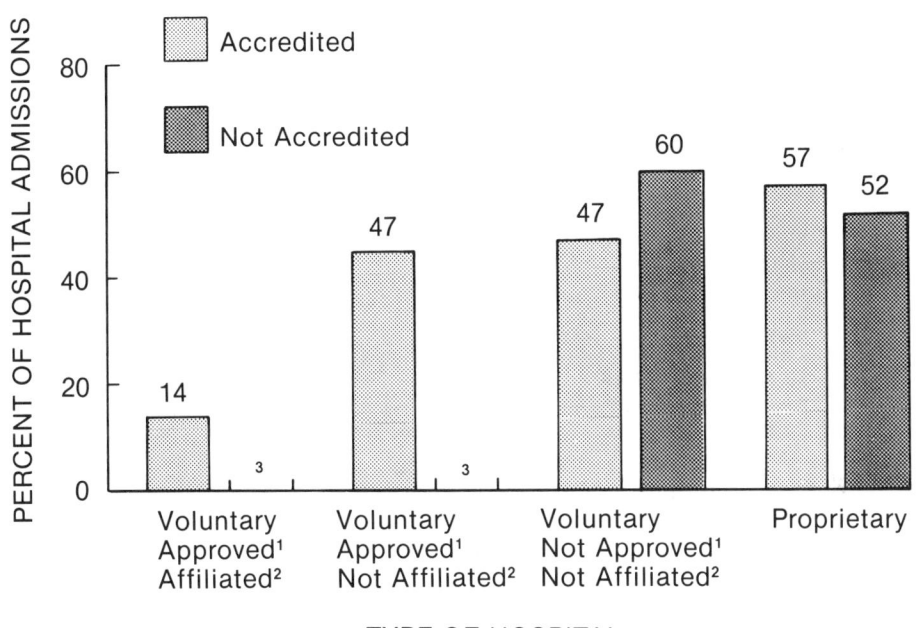

[1] Approved for residency and for internship.

[2] Affiliated with a medical school.

[3] No non-accredited hospital in this category.

SOURCE: Personal communication from M.A. Morehead, based on data from: Morehead, M.A. and R.S. Donaldson, *A Study of the Quality of Hospital Care Secured by a Sample of Teamster Family Members in New York City*, Columbia University, School of Public Health and Administrative Medicine, New York, 1964.

Quality of Care

Chart G-28

Percent of Hospital Admissions Judged to Have Received "Less Than Optimal" Care, by Type of Hospital and by Physician Qualification (Teamster Family Members, New York City, 1962).

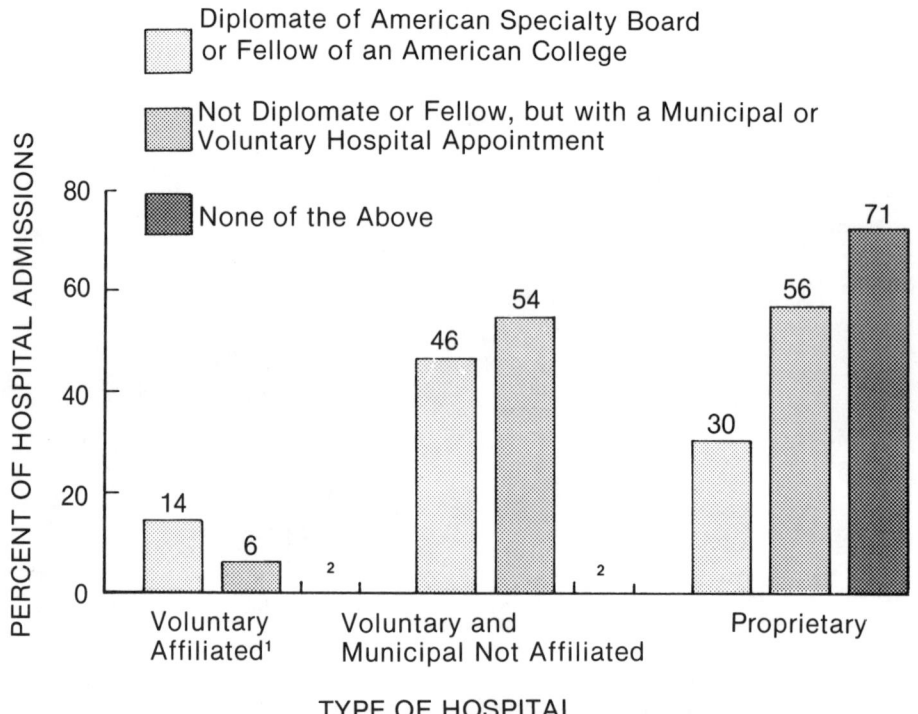

[1] Affiliated with a medical school.

[2] No physicians without special qualifications in hospitals in these categories.

SOURCE: Morehead, M.A. and R.S. Donaldson, *A Study of the Quality of Hospital Care Secured by a Sample of Teamster Family Members in New York City*, Columbia University, School of Public Health and Administrative Medicine, New York, 1964.

Quality of Care

Chart G-29 Percent of Surgical and Non-Surgical Admissions Under Care of a Board Certified Physician, and Percent Judged as Having Received Optimal Medical Care (Teamster Family Members, New York City, 1962).

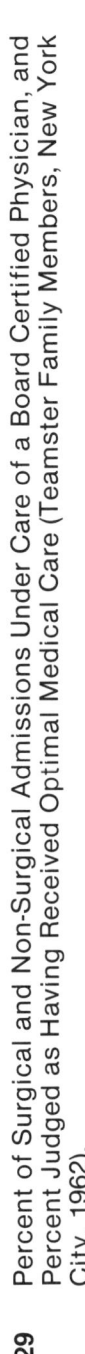

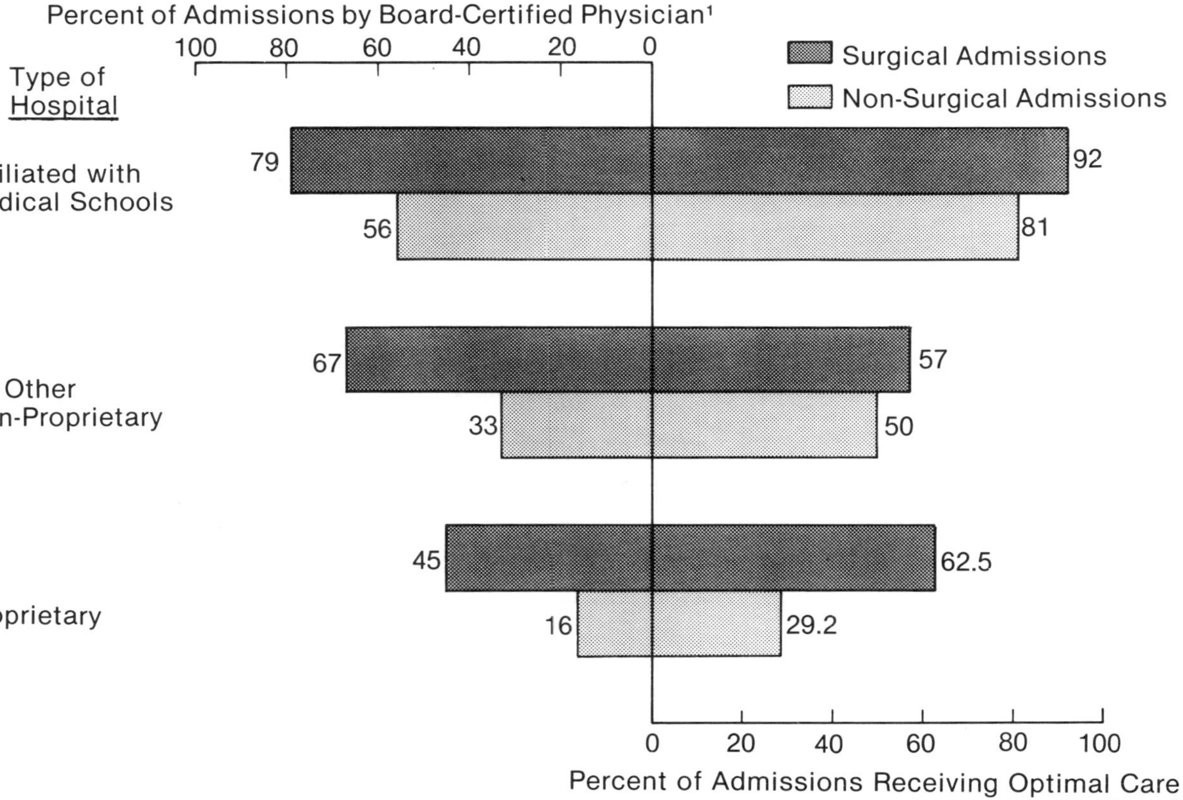

Type of Hospital	Percent of Admissions by Board-Certified Physician[1]		Percent of Admissions Receiving Optimal Care	
	Surgical Admissions	Non-Surgical Admissions	Surgical Admissions	Non-Surgical Admissions
Affiliated with Medical Schools	79	56	92	81
All Other Non-Proprietary	67	33	57	50
Proprietary	45	16	62.5	29.2

[1]Diplomates of an American Specialty Board or Fellows of an American College.

SOURCE: Morehead, M.A. and R.S. Donaldson, *A Study of the Quality of Hospital Care Secured by a Sample of Teamster Family Members in New York City*, Columbia University, School of Public Health and Administrative Medicine, New York, 1964, Table 5, p. 49 and Table 6, p. 60.

Chart G-30 Physician Performance Index[1] and Percent of Cases that Are Appropriately Admitted and Have an Appropriate Length of Stay, According to Specialist Status of Physician[2] and Size of Hospital,[3] in a Representative Sample of Hospital Discharges, 16 Diagnostic Categories (Hawaii, 1968).

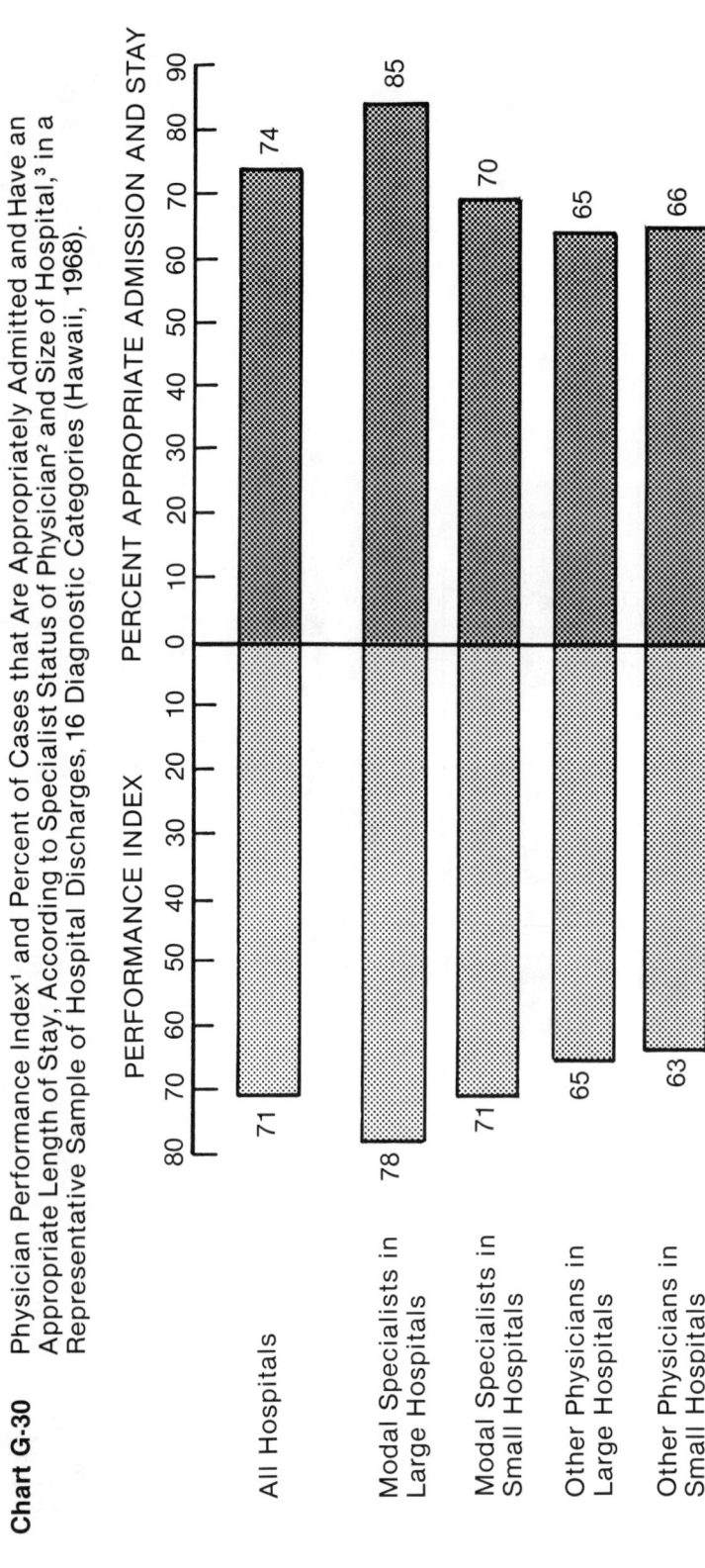

[1] The Performance Index is actual score as a percent of perfect score determined by 8 panels of "outstanding practitioners" in Hawaii according to specified standards of care, admission and length of stay for each diagnosis.

[2] The modal specialist is the one who characteristically cares for each particular diagnosis.

[3] Large hospitals are those that have annual discharges of 4,000 or more.

SOURCE: Payne, B.C. and T.F. Lyons, *Method of Evaluating and Improving Medical Care Quality: Episode of Illness Study*, Ann Arbor, Michigan, The University of Michigan School of Medicine, February 1972, p. 38.

Quality of Care

Chart G-31 Physician Performance Index[1] and Percent of Cases That are Appropriately Admitted and Have Appropriate Length of Stay, by Type of Practice[2] in a Representative Sample of Hospital Discharges in 16 Diagnostic Categories (Hawaii, 1968).

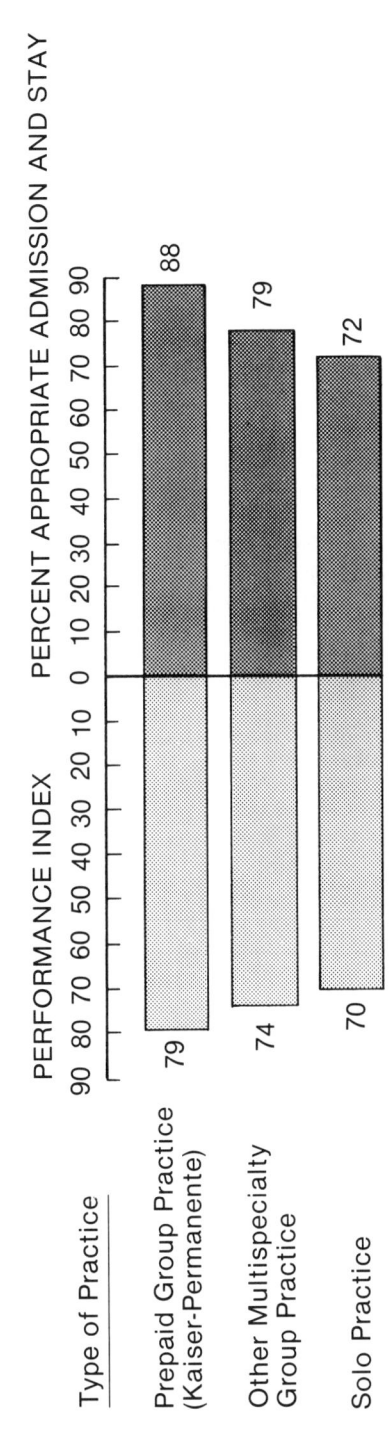

[1] The Performance Index is actual score as a percent of perfect score determined by 8 panels of "outstanding practitioners" in Hawaii according to specified standards of care, admission and length of stay for each diagnosis.

[2] Differences were virtually eliminated when comparison was continued to cases cared for by "modal specialist" in hospitals that had 4000 or more annual discharges.

SOURCE: Payne, B.C. and T.F. Lyons, *Method of Evaluating and Improving Medical Care Quality: Episode of Illness Study*, Ann Arbor, Michigan, The University of Michigan School of Medicine, February 1972, p. 38.

Quality of Care

Chart G-32

Standardized Physician Performance Scores for Episodes of Care that Included Hospitalization, for 15 Diagnostic Categories, by Specialty Status and Domain of Practice, General Hospitals, (Hawaii, Care Initiated in 1968).[1]

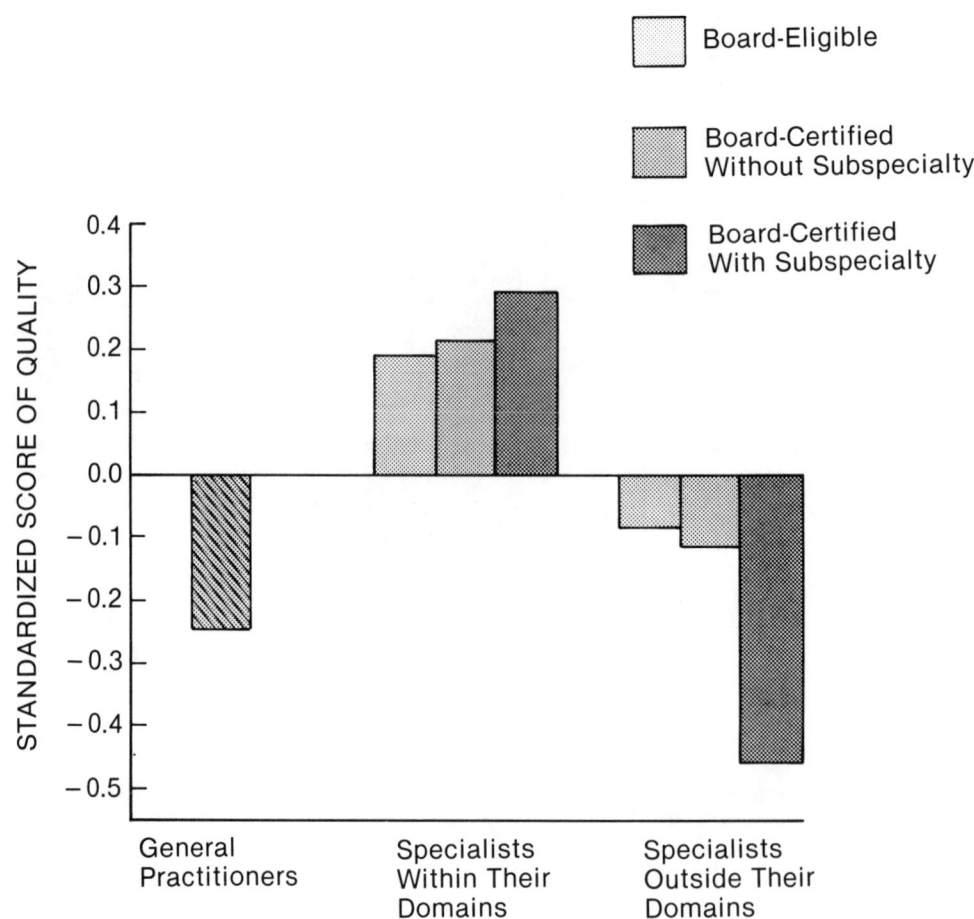

[1]Scores are standard deviations from the mean Performance Index for all cases and all physicians. The Performance Index is the percent of diagnosis-specific criteria complied with, as shown in the record. Criteria are weighted according to judged importance. "Domain" is the area of practice for which a specialist is specifically qualified. Generalists are considered not to have a distinctive "domain."

SOURCE: Rhee, S., *Relative Influence of Specialty Status, Organization of Office Care and Organization of Hospital Care on the Quality of Medical Care: A Multivariate Analysis*, Doctoral Dissertation, Ann Arbor, Michigan, The University of Michigan, 1975, Table IV-2, p. 79 and Table IV-4, p. 89.

Quality of Care

Chart G-33

Standardized Physician Performance Scores, for Episodes of Care That Included Hospitalization, for 15 Diagnostic Categories, by Type of Office Practice, Specialty Status and Domain of Practice, General Hospitals (Hawaii, Care Initiated in 1968).[1]

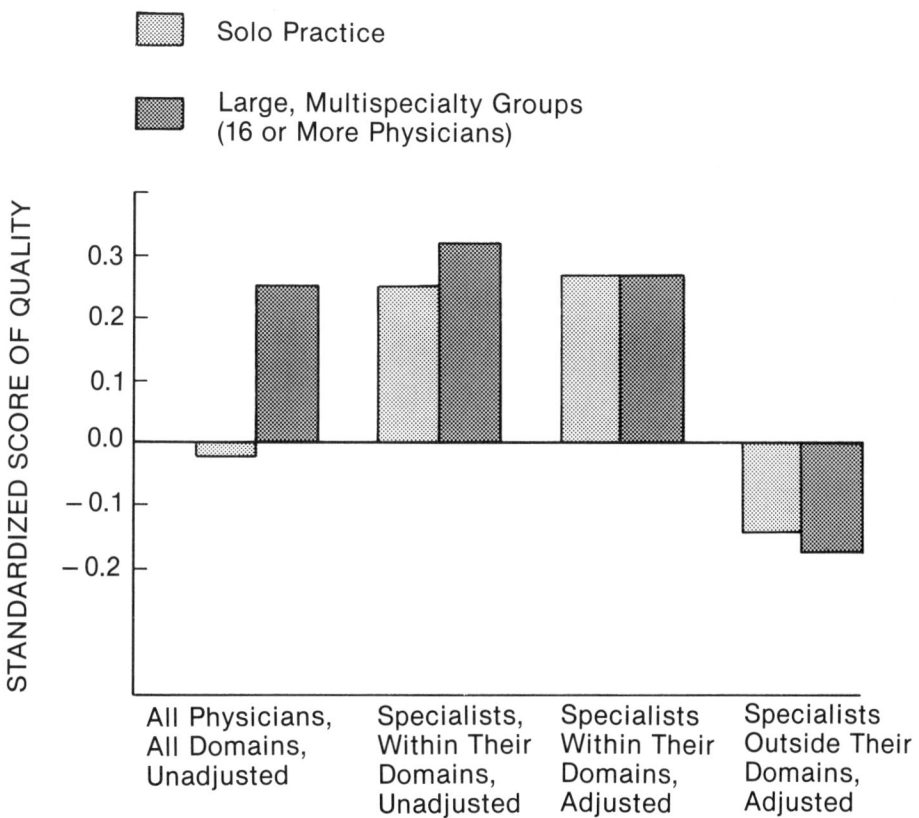

[1]Scores are standard deviations from the mean Performance Index for all cases and all physicians. The Performance Index is the percent of diagnosis—specific criteria complied with, as shown in the record. Criteria are weighted according to judged importance. "Domain" is the area of practice for which a specialist is specifically qualified. Generalists are considered not to have a distinctive "domain." Adjustment is for categories of medical school, length of practice, specialty status and type of hospital.

SOURCE: Rhee, S., *Relative Influence of Specialty Status, Organization of Office Care and Organization of Hospital Care on the Quality of Medical Care: A Multivariate Analysis*, Doctoral Dissertation, Ann Arbor, Michigan, The University of Michigan, 1975, Table V-5, p. 115 and Table V-6, p. 120.

Chart G-34

Standardized Physician Performance Scores, for Episodes of Care That Included Hospitalization, for 15 Diagnostic Categories, by Type of Hospital, General Hospitals (Hawaii, Care Initiated in 1968).[1]

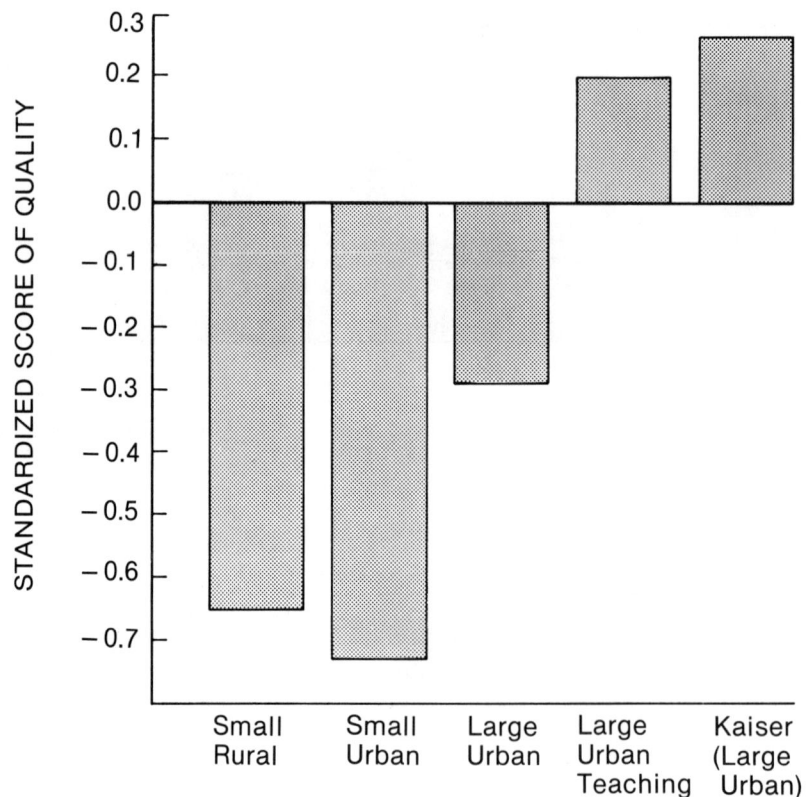

[1]Scores are standard deviations from the mean Performance Index for all cases and all physicians. The Performance Index is the percent of diagnosis-specific criteria complied with, as shown in the record. Criteria are weighted according to judgment of importance. Small hospitals have 52 beds or less. Large hospitals, with one exception have 100 beds or more.

SOURCE: Rhee, S., *Relative Influence of Specialty Status, Organization of Office Care and Organization of Hospital Care on the Quality of Medical Care: A Multivariate Analysis*, Doctoral Dissertation, Ann Arbor, Michigan, The University of Michigan, 1975, Table VI-5, p. 150.

Quality of Care

Chart G-35

Standardized Physician Performance Scores, for Episodes of Care That Included Hospitalization, for 15 Diagnostic Categories, by Type of Hospital and Level of Training of Physician, General Hospitals (Hawaii, Care Initiated in 1968).[1]

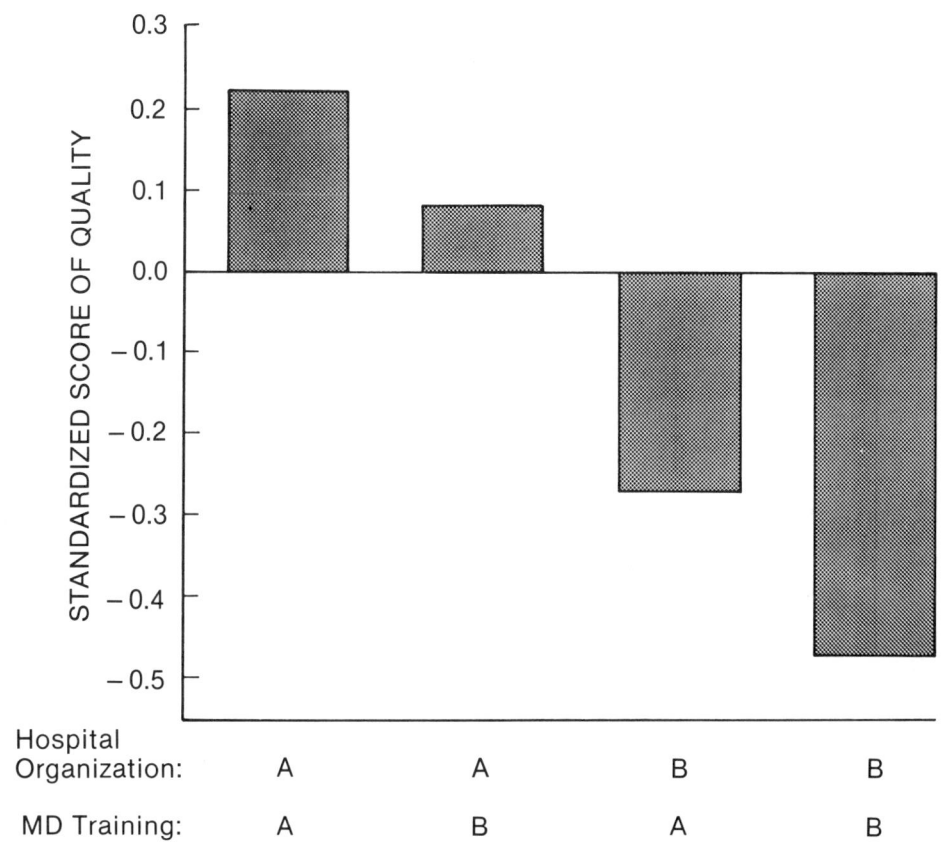

(A = High, and B = Low Hospital Organization or MD Training)

[1] Scores are standard deviations from the mean Performance Index for all cases and all physicians. The Performance Index is the percent of diagnosis-specific criteria complied with, as shown in the record. Criteria are weighted according to judged importance. The category of "highly organized" hospitals comprises teaching hospitals and the Kaiser Foundation Hospital, and that of "less organized" hospitals consists of all the rest. "Highly trained" physicians are those at least eligible for Board certification, all others are in the "low" category of training.

SOURCE: Rhee, S., *Relative Influence of Specialty Status, Organization of Office Care and Organization of Hospital Care on the Quality of Medical Care: A Multivariate Analysis*, Doctoral Dissertation, Ann Arbor, Michigan, The University of Michigan, 1975, Table VII, p. 182.

Chart G-36

Assessment of the Quality of Practice of a Representative Sample of General Practitioners (North Carolina, 1953-1954).[1]

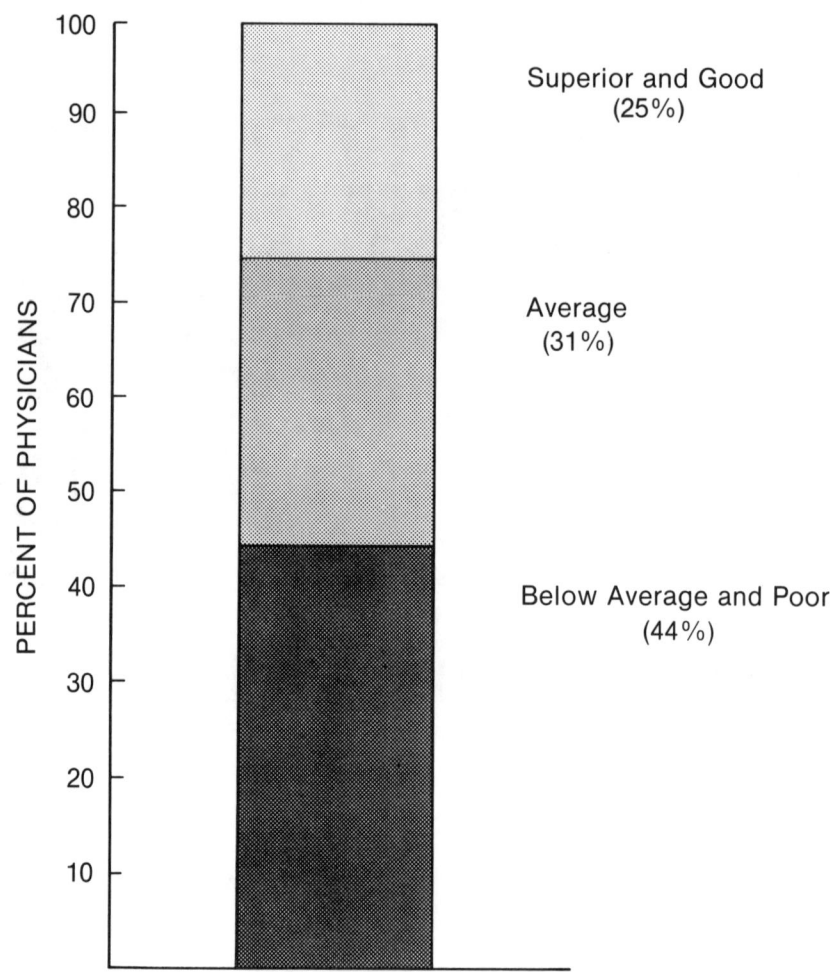

[1]Based on an assessment of individual practices with respect to clinical history, physical examination, use of laboratory aids, preventive medicine, and clinical records.

SOURCE: Peterson, O.L., et. al., "An Analytical Study of North Carolina General Practice, 1953-1954," *Journal of Medical Education*, Vol. 31, December 1956, Part 2.

Quality of Care

Chart G-37

Percent of General Practitioners Who Failed to Perform Specified Procedures or Performed Them Inadequately (North Carolina, 1953-1954).[1]

Procedure	Percent of Physicians
A. Physical Examination	
Disrobing of Patient for Examination	45
Percussion of Lungs	60
Auscultation of Lungs	23
Physical Examination of Heart	65
Examination of Abdomen	16
Rectal Examination	83
Ophthalmoscopy	66
B. Diagnostic Tests	
Urine	11
Hemoglobin	26
White Blood Cell Count	45
X-rays	18
Electrocardiograms	45
C. Treatment	
Use of Antibiotics	67
Treatment of Anemia	85
Treatment of Hypertension	57
Treatment of Congestive Heart Failure	39

[1] Data based on a survey of a representative sample of general practitioners.

SOURCE: Peterson, O.L. et. al., "An Analytical Study of North Carolina General Practice, 1953-1954," *Journal of Medical Education*, Vol. 31, December 1956, Part 2.

Quality of Care

Chart G-38

Assessment of the Quality of Practice of a Representative Sample of General Practitioners (Ontario, July 1956–October 1957 and Nova Scotia, December 1958–February 1960, Canada).

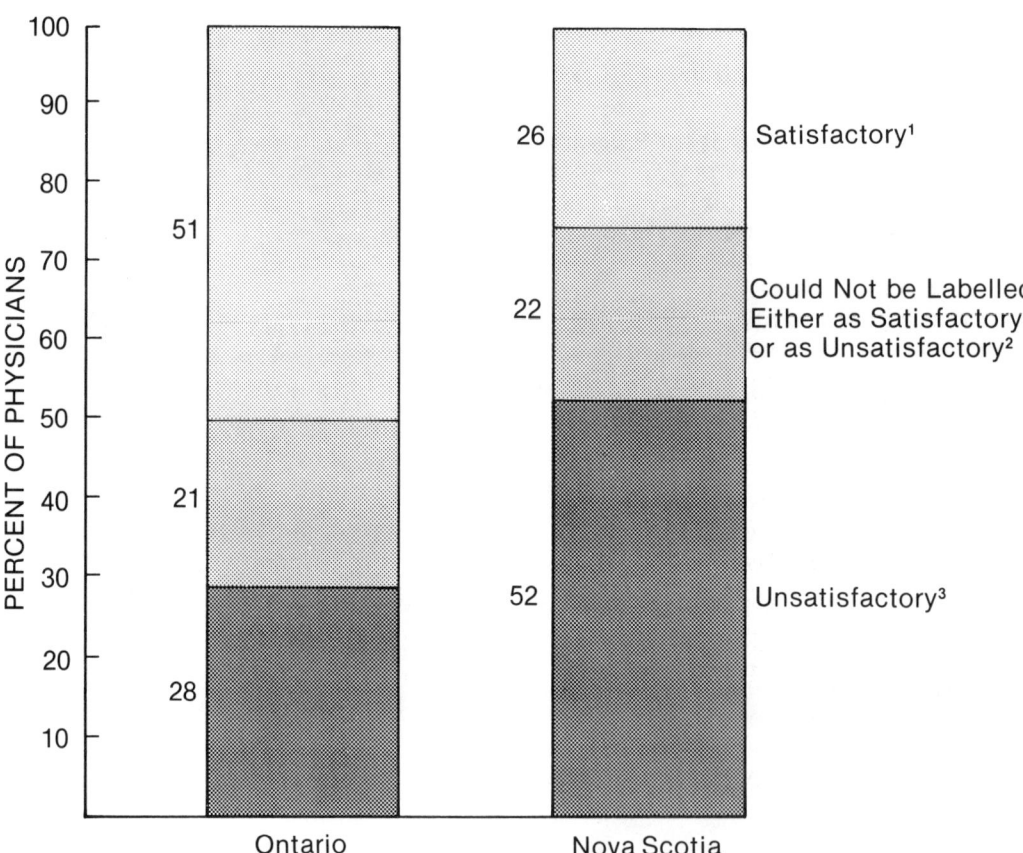

[1]"It appeared that the deficiencies of these men were not likely to have serious consequences for their patients, especially as they were likely to seek the help of a specialist ... some of these practices were of outstanding quality."

[2]"These doctors ... constituted a group about whom the observers were in some doubt."

[3]"(these physicians) caused the observers grave misgivings. The deficiencies in these men's practices were thought likely to expose their patients to serious risk."

SOURCE: Clute, K.F., *The General Practitioner—A Study of Medical Education and Practice in Ontario and Nova Scotia*, University of Toronto Press, Toronto, 1963, pp. 313–314.

Quality of Care

Chart G-39

Average Percent of Preformulated Explicit Criteria of Good Care that were Complied With in a Study of Ambulatory Patients Classified by Diagnosis, Specialty Status of the Physician, and Site of Care (New Haven and Hartford Metropolitan Areas, Connecticut, 1974–1975).

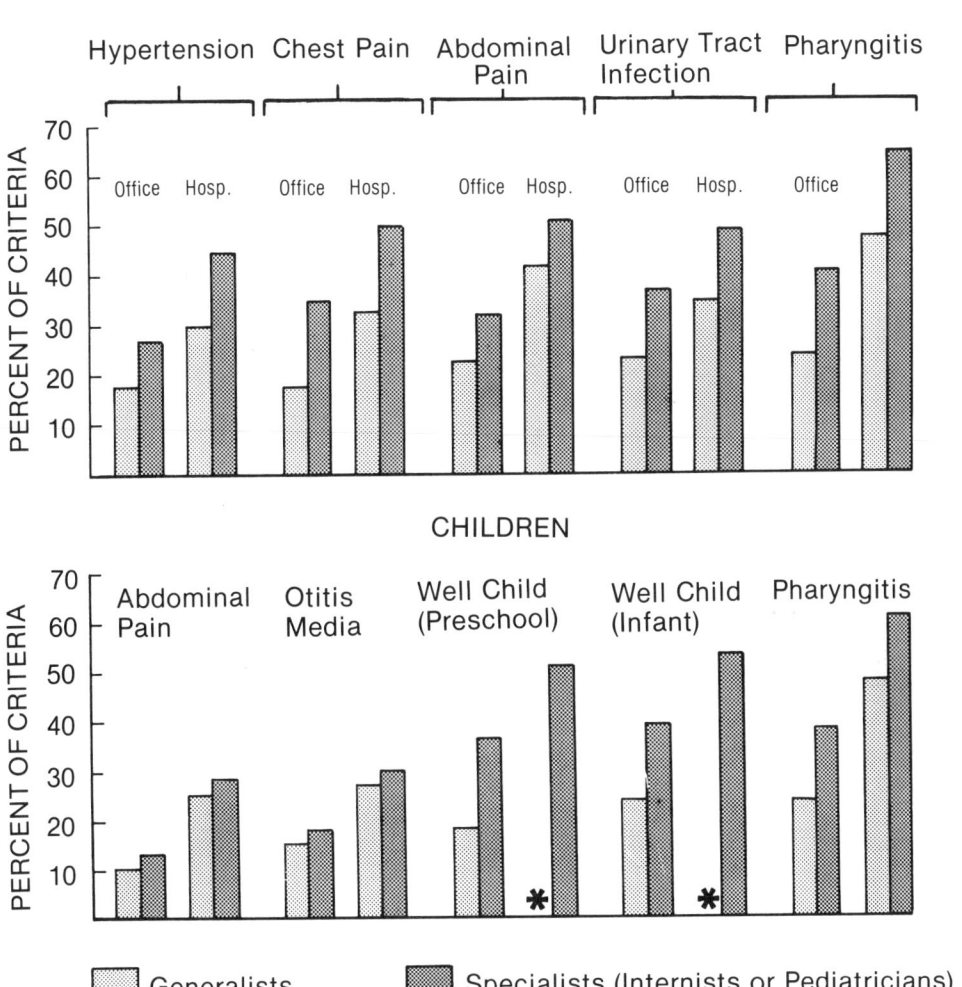

NOTE: Criteria are items of care considered significant by a panel of physicians. Compliance is determined by review of the record of care. Asterisks indicate missing categories. All differences are statistically significant except for the comparison of generalists and specialists in abdominal pain of children.

SOURCE: Riedel, Ruth L. and Donald E. Reidel, *Practice and Performance: An Assessment of Ambulatory Care*, Health Administration Press, Ann Arbor, Michigan, 1979, Tables 7.2a–7.10a, pp. 130–139.

Chart G-40

Scores of the Quality of Care Based on Reviews of Patient Records, According to Institutional Source and Category of Care (U.S.A., cirica 1968).[1]

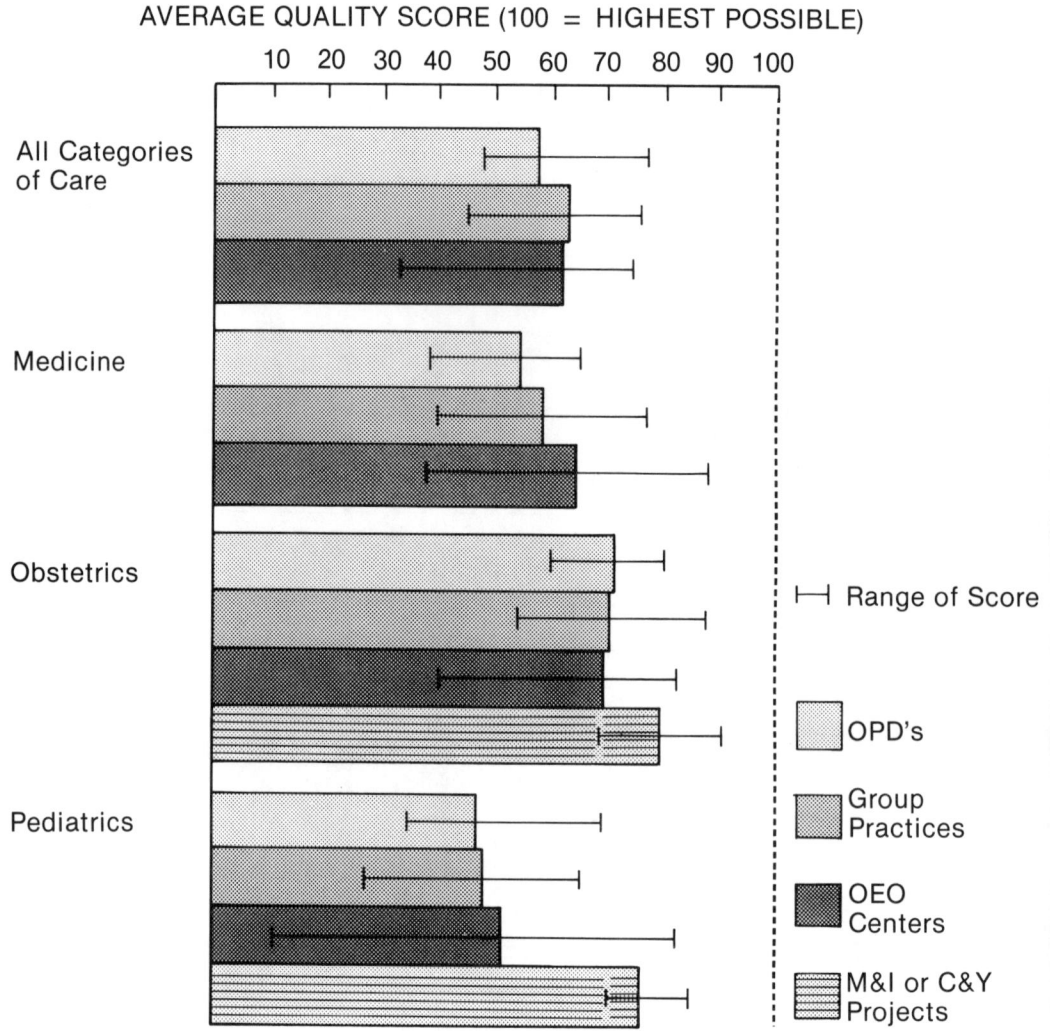

[1]There were 10 outpatient departments (OPD) of hospitals affiliated with medical schools, 7 group practices with various forms of financing, 35 OEO neighborhood health centers, 6 Maternal and Infant Care (M&I) programs and 4 Children and Youth (C&Y) programs. Only the 35 out of 50 OEO Centers are considered representative of their category.

SOURCE: Communication from M.A. Morehead, Also see *American Journal of Public Health*, Vol. 61, July 1971, pp. 1294-1306.

Quality of Care

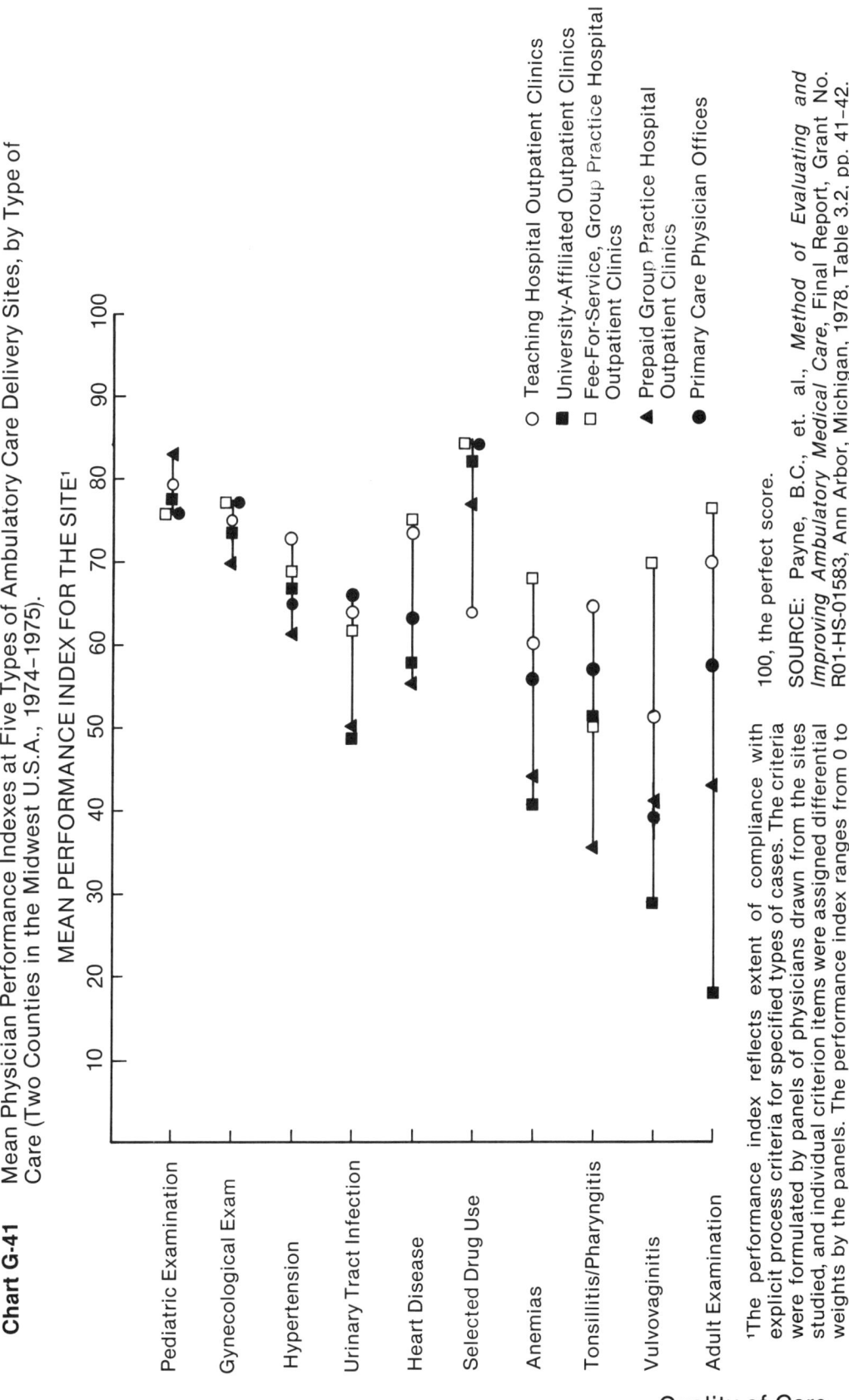

Chart G-41 Mean Physician Performance Indexes at Five Types of Ambulatory Care Delivery Sites, by Type of Care (Two Counties in the Midwest U.S.A., 1974–1975).

[1] The performance index reflects extent of compliance with explicit process criteria for specified types of cases. The criteria were formulated by panels of physicians drawn from the sites studied, and individual criterion items were assigned differential weights by the panels. The performance index ranges from 0 to 100, the perfect score.

SOURCE: Payne, B.C., et. al., *Method of Evaluating and Improving Ambulatory Medical Care*, Final Report, Grant No. R01-HS-01583, Ann Arbor, Michigan, 1978, Table 3.2, pp. 41–42.

Chart G-42 Number of Injections Billed per 100 Ambulatory Visits and Number and Percent of Injections Approved and Not Approved for Payment by Medical Peer Review, by Type of Physician (Medicaid Program, New Mexico, September 1971–August 1973, Inclusive).

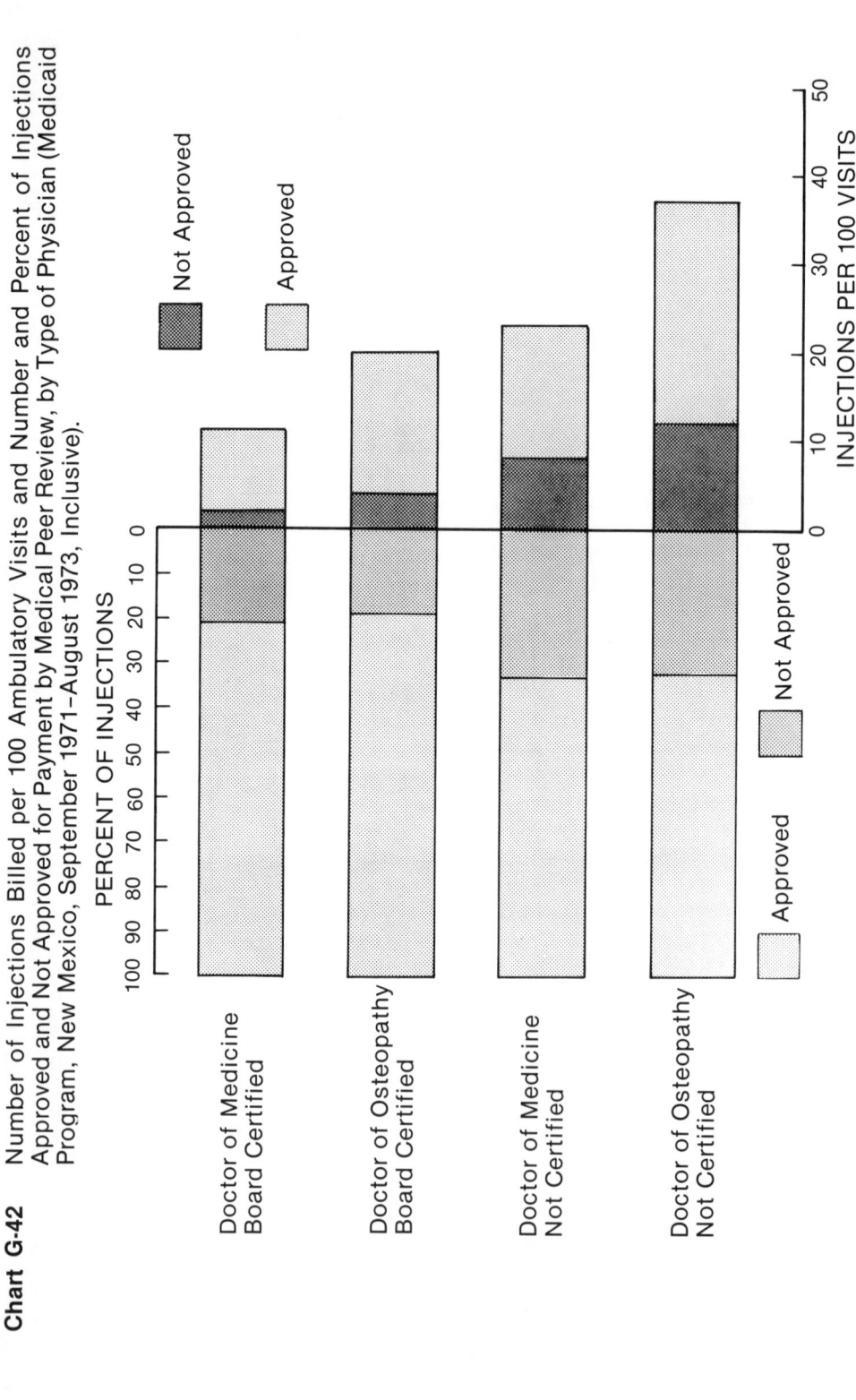

NOTE: Differences between provider types and certification status groups are significant at p 0.05 or less, by the chi square test.

SOURCE: Brook, R.H. and K.N. Williams, "Evaluation of the New Mexico Peer Review System, 1971 to 1973," *Medical Care*, Vol. 14, Supplement, December 1976, Table 6.10, p. 71.

Chart G-43

Percent of Patients Who Were Seen in the Emergency Room With Nonemergency Gastrointestinal Symptoms and Referred for X-Ray Examination, by Specified Subsequent Events in the Course of Management (Baltimore City Hospital Emergency Room, April–June, 1969).[1]

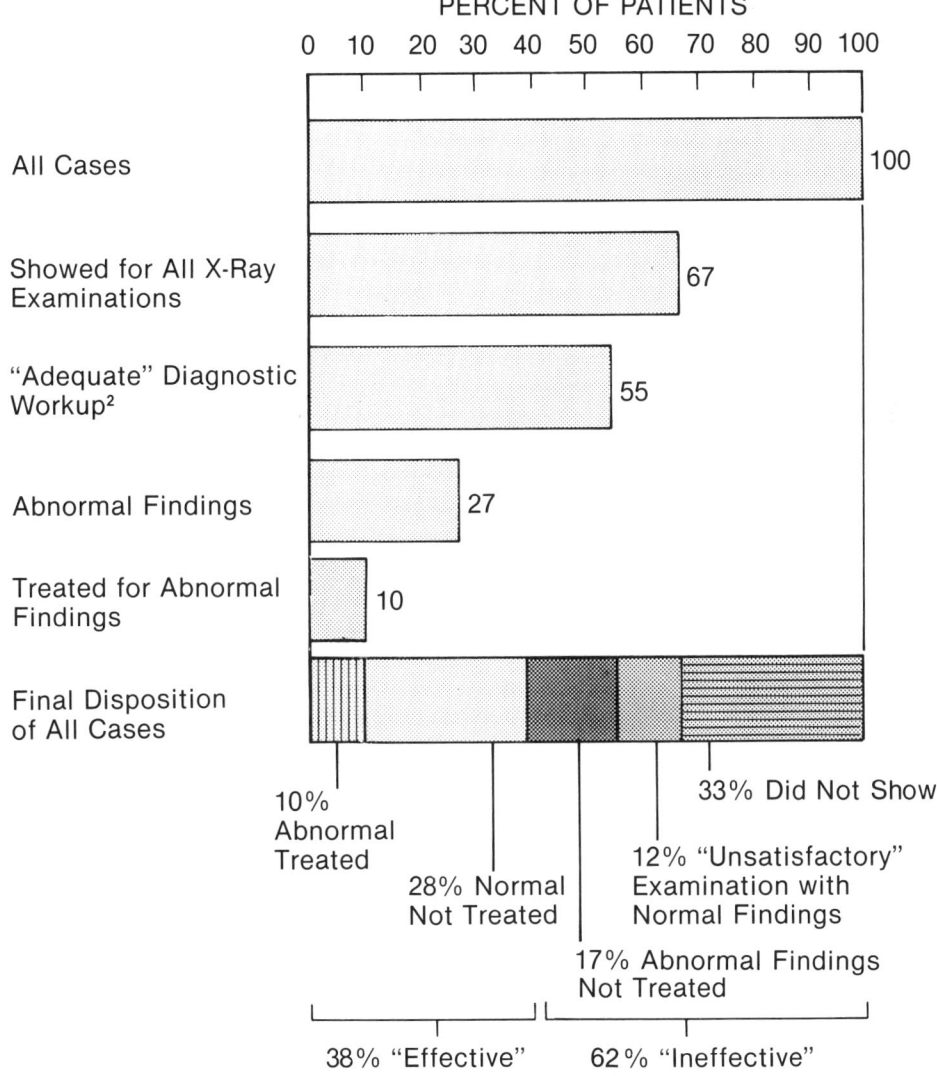

[1]The study was conducted in an emergency room staffed by interns and residents. "Ninety to ninety-five percent of the medical resident staff, an integral part of Johns Hopkins University School of Medicine, are graduates of American Medical Schools."

[2]"The minimal criteria selected were . . . completion of x-ray studies by the patient; production of an x-ray film of adequate quality to eliminate treatable lesions; and sigmoidoscopy of all patients who received a barium-enema examination."

SOURCE: Brook, R.H. and R.L. Stevenson, "Effectiveness of Patient Care in an Emergency Room," *New England Journal of Medicine,* Vol. 283, 1970, pp. 904–907.

Quality of Care

Chart G-44 Number and Percent Distribution of Cases that Were Judged to Have Had Specified Deficiencies in Care, Categorized by "Problem Status Outcome" One Month After Care was Provided (Columbia Medical Plan, Columbia, Maryland, 1974).

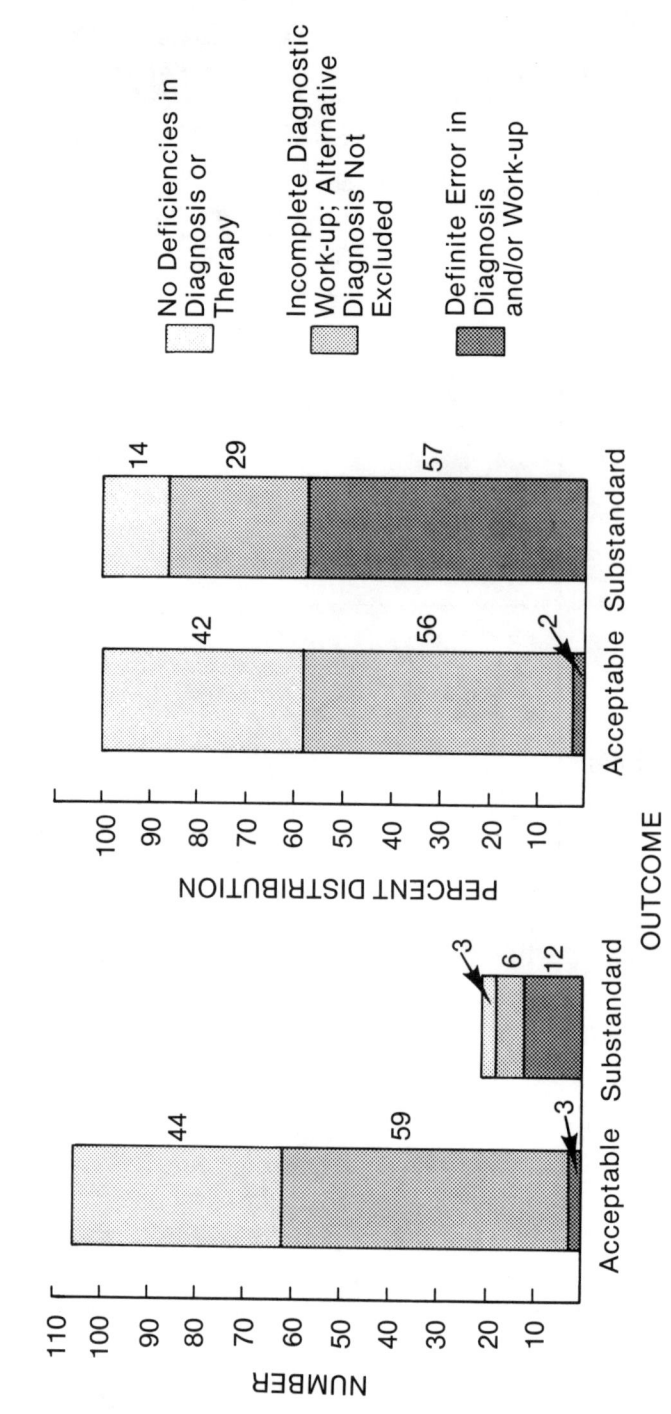

NOTE: Ambulatory patients with upper respiratory tract infection, sore throat and urinary tract infection were questioned one month later about the status of their "problem." Errors in management were determined by independent chart review using explicit criteria supplemented by the reviewer's judgment.

SOURCE: Mushlin, A. J., F. A. Appel and D. M. Barr, "Quality Assurance in Primary Care: A Strategy Based on Outcome Assessment," *Journal of Community Health*, Summer 1978, pp. 242–305.

Chart G-45

Percent of Cases with Different Levels of Compliance with Explicit Criteria, Judged by Implicit Criteria to Have Received Care of Specified Quality, Four Conditions, Office Practice of Selected Internists (North Carolina, 1975–1977).

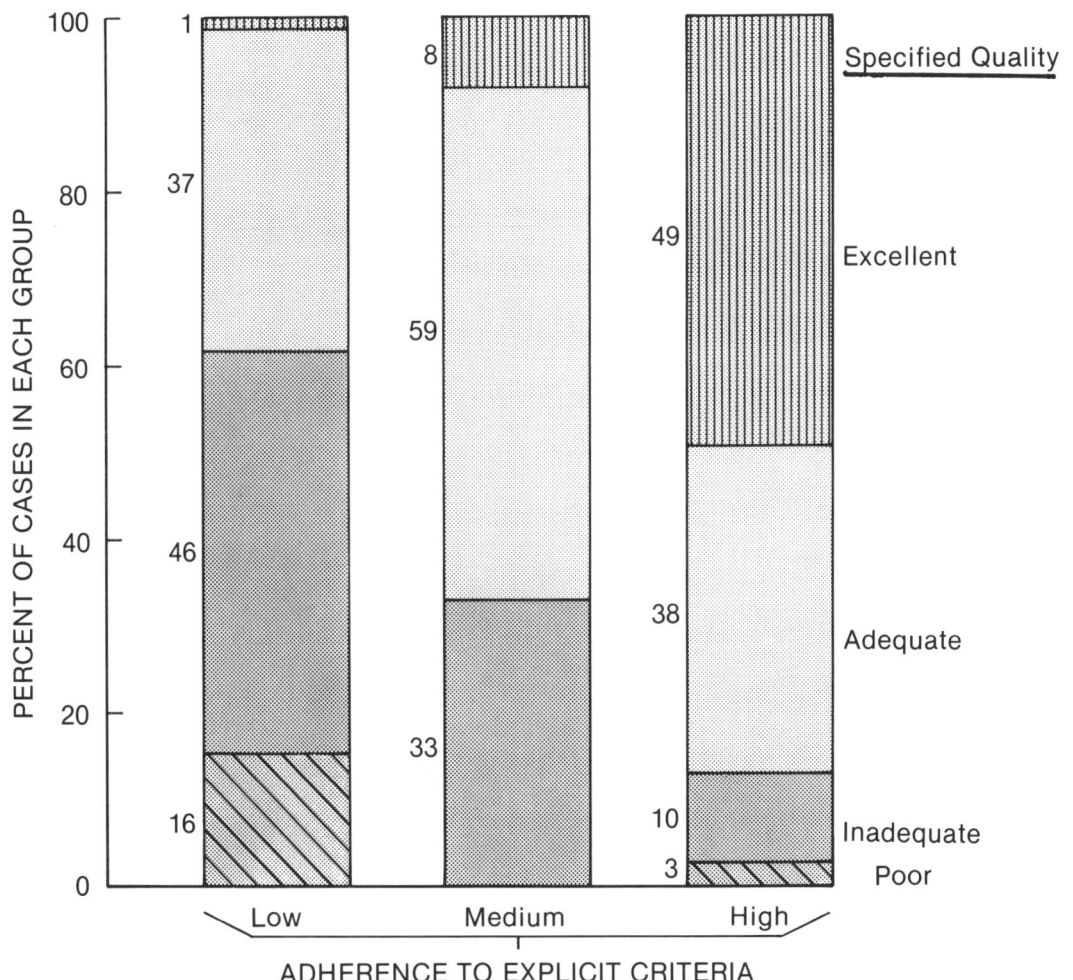

SOURCE: Hulka, Barbara S., et al., "Peer Review in Ambulatory Care: Use of Explicit Criteria and Implicit Judgments," *Medical Care*, Vol. 17, March 1979, Supplement, Table 43, p. 57.

Quality of Care

Chart G-46

Interns Ranked by Overall Clinical Capability and by Cost of Laboratory Tests Requested During the First Three Days of Care of Uncomplicated Acute Myocardial Infarction (Coronary Care Unit, George Washington University Hospital, 1971–1972).

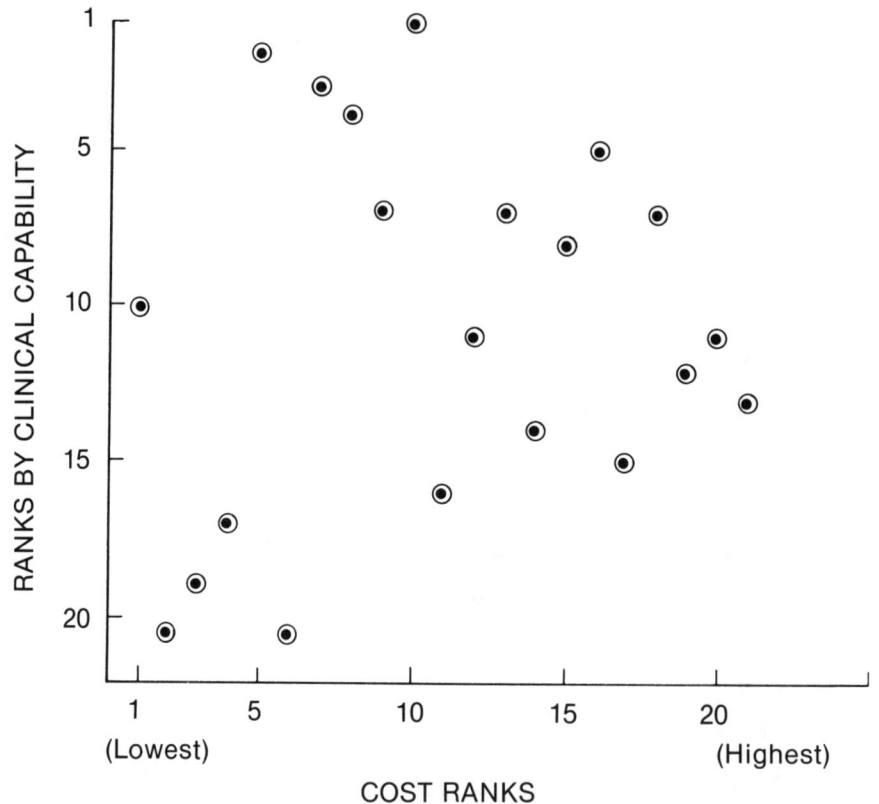

NOTE: Interns were ranked independently by each of 5 faculty internists at the end of the internship year. Rank 1 means highest competence and rank 21 lowest. For cost, rank 1 means lowest and 21 means highest cost. $r_s = -0.13$, not significant.

SOURCE: Schroeder, S. A., et al., "Variation Among Physicians in Use of Laboratory Tests: Relation to Quality of Care," *Medical Care*, Vol. 12, August 1974, Fig. 1, p. 710, plus data from author.

Quality of Care

Chart G-47

Percent of Patients Who Received Diagnostic X-Ray Examinations, by Type of Physician Responsible for the Case[1] and Percent of Chest X-Ray Examinations That Were of Specified Kind, by Type of Physician Performing the Examination (Recipients of Old Age Assistance, Alameda County, California, September 1965–January 1966, Inclusive).[2]

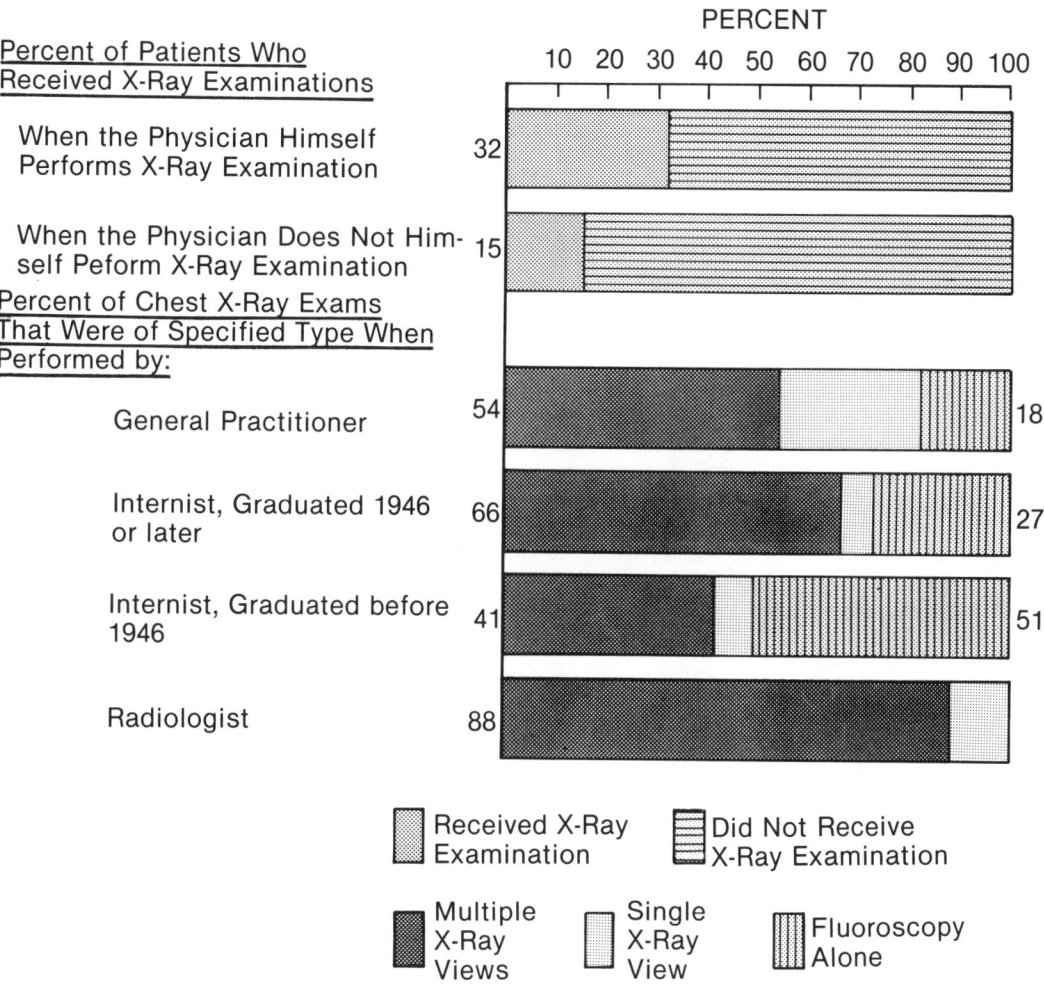

[1]Patients who were seen by more than one type of physician were assigned to the physician who himself provided x-ray services.

[2]90 percent of persons were eligible throughout the period of 6 months.

SOURCE: Childs, A.W. and E.D. Hunter, "Non-Medical Factors Influencing Use of Diagnostic X-Ray by Physicians," *Medical Care*, Vol. 10, July to August, 1972, pp. 323–335.

Quality of Care

Chart G-48

Percent of Cases in Which Antibiotics Were Judged to Have Been Apprroprietely Used Before and After the Institution of a Medical Audit and Education Program, as Compared to Opinion About Current Practice, Knowledge About Antibiotic Usage, and Minimum Acceptable Practice (Chestnut Hill Hospital, Philadelphia, 1970).

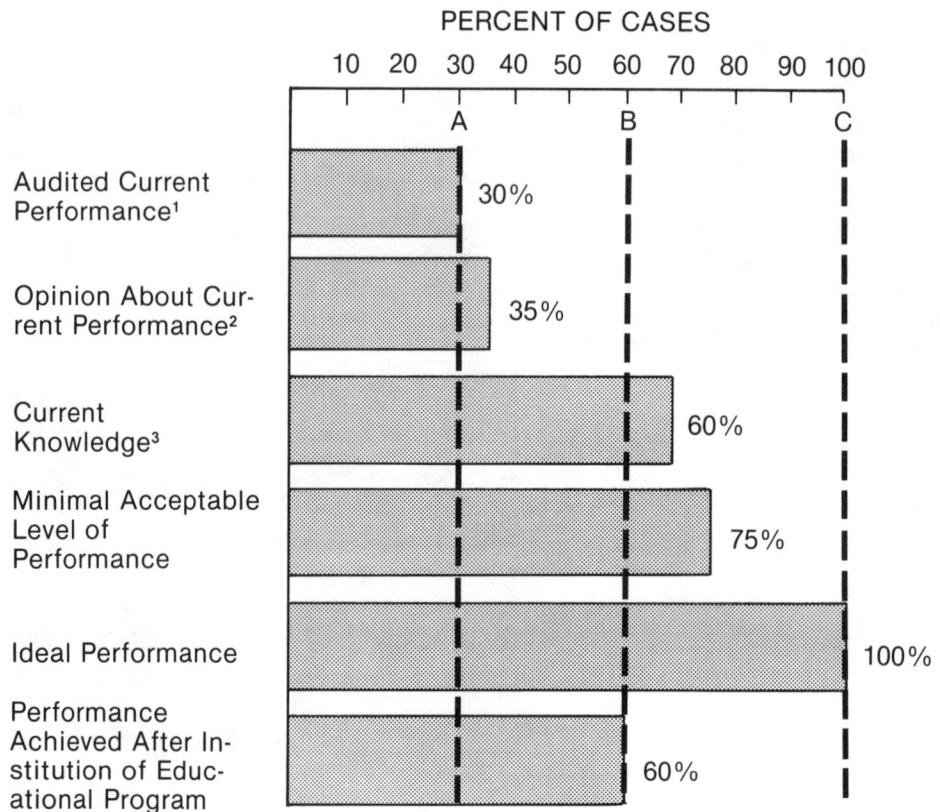

[1] A panel of staff physicians on the audit committee reviewed 50 consecutive records of patients on the medical service.

[2] Medical Department staff estimate of what audit results would be.

[3] Determined by a written examination taken by medical staff based on 16 of 50 cases audited.

SOURCE: Brown, C.R. and S.M. Uhl, "Mandatory Continuing Education: Sense or Nonsense?" *Journal of the American Medical Association,* Vol. 213, September 7, 1970, pp. 1660–1668.

Chart G-49

Mean Percent of Highest Possible Performance Score Obtained by a Sample of Community Pharmacists, by Activity Category and by Location of Pharmacy (A Metropolitan Area, Ohio, Undated).

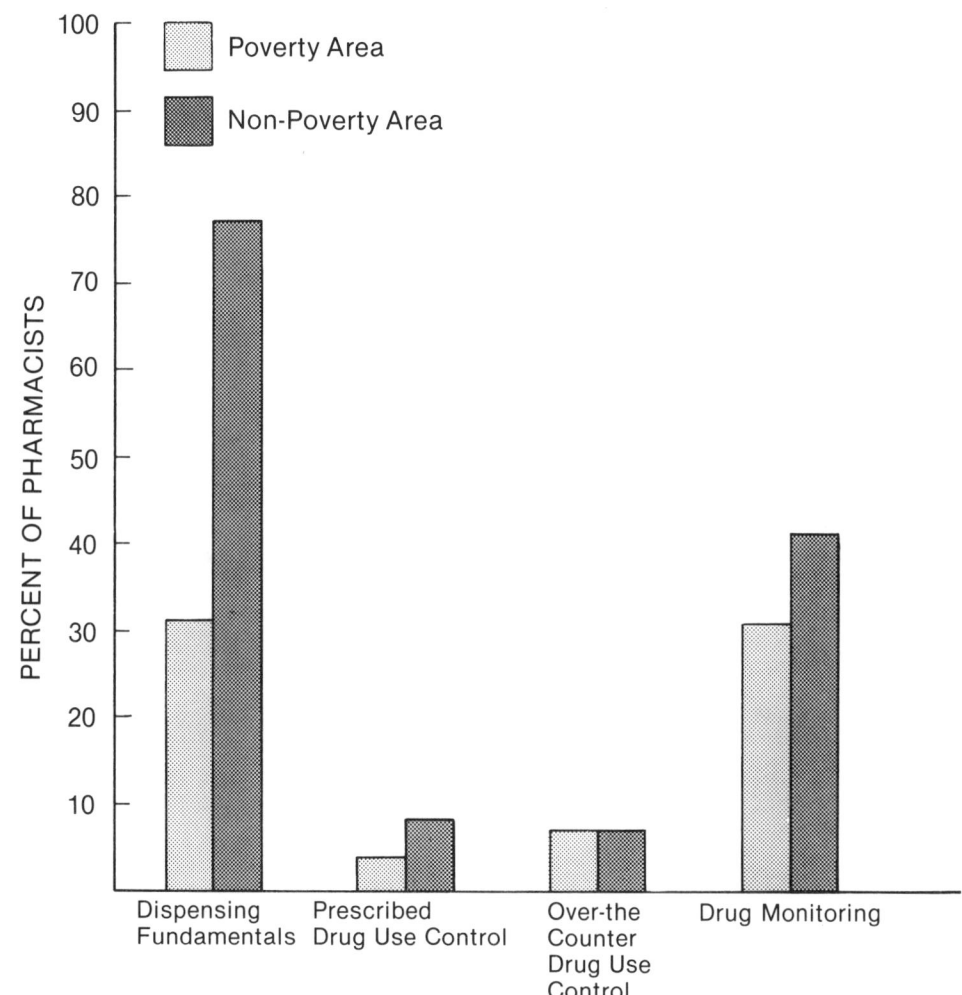

NOTE: The activity categories consisted of the following:
Dispensing fundamentals: providing accurately prepared and labeled prescriptions.
Prescribed drug use control: assuring good drug therapy through checking patient comprehension, explaining dosage, cautions and storage conditions, and by entering on the family medication record.
Over-the-counter drug usage control: advising on choice of product and limitations of self-therapy, referral to appropriate sources of care, and entering on family medication record.
Drug monitoring: detecting and solving problems involving drug incompatabilities and adverse reactions.
SOURCE: Jang, R., D.A. Knapp and D.E. Knapp, "An Evaluation of the Quality of Drug-related Services in Neighborhood Pharmacies," *Drugs in Health Care*, Winter 1975, Table 9, p. 30.

Quality of Care

Chart G-50

Community Pharmacists by Quality of Professional Performance[1] and by Charge Per Prescription (Northern Mississippi, circa 1973).

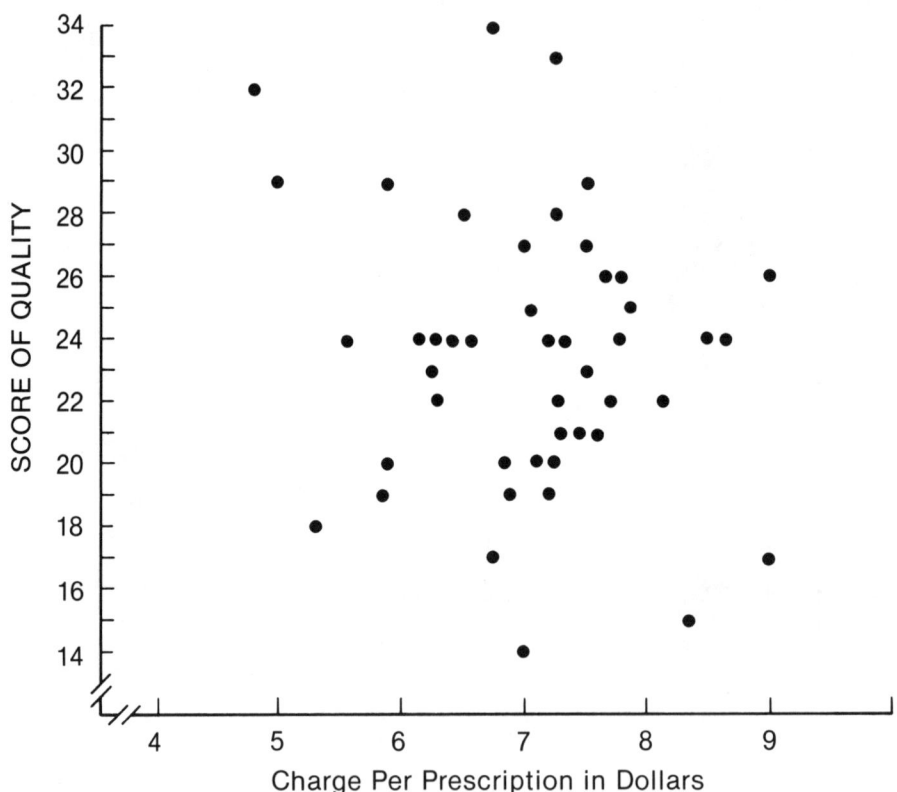

[1]Quality was judged on the basis of performance of 13 professional functions in connection with filling prescriptions for, and responding to preformulated questions by, trained "shoppers."

SOURCE: Jackson, R.A. and M.C. Smith, "Relations Between Price and Quality in Community Pharmacy," *Medical Care*, Vol. 12, January 1974, Table 4, p. 36.

Quality of Care

Chart G-51

Percent of Patient Care Records Judged to Represent Nursing Care of Specified Quality, by Aspect of Care (500 Recipients of Care From 20 Agencies, Greater New York Area, circa 1967).

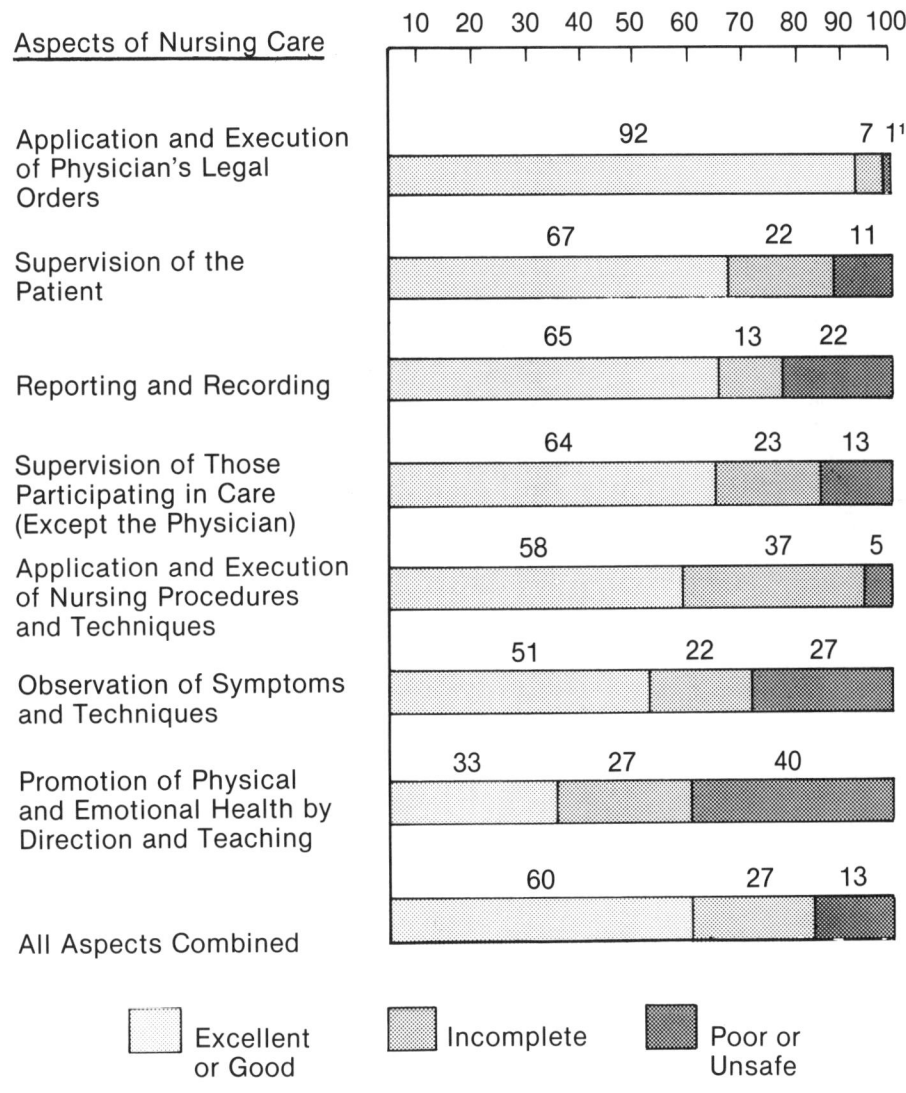

[1] Poor or unsafe care.

SOURCE: Phaneuf, M.C., "Analysis of a Nursing Audit," *Nursing Outlook*, Vol. 16, January 1968, pp. 56–59.

Quality of Care

Chart G-52

Percent of Children Needing Glasses, and Judgment of Glasses Used (Washington, D.C., 1971).

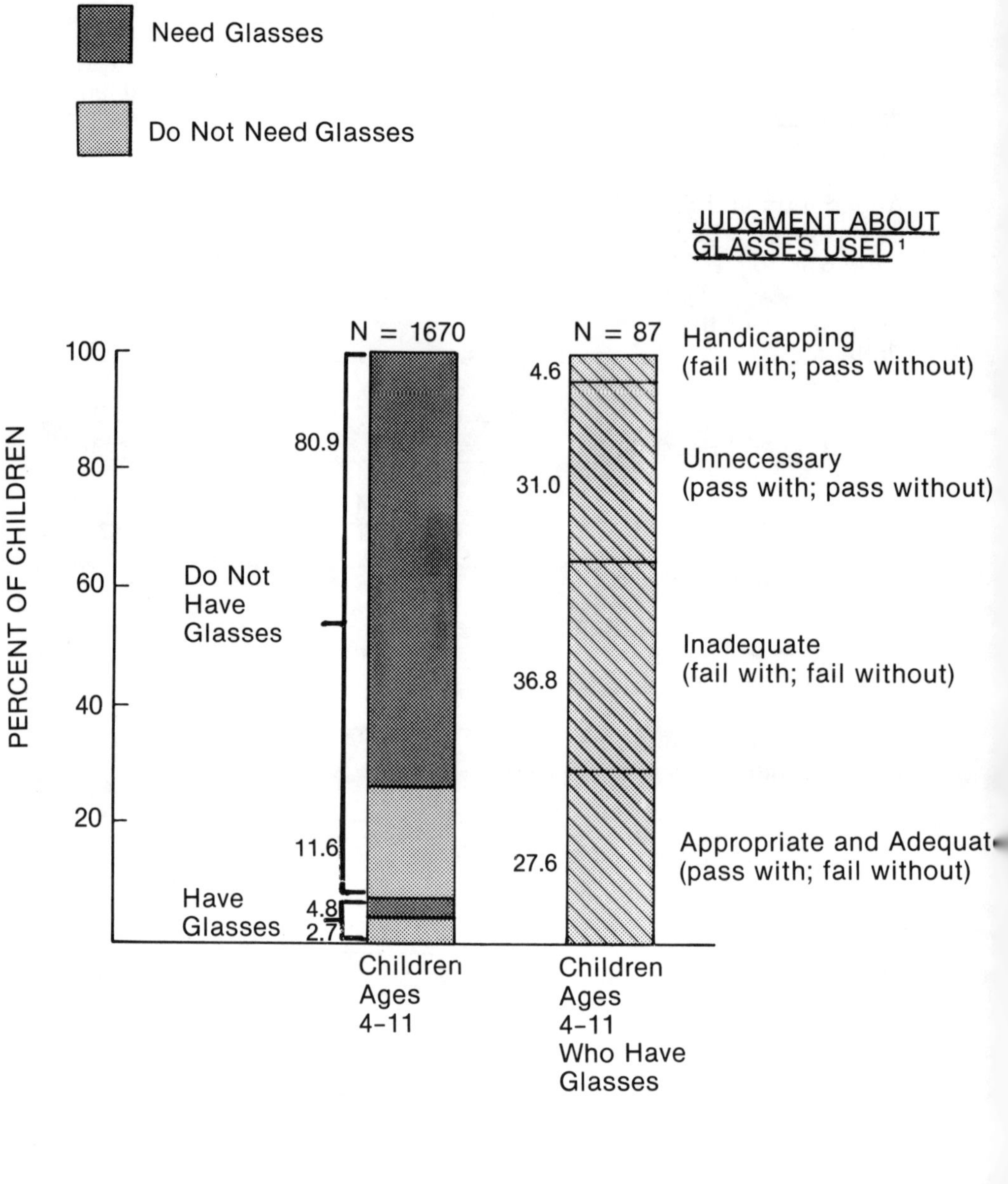

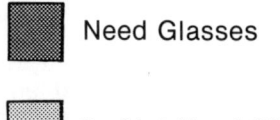

Need Glasses
Do Not Need Glasses
JUDGMENT ABOUT GLASSES USED[1]
PERCENT OF CHILDREN
100
80
60
40
20
N = 1670
80.9
Do Not Have Glasses
11.6
Have Glasses
4.8
2.7
Children Ages 4–11
N = 87
4.6
31.0
36.8
27.6
Children Ages 4–11 Who Have Glasses
Handicapping (fail with; pass without)
Unnecessary (pass with; pass without)
Inadequate (fail with; fail without)
Appropriate and Adequate (pass with; fail without)

[1]Results of visual acuity test with and without glasses.

SOURCE: Kessner, D.M., C.K. Snow, and J. Singer, *Assessment of Medical Care for Children*, Institute of Medicine, National Academy of Sciences, Washington, D.C., 1974, Table A-5, p. 174, Table B-1, p. 186, and Table B-4, p. 188.

Chart G-53 Percent of Optometric Patients Receiving Unsatisfactory Care, and Deficiencies in Care for Those Receiving Unsatisfactory Care (New York City, 1969).

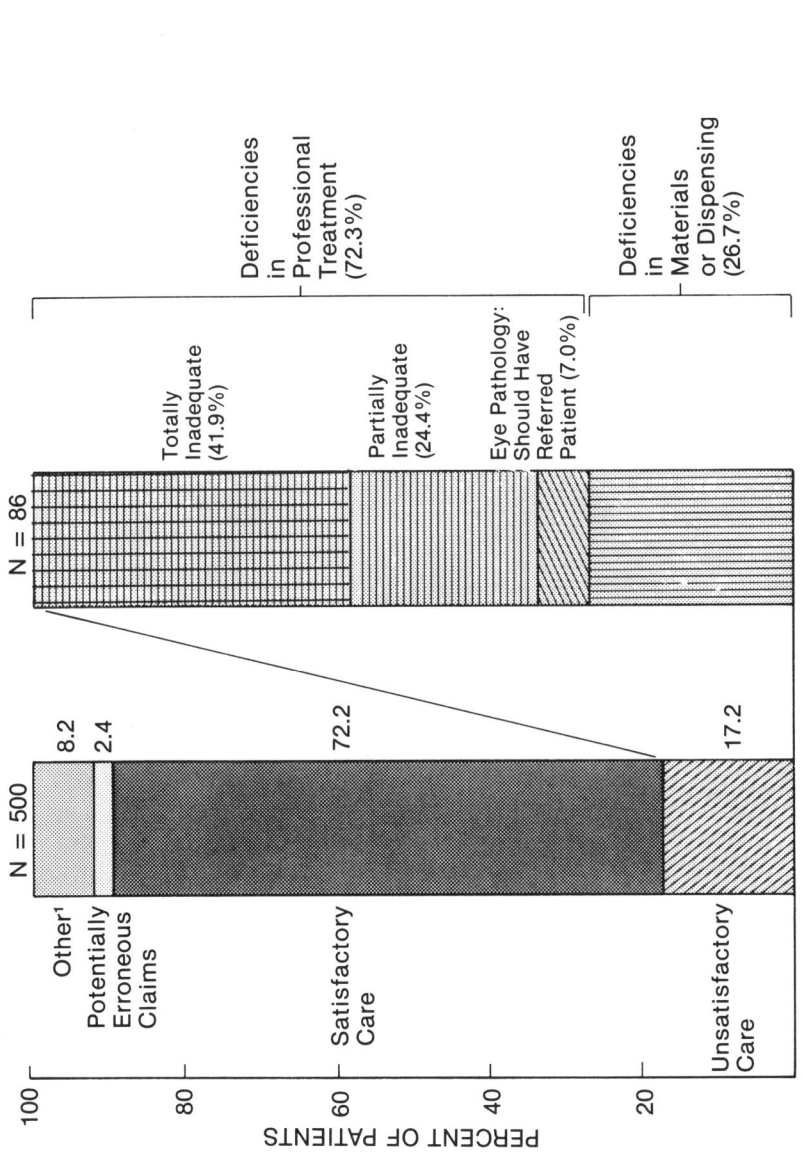

[1]Includes "professional discretion" (5.0%) and "visual training evaluation indicated" (3.2%).

SOURCE: Bellin, L.E. and F. Kavaler, "Policing Publicly Funded Health Care for Poor Quality, Overutilization, and Fraud — the New York City Medicaid Experience," *American Journal of Public Health*, Vol. 60, May 1970, Table 1, p. 814.

Chart G-54

Hebdomadal Death Rates[1] in One Hospital Before and After the Introduction by the Health Department of a System of Reporting, Review and Corrective Action ("Alerter" System)[2] (Chicago, 1953–1954).

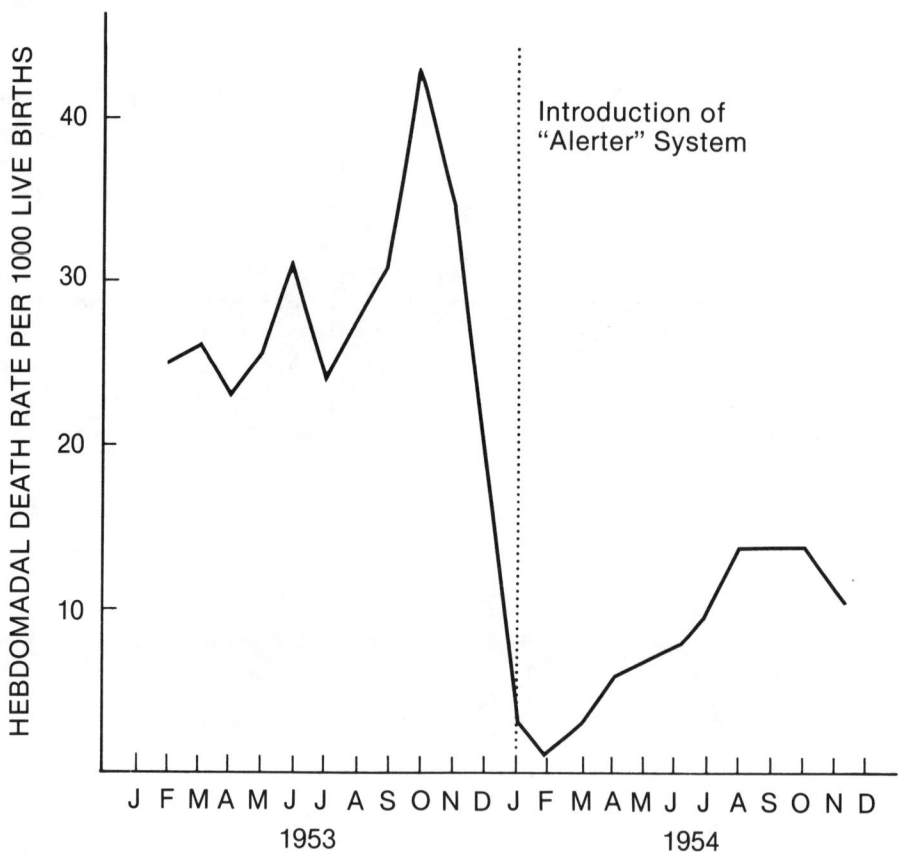

[1] Three-month moving average computed on the assumption that the number of births remained constant.

[2] The "Alerter" system was introduced January, 1954.

SOURCE: Bundesen. H.N., "Effective Reduction of Needless Hebdomadal Deaths in Hospitals," *Journal of the American Medical Association*, Vol. 157, April 16, 1955, Figure 8, p. 1393.

Chart G-55

Number of Justified and Criticized Operations on Uterus, Ovary, and Fallopian Tubes that Resulted in Sterilization or Castration
(One Hospital, U.S.A., circa 1954).

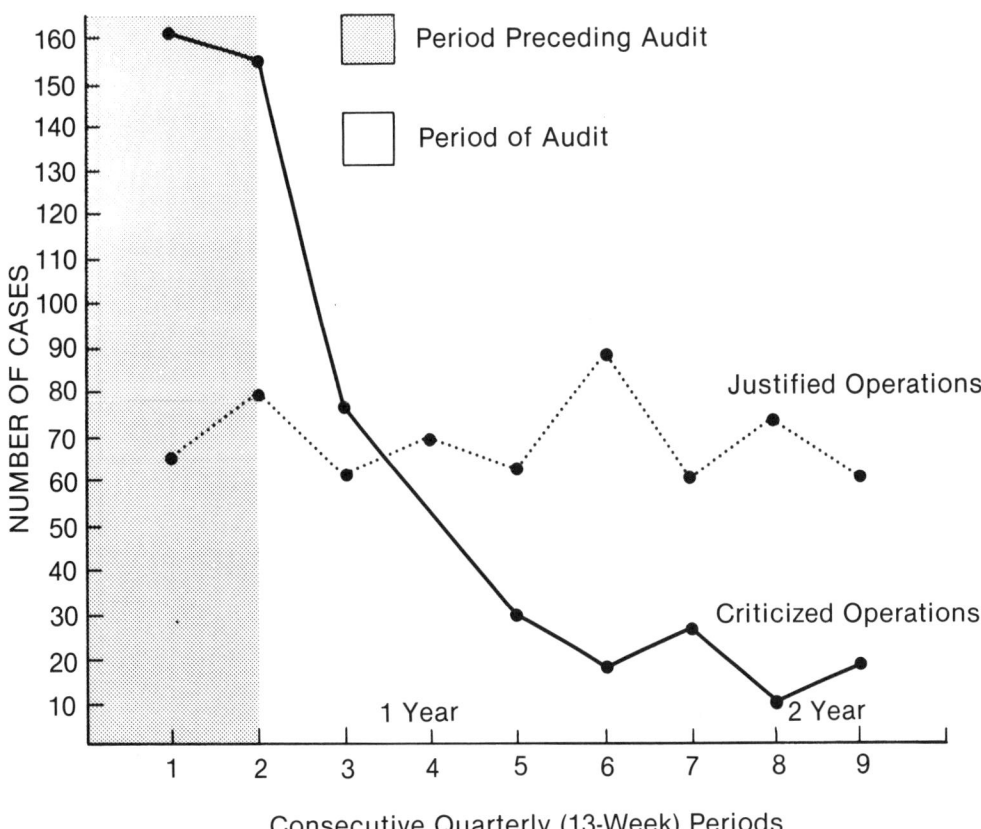

SOURCE: Lembcke, P.A., "Medical Auditing by Scientific Methods," *Journal of the American Medical Association*, Vol. 162, October 13, 1956, pp. 646–655.

Chart G-56

Relative Frequency[1] of Specified Pathological Diagnosis in Appendectomies Performed Before and After the Institution of a Tissue Committee in One Hospital (St. Louis, Missouri, 1952-1956).

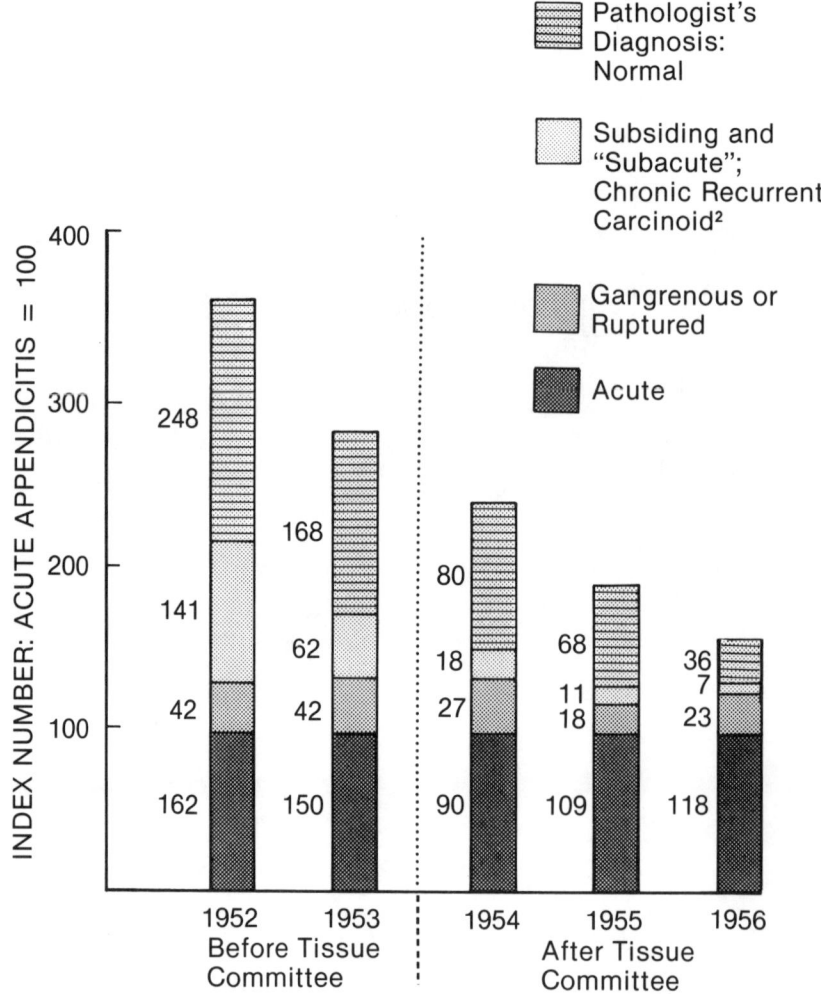

[1]On the assumption that appendectomies are appropriate and not unduly delayed if the pathologist reports acute inflammation, the number of such appendectomies performed each year has been used as the standard against which the frequency of other diagnoses is measured. This procedure is adopted because the absence of a population base does not permit the computation of incidence rates.

[2]Carcinoid was the pathological diagnosis in only 5 out of 1620 operations.

NOTE: Numbers to the left of bars refer to actual number of cases in each category.

SOURCE: Verda, D.J. and W.R. Platt, "The Tissue Committee Really Gets Results," *The Modern Hospital,* Vol. 91, September 1958, pp. 74-75.

Chart G-57

Percent of Abnormal Laboratory Findings That Evoked Physician Responses as Judged by Entries in the Record, Three Time Periods (Rockford Memorial Hospital, Rockford, Illinois, 1963, 1964 and 1965).

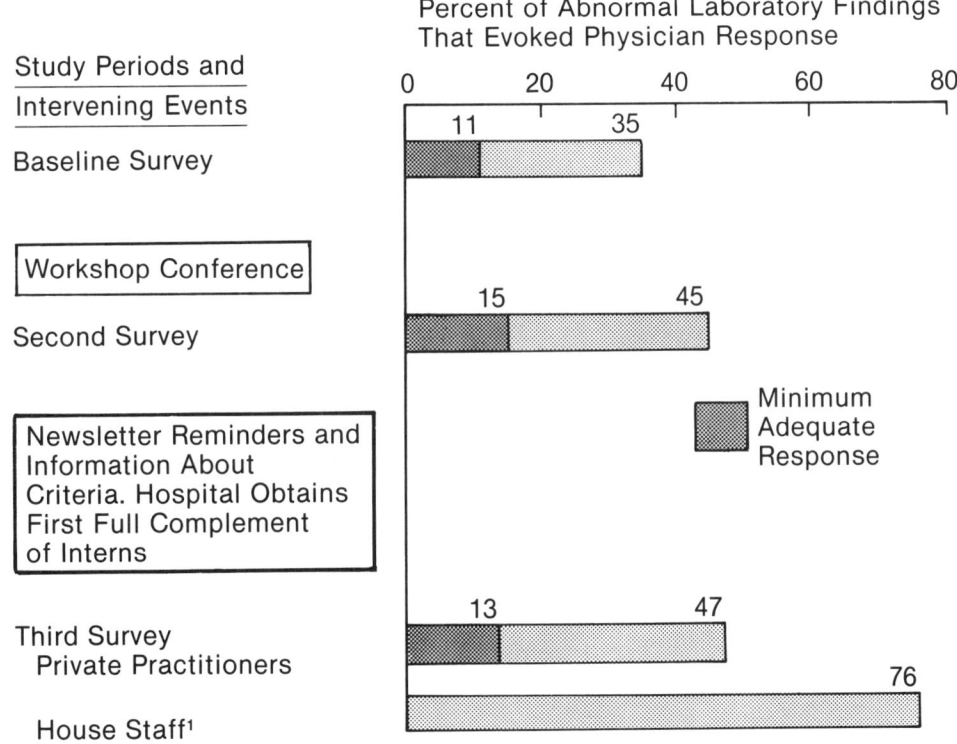

[1]Hospital had no house staff at the time of the two previous surveys.

SOURCE: Williamson, J.W., M. Alexander, and G.E. Miller, "Continuing Education and Patient Care Research," *Journal of the American Medical Association,* Vol. 201, September 18, 1967, pp. 118–122.

Chart G-58

Percent of 87 Studies of Outcome Using the Health Accounting Method Which Revealed Significant Deficiencies and Progressed through Specified Steps to Demonstrated Improvement (23 Sites in the U.S., 1963-1973).

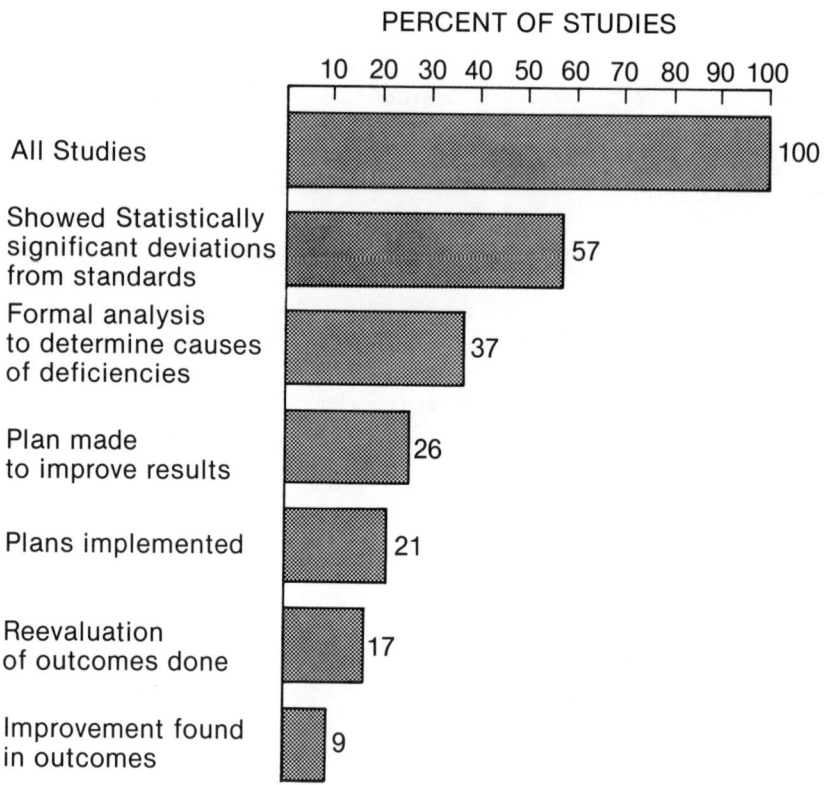

SOURCE: Williamson, J. W., *Assessing and Improving Health Care Outcomes*, Cambridge, Massachusetts, 1978, p. 150.

Chart G-59

Percent of Hospital Cases Discharged Which Exceeded Length of Stay Limits According to AID[1] Standards, Before and After Implementation of the AID Hospital Use Certification Program (New Jersey, 1964-1966).

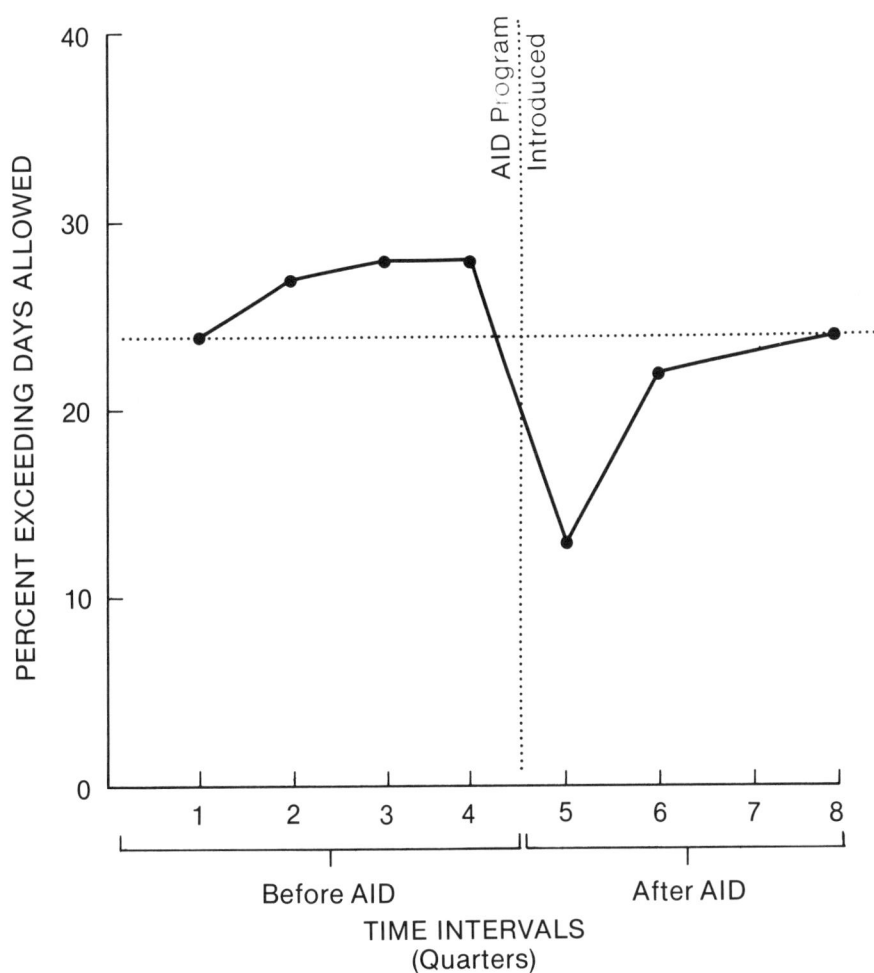

[1] "Approval by Individual Diagnosis Program," a Blue Cross instituted program of variable-interval hospital certification. Under the AID system, the number of benefit days initially approved for a patient's hospitalization is dependent on the admitting diagnosis.

SOURCE: Bailey, D.R. and D.C. Riedel, "Recertification and Length of Stay: the Impact of New Jersey's AID Program on Patterns of Hospital Care," *Blue Cross Reports,* Vol. 6, July 1968, and personal communication.

Quality of Care

Chart G-60

Percent Change in Adjusted Length of Stay Before and After the Introduction of a Predischarge Utilization Review Program (PDUR) in Selected Hospitals, Compared with Hospitals Without PDUR
(Allegheny County, Pa., July 1, 1971–June 1, 1974).

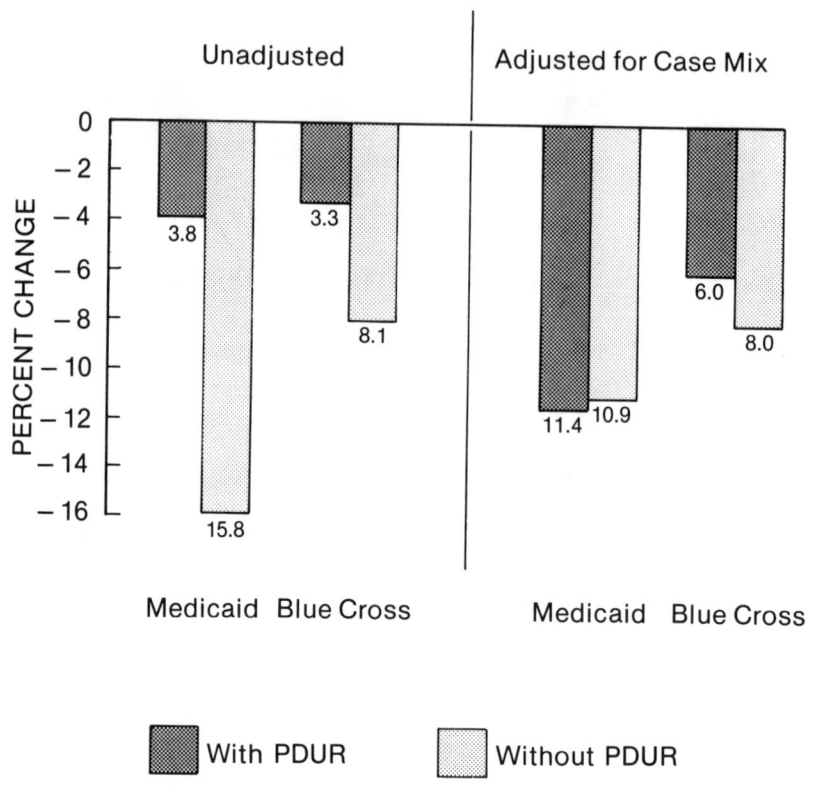

SOURCE: Lave, J. P. and S. Leinhardt, "An Evaluation of a Hospital Stay Regulatory Mechanism," *American Journal of Public Health*, Vol. 66, October 1976, pp. 959–967.

Quality of Care

Chart G-61

Discharge Ratio by Days Since Admission for Patients 65 Years and Older, Pre- and Post-Medicare (U.S.A., January–December 1965 and October 1966–June 1967).

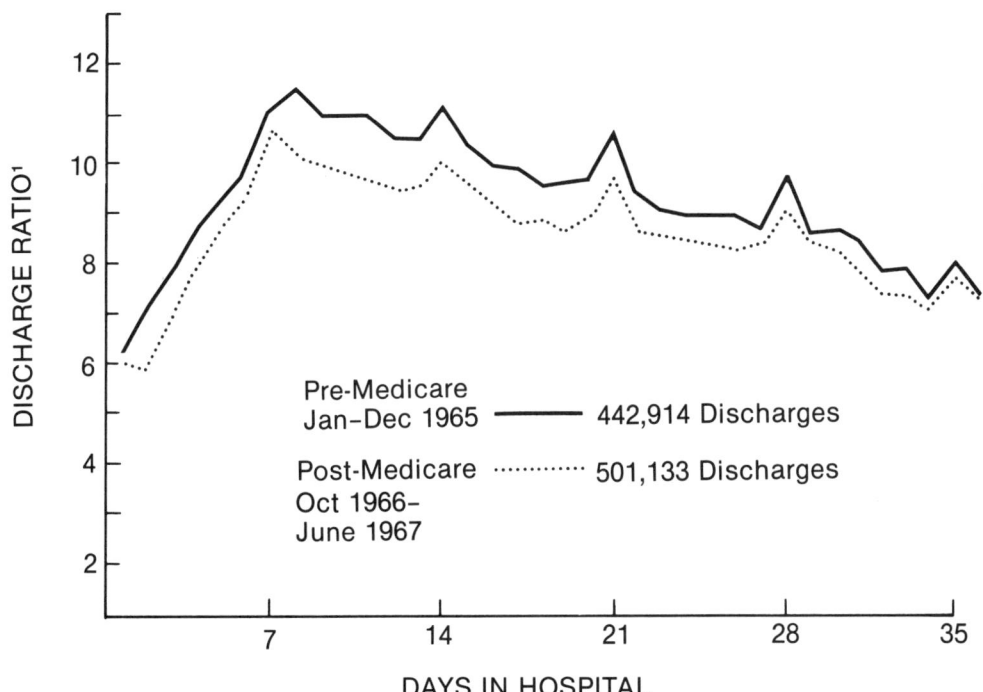

[1] Discharge Ratio defined as "the ratio of the number of discharges on a specific day to the number not yet discharged, multiplied by 100."

NOTE: Reproduced with the permission of the Commission on Professional and Hospital Activities.

SOURCE: Commission on Professional and Hospital Activities, *PAS Reporter,* Volume 9, No. 2, Illustration #2.

Chart G-62

Percent of Diagnostic Categories Treated Medically, by Length of Stay Approved at Admission, AID Program (New Jersey, 1965).

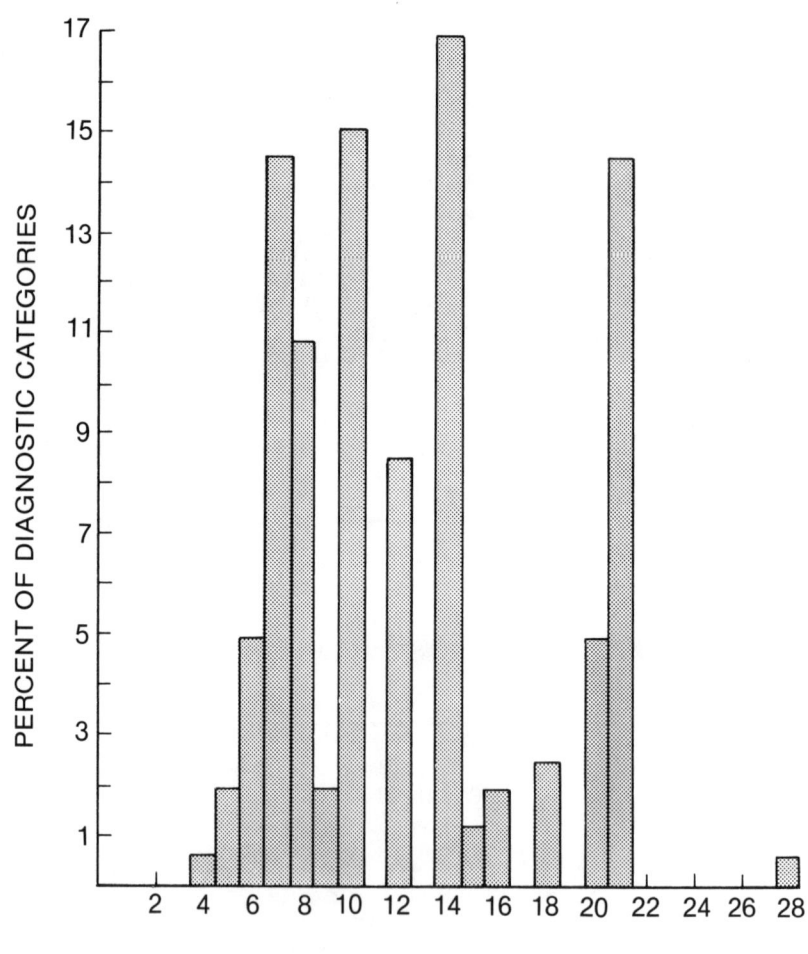

SOURCE: Donabedian, A., "The Numerology of Utilization Control," *Inquiry,* Vol. II, 1974, Fig. 1, p. 230.

Chart G-63 Percent of Judgments of Appropriateness of Hospital Stay Made During Specified Intervals After Admission that were Negative or Uncertain, by Type of Service (Strong Memorial Hospital, Rochester, N.Y., January 1968–August 1970).[1]

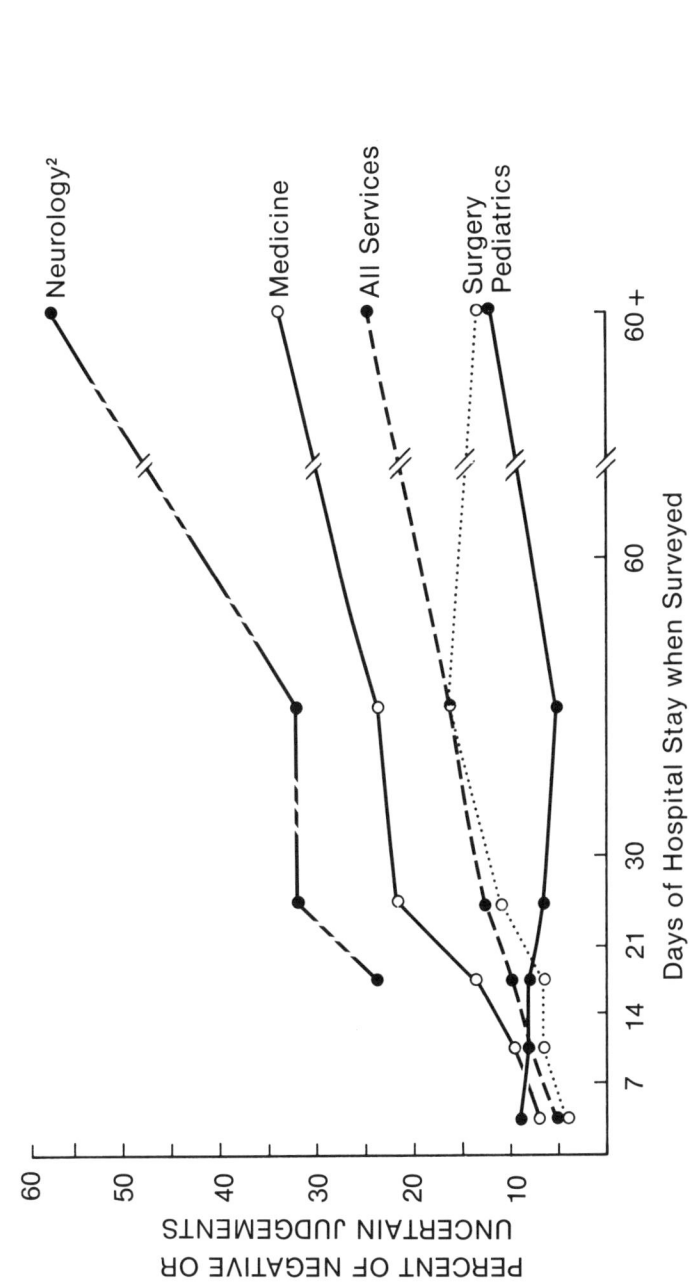

[1] Judgments were made by physicians using implicit criteria after review of all patient records and talking with staff and patients if necessary. There were 8,064 observations on 3,369 patients.

[2] Shown in part.

SOURCE: Zimmer, J. G., "Length of Stay and Hospital Misutilization," *Medical Care*, Vol. 12, May 1974, Table 1, p. 456.

Quality of Care

Chart G-64 Percent of Medicare and Medicaid Cases on Each Day Since Admission that were Judged Not to Require Acute Hospital Care, and Percent Distribution of All Cases Judged Not to Require Such Care, by Day Since Admission (Herrick Memorial Hospital, Berkeley, California, October 15, 1973–August 15, 1974).

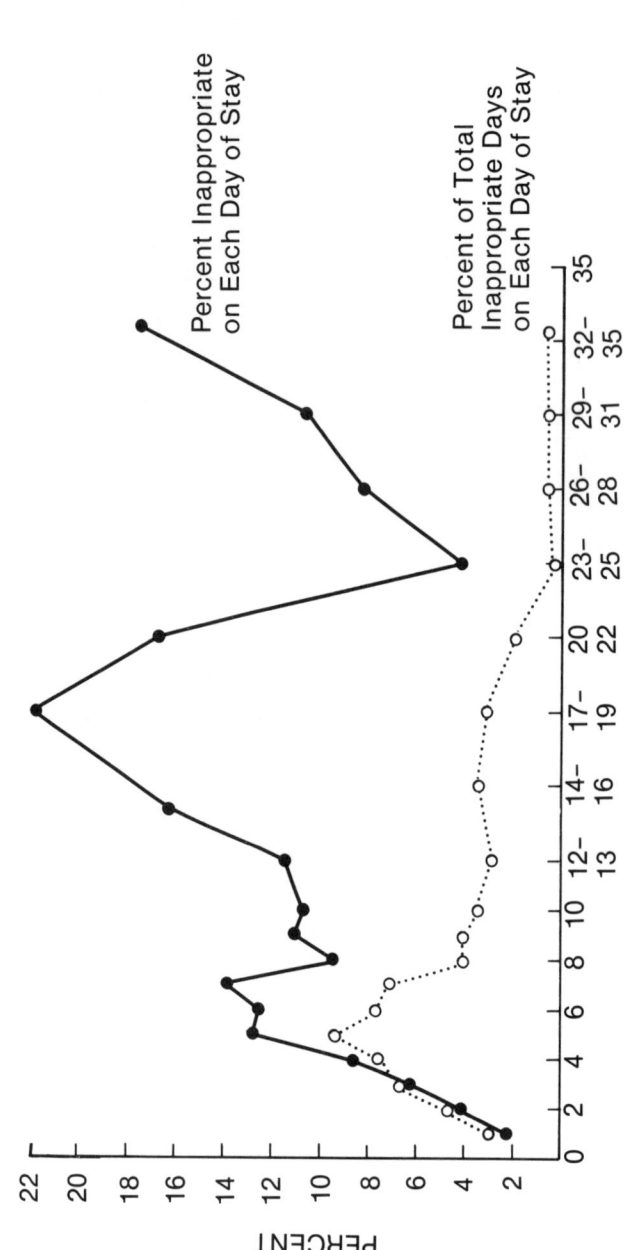

SOURCE: Restuccia, J.D. and D.C. Holloway, "Barriers to Appropriate Utilization of an Acute Facility," *Medical Care*, Vol. 14, July 1976, Table 1, pp. 566–567.

Chart G-65 Professional Standards Review Organization Structure and Activities (U.S.A., 1980).

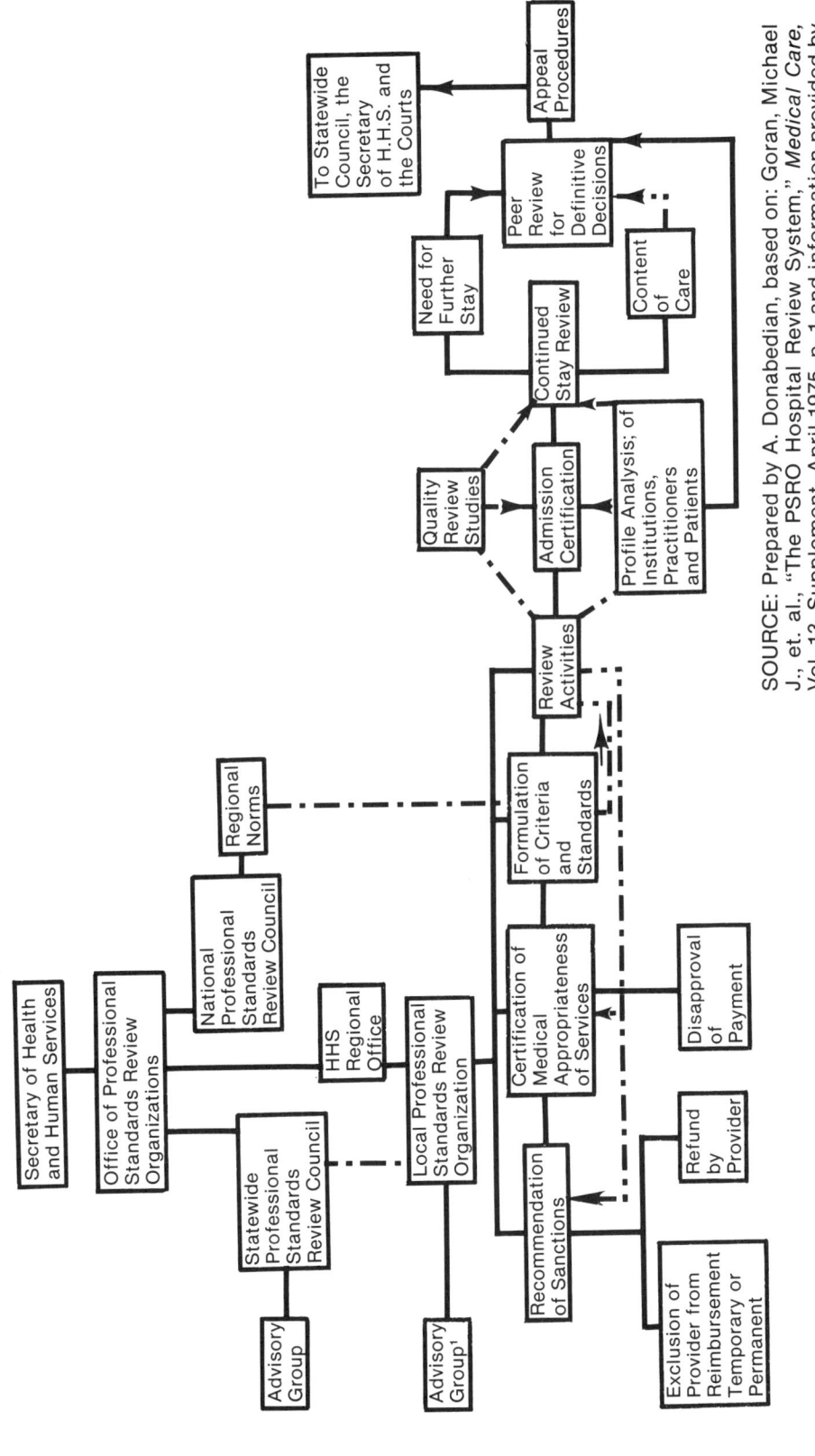

SOURCE: Prepared by A. Donabedian, based on: Goran, Michael J., et. al., "The PSRO Hospital Review System," *Medical Care*, Vol. 13, Supplement, April 1975, p. 1 and information provided by D.F. Siebert and Alan Reider, Office of Professional Standards Review Organizations, June 1980.

[1] When there is no statewide council.

NOTE: Dotted lines indicate influences among components.

Chart G-66 Certification of Admission and Stay Under Professional Standards Review Organization (U.S.A., 1980).

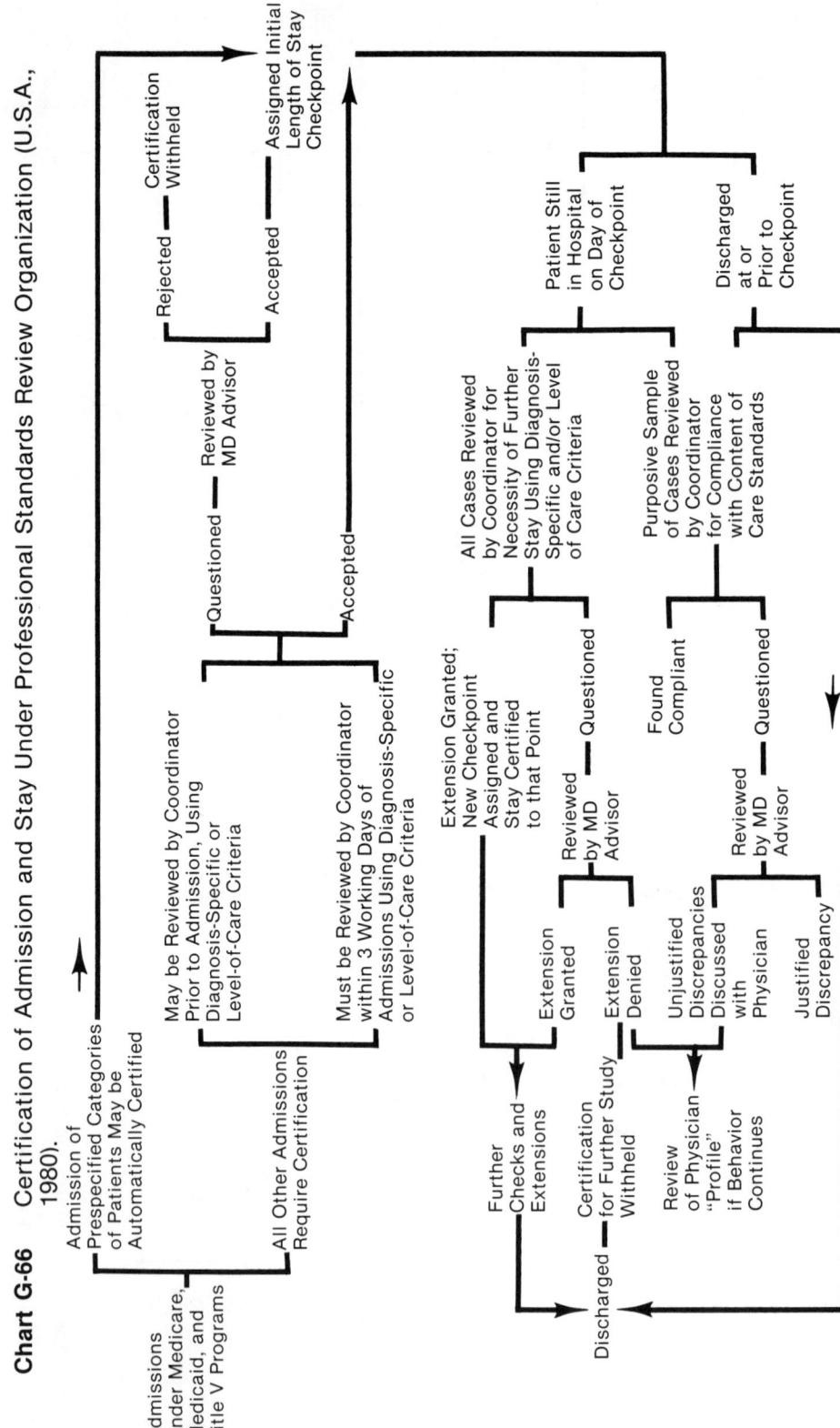

SOURCE: Prepared by A. Donabedian, based on: Goran, Michael J., et al., "The PSRO Hospital Review System," *Medical Care*, Vol. 13, Supplement, April 1975, p. 1 and information provided by D. F. Siebert and Alan Reider, Office of Professional Standards Review Organizations, June 1980.

Chart G-67

Number of Areas in the United States with Planning and Conditional Professional Standards Review Organizations (PSRO s) and with no Funded PSRO s (1974-1979).

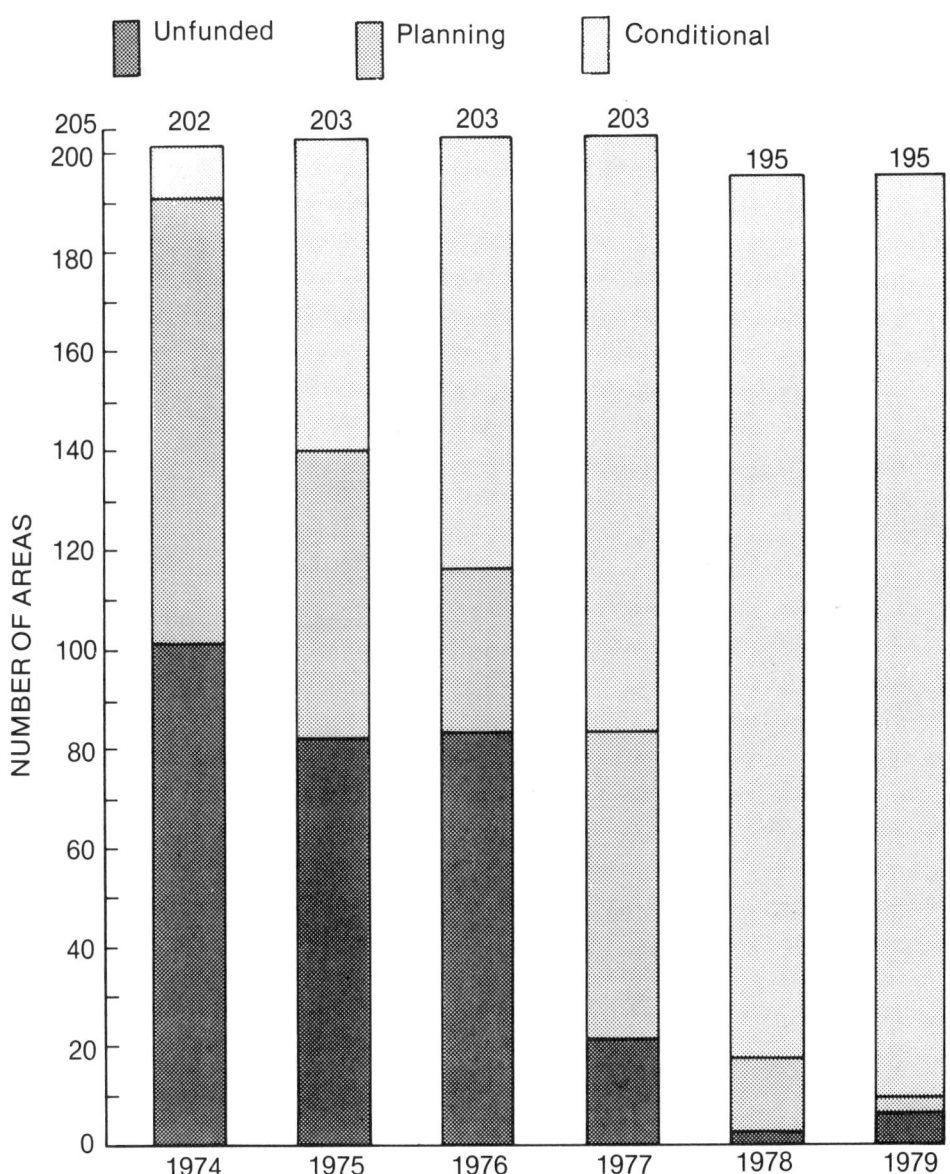

NOTE: The United States was originally divided into 202 PSRO areas. Subsequent redefinition of areas resulted in the number of areas changing to 203 in 1975, and to 195 in 1978.

SOURCE: Health Care Financing Administration, *Health Care Financing Research Report, Professional Standards Review Organization, 1979 Program Evaluation,* Office of Research, Demonstrations, and Statistics, Baltimore, Maryland, May 1980, Table 89, p. 159.

Quality of Care

Chart G-68

Percent Distribution of Professional Standards Review Organization (PSRO) Areas with Programs for Conducting Review of Care, Percent of Hospitals in PSRO Conditional Areas Under Review, and Percent of Hospitals Under Fully and Partially Delegated Review (U.S.A., 1979).

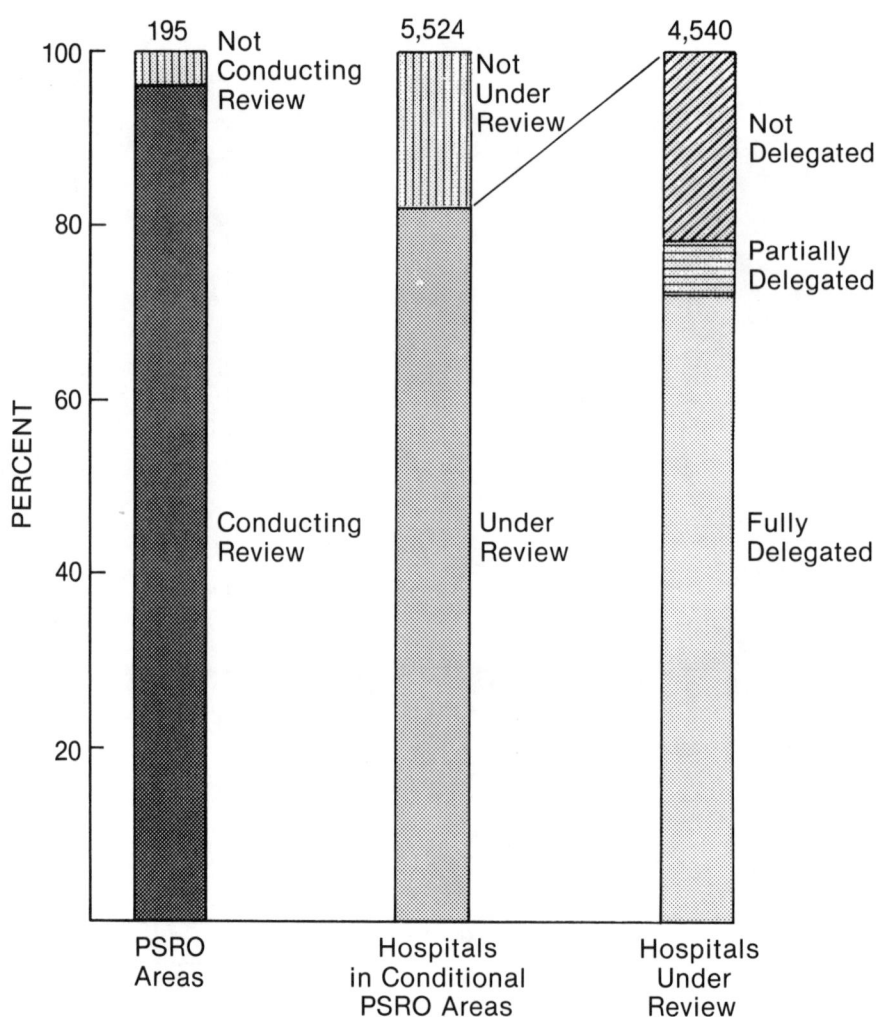

NOTE: Actual numbers shown on top of bars.

SOURCE: Health Care Financing Administration, *Health Care Financing Research Report, Professional Standards Review Organization, 1979 Program Evaluation,* Office of Research, Demonstrations, and Statistics, Baltimore, Maryland, May 1980, Table 85, p. 156.

Quality of Care

Chart G-69

Medicare Total Days of Care and Discharges per 1,000 Aged Enrollees, and Average Length of Stay for Active and Inactive PSROs (U.S.A., 1974-1977).

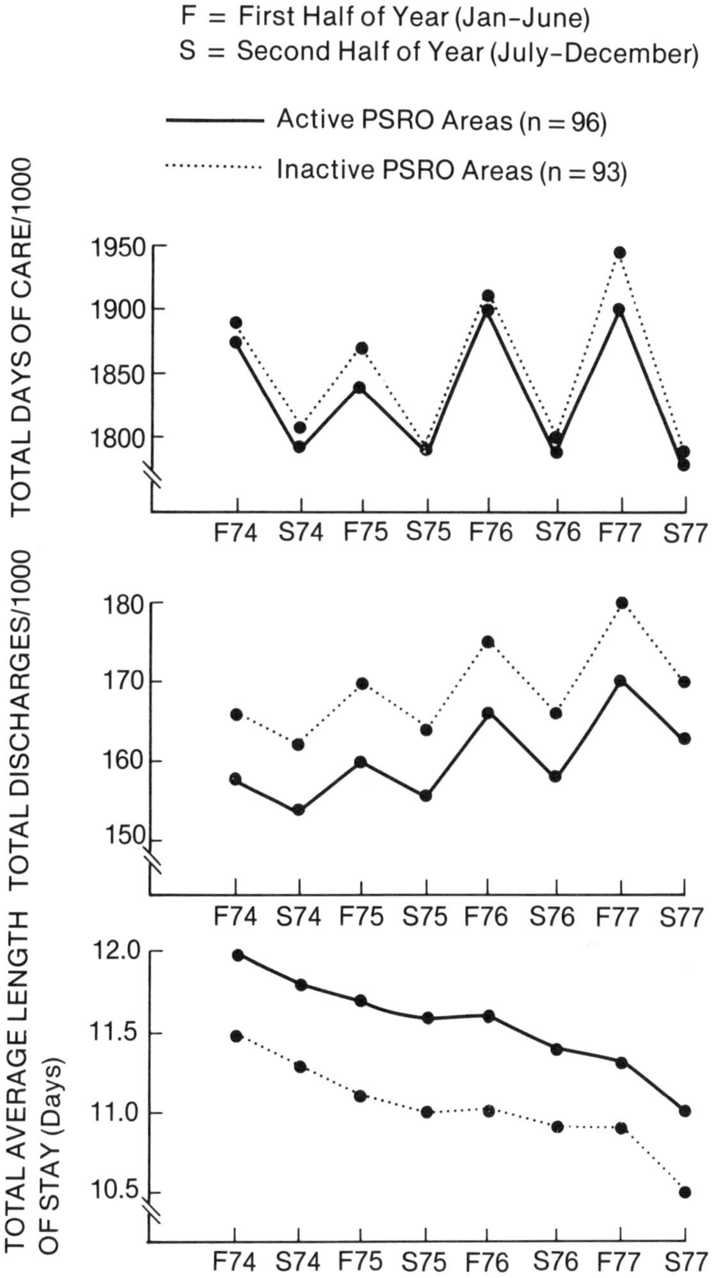

F = First Half of Year (Jan-June)
S = Second Half of Year (July-December)

——— Active PSRO Areas (n = 96)
······· Inactive PSRO Areas (n = 93)

SOURCE: Health Care Financing Administration, *Professional Standards Review Organization, 1978 Program Evaluation*, DHEW, January 1979, Table 1, p. 20.

Chart G-70

Incidence of Rheumatic Fever Prior to the Establishment of a Comprehensive Care Program and During its Operation, Eligible and Non-eligible Populations (Baltimore, predominantly Black Census Tracts, 1960–1970).

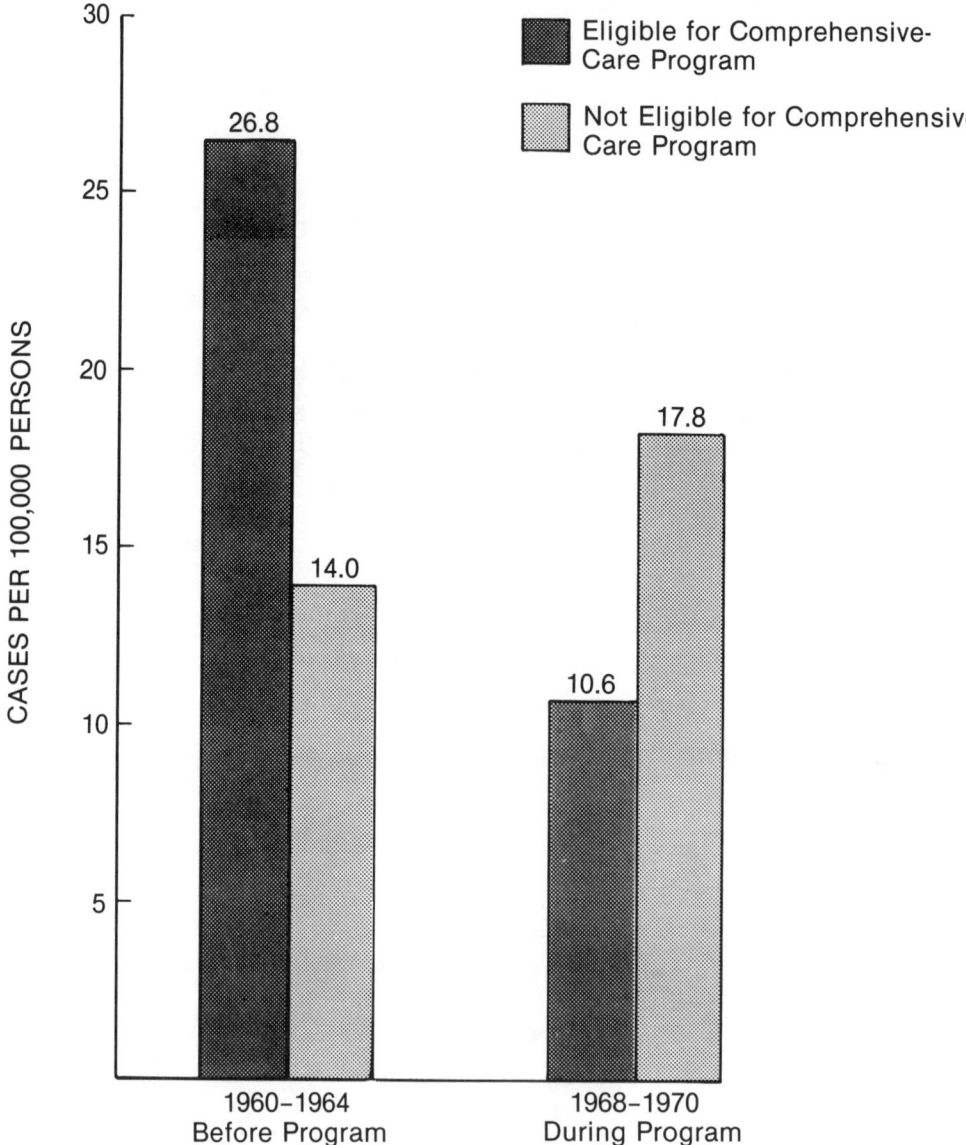

SOURCE: Gordis, Leon, "Effectiveness of Comprehensive-Care Programs in Preventing Rheumatic Fever," *New England Journal of Medicine,* Vol. 289, No. 7, August 16, 1973, Table 3, p. 333.

Quality of Care

Chart G-71

Percent of Persons with Urinary Symptoms Who Experienced Specified Events During 2 Subsequent Years; Recipients of Public Assistance Who Were Invited to Receive Care in a Hospital-Based, Comprehensive Care Project Compared to Those Who Continued as Usual (Yorkville Welfare District, New York City, 1961–1964).

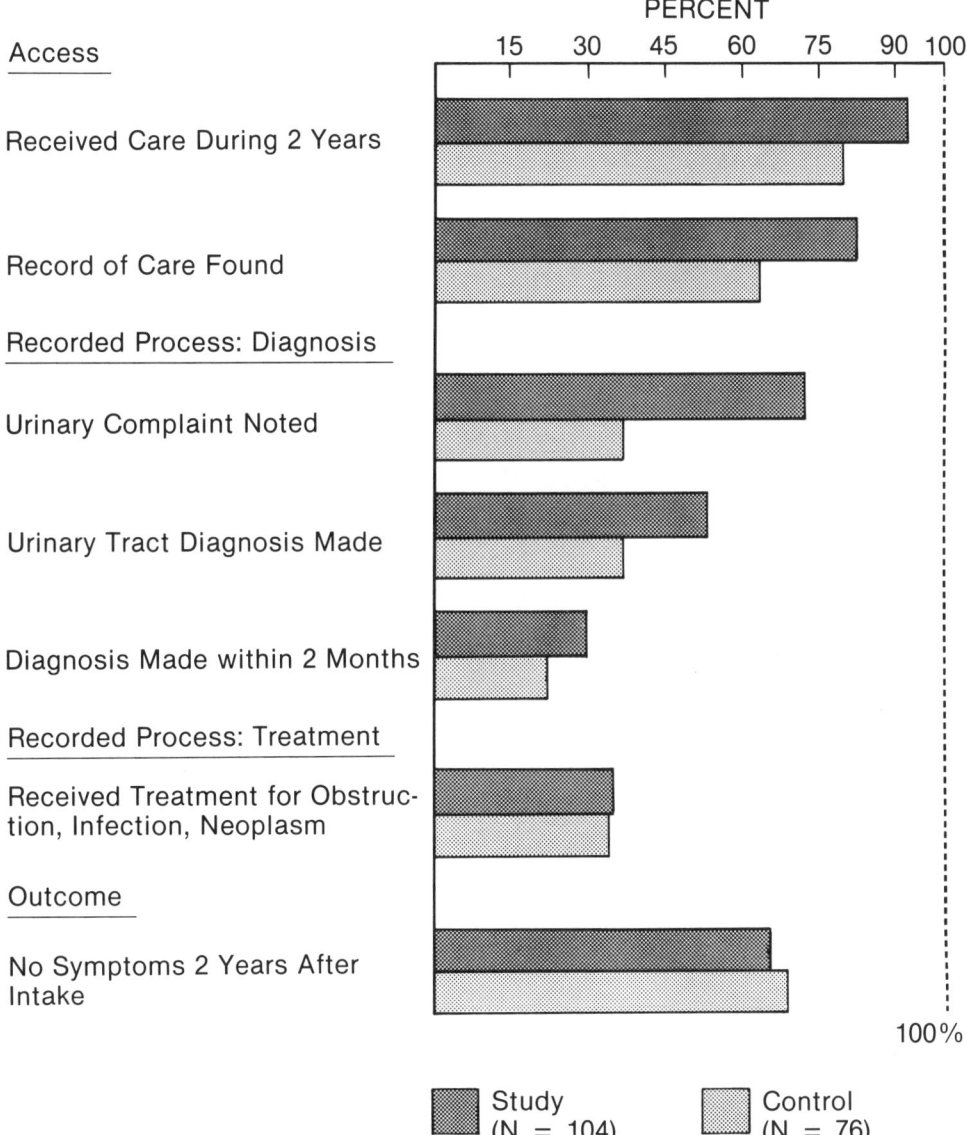

NOTE: In this study the characteristics of the two settings for care (study and control) represent "structure." Data on "outcome" are clouded by losses to the two samples and by inconsistencies in reported presence of symptoms at intake when compared to recall two years later. Not shown is a much higher degree of satisfaction in the study group.

SOURCE: Goodrich, C.H., M.C. Olendzki, and G.G. Reader, *Welfare Medical Care: An Experiment*, Cambridge, Mass., Harvard University Press, 1970, pp. 180–186.

SECTION H
Tax-Supported Programs

Chart H-1

Social Welfare Expenditures Under Public Programs, and National Health Expenditures as Percent of Gross National Product (U.S.A., Selected Years, 1950–1978).[1]

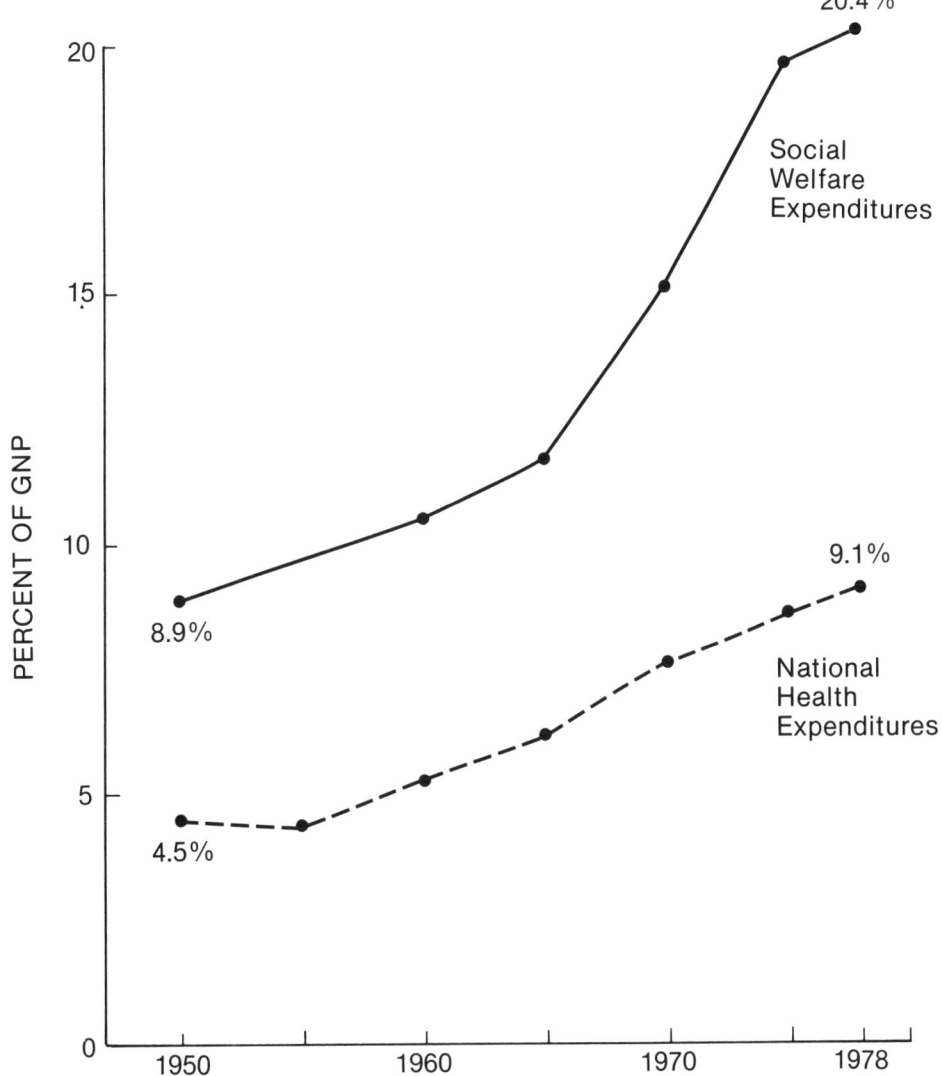

[1]Social Welfare Expenditures under public programs include public outlays for social insurance, public aid, health and medical programs, veterans' programs, education, and housing.

SOURCES: U.S. Department of Commerce, Bureau of the Census, *Statistical Abstract of the United States, 1979*, Washington, D.C., 1979, Table 521, p. 325; Gibson, R.M., "National Health Expenditures, 1978," *Health Care Financing Review*, Summer 1979, Table 1, p. 22.

Tax-Supported Programs

Chart H-2

Federal Health Expenditures as a Percent of Total Federal Expenditures (U.S.A., Fiscal Years 1965, 1970, 1975, and 1979).

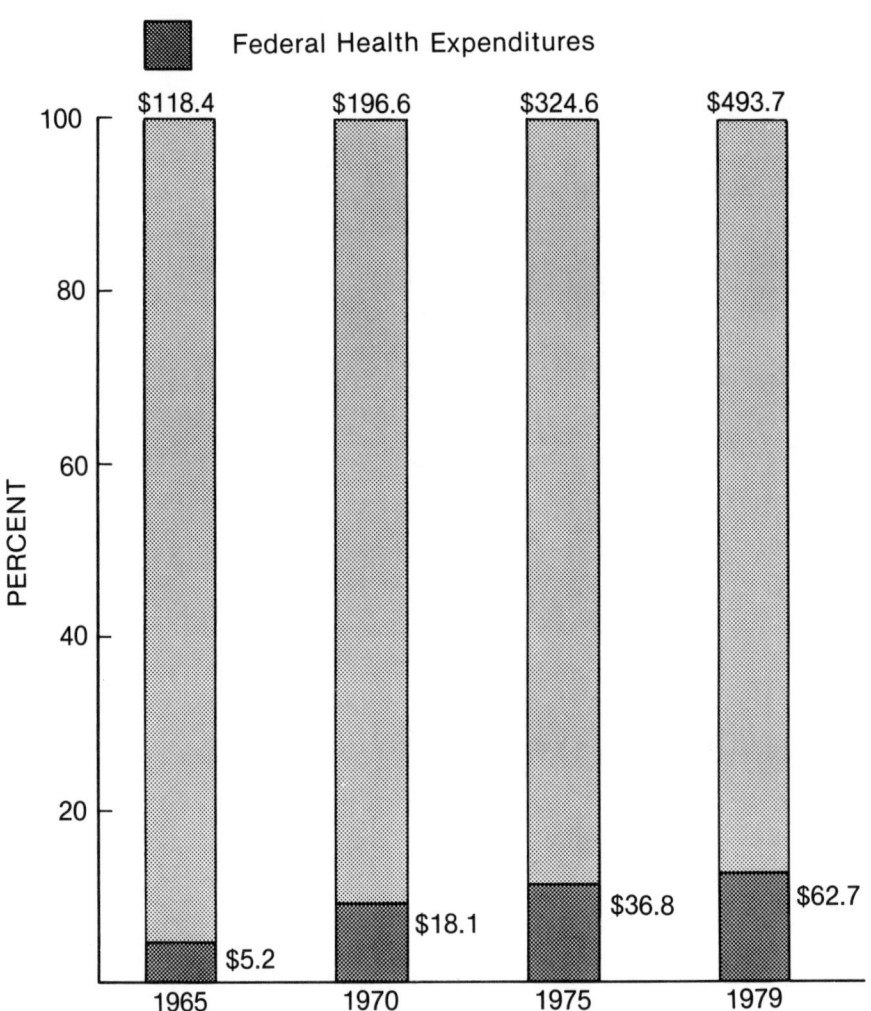

NOTE: Dollar amounts in billions.

SOURCES: *Special Analyses Budget of the United States Government,* Office of Management and Budget, Washington, D.C., U.S. Government Printing Office; for 1965: Special Analyses for Fiscal Year 1975, Table J-1, p. 136; for 1970: Special Analyses for Fiscal Year 1972, Table K-1, p. 149; for 1975: Special Analyses for Fiscal Year 1977, Table K-1, p. 192; for 1979: Special Analyses for Fiscal Year 1981, Table A-13, p. 45, and data provided by B. Clendenin, Office of Management and Budget; Washington, D.C., April 1980.

Chart H-3

Federal Health Expenditures as a Percent of National Health Expenditures (U.S.A., Fiscal Years 1965, 1970, 1975, and 1977).

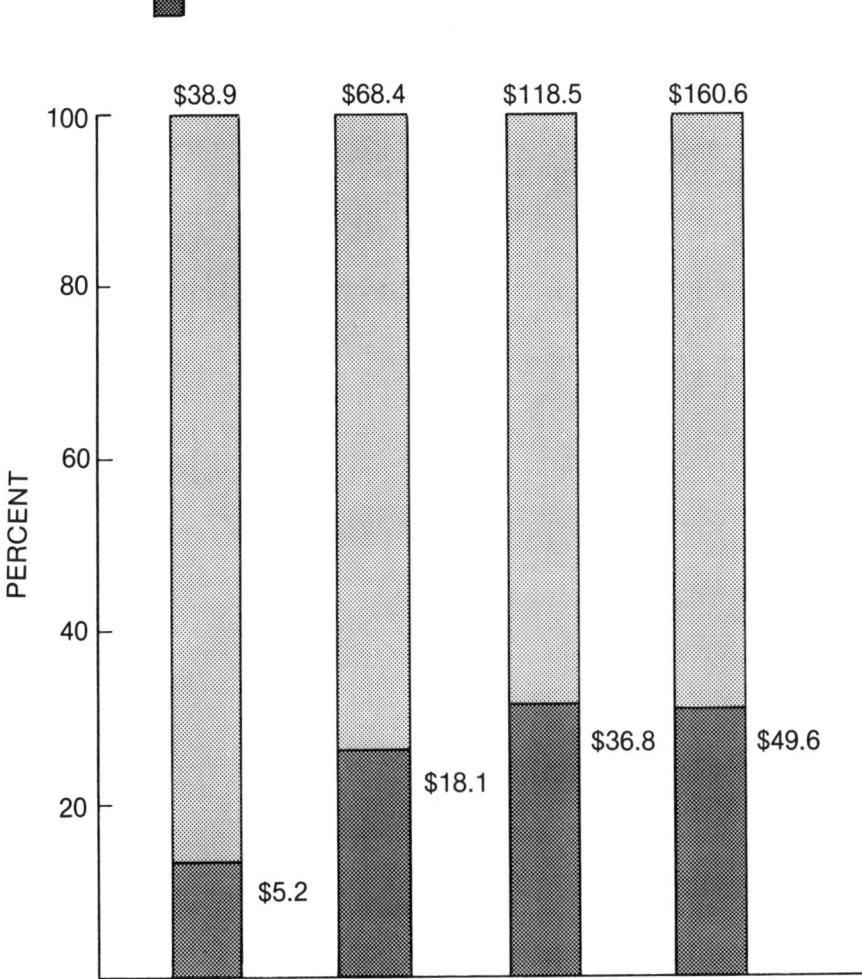

NOTE: Dollar amounts in billions.
SOURCES: *Special Analyses Budget of the United States Government,* Office of Management and Budget, Washington, D.C., U.S. Government Printing Office; for 1965: Special Analyses for Fiscal Year 1977, Graph K-3, p. 193 and Special Analyses for Fiscal Year 1974, Table J-1, p. 135; for 1970 and 1977; Special Analyses for Fiscal Year 1979, Table L-1, p. 242 and Graph: Public and Private Health Expenditures, p. 243; for 1975: Special Analyses for Fiscal Year 1977, Graph K-3, p. 193 and Special Analyses for Fiscal Year 1979, Table L-1, p. 242.

Chart H.-4 Percent Distribution of Federal Health Expenditures, by Type of Expenditure (U.S.A., Selected Years, 1965–1979).

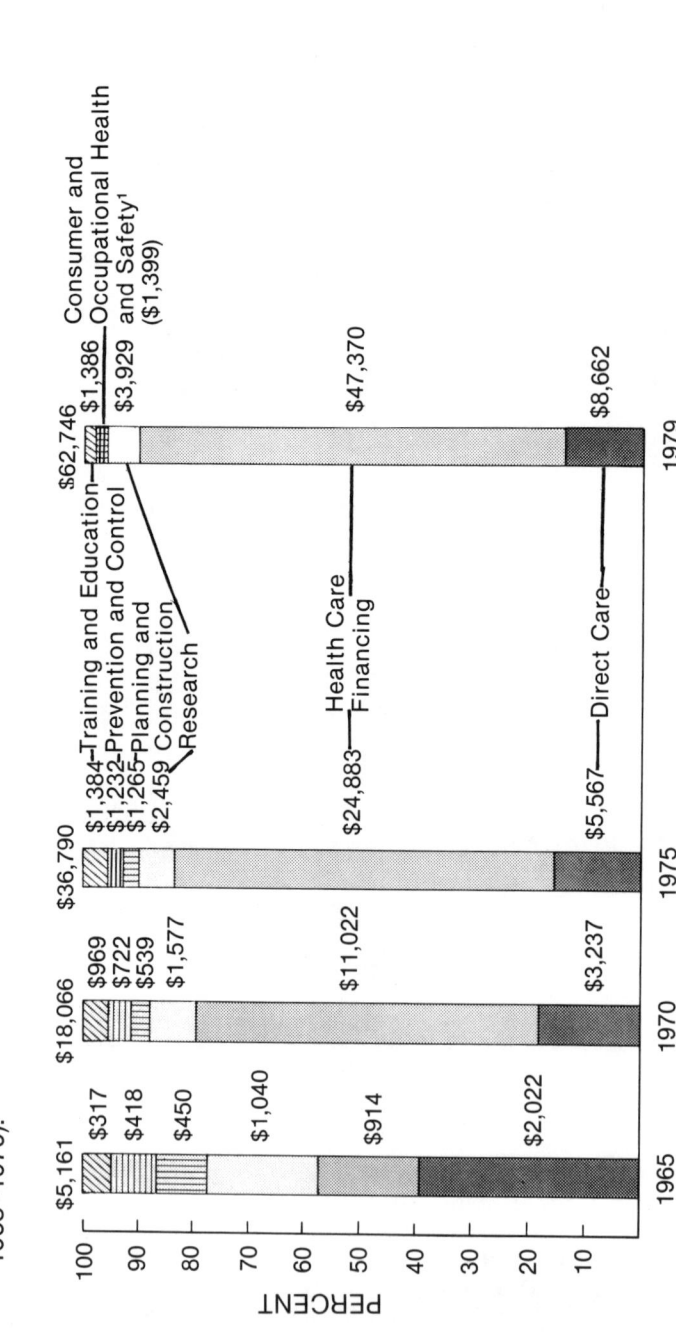

[1] In 1979 the categorization of federal health expenditures was changed. The new category of "consumer and occupational health and safety" includes expenditures formerly listed under "prevention and control," while expenditures for "planning and construction" were incorporated in the "direct care" and the "health care financing" categories.

NOTE: All dollar amounts shown are in billions.

SOURCES: For 1965 and 1970: Office of Management and Budget, *Special Analysis Budget of the United States Government, Fiscal Year 1972, Special Analysis K: Federal Health Programs,* Table K-14, p. 170 and Table K-15, p. 171; for 1975: Office of Management and Budget, *Special Analysis Budget of the United States Government, Fiscal Year 1977, Special Analysis K: Federal Health Programs,* Table K-28, p. 215; for 1979: Data provided by B. Clendenin, Office of Management and Budget, Washington, D.C., April 1980.

Tax-Supported Programs

Chart H-5

Distribution of Federal Health Expenditures, by Agency (U.S.A., 1979).

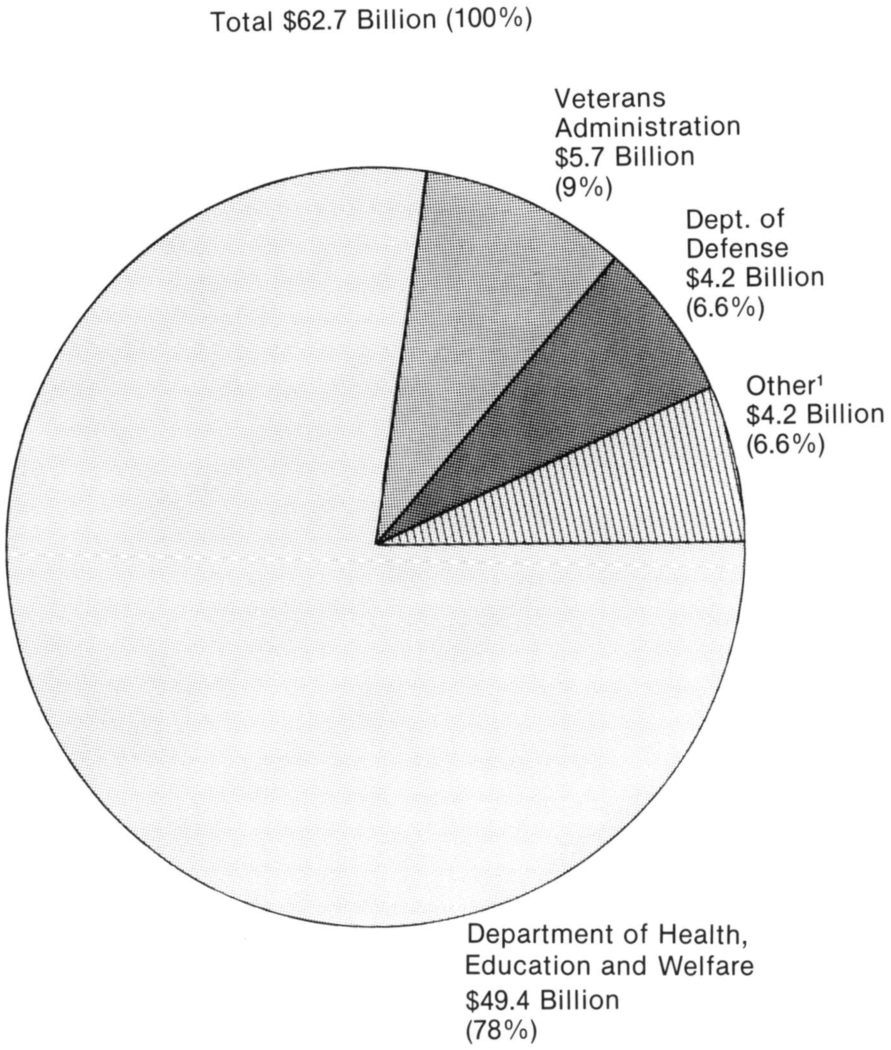

Total $62.7 Billion (100%)

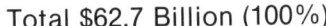

Veterans Administration
$5.7 Billion
(9%)

Dept. of Defense
$4.2 Billion
(6.6%)

Other[1]
$4.2 Billion
(6.6%)

Department of Health, Education and Welfare
$49.4 Billion
(78%)

[1]"Other" includes: Departments of Housing and Urban Development, Agriculture, Energy, Labor, State, Interior, Transportation, Justice; other agencies; and agency contributions to employee health funds.

SOURCE: Data provided by B. Clendenin, Office of Management and Budget, Washington, D.C., April 1980.

Tax-Supported Programs

Chart H-6 Major Programs Dealing with Important Causes of Dependency (U.S.A., 1980).

CAUSES OF DEPENDENCY	PUBLIC SECTOR PROGRAMS					PRIVATE SECTOR PROGRAMS
	Social Security Act Programs		Other Governmental Programs			
	Insurance	Assistance	Insurance	Assistance		
Unemployment	Unemployment Insurance	Aid to Families with Dependent Children (if father is unemployed)(AFDC)		General Assistance		Supplemental Unemployment Benefits
Old Age	"OA" provisions of O̲ASDHI[1]	Supplemental Security Income (SSI)	Veterans Administration; Public Employees Retirement Plans	General Assistance		Private pension plans
Premature Death of Breadwinner	"S" provisions of OA̲S̲DHI	Aid to Families with Dependent Children (AFDC)		General Assistance		Life Insurance
Illness: Loss of Income	"D" provisions of OAS̲D̲HI	Supplemental Security Income (SSI)	Workers' Compensation; State Disability Insurance (5 States); Veterans Administration	General Assistance		Temporary disability insurance; ("accident and health insurance")
Illness: Costs of Medical Care[2]	"H" provisions of OASD̲H̲I̲	Medicaid	Workers' Compensation; State Temporary Disability Insurance (In California and New York only)	General Assistance		Medical care insurance

[1]O.A.S.D.H.I. = Old Age, Survivors, Disability and Health Insurance.

[2]Not including programs providing medical care for Federal beneficiaries (Native Americans, merchant seamen, veterans, members of armed forces and their dependents, and Federal employees).

SOURCE: Prepared by S.J. Axelrod, The University of Michigan, June 1980.

Tax-Supported Programs

Medical Care Chartbook

Chart H-7 Percent Distribution of Cash Benefit Payments Under Public Income Maintenance Programs, by Type of Program (U.S.A., Selected Years, 1940–1978).

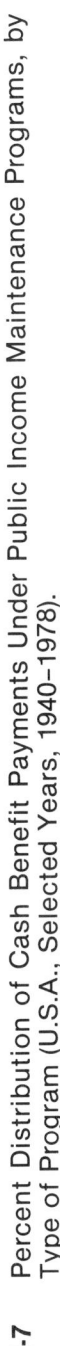

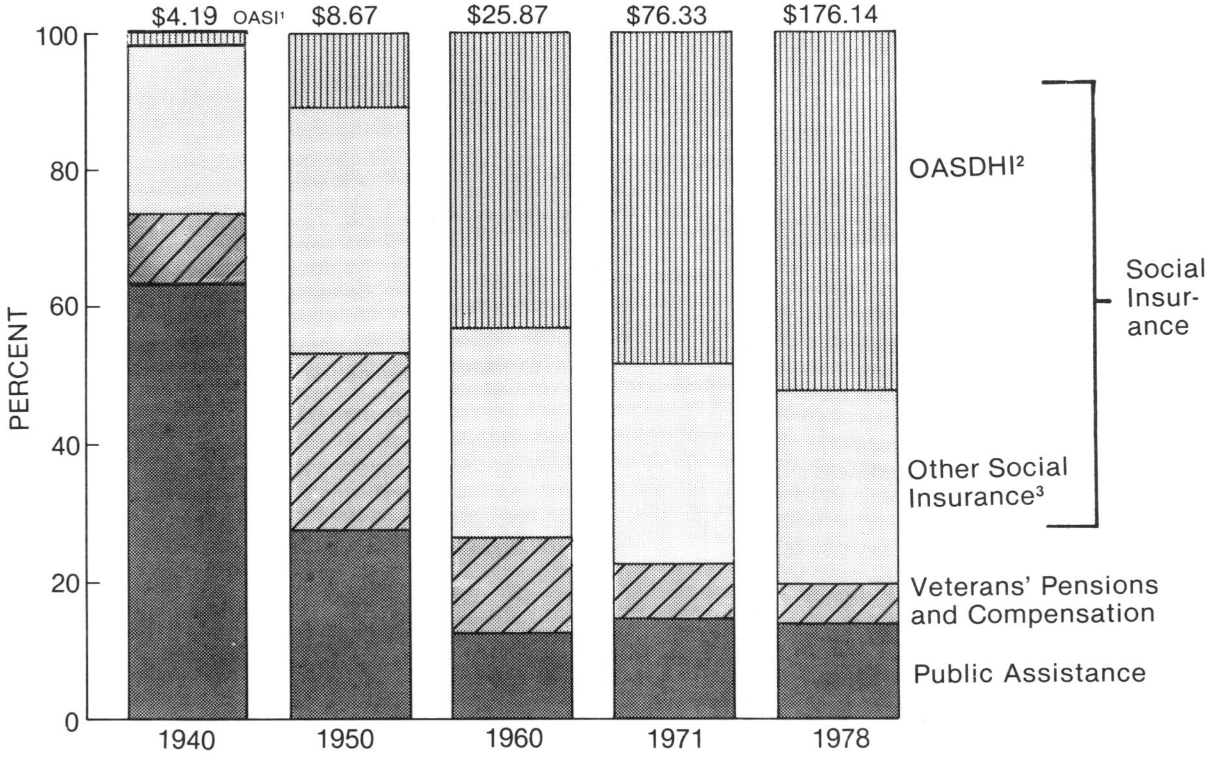

[1] Old Age and Survivors Insurance.

[2] Old Age, Survivors, Disability, and Health Insurance.

[3] Includes Railroad Retirement, public employee retirement, unemployment insurance, Workers' Compensation (net of medical) and temporary disability insurance (net of medical).

NOTE: Dollar amounts in billions.

SOURCES: For 1940–1960: Social Security Administration, *Social Security Programs in the United States*, DHEW, Washington, D.C., January 1973, Table 2, p. 16; for 1978: Unpublished data from the Department of Health, Education, and Welfare provided by Ann K. Bixby of the Office of Research and Statistics, Social Security Administration, May 1980.

Tax-Supported Programs

Chart H-8 Number of Persons Aged 65 and Over and Number Covered by Specified Social Insurance and Assistance Programs (U.S.A., 1940–1978).

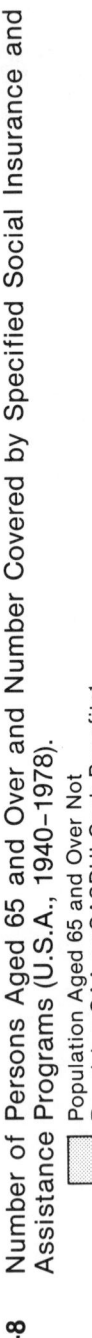

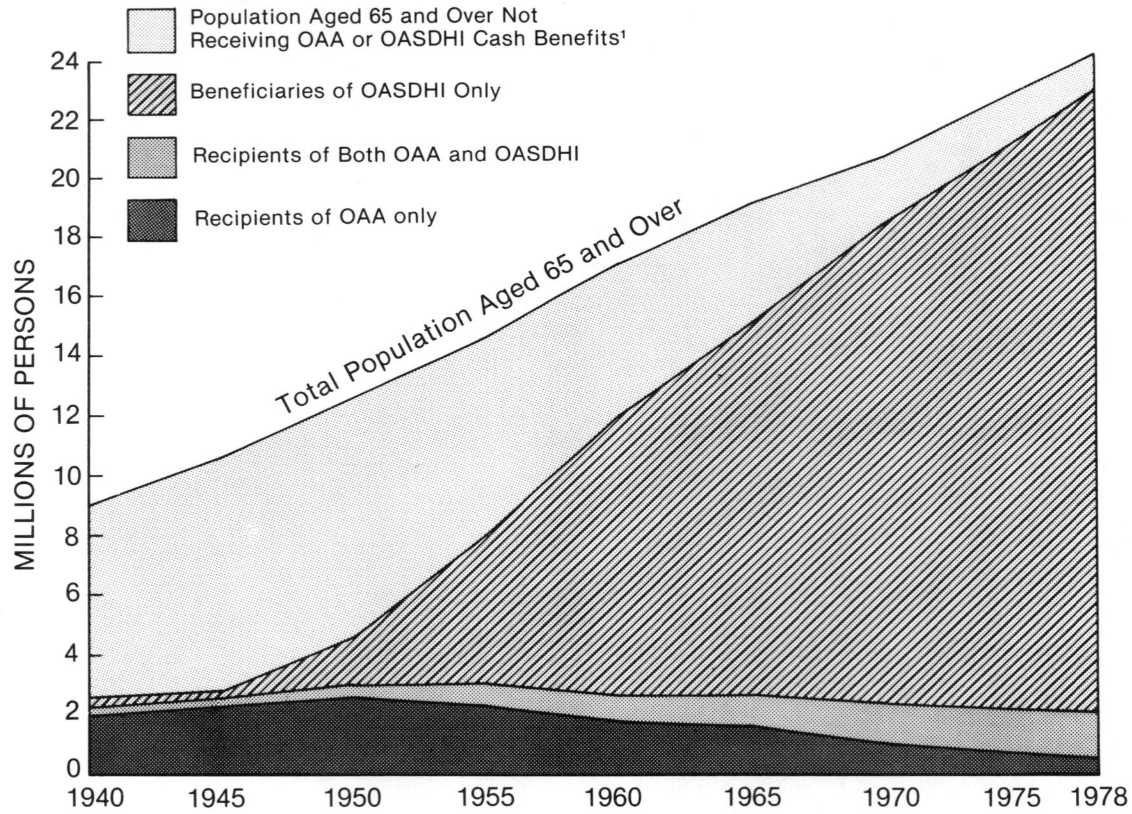

- Population Aged 65 and Over Not Receiving OAA or OASDHI Cash Benefits[1]
- Beneficiaries of OASDHI Only
- Recipients of Both OAA and OASDHI
- Recipients of OAA only

[1] OAA = Old Age Assistance; OASDHI — Old Age, Survivors, Disability, and Health Insurance.

NOTE: In 1974 the three adult categories in public assistance, OAA, Aid to the Blind, and Aid to the Totally and Permanently Disabled, were consolidated under the new federal Supplemental Security Income (SSI) program. The number of OAA recipients shown for the period following 1974 corresponds to the old-age

SOURCES: For 1940–1971: Social Security Administration, *Social Security Programs in the United States*, DHEW, Washington, D.C., January 1973, Chart 3, p. 19; for 1978: Data provided by Ann K. Bixby, Department of Health, Education, and Welfare, Social Security Administration, Office of Research and Statistics, May 1980.

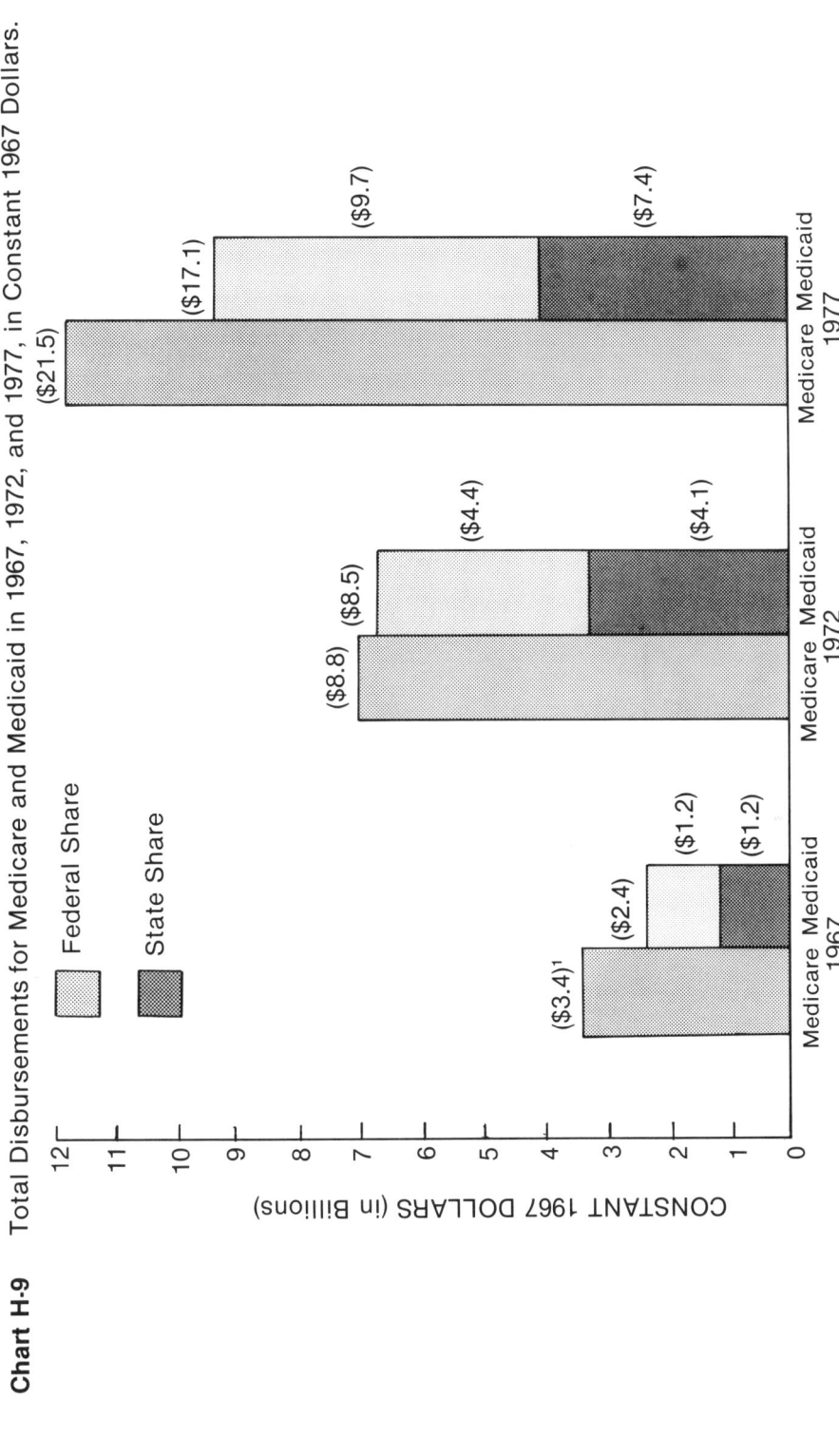

Chart H-9 Total Disbursements for Medicare and Medicaid in 1967, 1972, and 1977, in Constant 1967 Dollars.

[1]Other plans include health maintenance organizations, community plans, employer-employee-union plans, private group clinics, and dental service corporations.

SOURCES: For Consumer Price Indexes: *Social Security Bulletin*, Vol. 41, No. 6, June 1978, Table M-45, p. 69; for Medicaid: Appendices to the Federal Budgets: 1969, p. 465, 1974, p. 442, 1979, p. 416; for Medicare: 1979 Annual Report of the Board of Trustees of the Federal Hospital Insurance Trust Fund, Table 5, p. 13, 1979 Annual Report of the Board of Trustees of the Federal Supplemental Medical Insurance Trust Fund, Table 5, p. 10 as cited by Mr. David Gibson of the Office of Statistics and Data Management, Health Care Financing Administration.

Chart H-10

Percent of Total Medicare Income and of the Income of Medicare Component Trust Funds Which derives from General Revenue Funds (U.S.A., Calendar Years, 1967–1978).

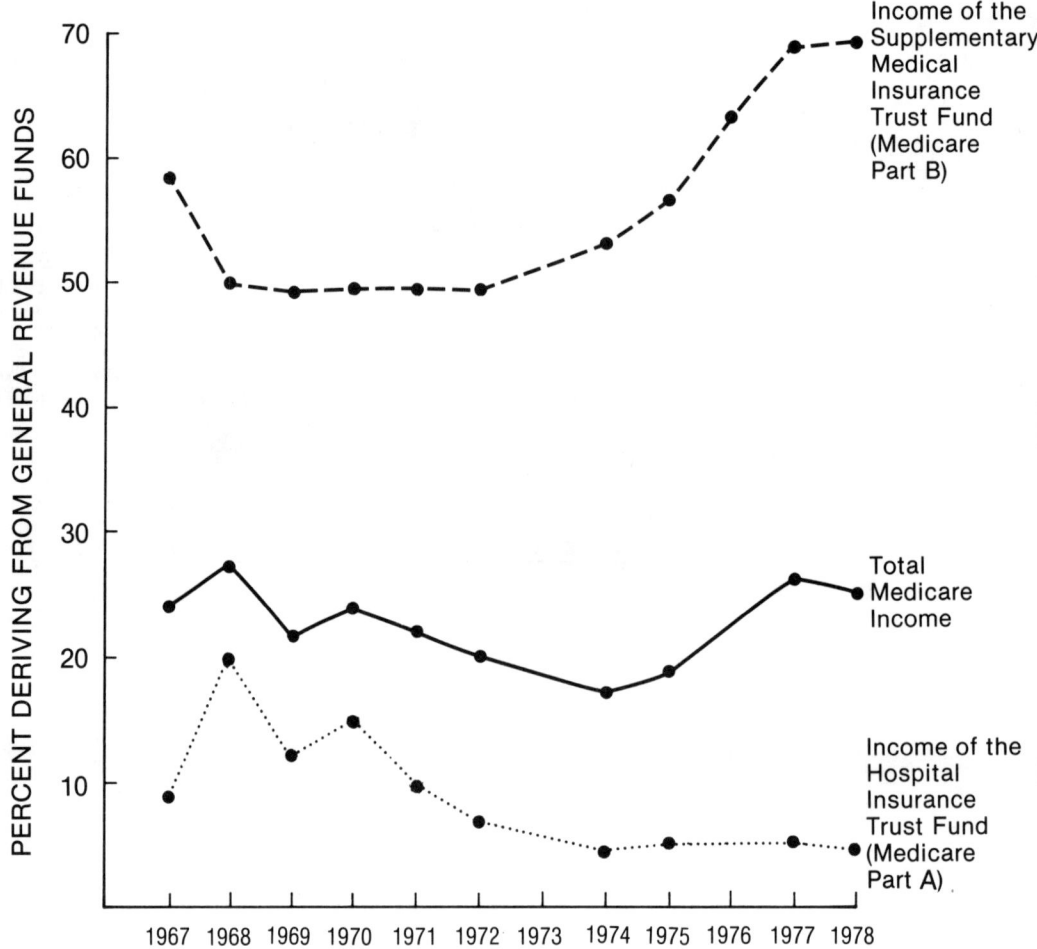

NOTE: In 1976 and 1977 changes were made in the schedule of dates on which funds are transferred from certain general revenue accounts into the Hospital Insurance Trust Fund, resulting in smaller transfers in one year followed by larger ones the next. To compensate for those changes, the data used for 1977 and 1978 include an adjustment to reflect only those transfers that would have been made over a regular 12-month period. Since such an adjustment could not be made for 1976, the data for that year are not shown for total Medicare income and for the Hospital Insurance Trust Fund income.

SOURCES: *1979 Annual Report of the Board of Trustees of the Federal Supplementary Medical Insurance Trust Fund*, 96th Congress, First Session, April 24, 1979, House of Representatives Document No. 96-103, Table 6, p. 11 and Document No. 96-102, Table 6, p. 14.

Medical Care Chartbook

Chart H-11

Percent Distribution of Public Expenditures under Medicare for Persons Age 65 and Older, by Type of Expenditure (U.S.A., Fiscal 1977).

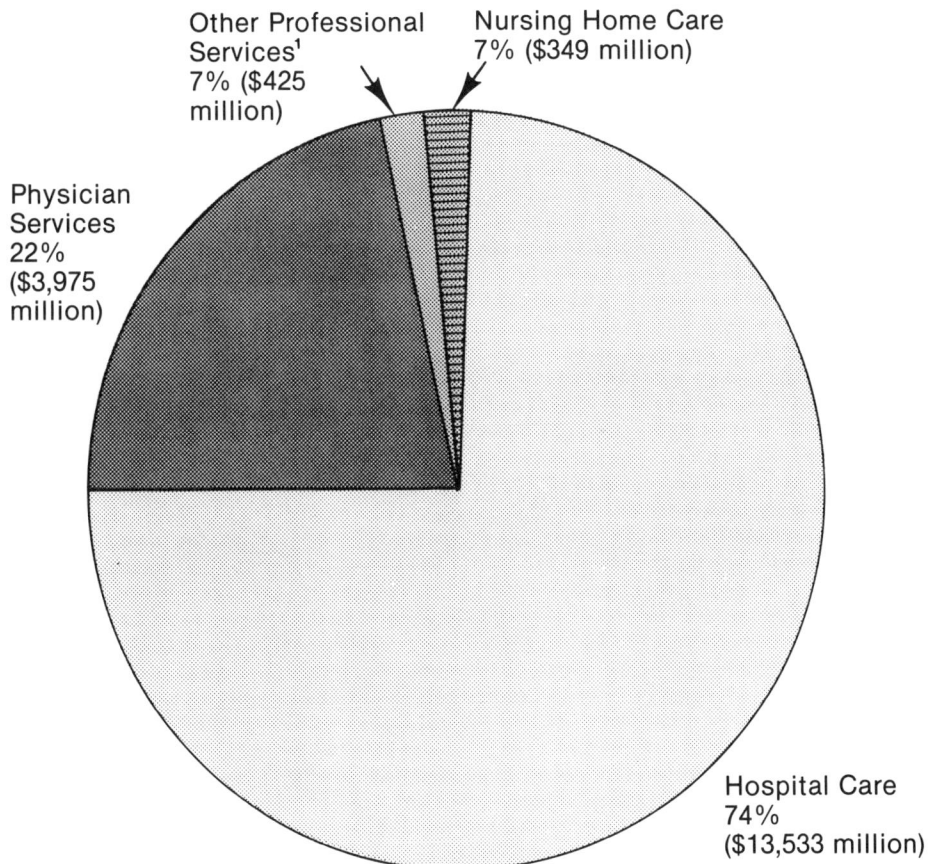

Total $18,282 Million

Other Professional Services[1] 7% ($425 million)

Nursing Home Care 7% ($349 million)

Physician Services 22% ($3,975 million)

Hospital Care 74% ($13,533 million)

[1]Includes home health and services provided by health professionals other than physicians and dentists such as private duty nurses, optometrists, chiropractors, and physical and speech therapists. Of the $425 million spent on such services, approximately $380 million, 90% of the total, was for home health services.

SOURCE: Gibson, R.M. and C.R. Fisher, "Age Differences in Health Care Spending, Fiscal Year 1977, "*Social Security Bulletin,* Vol.42, No.1, January 1979, Table 6, p.14, and data provided by Charles Fisher, Office of Policy, Planning, and Research, Financial and Actuarial Analysis, Health Care Financing Administration, July 1980.

Tax-Supported Programs

Chart H-12 Relative Growth in Amounts Reimbursed for Medicare Parts A and B, for Part A Only, and for Inpatient Services, Skilled Nursing Services, and Home Health Care Facilities Under Part A (U.S.A., 1967, 1970 and 1979).

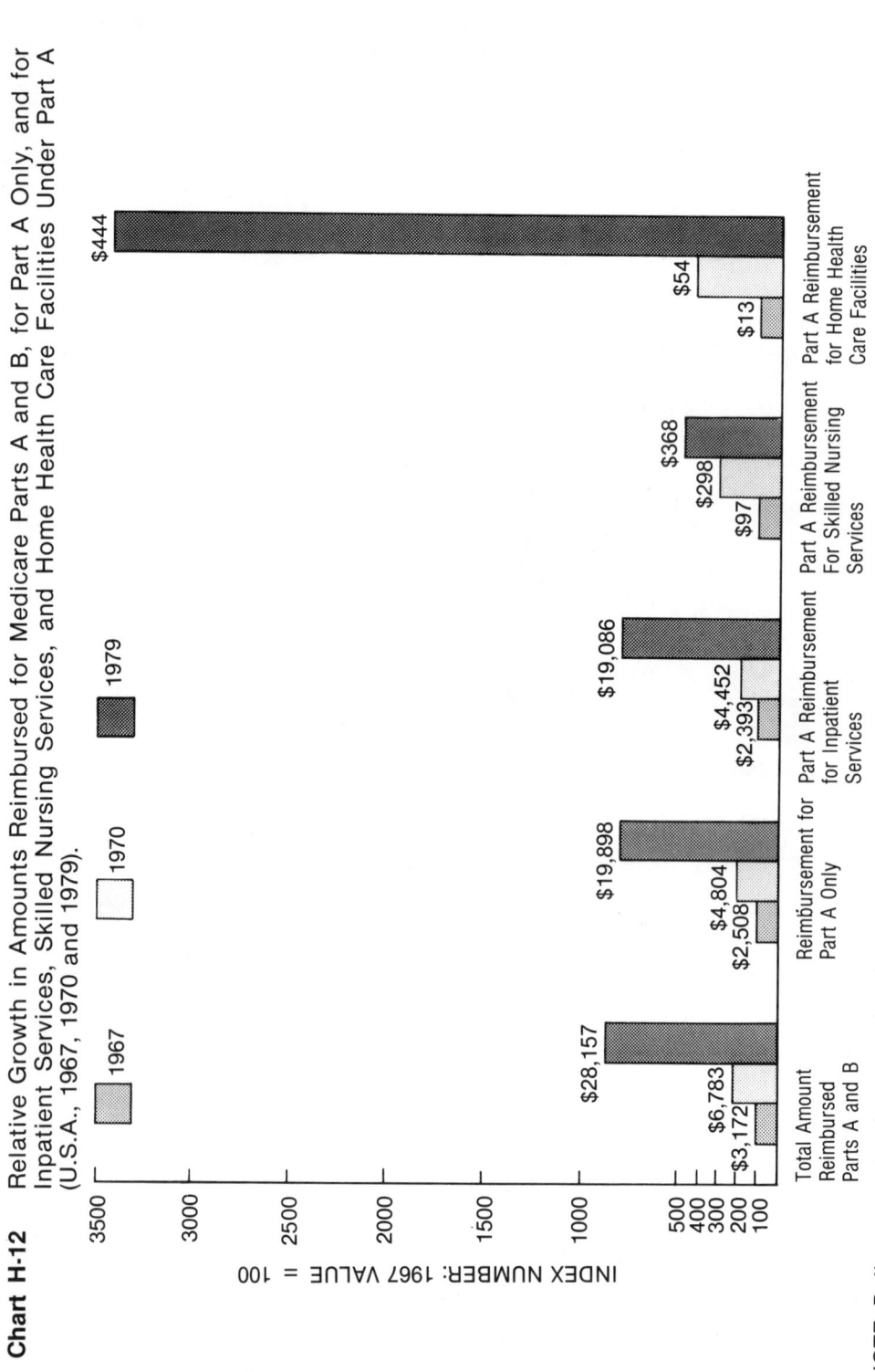

NOTE: Dollar amounts shown are in millions.

SOURCE: Department of Health and Human Services, Health Care Financing Administration, data provided by David Gibson, Office of Statistics and Data Management, May 1980.

Chart H-13

Percent Distribution of Physicians' Services Covered by the Supplementary Medical Insurance Program of Medicare (Part B), by Place of Service (U.S.A., 1974).

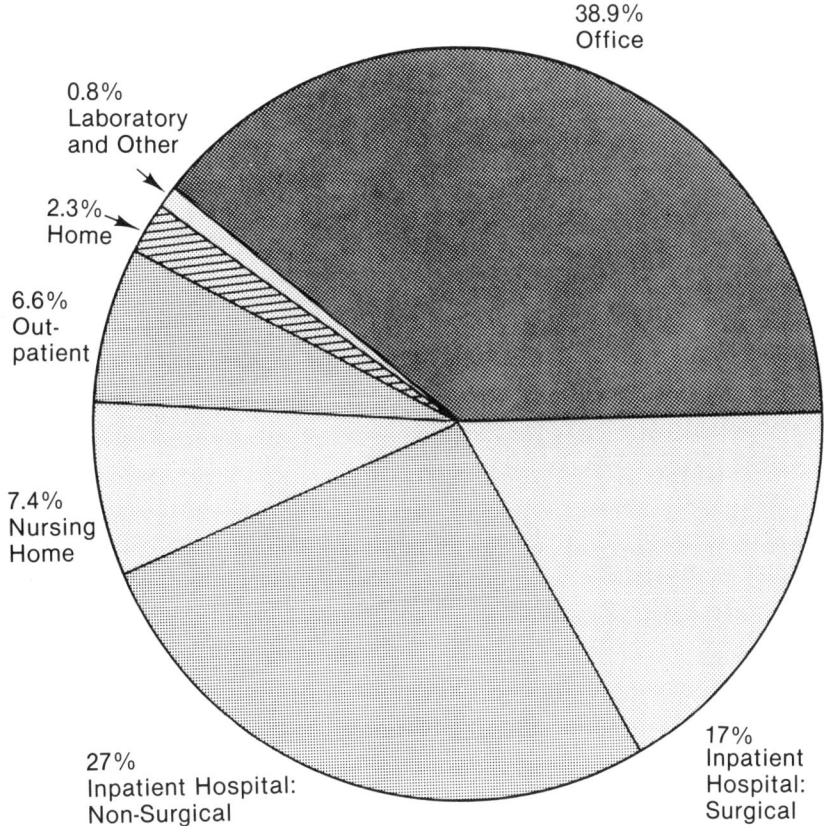

SOURCE: U.S. Department of Health, Education, and Welfare, Health Care Financing Administration, Office of Policy, Planning and Research, *Research Statistics Note No. 1, Current Medicare Survey Report, Supplementary Medical Insurance Utilization and Charges for the Aged, 1974*, June 1978, Table 7.

Chart H-14

Relative Number of Hospital Discharges per 1,000, Days of Hospital Care per 1,000, and Average Length of Hospital Stay, Before and After the Implementation of Medicare and Medicaid, by Age (U.S.A., Civilian Non-institutioinalized Population, 1963-1978).[1]

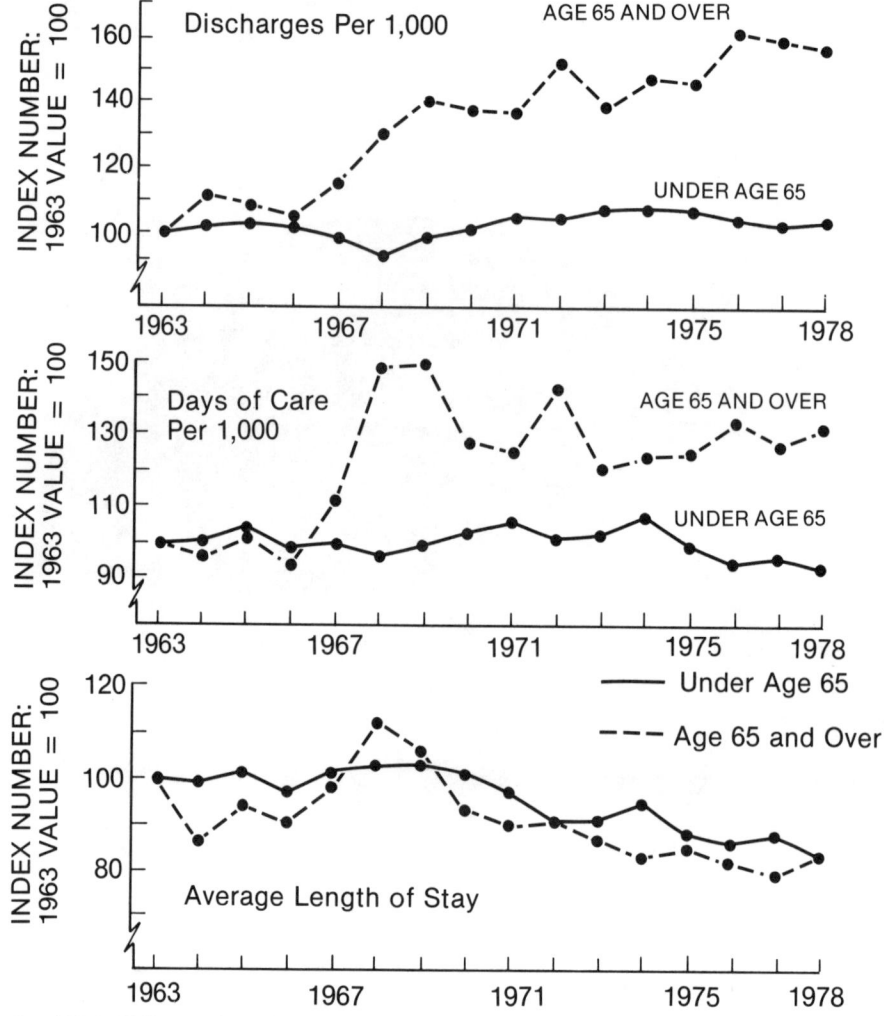

[1]Data for 1963-1967 are for fiscal years.

NOTE: Title XVIII and XIX of the Social Security Act establishing the Medicare and Medicaid programs were enacted into law in 1965. The Medicaid program went into effect on January 1, 1966; the Medicare program became effective July 1, 1966.

SOURCES: For 1963-1970: Pettengill, J., "Trends in Hospital Use by the Aged," *Social Security Bulletin,* Vol. 35, No. 7, Table A, p. 12; for 1970-1978: U.S. National Center for Health Statistics, *Current Estimates from the Health Interview Survey, United States,* DHEW, Public Health Service, Office of Health Research, Statistics, and Technology, Hyattsville, Maryland, Series 10, No. 79, Table 13, p. 20, Series 10, No. 85, Table 13, p. 20, Series 10, No. 95, Table 13, p. 20, Series 10, No. 100, Table 13, p. 20, Series 10, No. 115, Table 13, p. 23, Series 10, No. 119, Table 15, p. 25, Series 10, No. 126, Table 15, p. 25, and Series 10, No. 130, Table 15, p. 25.

Tax-Supported Programs

Chart H-15

Relative Change in Days of Short-Stay Hospital Care Per 100 Persons, by Selected Personal Characteristics, After the Implementation of Medicare and Medicaid, Persons 65 years of Age and Over (U.S.A., 1965 and 1967).

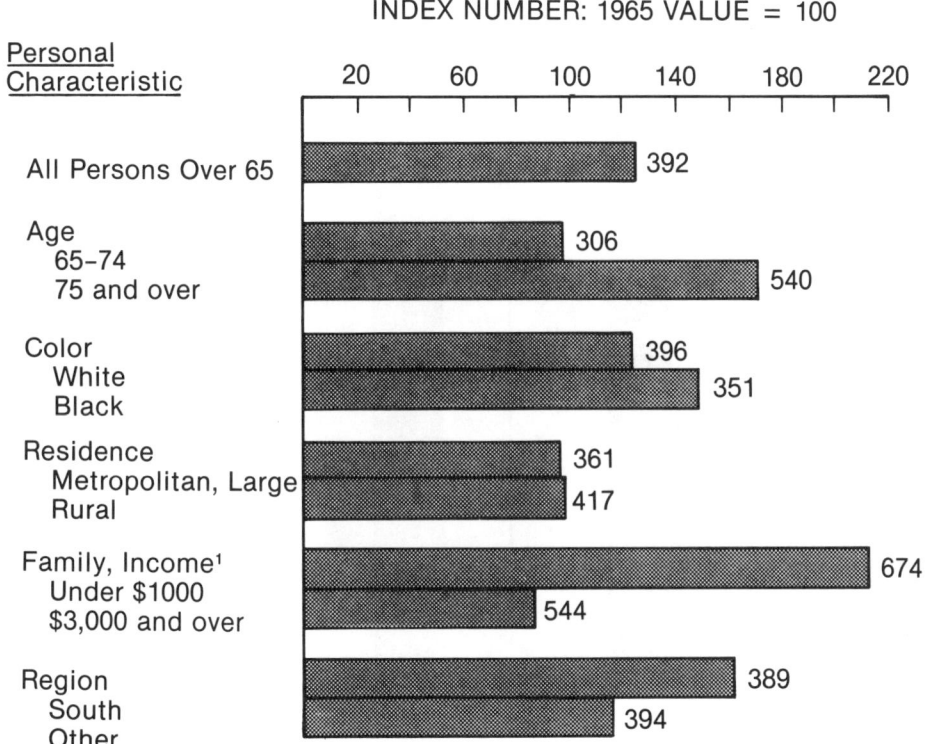

[1] One-person families only.

NOTE: Numbers to the right of bars are actual days of care per 100 persons 65 and over in 1967.

SOURCE: Loewenstein, Regina, "Early Effects of Medicare on the Health Care of the Aged," *Social Security Bulletin*, Vol. 34, April 1971, Table 2, p. 7.

Chart H-16

Relative Change in Percent of Persons With Reported Ambulatory Medical Visits by Place of Visit, After the Implementation of Medicare and Medicaid (U.S.A., 1965 and 1967).

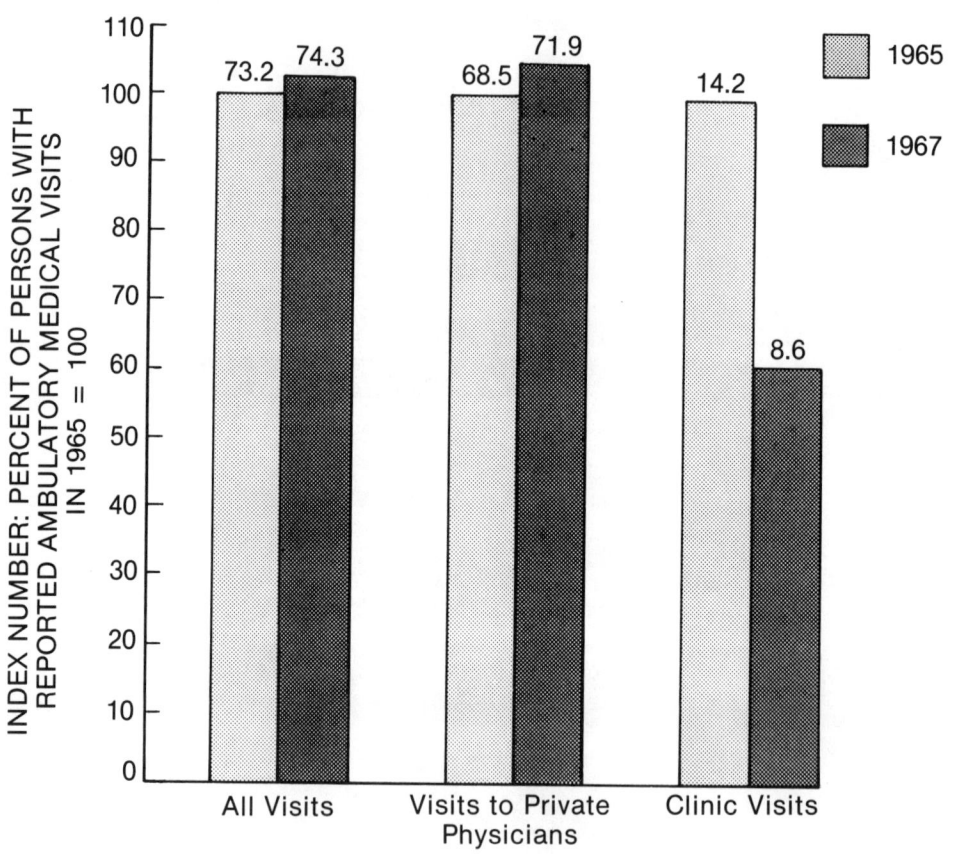

NOTE: Numbers above bars are percent of persons with reported visits.

SOURCE: Loewenstein, Regina, "Early Effects of Medicare on the Health Care of the Aged," *Social Security Bulletin*, Vol. 34, April 1971, Table 9, p. 14.

Tax-Supported Programs

Chart H-17

Percent of Payments for Selected Medical Services Which are Out-of-Pocket Before and After Medicare, Persons 65 and Over (U.S.A., 1965 and 1967).

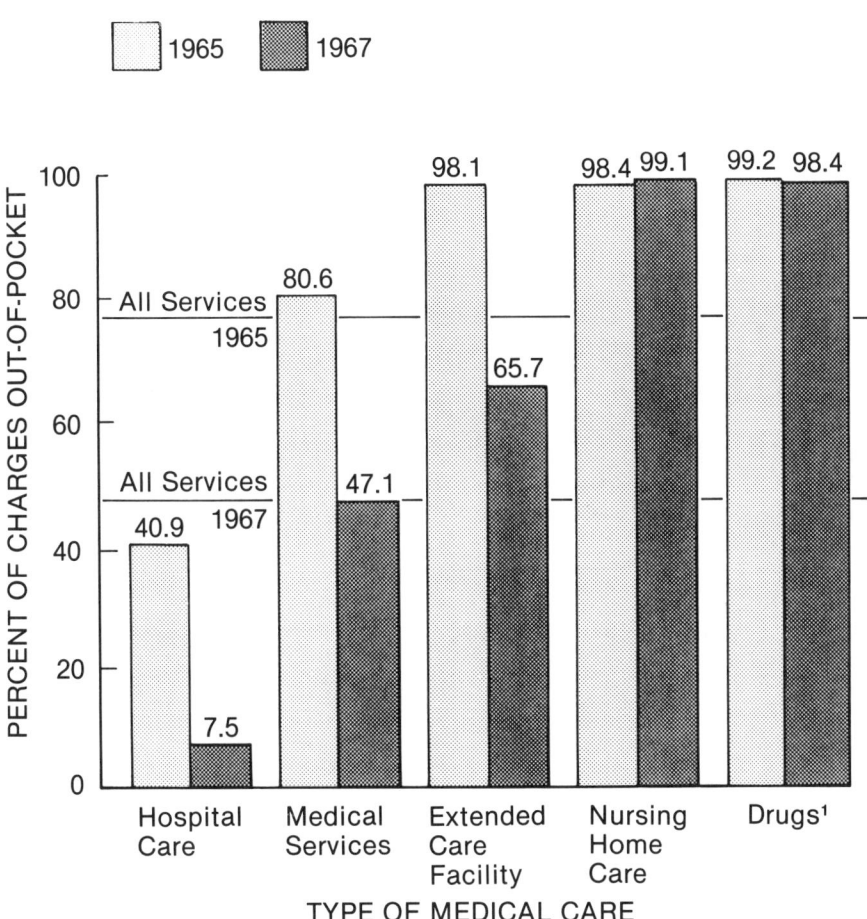

[1] Prescribed and non-prescribed drugs.

SOURCE: Loewenstein, Regina, "Early Effects of Medicare on the Health Care of the Aged," *Social Security Bulletin*, Vol. 34, April 1971, Table 8, p. 12 and Table 11, p. 16.

Chart H-18

Percent Distribution of Personal Health Care Expenditures for Persons 65 and Over, by Source of Funds (U.S.A., Fiscal Years 1966–1977).

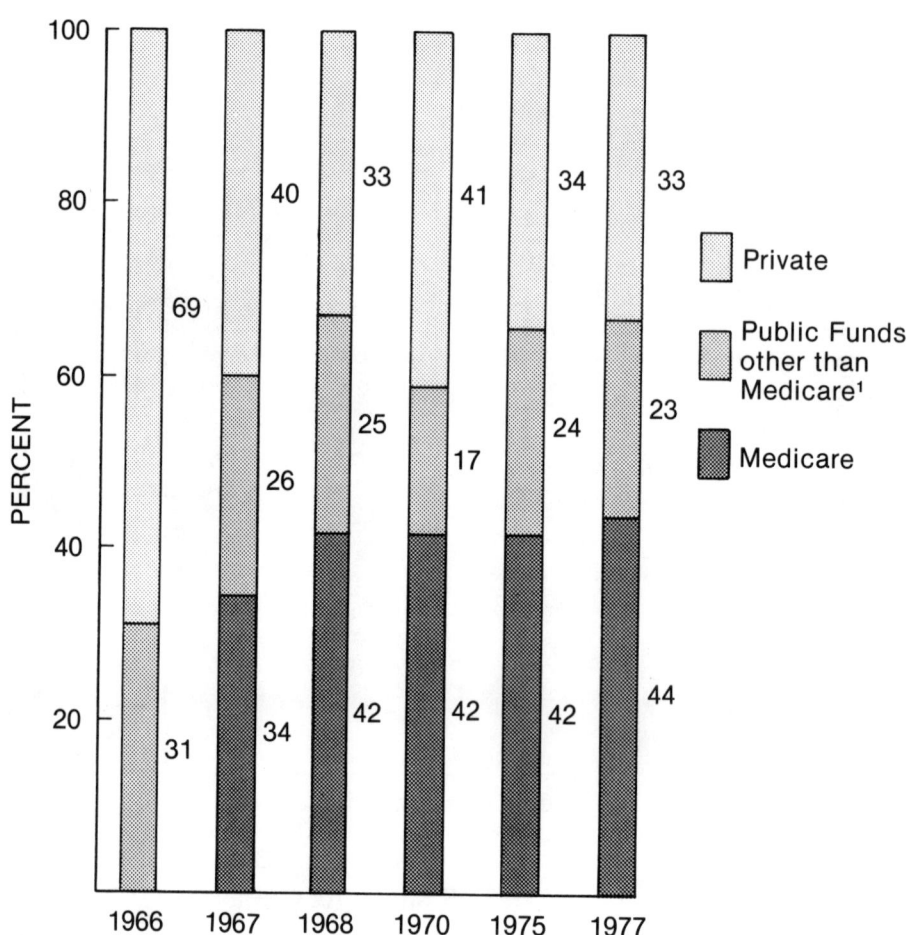

[1]Predominantly public assistance vendor medical payments; since 1967 those payments have come primarily from Medicaid funds.

SOURCES: For 1966–68: Cooper, B.S. and M.F. McGee, "Medical Care Outlays for Three Age Groups: Young, Intermediate, and Aged," *Social Security Bulletin,* Vol. 34, May 1971, Table 6, p. 12 and Table 8, p. 13; for 1970–77: Gibson, R.M. and C.R. Fisher, "Age Differences in Health Care Spending, Fiscal Year 1977," *Social Security Bulletin,* Vol. 42, No. 1, January 1979, Table 5, p. 12.

Tax-Supported Programs

Chart H-19

Percent Distribution and Amount of Average Personal Health Care Expenditures for a Person 65 Years of Age or Older, by Source of Funds (U.S.A., 1970, 1975 and 1977).

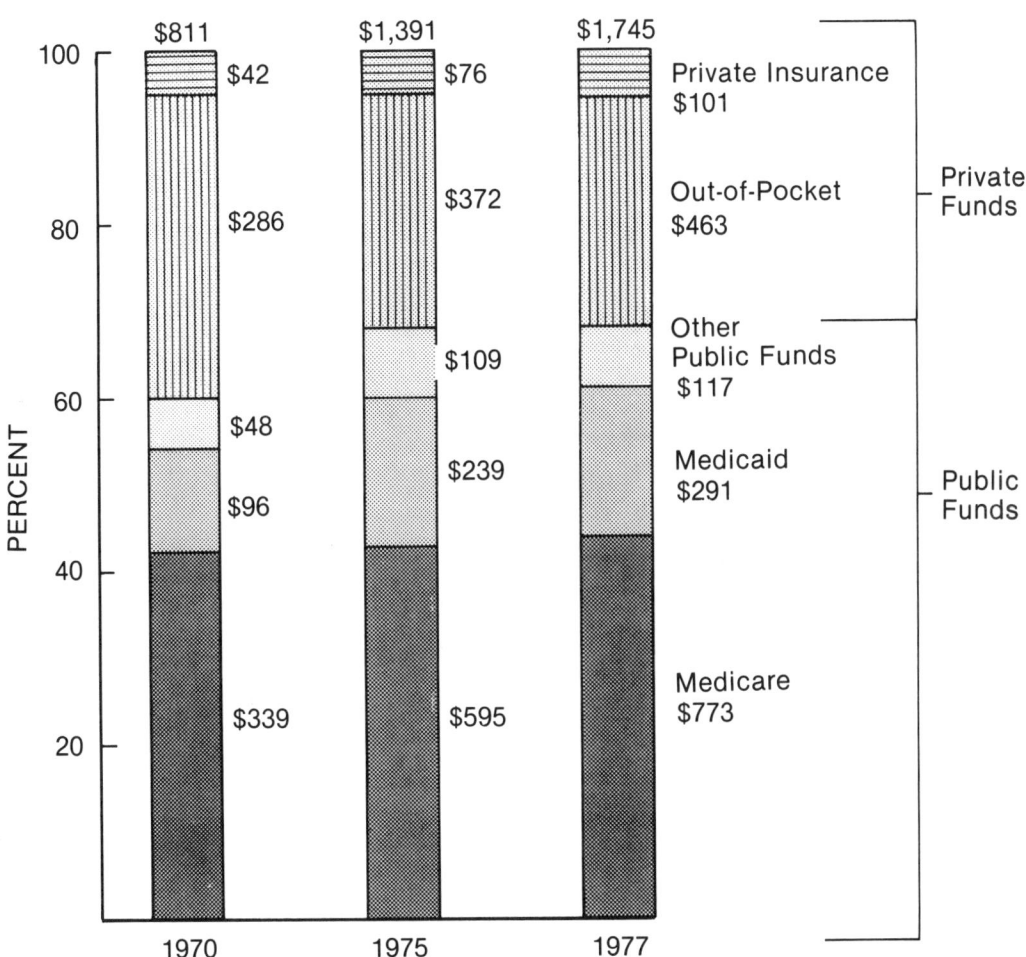

NOTE: Numbers to the right of bars are actual dollar amounts.
SOURCE: *National Health Insurance Report*, Vol. 9, No. 2, January 15, 1979, p. 5.

Tax-Supported Programs

Chart H-20

Premiums and Deductibles for Medicare Part A (Hospital Benefits) and Part B (Supplementary Medical Insurance) (U.S.A., 1966–1978).

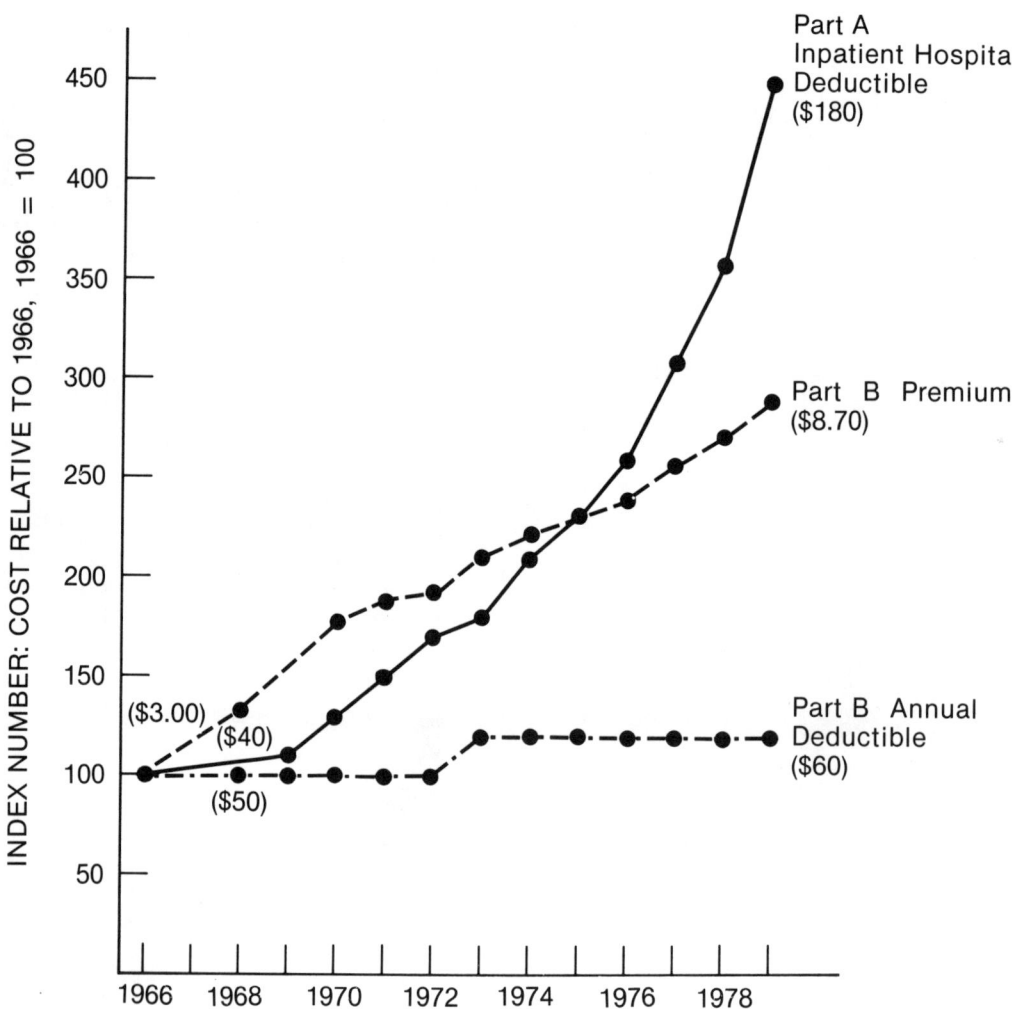

SOURCE: *Social Security Bulletin: Annual Statistical Supplement, 1976,* Social Security Administration, Office of Research and Statistics, DHEW, 1980, p. 31.

Chart H-21

Percent Distribution of Enrollees and Charges, Medicare Part B (Supplementary Medical Insurance Program), by the Nature of the Liability Assumed by the Program (U.S.A., 1974).

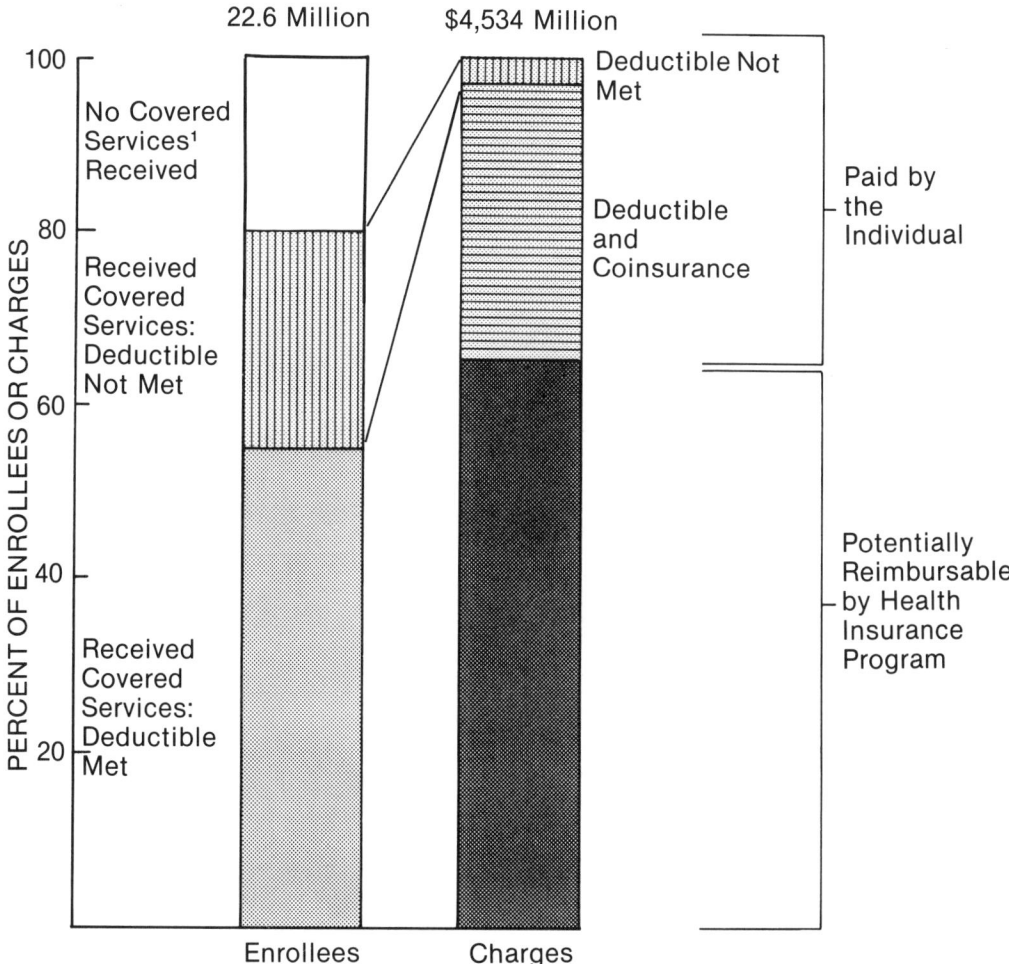

[1]Covered services are those medical services and supplies which are potentially reimbursable under the Supplementary Medical Insurance Program of Medicare.

SOURCE: U.S. Department of Health, Education, and Welfare, *Research and Statistics Note, No. 1—Current Medicare Survey Report*, Health Care Financing Administration, Office of Policy, Planning, and Research, June 1978, Table 3 and Table 4.

Tax-Supported Programs

Chart H-22

Physicians' Perceived Effects of Medicare Immediately Following the Implementation of Medicare and Six to Ten Months Later (New York, May–June 1966 and January–April 1967).

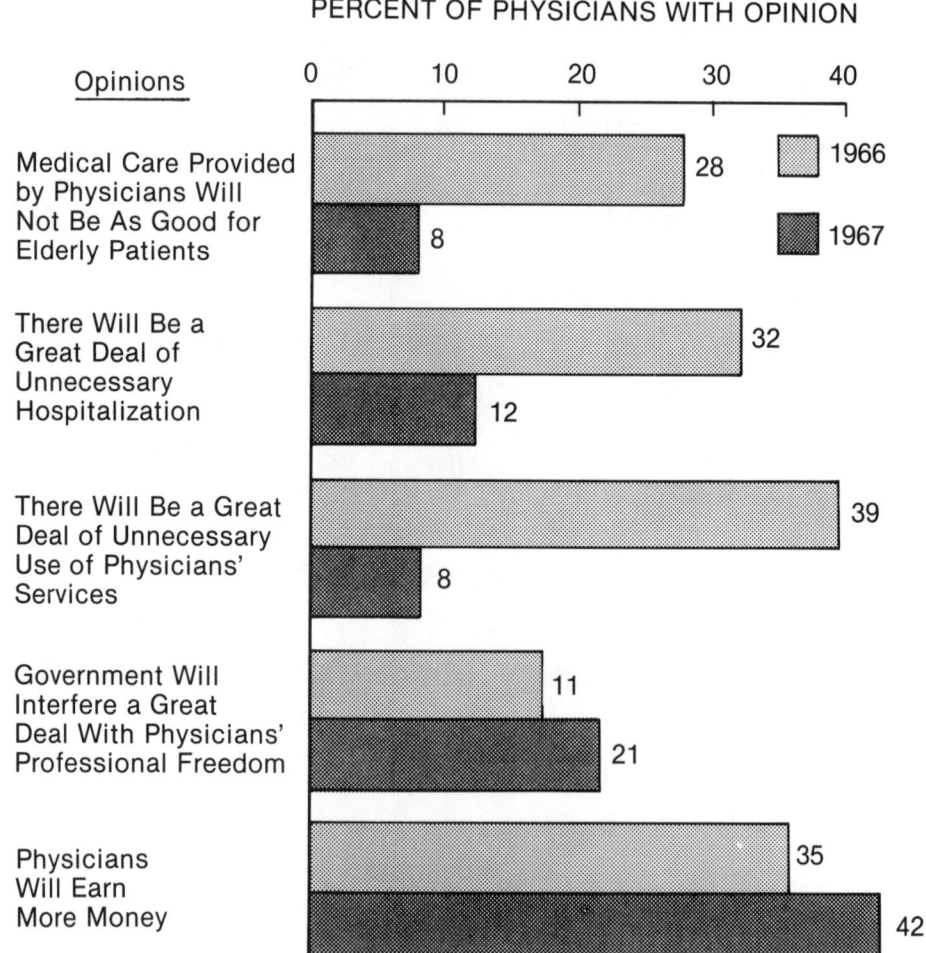

SOURCE: Colombotos, John, "Physicians and Medicare: a Before-After Study of the Effects of Legislation on Attitudes," *American Sociological Review,* Vol. 34, June 1969, Table 4, p. 328.

Chart H-23

Percent Distribution of Expenditures Under Medicare and of Medical Vendor Payments Under Medicaid, by Specified Type of Service (U.S.A., Fiscal 1977).

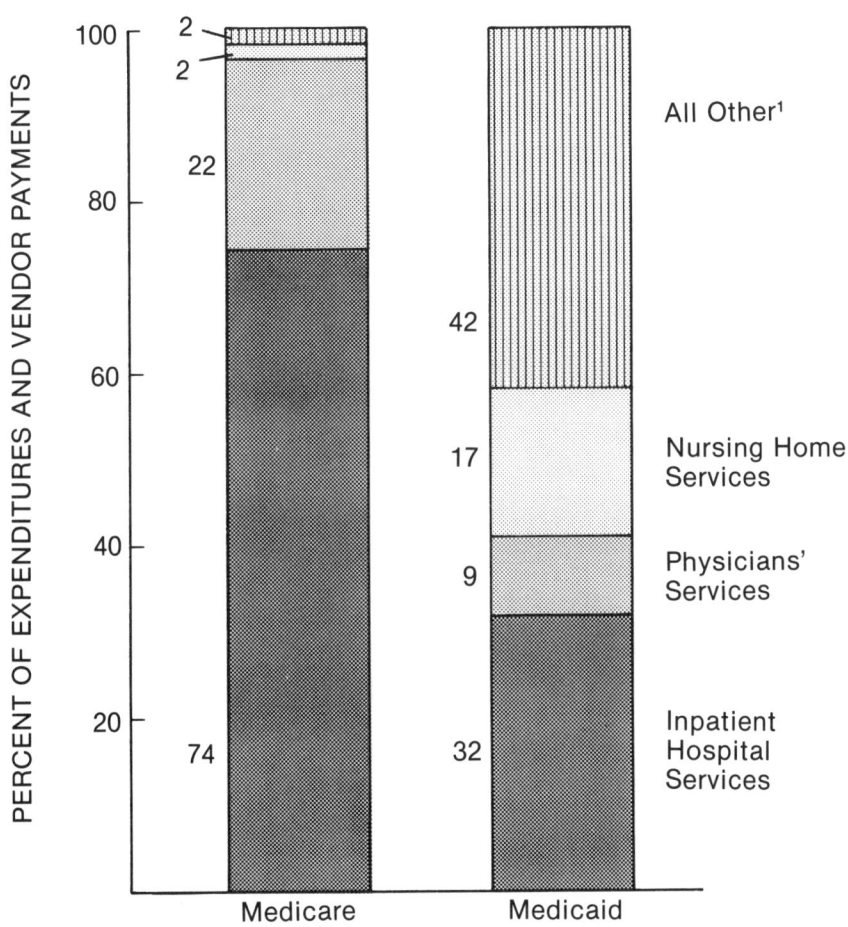

[1] For Medicaid, "all other" includes intermediate care facility services (22%), dental services (2.5%), outpatient hospital services (5.2%), clinic services (1.1%), laboratory and x-ray services (1%), home health services (1.1%), prescribed drugs (6.2%), and other care (3%).

SOURCES: For Medicare: Gibson, R. and C. Fisher, "Age Differences in Health Care Spending, Fiscal Year 1977," *Social Security Bulletin,* Vol. 42, No. 1, Table 6, p. 14; for Medicaid: "HCFA Program Statistics," *Health Care Financing Review,* Vol. 1, No. 2, Fall 1979, Table 5, p. 74.

Chart H-24

Percent Distribution of Recipients of Medicaid and Percent Distribution of Payments, by Basis of Eligibility (U.S.A., Fiscal 1978).

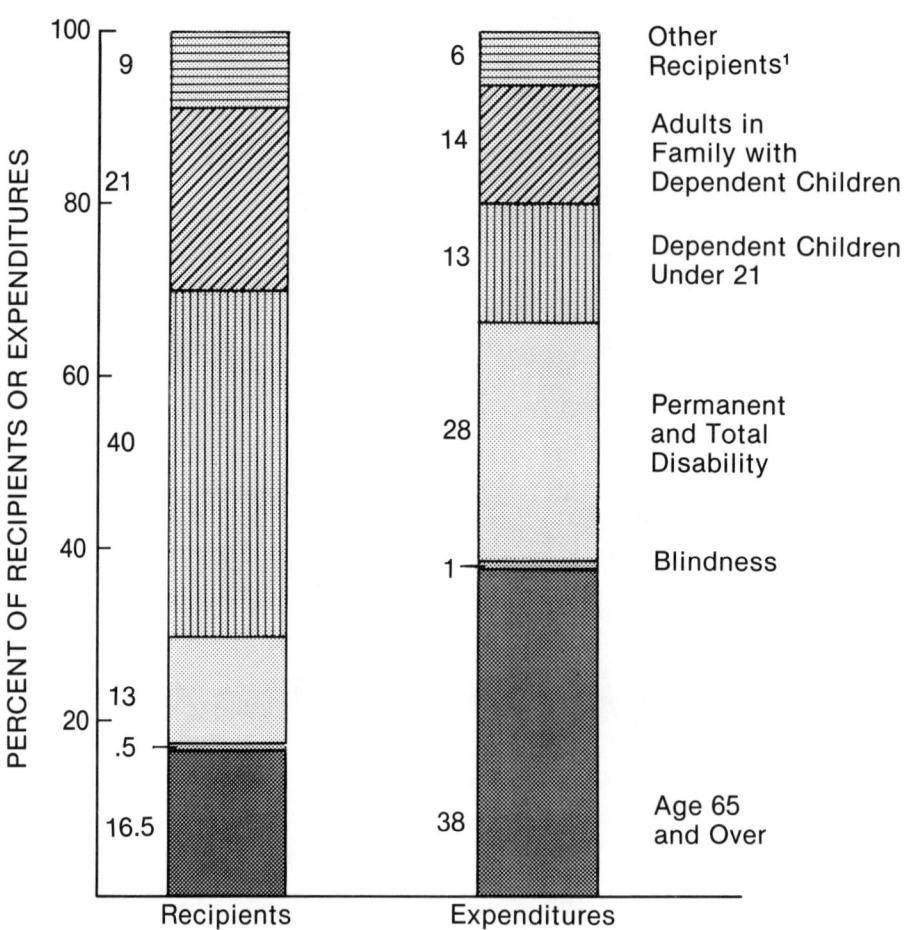

[1] Includes persons who do not qualify for any of the other categories listed, and are therefore not eligible for money payments, but who are eligible for medical assistance under Medicaid.

SOURCE: "HCFA Program Statistics," *Health Care Financing Review,* Vol. 1, No. 2, Fall 1979, Table 6, p. 75 and Table 7, p. 76.

Tax-Supported Programs

Chart H-25

Percent of Medicaid Expenditures, by Eligibility Categories and Receipt of Public Assistance (U.S.A., 1978).

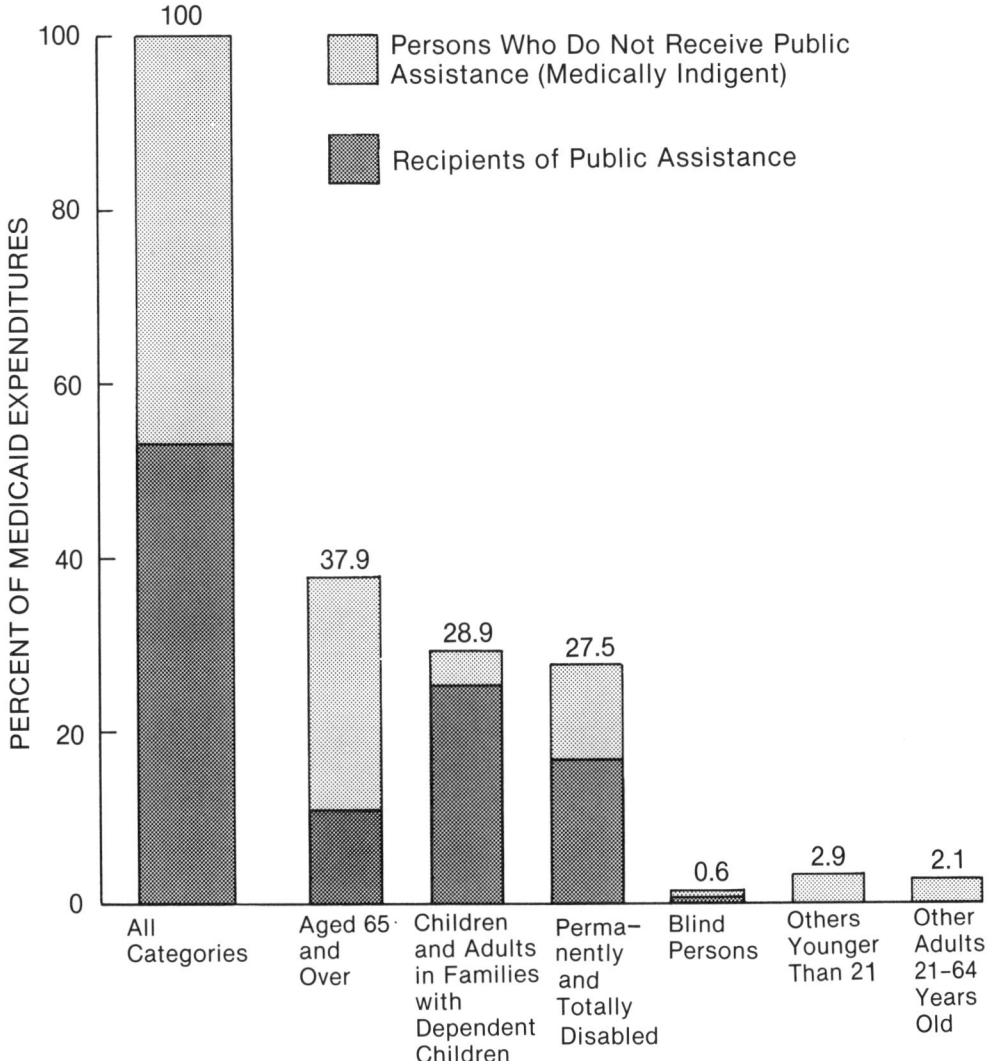

SOURCE: Department of Health, Education, and Welfare, Health Care Financing Administration, Office of Policy, Planning and Research, *Medicaid Statistics, January 1978: Medical Assistance (Medicaid) Financed Under Title XIX of the Social Security Act*, DHEW, August 1978, pp. 2–3.

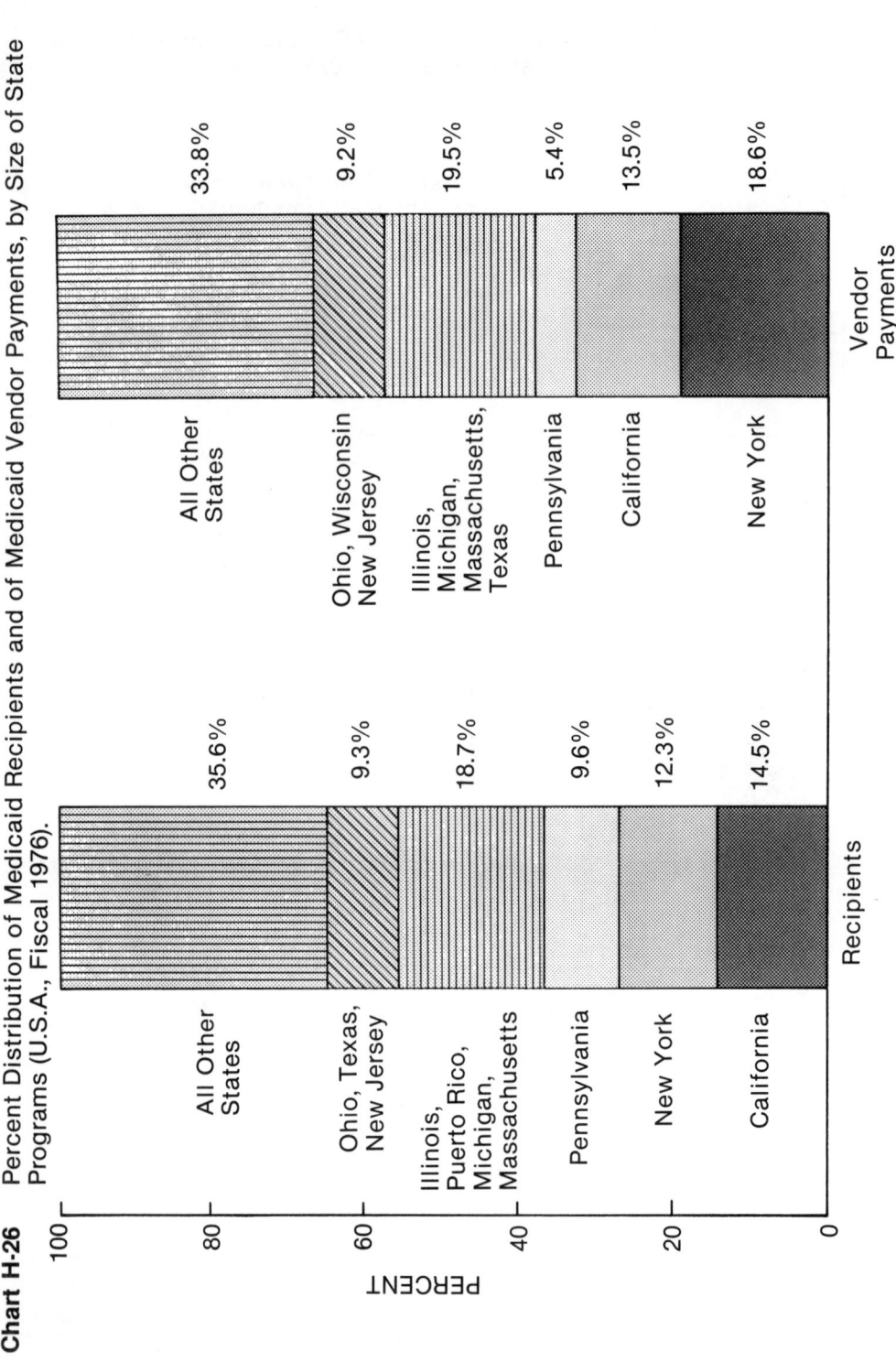

Chart H-26 Percent Distribution of Medicaid Recipients and of Medicaid Vendor Payments, by Size of State Programs (U.S.A., Fiscal 1976).

SOURCE: Health Care Financing Administration, *Data on the Medicaid Program: Eligibility, Services, Expenditures, 1979 Revised Edition,* Baltimore, Maryland, 1979, Table 27, p. 54 and Table 30, p. 57.

Tax-Supported Programs

Chart H-27

States by Net Medicaid Benefits per Household[1] and by Average Income per Household (States with Medicaid Programs, Fiscal Year, 1968).

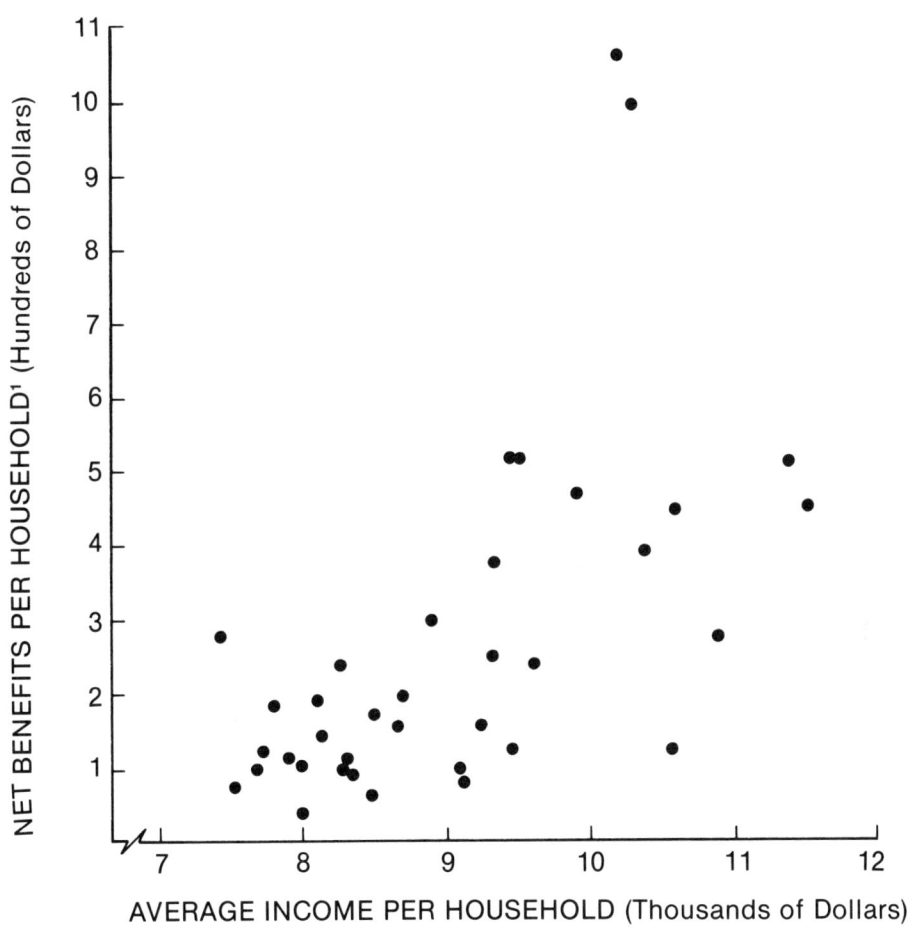

[1]Net Benefits per Household is defined as federal expenditures for Medicaid benefits per household with income under $3,000, minus Medicaid-related tax burden per household with income under $3,000 attributed to that income class.

SOURCE: Stuart, B.C., *The Impact of Medicaid on Interstate Income Differentials*, Michigan Department of Social Services, Research and Program Analysis Division, Lansing, Michigan, January 1971, Research Paper No. 3, Table 5, pp. 28-29.

Chart H-28

Percent of Children by Whether Enrolled in Medicaid and by Source of Medical Care[1] (Rochester, New York, 1967 and 1969).

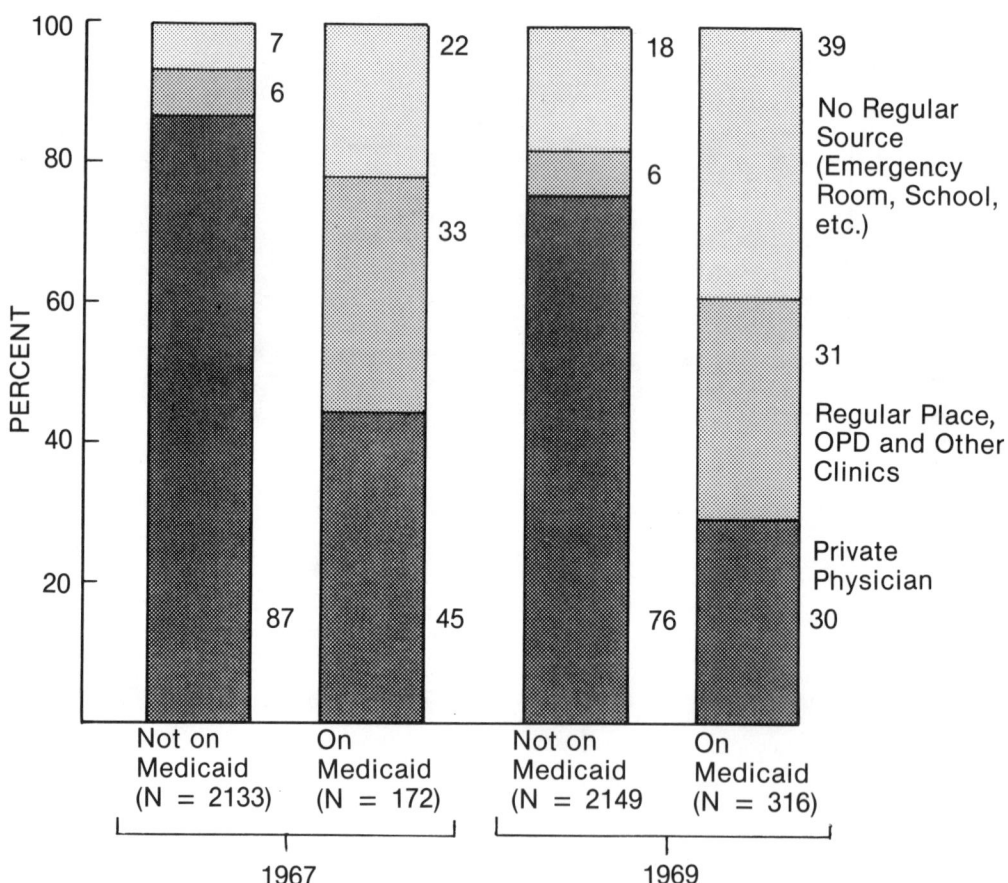

[1]Based on representative sample of families with children under 18.

NOTE: Medicaid legislation was enacted in the spring of 1966 and the 1967 survey was conducted less than one year later.

SOURCE: Roghmann, K. J., R.J. Haggerty and R. Loren, "Anticipated and Actual Effects of Medicaid on the Medical-Care Pattern of Children," *New England Journal of Medicine*, Vol. 285, November 4, 1971, pp. 1053–1057.

Chart H-29

Average Monthly Expenditures per Eligible Person, Before, During, and After Announced Cutbacks in Payments for Selected Services, Medi-Cal Recipients (California, 1967).

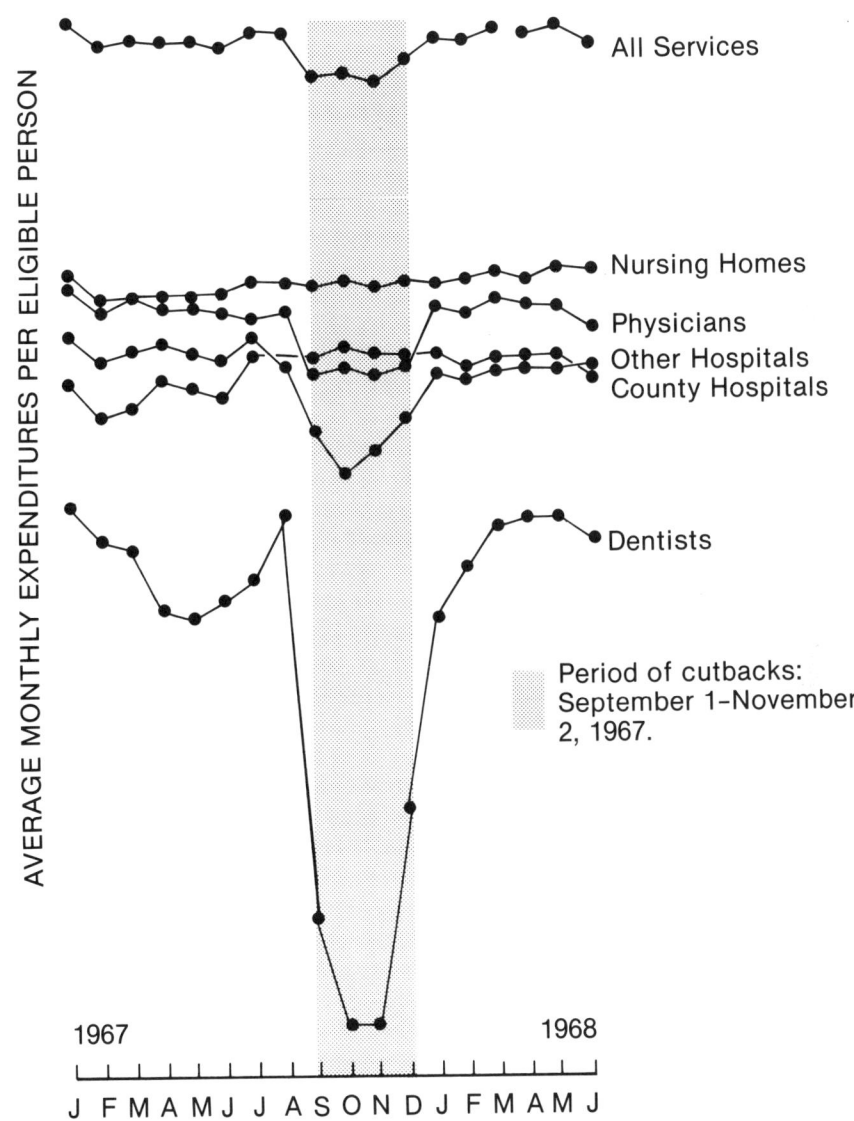

SOURCE: Gartside, F., "Medi-Cal Cutbacks of 1967 Revisited," *Medical Care*, Vol. IX, No. 1, January–February 1971, Table 3, p. 13.

SECTION I
Medical Care Insurance

Glossary of Selected Terms Used in Section I

Prepaid Health Plans, Health Maintenance Organizations, and *Prepaid Plans* are used as equivalent terms that refer to a medical care delivery system which has four basic attributes: (1) an organized system of health care in a geographic area; (2) a specified set of comprehensive health maintenance and treatment services; (3) a voluntarily enrolled group of persons; and (4) a predetermined and fixed period prepayment made by or on behalf of each person or family enrolled without regard to the amount of service provided a particular person or family unit.

The legal definition of a Health Maintenance Organization (HMO) set forth in the HMO Act of 1973 (Public Law 93-222), as amended in 1976 and 1978, encompasses two distinct organizational forms:

1. The *Medical Group* model (also known as *Prepaid Group Practice Plan* or *Prepaid Group Health Plan*), which may be either (1) a group practice model HMO in which the HMO contracts with a medical group; or (2) a staff model HMO, in which the HMO employs a staff of physicians and other health care personnel to provide health care services.

2. The *Individual Practice Association* (IPA), also known as a *Medical Care Foundation*, in which the HMO contracts with an association of individual practitioners working out of their own offices who provide health care to HMO members.

A qualified HMO is one that has been certified by the Secretary of Health, Education and Welfare (now Health and Human Services) as complying with the requirements of the HMO Act of 1973, as amended in 1976 (Public Law 94-460) and in 1978 (Public Law 95-559). Requirements relate to staffing, benefits, payment for benefits and enrollment.

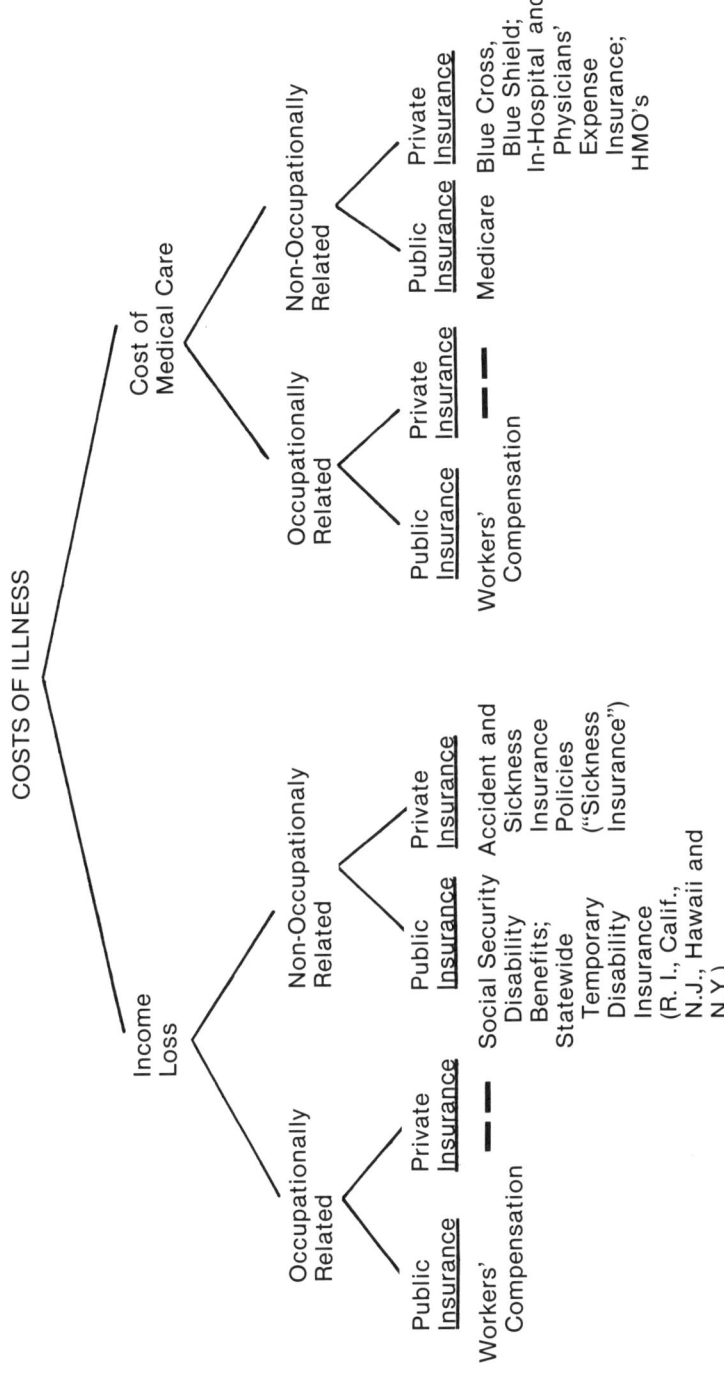

Chart I-1 Insurance Against Costs of Illness (U.S.A., 1980).

SOURCE: Prepared by S. J. Axelrod, The University of Michigan, June 1980.

366 Medical Care Chartbook

Chart I-2 Workers' Compensation Coverage, Types of Benefits, and Sources of Benefits (U.S.A., 1940 and 1975).

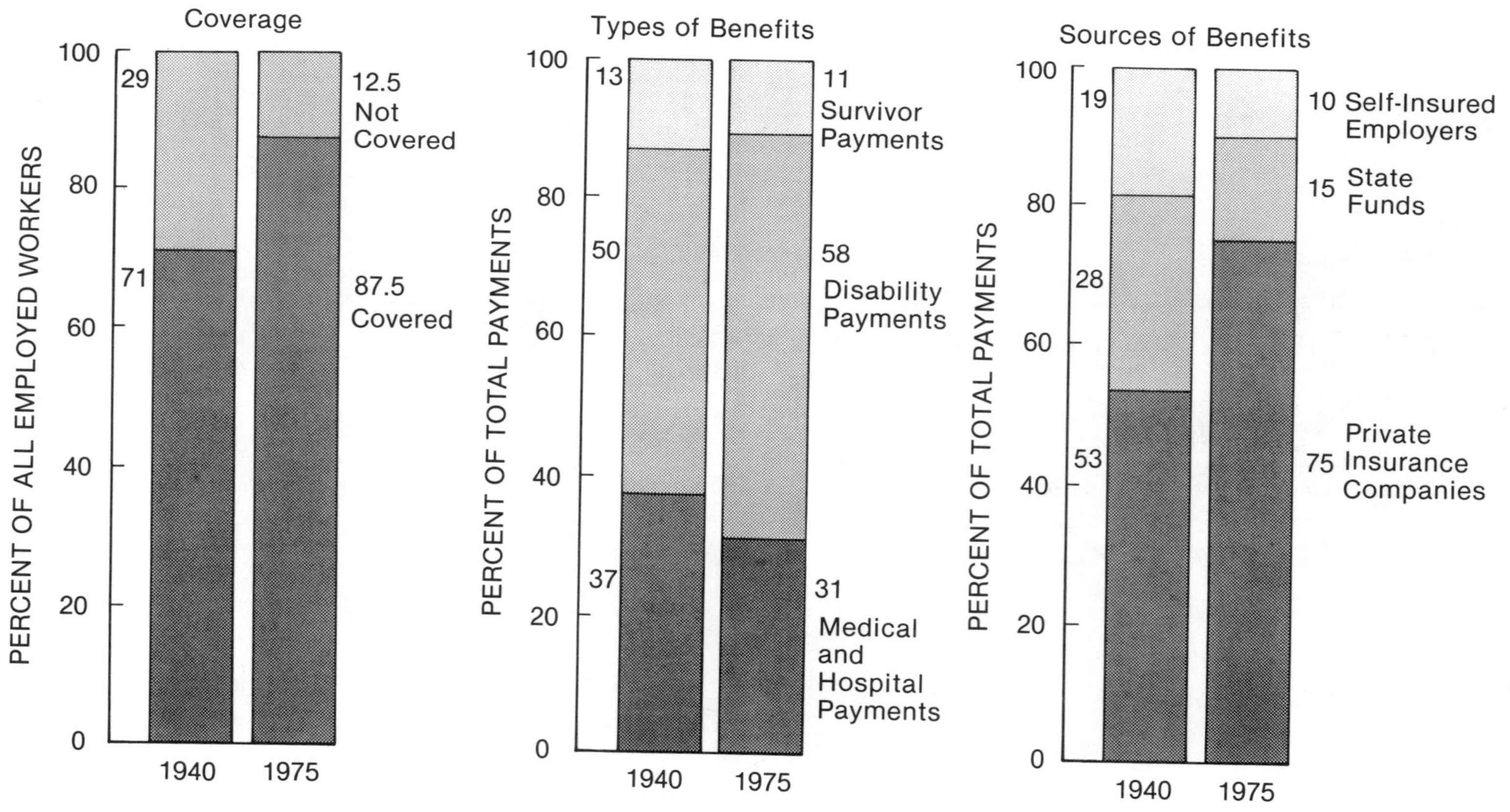

Coverage (Percent of All Employed Workers)
- 1940: 71 Covered, 29 Not Covered
- 1975: 87.5 Covered, 12.5 Not Covered

Types of Benefits (Percent of Total Payments)
- 1940: 37 Medical and Hospital Payments, 50 Disability Payments, 13 Survivor Payments
- 1975: 31 Medical and Hospital Payments, 58 Disability Payments, 11 Survivor Payments

Sources of Benefits (Percent of Total Payments)
- 1940: 53 Private Insurance Companies, 28 State Funds, 19 Self-Insured Employers
- 1975: 75 Private Insurance Companies, 15 State Funds, 10 Self-Insured Employers

SOURCES: For 1975: Price, Daniel N., "Workers' Compensation: Coverage, Payments, and Costs, 1975," *Social Security Bulletin*, Vol. 40, No. 1, January 1977, pp. 32–34; for 1940: Skolnik, Alfred M., "Twenty-five Years of Workmens' Compensation Statistics," *Social Security Bulletin*, Vol. 29, No. 10, October 1966, Table 1, p. 6, Tables 3 and 4, p. 9.

Medical Care Insurance

Chart I-3

Percent Distribution of Compensation Cases and Incurred Losses, by Injury Classification (Workers' Compensation, U.S.A., 1974).[1]

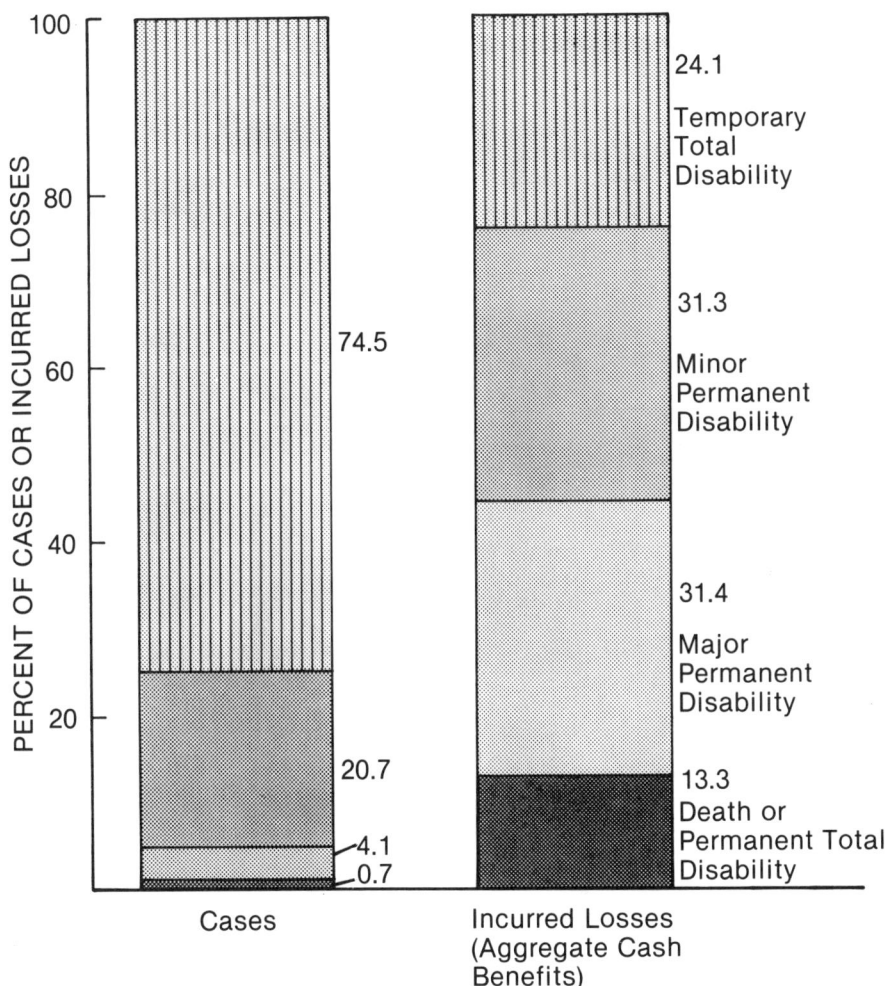

[1]Excludes cases receiving medical benefits only.
SOURCE: Price, Daniel N., "Workers' Compensation Programs in the 1970's," *Social Security Bulletin*, Vol. 42, May 1979, Table 5, p. 11.

Chart I-4

Percent of Income Loss From Short-term Sickness Covered by Insurance and Sick Leave in 1948, 1962, and 1976, and Percent Distribution of 1976 Benefits by Type of Protection (U.S.A.).[1]

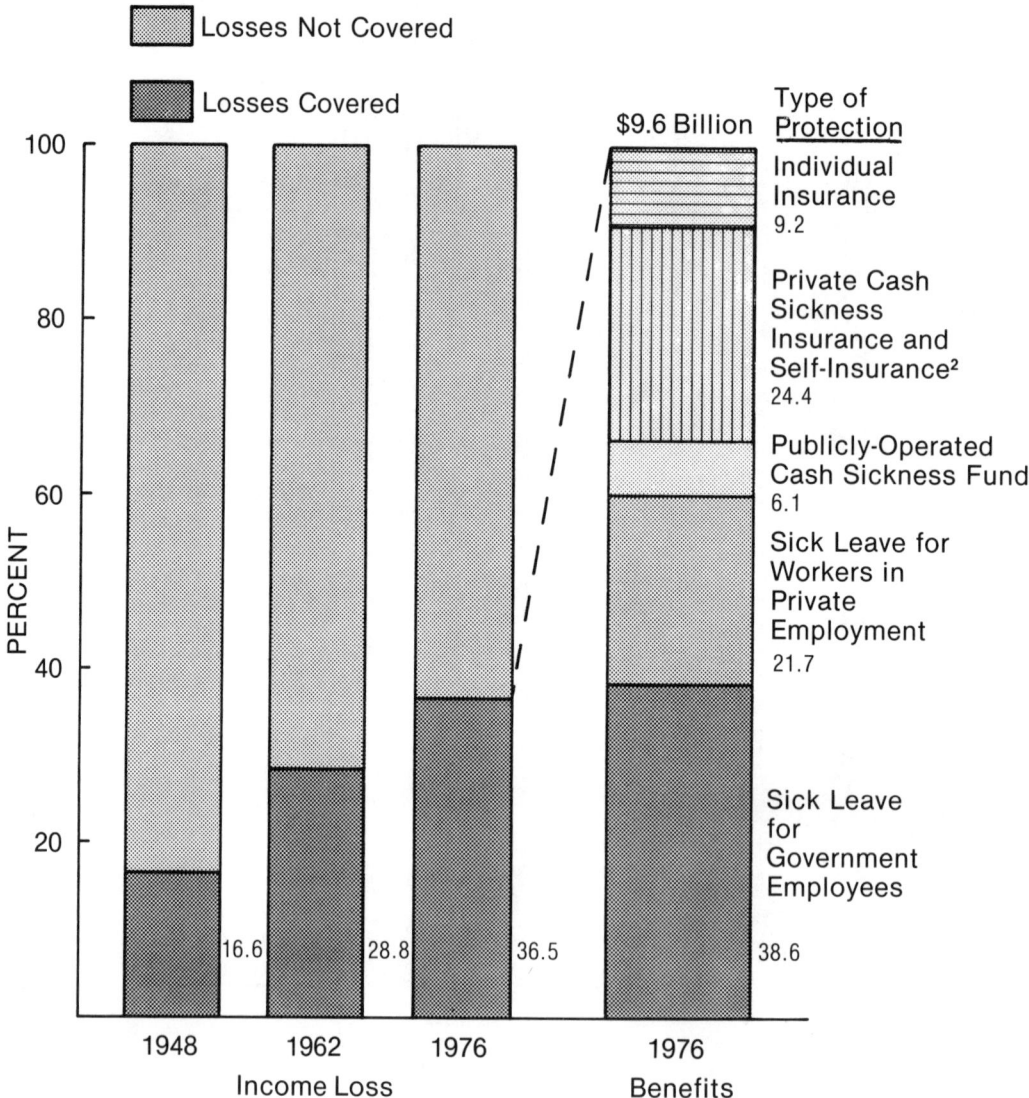

[1]The data shown are for losses incurred during the first six months of non-occupational illness or injury, including losses during the first six months of a long-term disability.

[2]Includes a small but undetermined amount of group disability insurance benefits paid to government workers and to self-employed persons through farm, trade, or professional associations.

SOURCE: Price, Daniel N., "Cash Benefits for Short-term Sickness, 1948–76," *Social Security Bulletin*, Vol. 41, No. 10, October 1978, Table 2, p. 4 and Table 4, p. 6.

Chart I-5 Number of Persons with Private Health Insurance Protection, by Type of Insurance (U.S.A., 1940–1977).

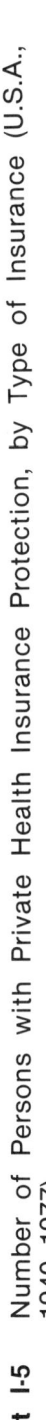

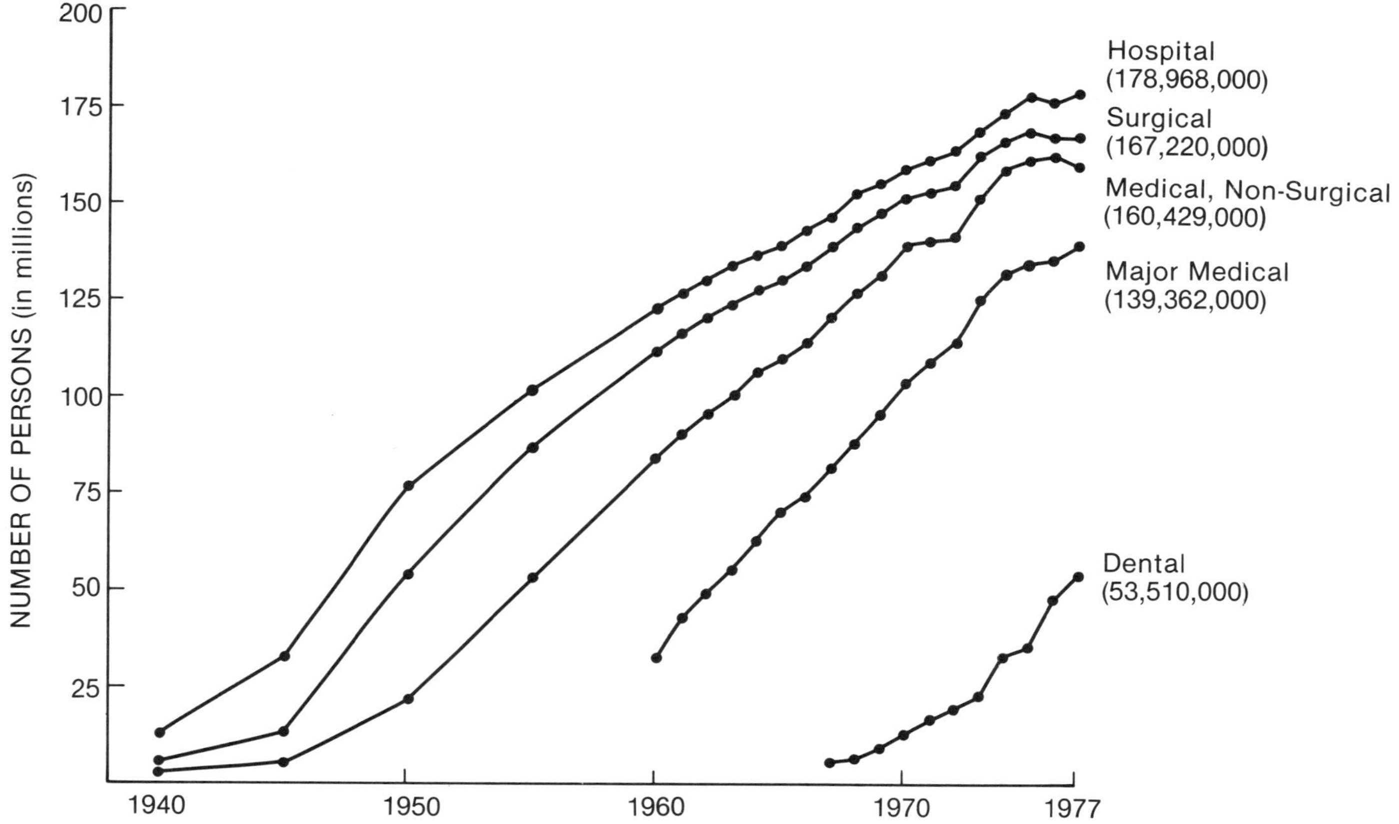

200
175
150
125
100
75
50
25
NUMBER OF PERSONS (in millions)
1940
1950
1960
1970
1977
Hospital
(178,968,000)
Surgical
(167,220,000)
Medical, Non-Surgical
(160,429,000)
Major Medical
(139,362,000)
Dental
(53,510,000)

NOTE: For 1975 and later, data include the number of persons covered in Puerto Rico and other U.S. territories and possessions. The numbers shown represent net totals: a person protected under more than one policy or by more than one company is counted only once.

SOURCE: Health Insurance Institute, *Source Book of Health Insurance Data 1978–79*, Washington, D.C., The Institute, 1979, Table 1.1, p. 9.

Chart I-6

Percent of Persons with Specified Insurance Benefits Under Private Health Insurance, Two Age Groups (U.S.A., 1960-1976).[1]

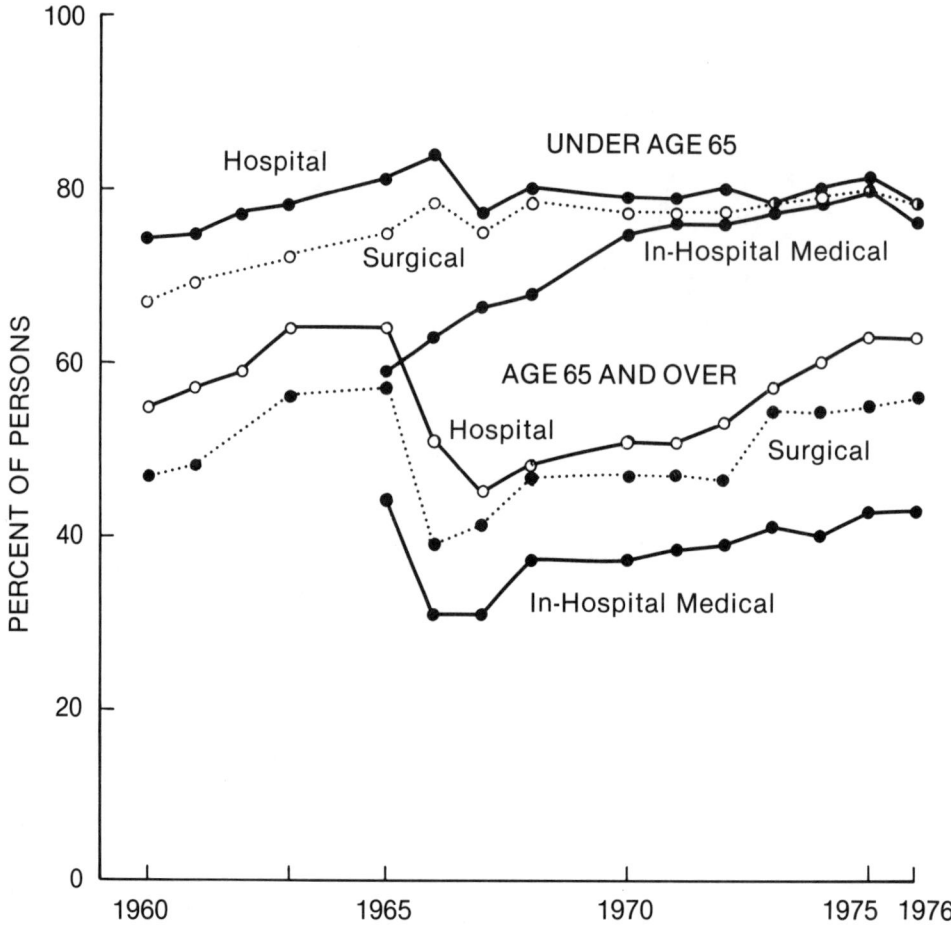

[1]Benefits include those of Blue Cross, Blue Shield, commercial, and other private plans.
SOURCES: For 1976: Carroll. Marjorie Smith, "Private Health Insurance Plans in 1976," *Social Security Bulletin*, Vol. 41, September 1978, Table 1, p.4; for 1975: Mueller, Marjorie Smith, "Private Health Insurance Plans in 1975," *Social Security Bulletin*, Vol. 40, June 1977, Table 1, p. 5.; for 1974: Mueller, Marjorie Smith and Paula A. Pino, "Private Health Insurance in 1974," *Social Security Bulletin*, Vol. 39, March 1976, Table 1, p. 4.; for 1973: Mueller, Marjorie Smith, "Private Health Insurance in 1973," *Social Security Bulletin*, Vol. 38, February 1975, Table 1, p. 22; for 1968-1972, Mueller, Marjorie Smith, "Private Health Care in 1972," *Social Security Bulletin*, Vol. 37, February 1974, Table 1, p. 2; for 1967 and previous years: Reed, Louis S. and William Carr, "Private Health Insurance in the U.S.," *Social Security Bulletin*, Vol. 32, February 1969, Table 7, p. 12.

Chart I-7

Percent of Persons with Private Hospital Insurance at Specified Intervals (U.S.A., 1940–1975).

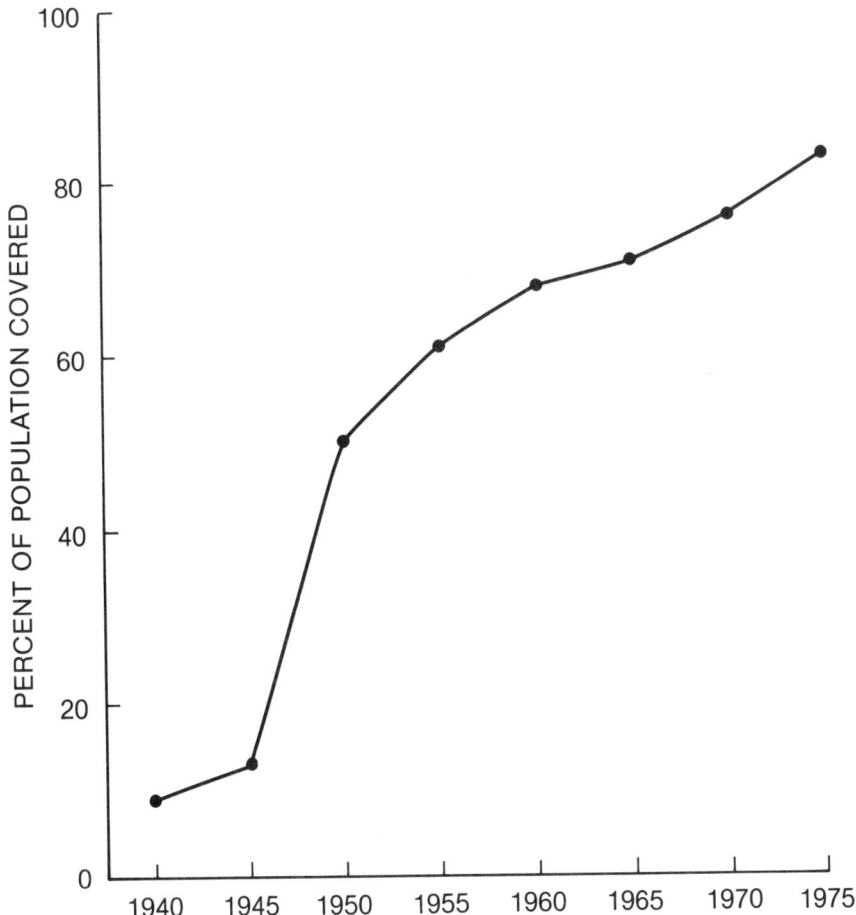

SOURCES: Estimated U.S. Resident Population: U.S. Department of Commerce, Bureau of the Census, *Statistical Abstract of the United States, 1979*, Table 2, p. 6; for Population Covered: Health Insurance Institute, *Source Book of Health Insurance Data, 1978-79*, Washington, D.C., The Institute, 1979, Table 1.1, p. 9.

Chart I-8

Percent of Persons Under 65 with Hospital Insurance Coverage, by Specified Population Characteristics (U.S.A., 1968 and 1974).

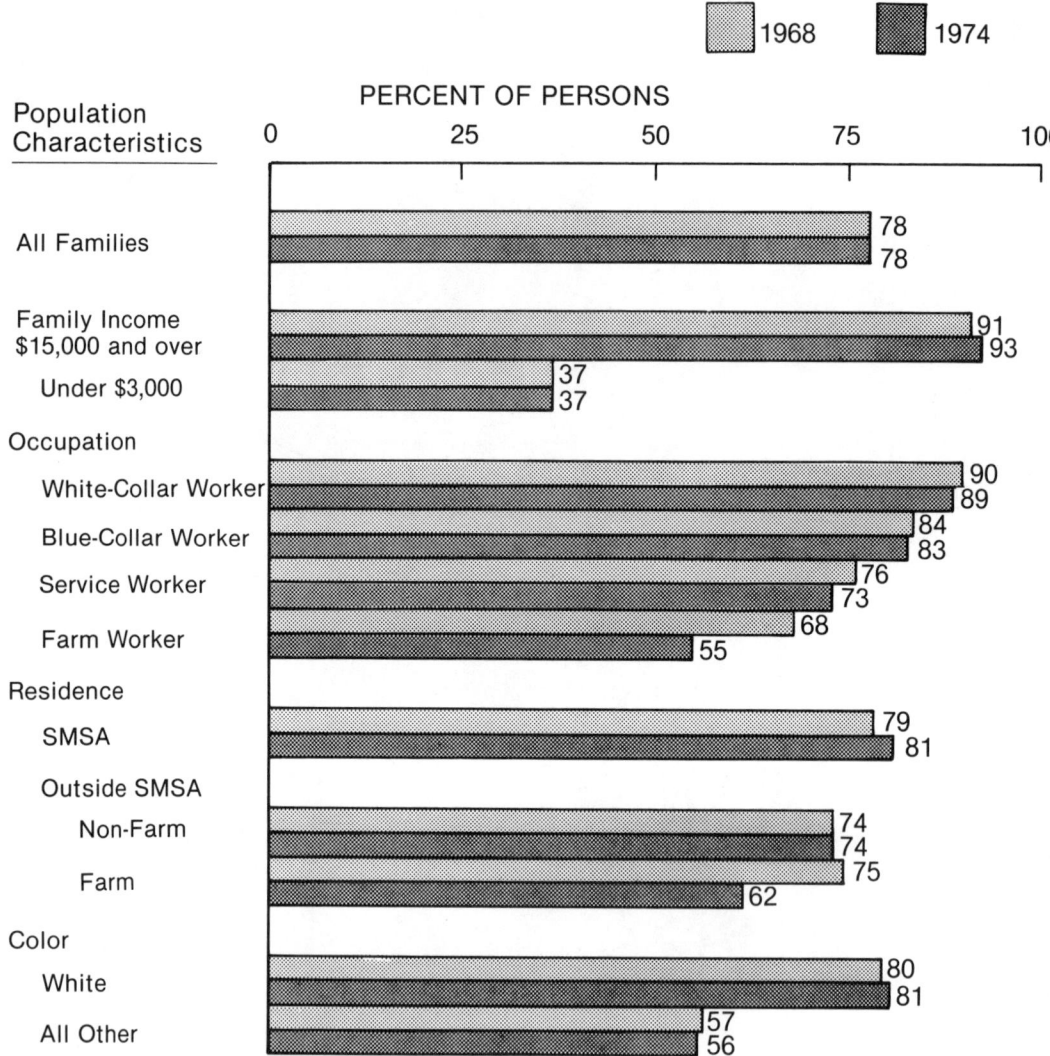

SOURCES: For 1974: U.S. National Center for Health Statistics, *Hospital and Surgical Insurance Coverage, United States, 1974*, DHEW, Public Health Service, Health Resources Administration, Hyattsville, Maryland, August 1977, Table D, p. 6 and Table 11, p. 22; for 1968: U.S. National Center for Health Statistics, *Hospital and Surgical Insurance Coverage, United States, 1968*, DHEW, Public Health Service, Health Services and Mental Health Administration, Rockville, Maryland, January 1972, Figure 1, p. 4, Table 3, p. 18, Table 10, p. 28 and Table 13, p. 33.

Chart I-9 Number of Persons With Hospital Expense Protection, by Type of Insurer (U.S.A., 1940–1977).

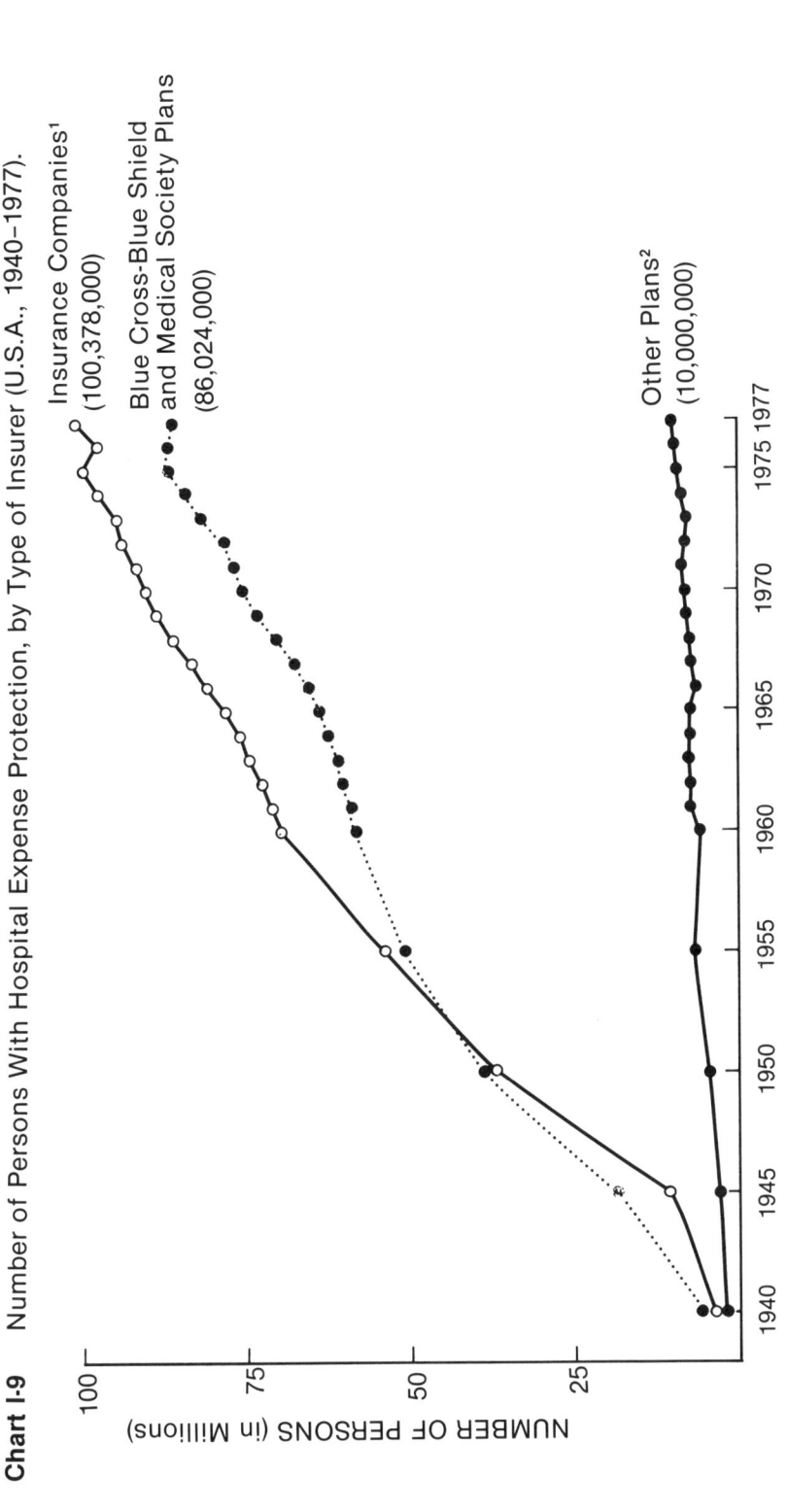

[1]The numbers shown represent net totals: a person protected under more than one policy or by more than one company is counted only once.

[2]Also designated "Independent Plans". Includes Health Maintenance Organizations (HMOs) and plans administered by employers, labor unions, communities and consumer cooperatives. The Figure of 10 million for 1977 is a preliminary estimate; of that number, approximately 7 million persons were enrolled in HMOs.

NOTE: For 1975 and later, data include the number of persons covered in Puerto Rico and other U.S. territories and possessions.

SOURCE: Health Insurance Institute, *Source Book of Health Insurance Data 1978–79*, Washington, D.C., The Institute, 1979, Table 1.2, p. 10.

Chart I-10

Number of Persons with Specified Types of Insurance, by Type of Insurer (U.S.A., 1945-1977).

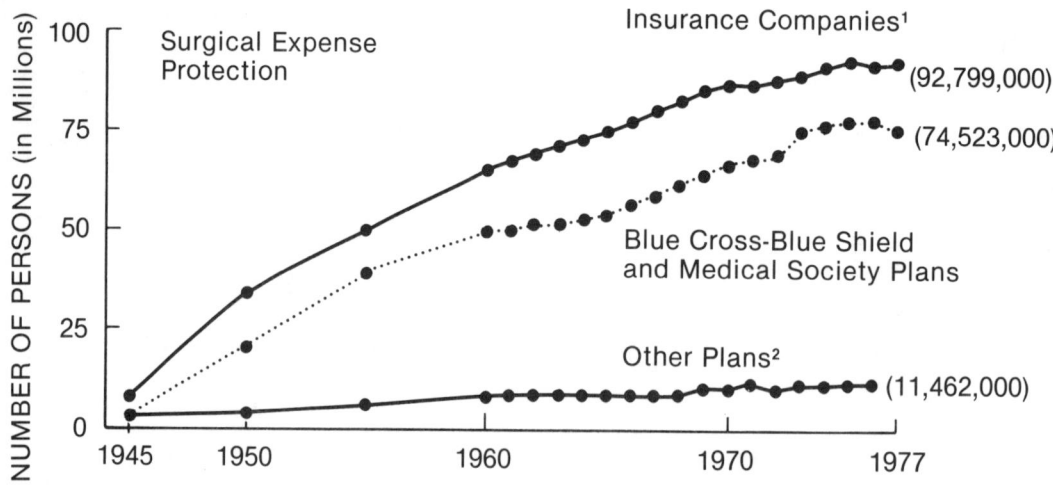

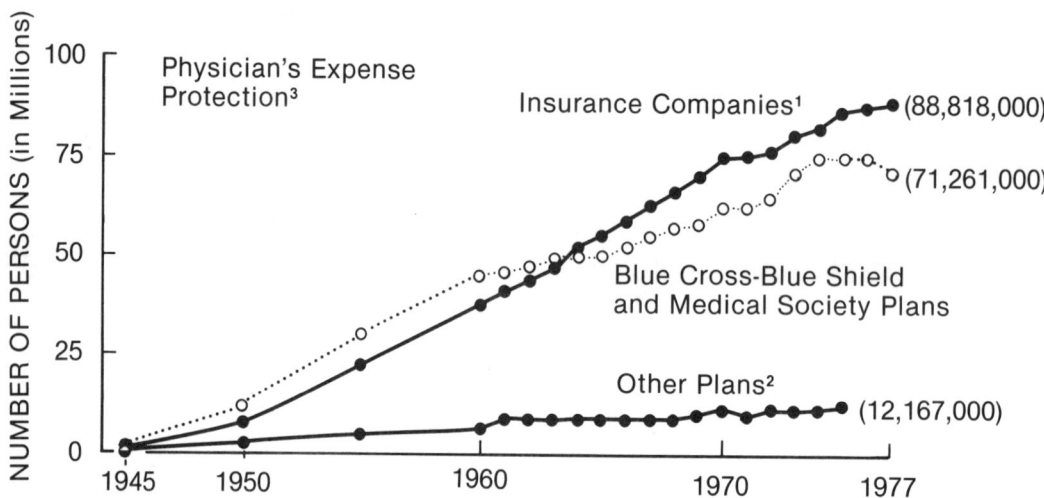

[1] The numbers shown represent net totals: a person protected under more the one policy or by more than one company is counted only once.
[2] Also designated "Independent Plans". Includes Health Maintenance Organizations (HMOs) and plans administered by employers, labor unions, communities and consumer cooperatives.
[3] Benefits toward physicians' fees for nonsurgical care given in the hospital, home, or at the physician's office.

NOTE: For 1975 and later, data include the number of persons covered in Puerto Rico and other U.S. territories and possessions.

SOURCE: Health Insurance Institute, *Source Book of Health Insurance Data 1978-79*, Washington, D.C., The Institute, 1979, Table 1.3, p. 11, and Table 1.4, p. 12.

Medical Care Insurance

Chart I-11

Percent Distribution of Persons with Private Health Insurance Protection, by Type of Benefit and by Insurer (U.S.A., 1977).[1]

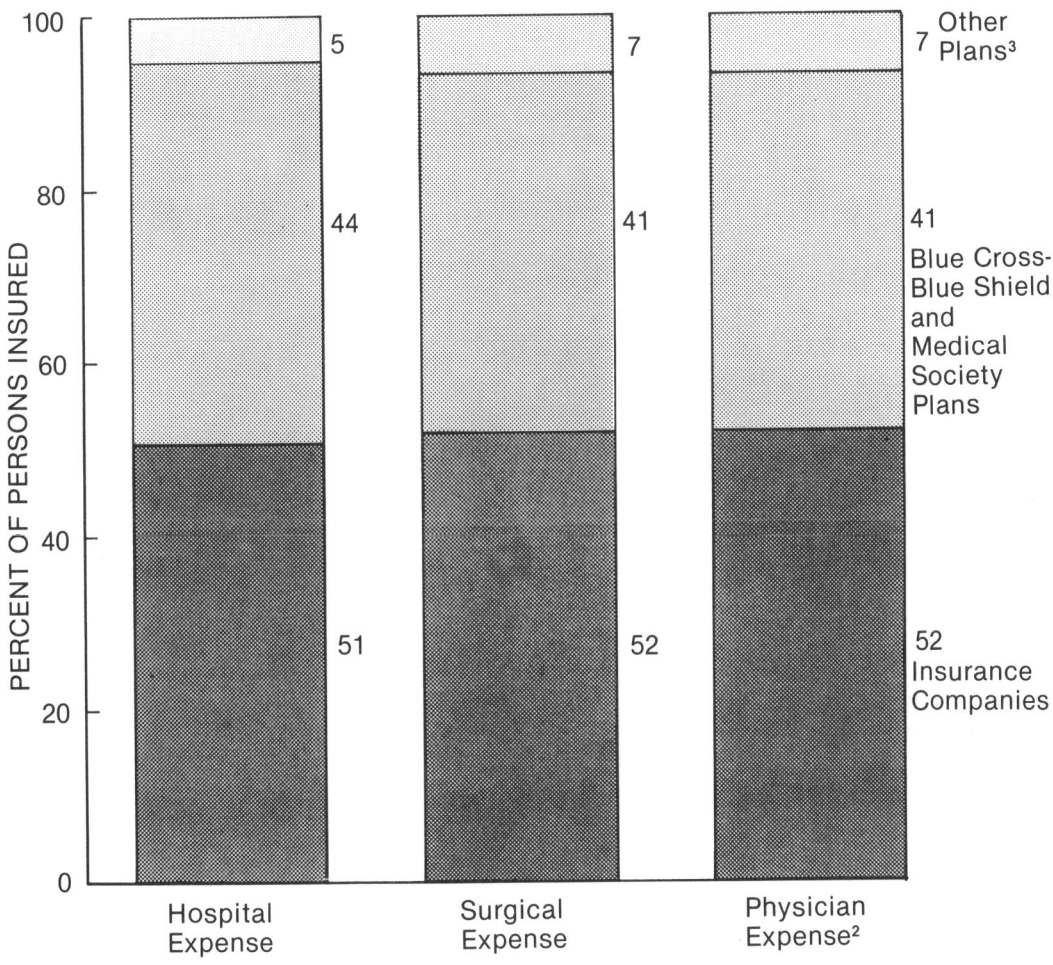

[1]The date refer to the net total of people protected, i.e., duplication among persons protected by more than one kind of insuring organization or more than one insurance company policy providing the same type of coverage has been eliminated.

[2]Benefits toward physicians' fees for nonsurgical care given in the hospital, home, or at the physician's office.

[3]Also designated "Independent Plans". Includes Health Maintenance Organizations (HMOs) and plans administered by employers, labor unions, communities and consumer cooperatives.

SOURCE: Health Insurance Institute, *Source Book of Health Insurance Data, 1978-79*, Washington, D.C., The Institute, 1979, Table 1.2, p. 10, Table 1.3, p. 11, and Table 1.4, p. 12.

Medical Care Insurance

Chart I-12

Percent of Persons with Private Health Insurance, by Type of Service Covered (U.S.A., 1976).[1]

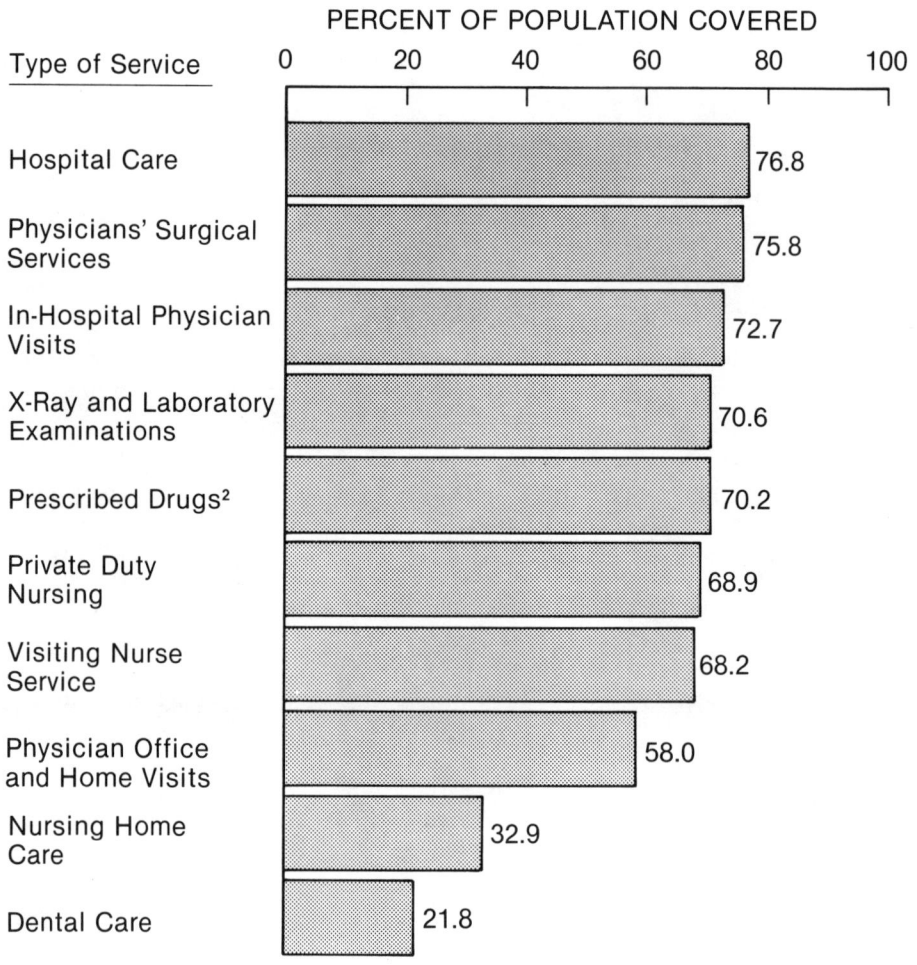

[1] Based on Bureau of Census estimate of 213,863,000 population as of January 1, 1977.
[2] Out-of-hospital.

SOURCE: Carroll, Marjorie Smith, "Private Health Insurance Plans in 1976: An Evaluation," *Social Security Bulletin*, Vol. 41, No. 9, September 1978, Table 1, p. 4.

Chart I-13

Percent of Wage and Salary Workers Covered by Employee-Benefit Plans, by Type of Benefit (U.S.A., 1950 and 1975).[1]

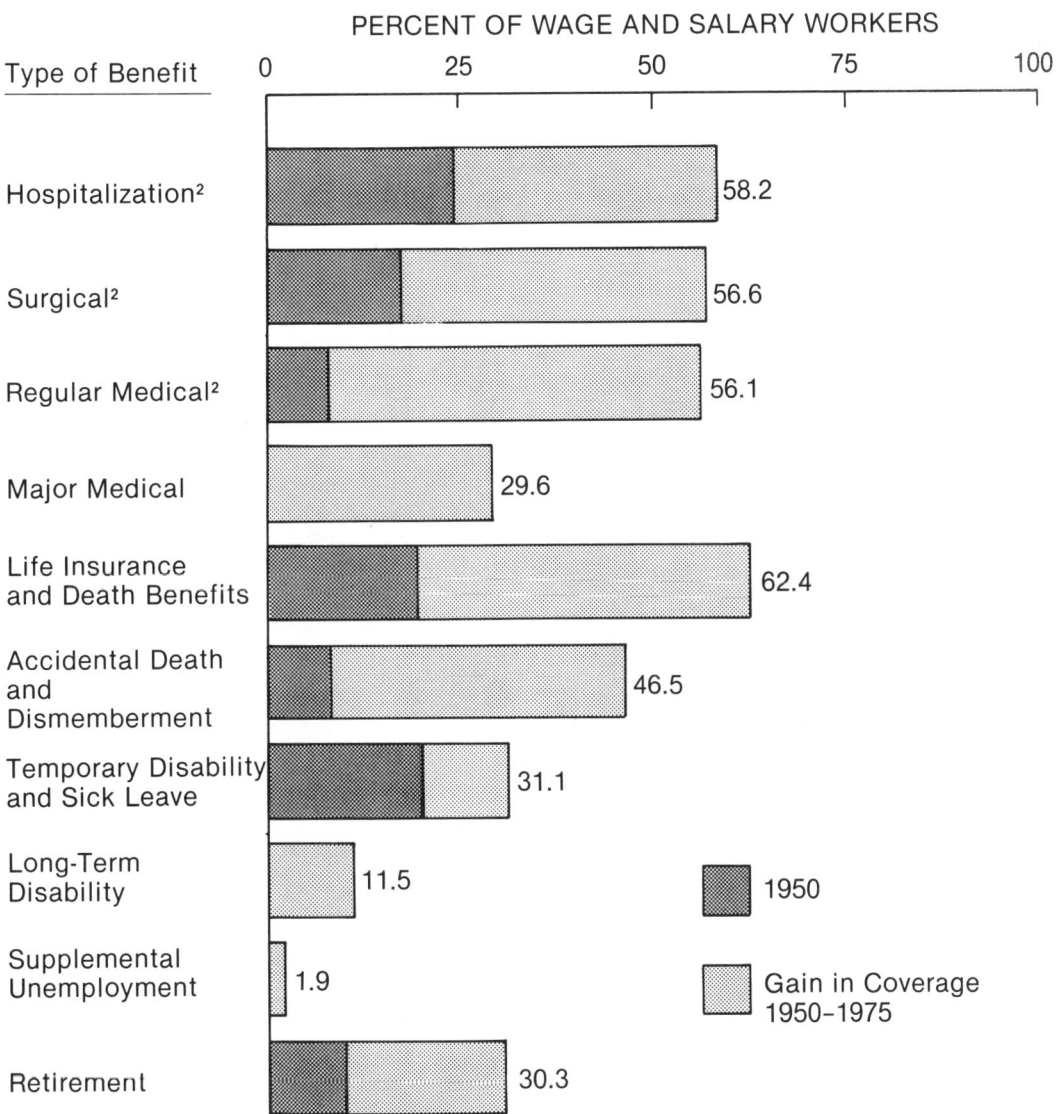

[1] Plans whose benefits flow from the employment relationship and are not underwritten or paid directly by the government (federal, state, or local). Excludes workers' compensation required by statute and employer's liability.

[2] Data modified to exclude participants not actively employed and to allow for duplication resulting in participation in more than one plan.

SOURCE: Yohalem, Martha Remy, "Employee Benefit Plans, 1975," *Social Security Bulletin*, Vol. 40, November 1977, Table 1, p. 20.

Chart I-14

Percent Distribution of Enrollees Under Federal Employees Health Benefits Program, by Type of Insurer and Level of Coverage Selected (U.S.A., 1976).

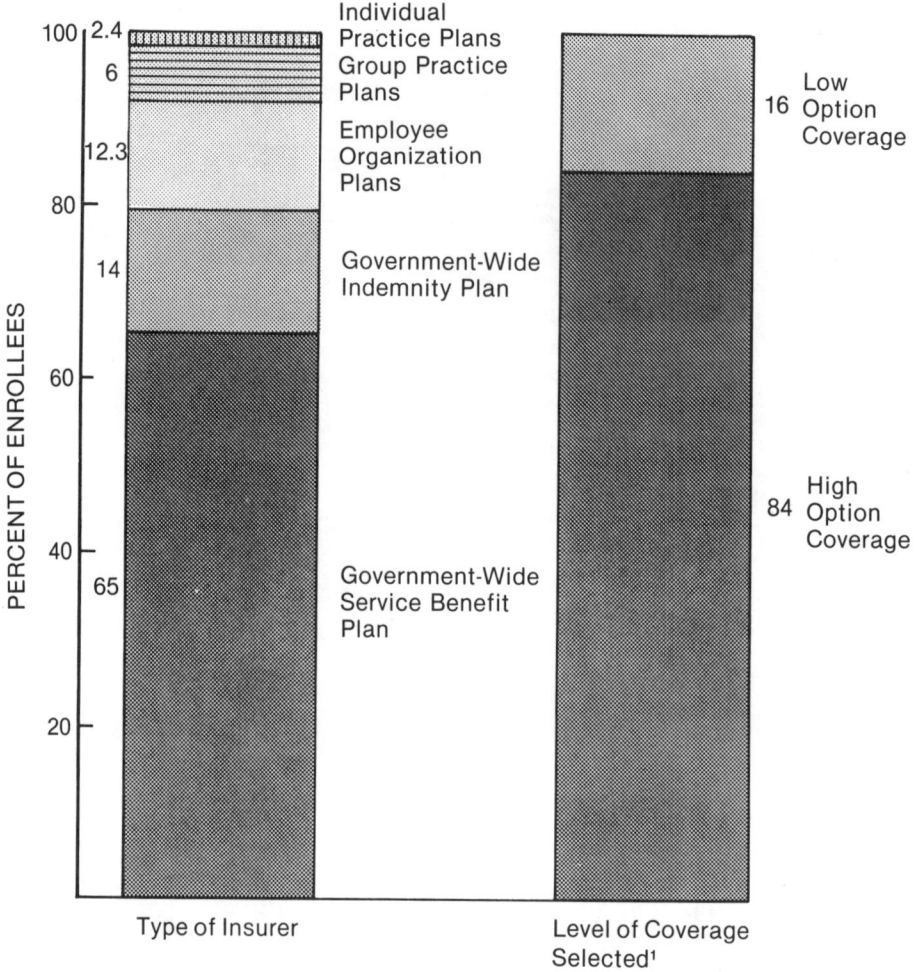

[1]Applies only to government-wide indemnity plan and to government-wide service benefit plan.

SOURCE: U.S. Civil Service Commission, *Federal Fringe Benefit Facts, 1977*, Office of Retirement, Insurance, and Occupational Health, Washington, D.C., 1978, Table D-4, p. 31, and Table D-6, p. 33.

Medical Care Insurance

Chart I-15
Percent of Consumer Expenditures for Personal Health Care Met by Private Insurance, by Type of Expenditure (U.S.A., 1950 and 1976).[1]

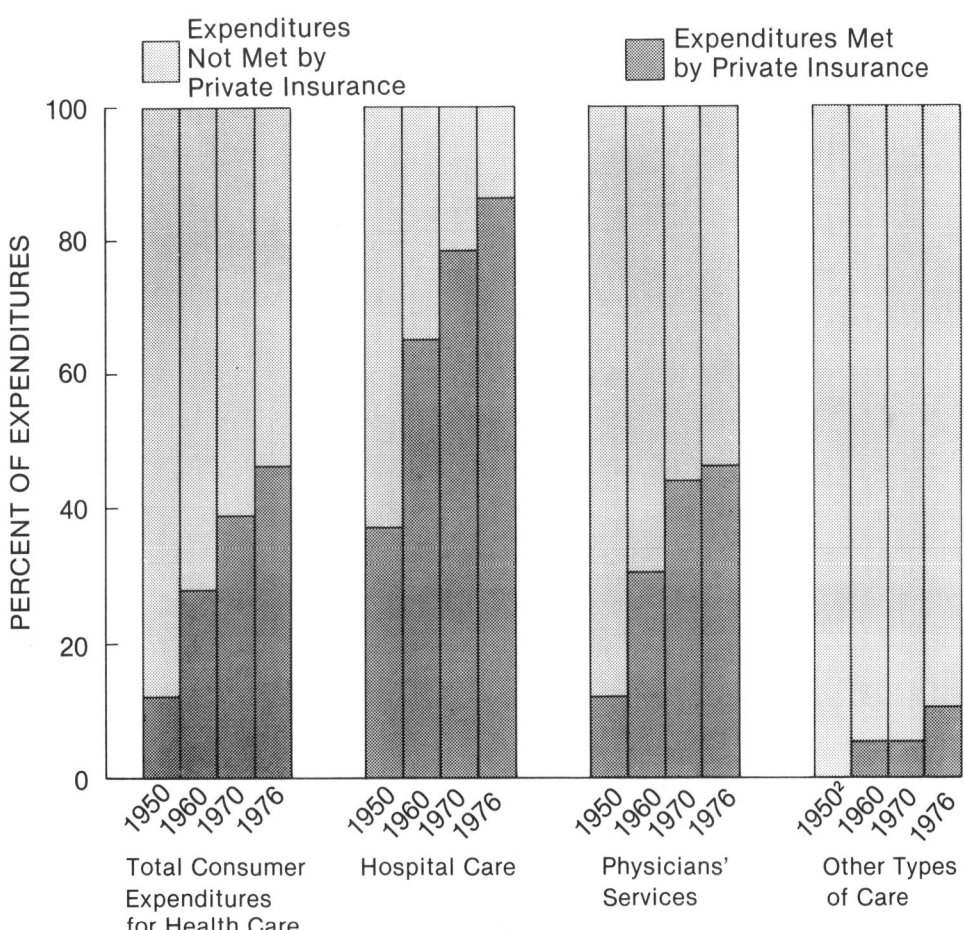

[1]Excludes net cost of insurance.

[2]Included in physicians' services in 1950.

SOURCE: Carroll, Marjorie Smith, "Private Health Insurance Plans in 1976," *Social Security Bulletin*, Vol. 41, No. 9, September 1978, p. 14.

Chart I-16 Percent of Premium Income of Private Health Insurance Organizations Returned to Subscribers as Benefits, ("Loss Ratio"), by Type of Organization and Type of Enrollment (U.S.A., 1976).

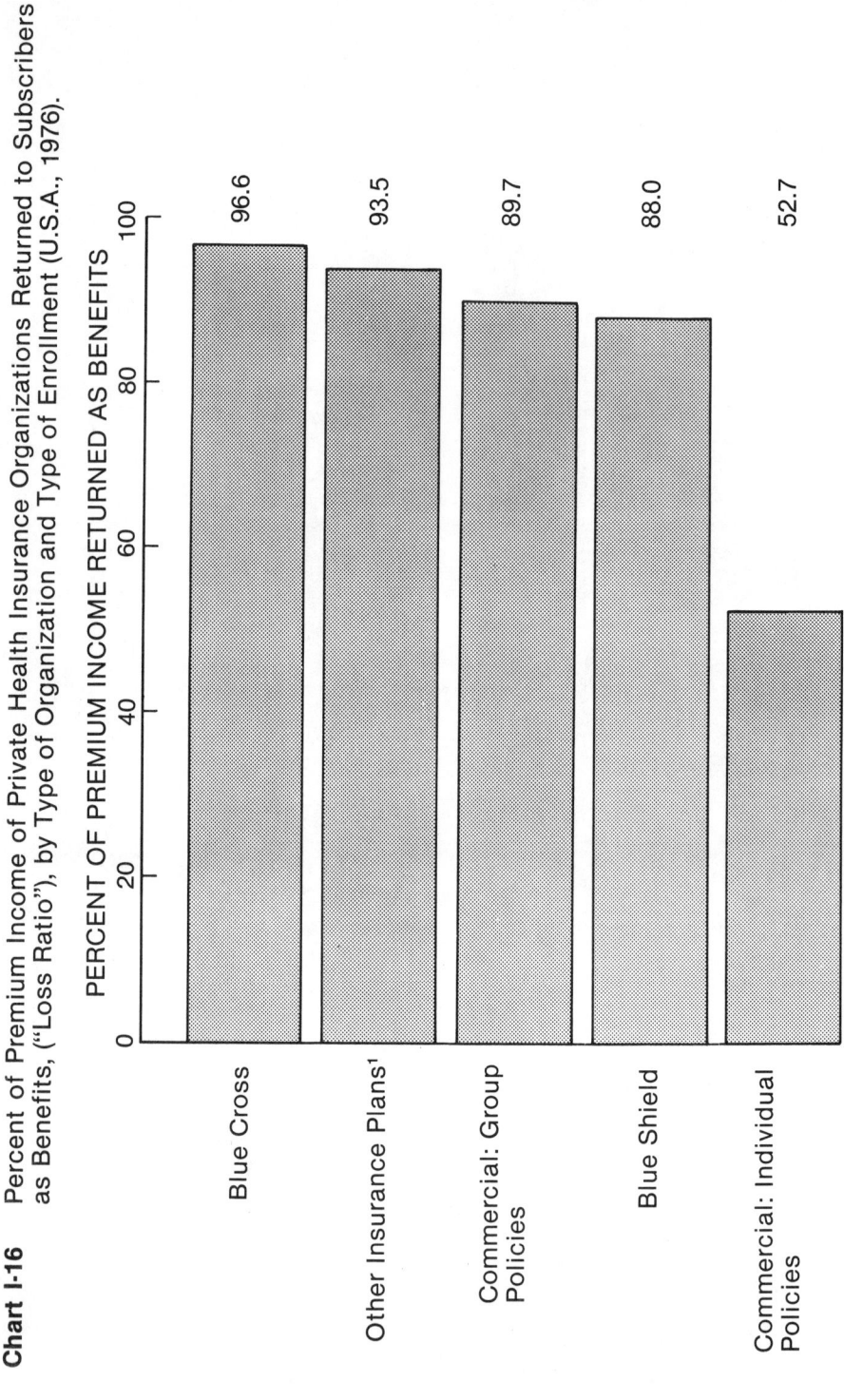

[1]Other plans include health maintenance organizations, community plans, employer-employee-union plans, private group clinics, and dental service corporations.

SOURCE: Carroll, Marjorie Smith, "Private Health Insurance Plans in 1976: An Evaluation," *Social Security Bulletin*, Vol. 41, No. 9, September 1978, Table 8, p.10.

Chart I-17

Patient Days of Hospital Care per 1000 Persons Enrolled in Blue Cross and per 1000 Persons in the United States (U.S.A., 1969–1978).

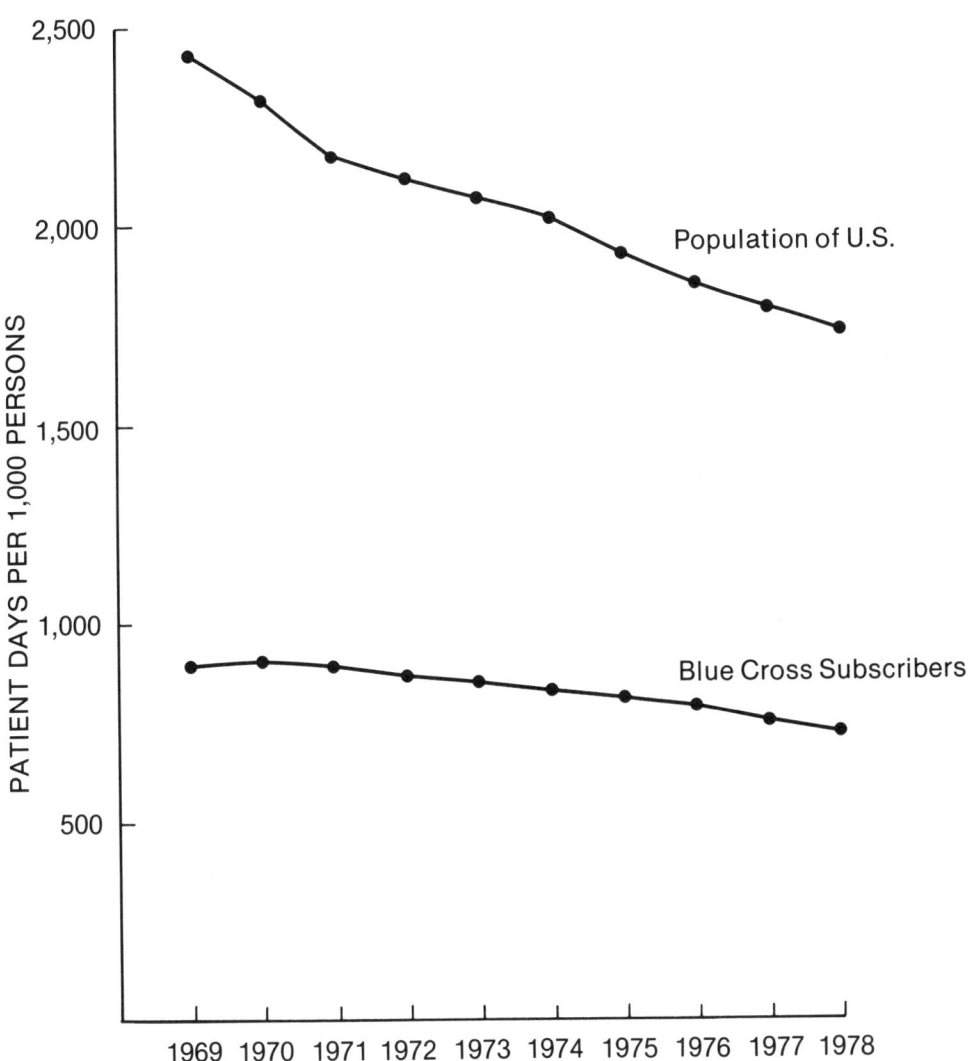

SOURCES: For Blue Cross subscribers: Blue Cross Association, *Enrollment and Utilization Report of the Blue Cross Plan, 4th Quarter and Year End 1979*, data provided by W. Elliott of the Blue Cross Association, June 1980; for United States: American Hospital Association, *Hospital Statistics, 1979*, Chicago, 1979, Table 1, p. 4.

Medical Care Insurance

Chart I-18 Hospital Admission Rates, Patient Days per 1000, and Outpatient Visits per 1000 Persons, by Type of Enrollment, Blue Cross Subscribers (U.S.A., 1979).[1]

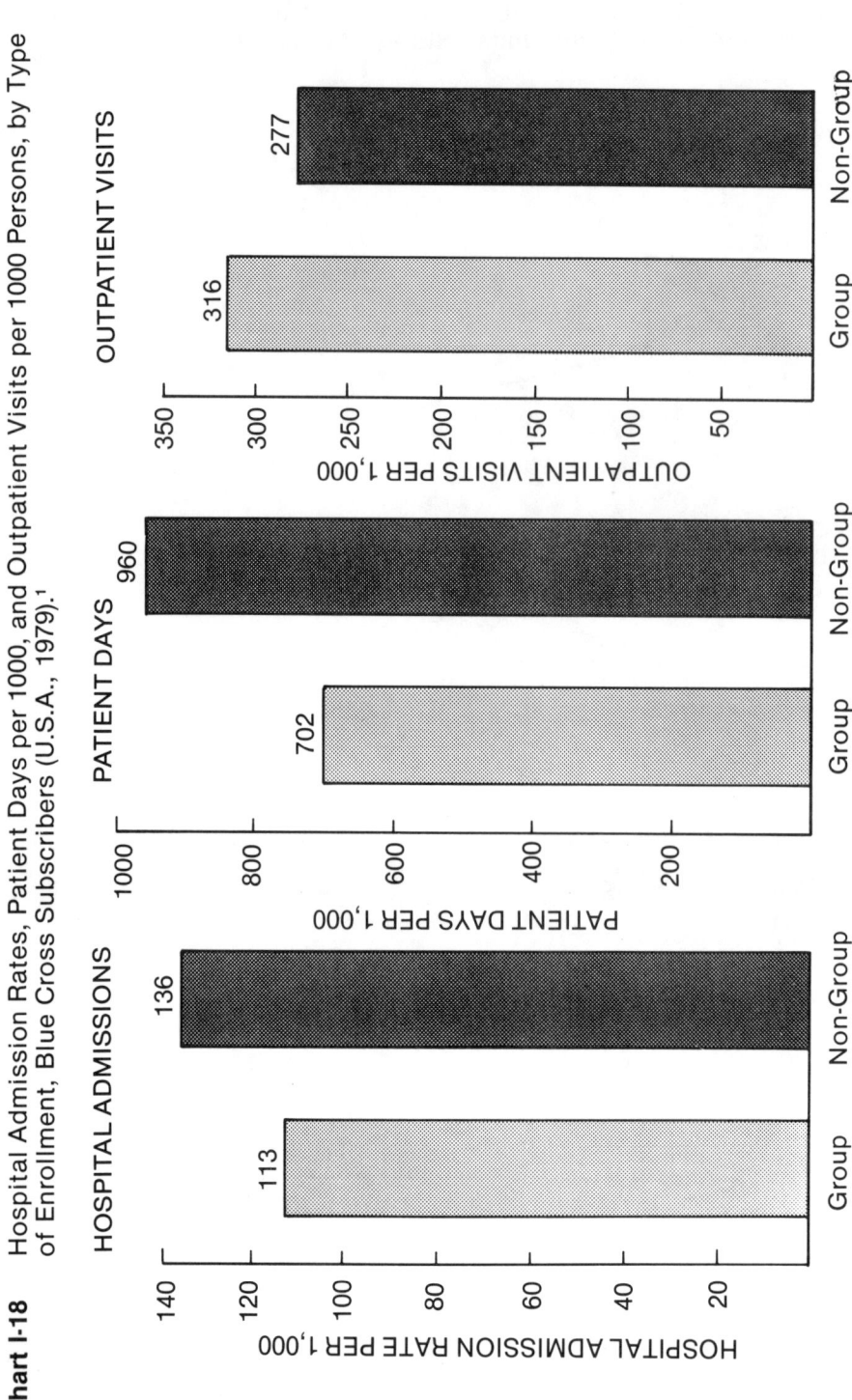

SOURCE: Blue Cross Association, *The Enrollment and Utilization Report of Blue Cross Plans*, Fourth Quarter and Year End 1979 Issue.

[1] Excludes utilization data for Puerto Rico and for members with coverage supplementing Medicare.

Chart I-19

Service Utilization Rates, by Duration of Enrollment (Group Health Insurance Program, New York and New Jersey, 1954–1967).

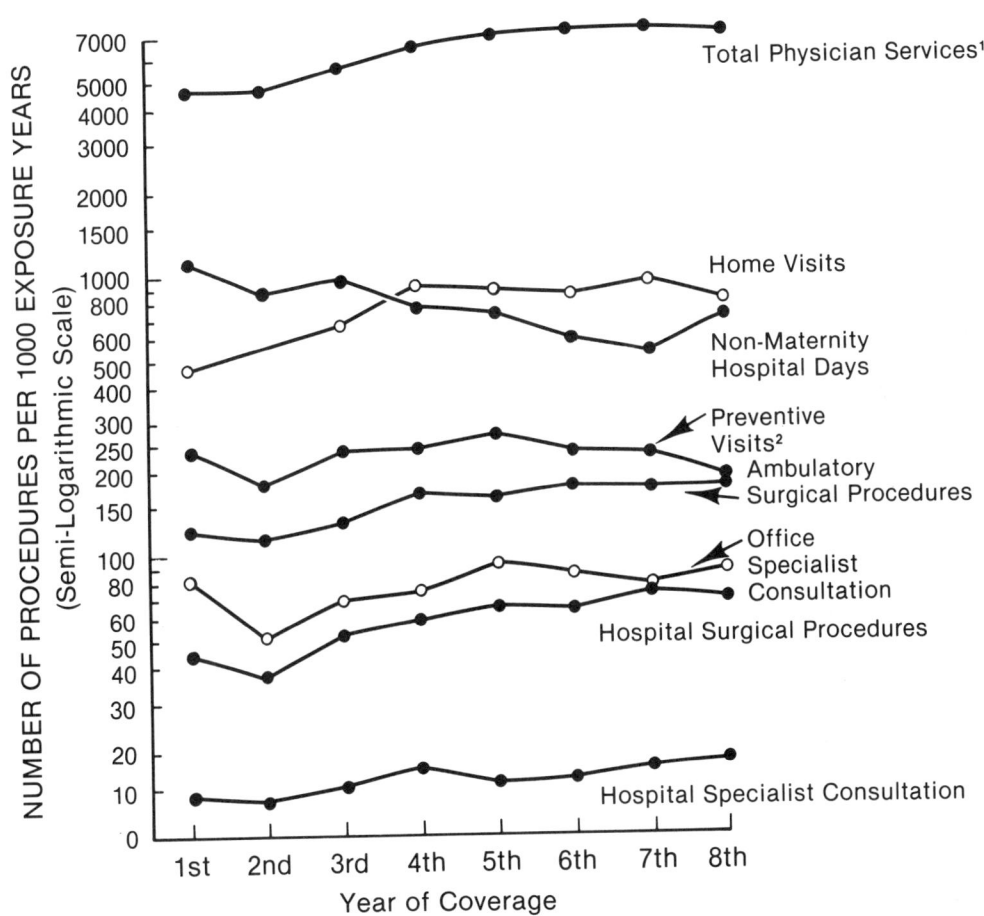

[1] Physician services include office calls and home calls, one physician service for each day of hospitalization, diagnostic x-rays and certain laboratory tests.

[2] Preventive visits include office services not associated with the diagnosis and treatment of specific illness.

SOURCE: Avnet, H.H., *Physicians Service Patterns and Illness Rates*, Group Health Insurance, Inc., United States, 1967, Table 66, p. 139, Table 74, p. 155, Table 78, p. 162, Table 84, p. 169, Table 108, p. 207, and Table 145, p. 397.

Medical Care Insurance

Chart I-20

Patient Visits per Person per Year,[1] by Duration of Membership in a Prepaid Group Health Plan (U.S.A., 1973).

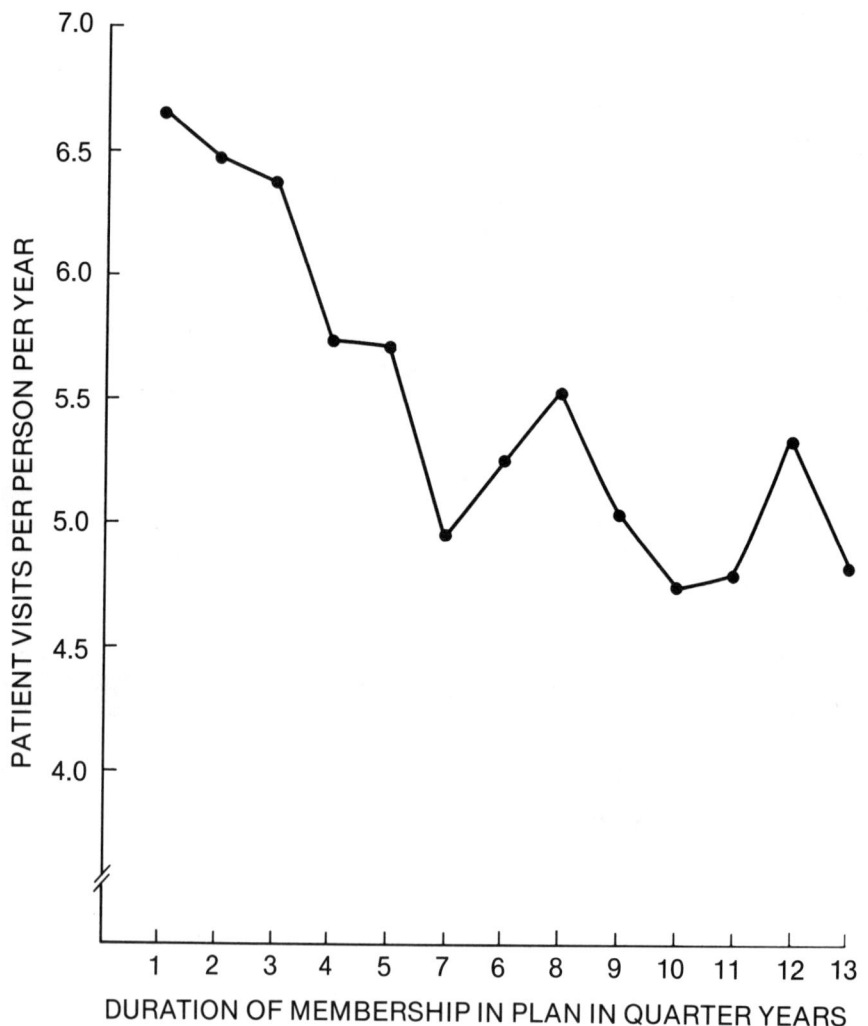

[1] Adjusted to eliminate seasonality and other confounding effects.
SOURCE: Yesalis, Charles E. and Philip D. Bonnet, "The Effect of Duration of Membership in a Prepaid Group Health Plan on the Utilization of Services," *Medical Care,* Vol. 14, No. 12, December 1976, Table 2, p. 1029.

Chart I-21

Number of Operational Prepaid Health Plans (Health Maintenance Organizations)[1] (U.S.A., 1970–1979).

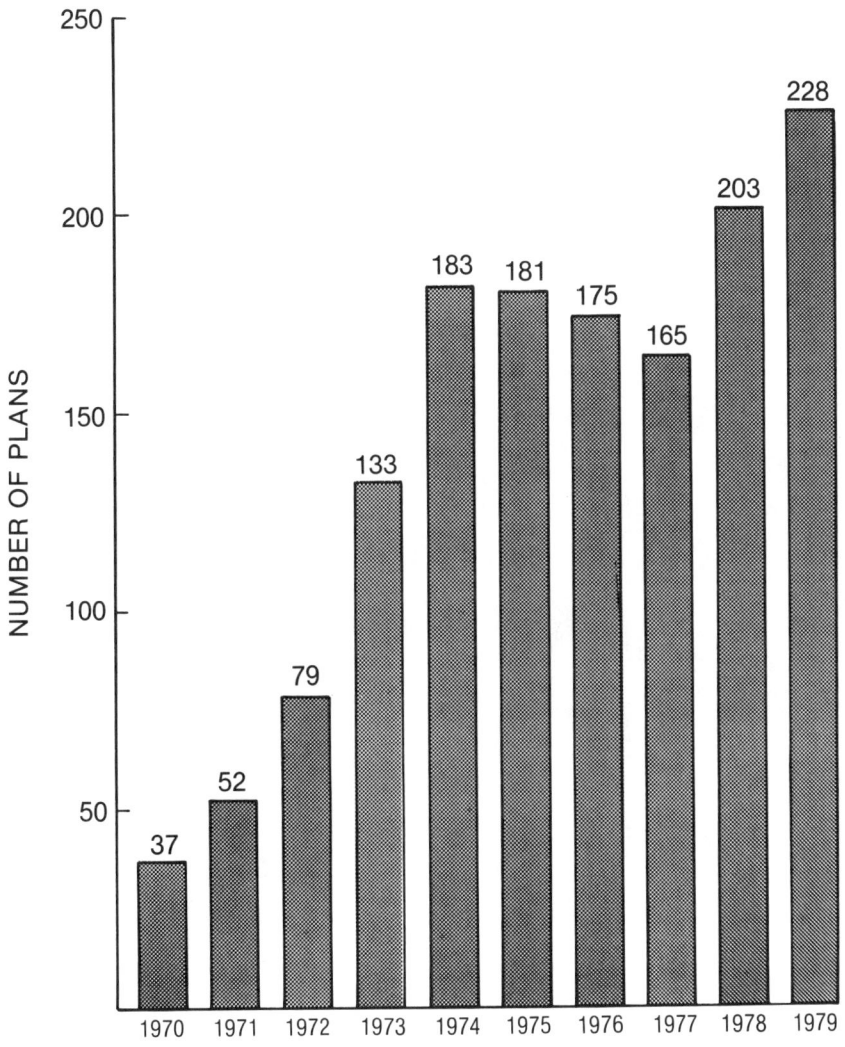

[1]Includes both federally qualified and not federally qualified plans.

SOURCE: "HMO Growth Most Dramatic 1970–1975," *Group Health News,* Vol. 21, May 1980, p. 4.

Chart I-22

Percent Distribution of Prepaid Health Plans (Health Maintenance Organizations) and Total Prepaid Enrollment by Federal Qualification Status (U.S.A., 1978).

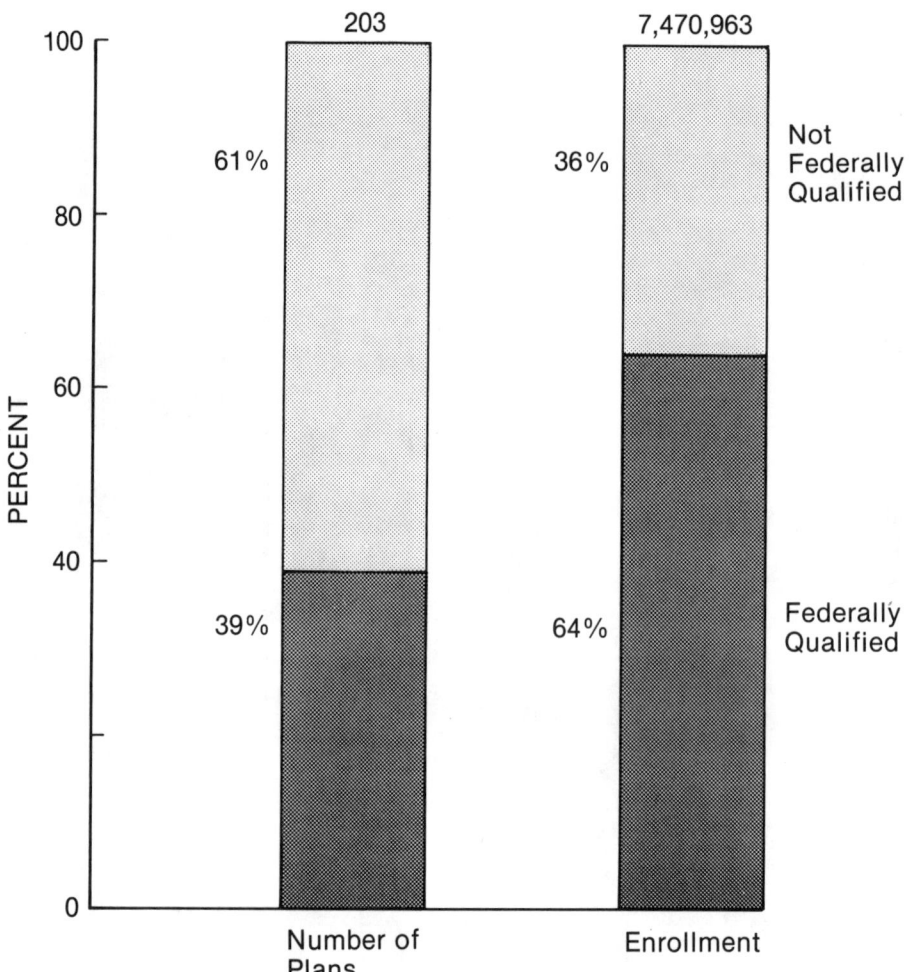

NOTE: Actual numbers are shown on top of bars.

SOURCE: U.S. Office of Health Maintenance Organizations, *National HMO Census of Prepaid Plans, 1978,* DHEW, Public Health Service, Rockville, Maryland, Table 4, p. 4.

Chart I-23

Percent Distribution of Prepaid Health Plans (Health Maintenance Organizations) and of Their Enrollees, by Size of Plan (U.S.A., 1978).

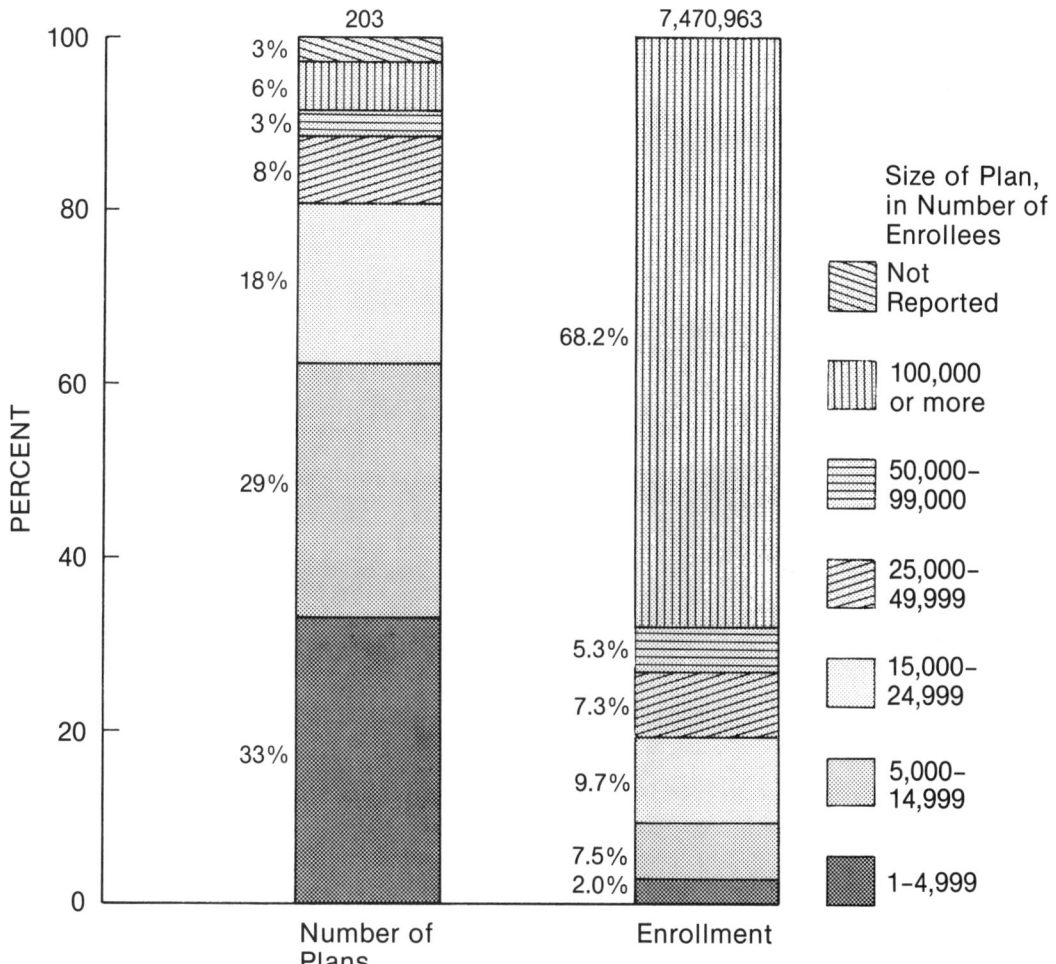

SOURCE: U.S. Office of Health Maintenance Organizations, *National HMO Census of Prepaid Plans, 1978*, DHEW, Public Health Service, Rockville, Maryland, Table 1, p. 3.

Chart I-24

Percent Distribution of Prepaid Health Plans (Health Maintenance Organizations) and of Total Prepaid Enrollment, by Type of Practice, (U.S.A., 1978).

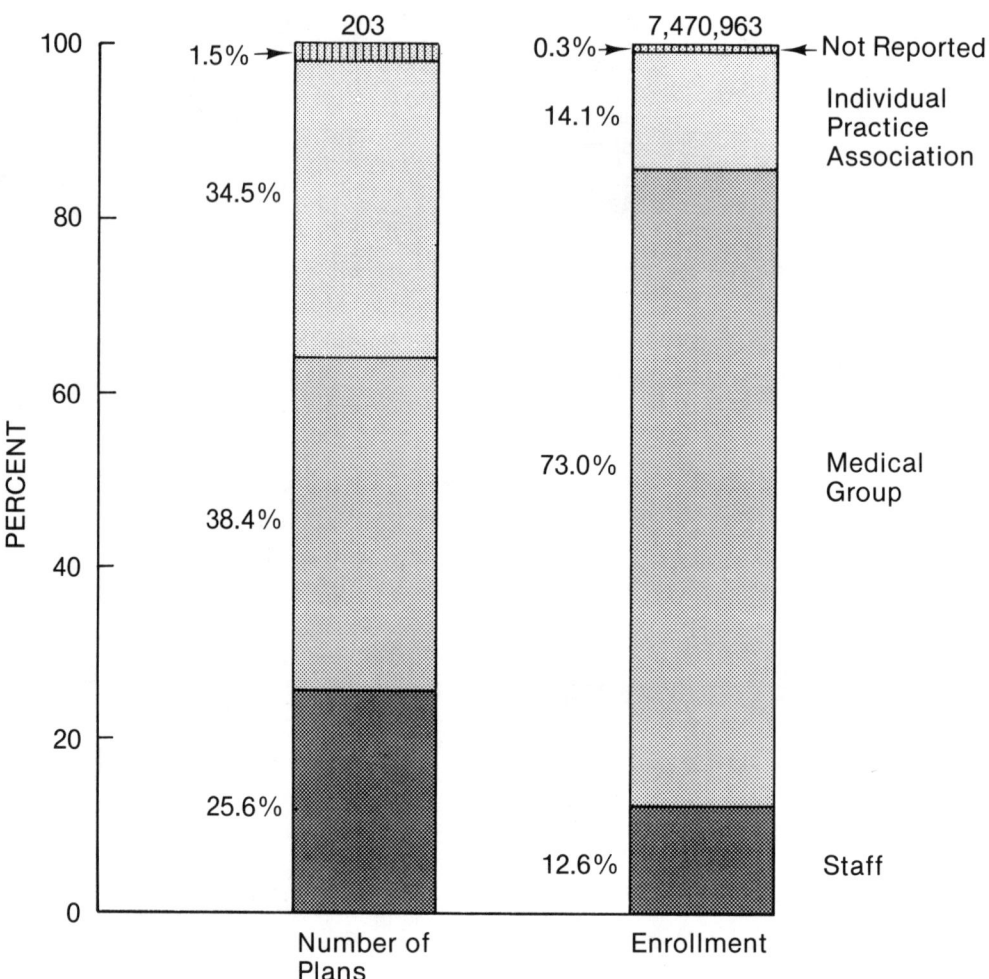

NOTE: Actual numbers are shown on top of bars.

SOURCE: U.S. Office of Health Maintenance Organizations, *National HMO Census of Prepaid plans, 1978*, DHEW, Public Health Service, Rockville, Maryland, Table 3, p. 4.

Chart I-25

Hospital Days per 1000 Members per Year in Prepaid Health Plans (Health Maintenance Organizations), by Type of Practice and Federal Qualification Status (U.S.A., 1978).

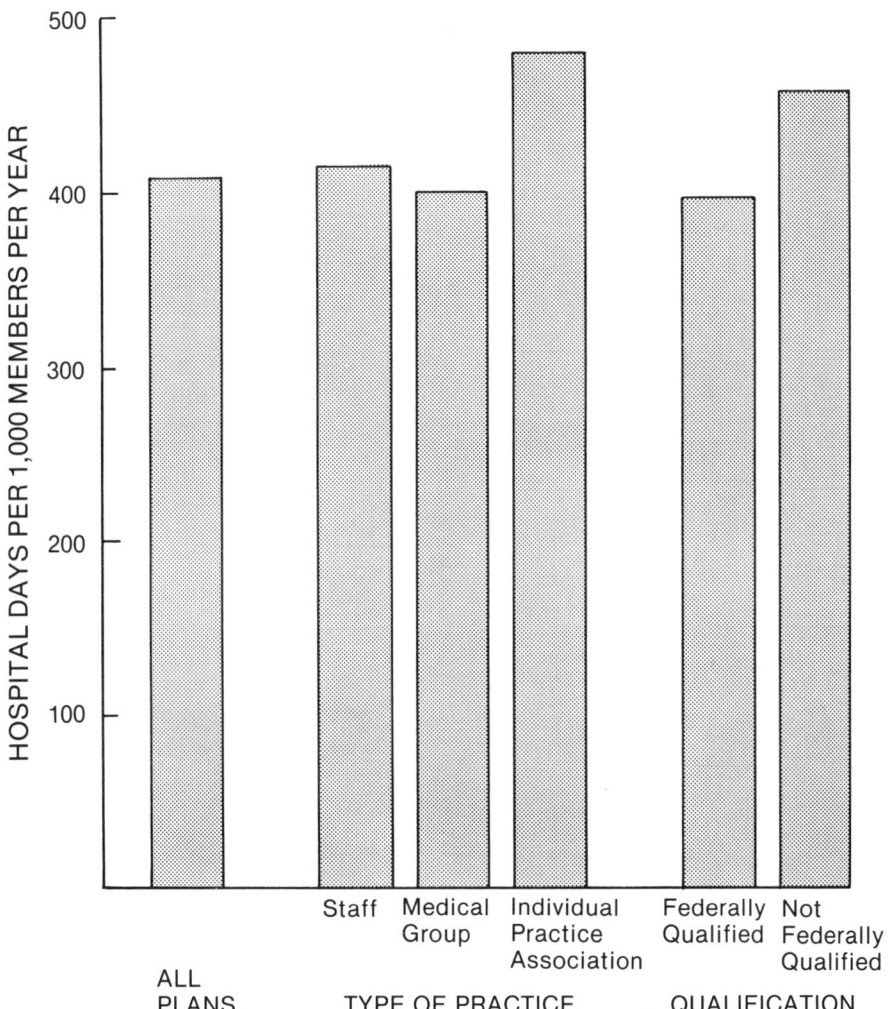

SOURCE: U.S. Office of Health Maintenance Organizations, *National HMO Census of Prepaid Plans, 1978*, DHEW, Public Health Service, Rockville, Maryland, Table 10, p. 8 and Table 11, p. 8.

Medical Care Insurance

Chart I-26

Relative Utilization of Health Services by Persons Under 65 Years of Age, by Type of Insurance Coverage (U.S.A., 1976).

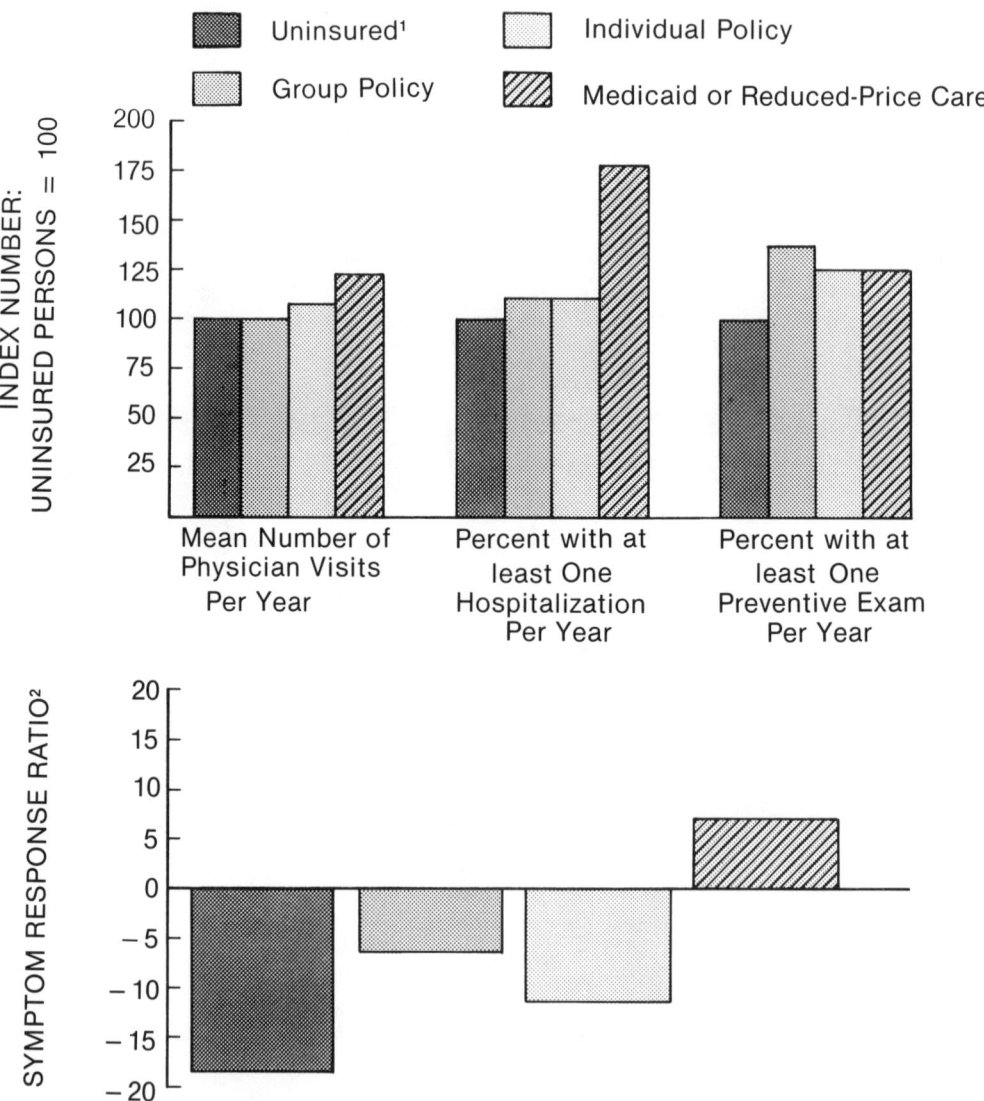

[1] Approximately 10% of the uninsured category had coverage through Medicare, Workmen's Compensation, Veterans' Administration, or private charity.

[2] Ratio is based upon a panel of physicians' judgments as to whether or not a person with a given symptom should see a physician. A positive score indicates that the population saw physicians more frequently than necessary, and a negative score indicates visits less frequently than necessary.

SOURCE: Aday, L. and R. Andersen, "Insurance Coverage and Access: Implications for Health Policy," *Health Services Research,* Vol. 13, No. 4, Winter 1978, Table 2, p. 374.

Chart I-27

Relative Utilization Rates,[1] by Type of Service and by Type of Insurance Plan, State Employees and Annuitants and Their Dependents (California, 1962–1963).[2]

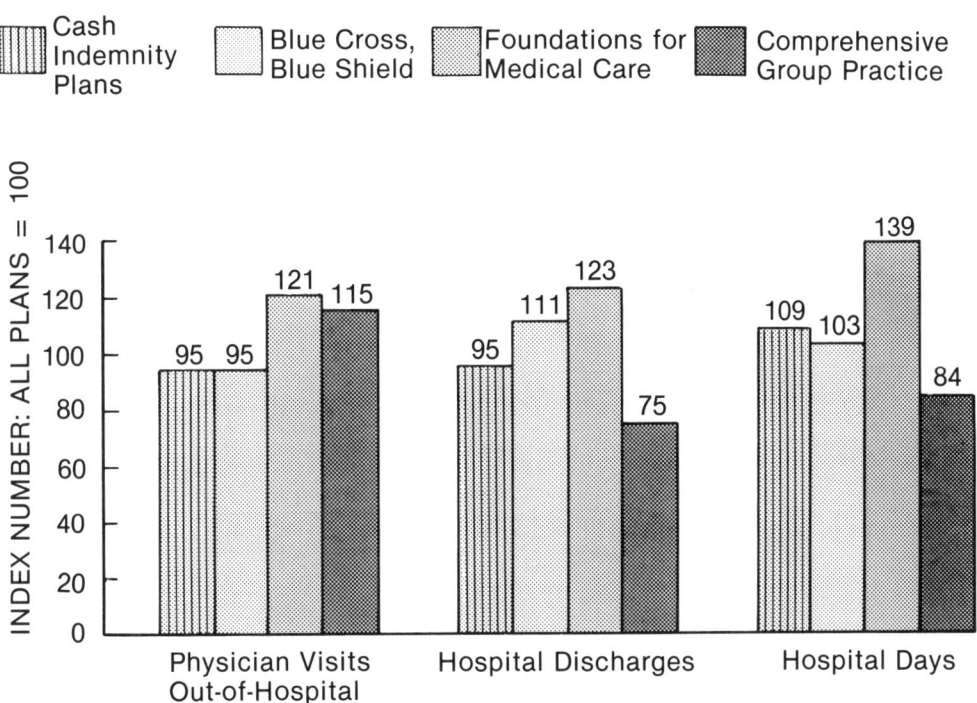

[1] Adjusted for age and sex.

[2] Out-of-hospital care between January 1 and March 31, 1963 and hospital care between July 1, 1962 and March 31, 1963.

SOURCE: Dozier, D., et al, *Final Report on the Survey of Consumer Experience under the State of California Employees' Hospital and Medical Care Act*, Sacramento, June 1968, Table 21, p. 52, Table 22, p. 53, and Table 23, p. 54.

Chart I-28

Relative Magnitude of Hospital Admission and Tonsillectomy Rates for Enrollees of the Health Insurance Plan of Greater New York as Compared With Similar Specified Populations (U.S.A., 1951, 1955, 1956–57, and 1958).

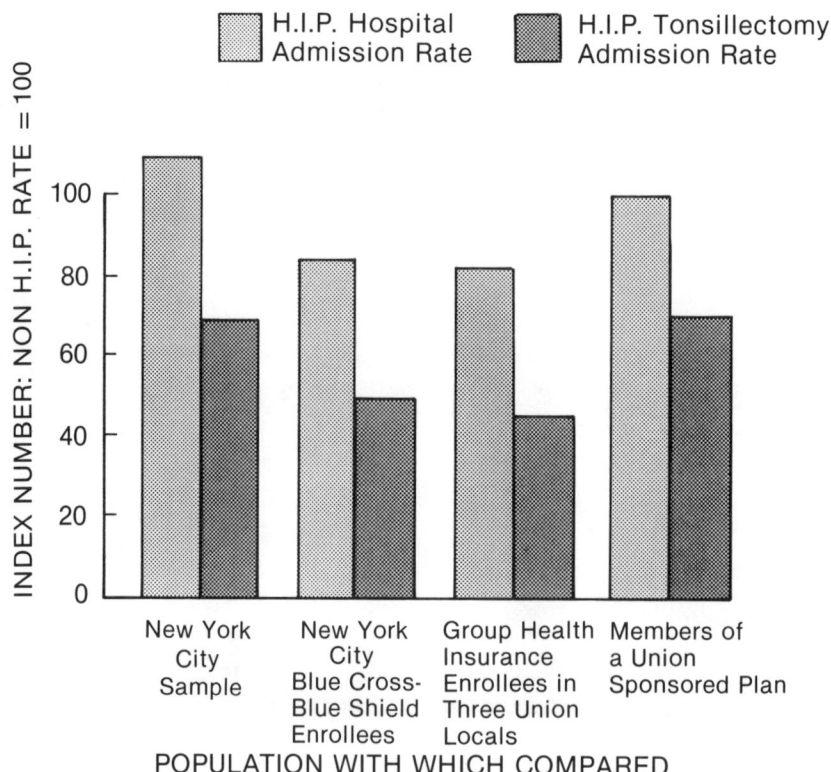

SOURCES: Committee for the Special Research Project on the Health Insurance Plan of Greater New York, *Health and Medical Care in New York City*, published for the Commonwealth Fund, Harvard University Press, 1957, pp. 149 and 159; Densen, P.M., E. Balamuth, and S. Shapiro, *Prepaid Medical Care and Hospital Utilization*, Hospital Monograph Series No. 3, American Hospital Association, Chicago, 1958, pp. 7 and 25; Densen, P.M., et al., "Prepaid Medical Care and Hospital Utilization in a Dual Choice Situation," *American Journal of Public Health*, Vol. 50, November 1960, pp. 1712 and 1719; Densen, P.M., et al., "Prepaid Medical Care and Hospital Utilization: Comparison of a Group Practice and Self-Insurance Situation," *Hospitals*, Vol. 36, November 16, 1962, Table 5.

Medical Care Insurance

Medical Care Chartbook

Chart I-29 Medicare Reimbursement Levels for Beneficiaries who Were Members of Group Practice Prepayment Plans and for Comparable Control Groups of Beneficiaries Receiving Fee-For-Service Care (U.S.A., 1970).

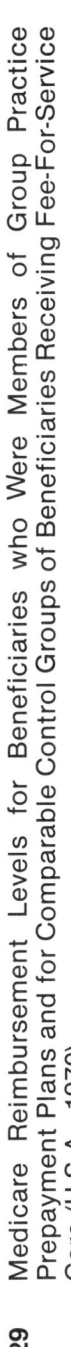

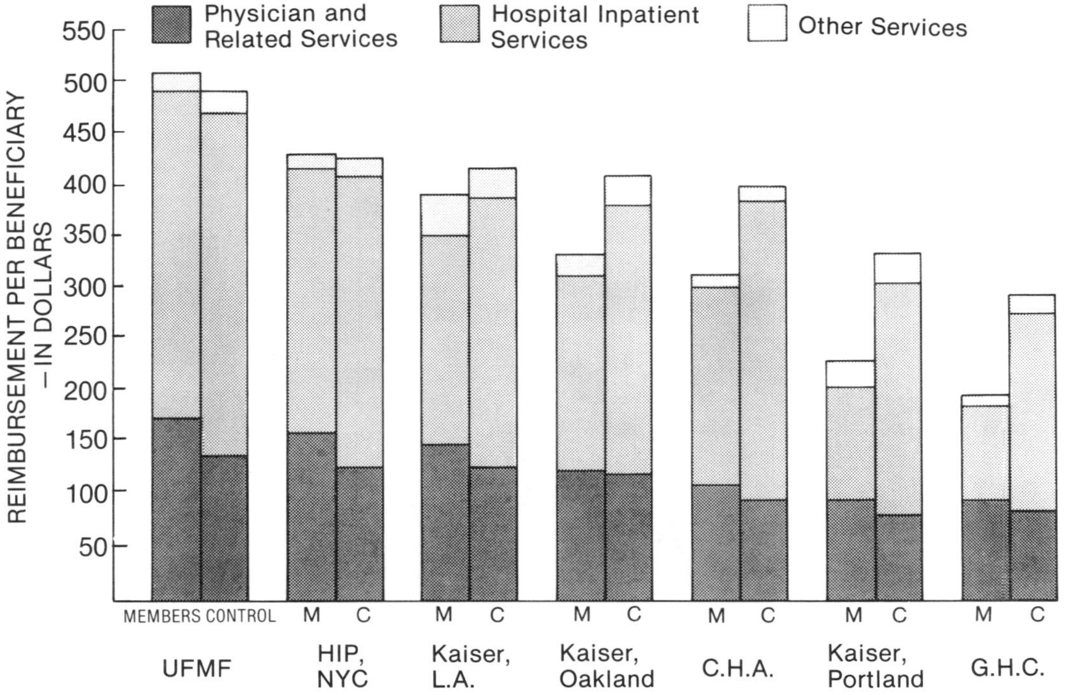

UFMF — Union Family Medical Fund of the Hotel Industry of New York City; HIP — Health Insurance Plan of Greater New York; Kaiser — Kaiser Foundation Health Plan — Los Angeles; Kaiser — Kaiser Foundation Health Plan — Oakland; C.H.A. — Community Health Association — Detroit; Kaiser — Kaiser Foundation Health Plan — Portland; G.H.C. — Group Health Cooperative of Puget Sound — Seattle.

NOTES: (1) The prepayment plans shown were participating in an incentive capitation program. Capitation payments covered "in-plan" physicians' services only. All other services were reimbursed through intermediaries using routine Medicare fee-for-service procedures. (2) Controls were a sample of non-plan member Medicare beneficiaries residing in the same counties as plan members. Plan members and Control groups were matched for age and sex distribution.

SOURCE: Corbin, M. and A. Krute, "Some Aspects of Medicare Experience with Group-Practice Prepayment Plans," *Social Security Bulletin*, Vol. 38, No. 3, March 1975, Table 1, p. 7.

Chart I-30

Hospital Days per 1000 Covered Persons, Excluding Maternity Days, by Type of Insurance Plan, Federal Employees Health Benefits Program (U.S.A.,1961–1972).

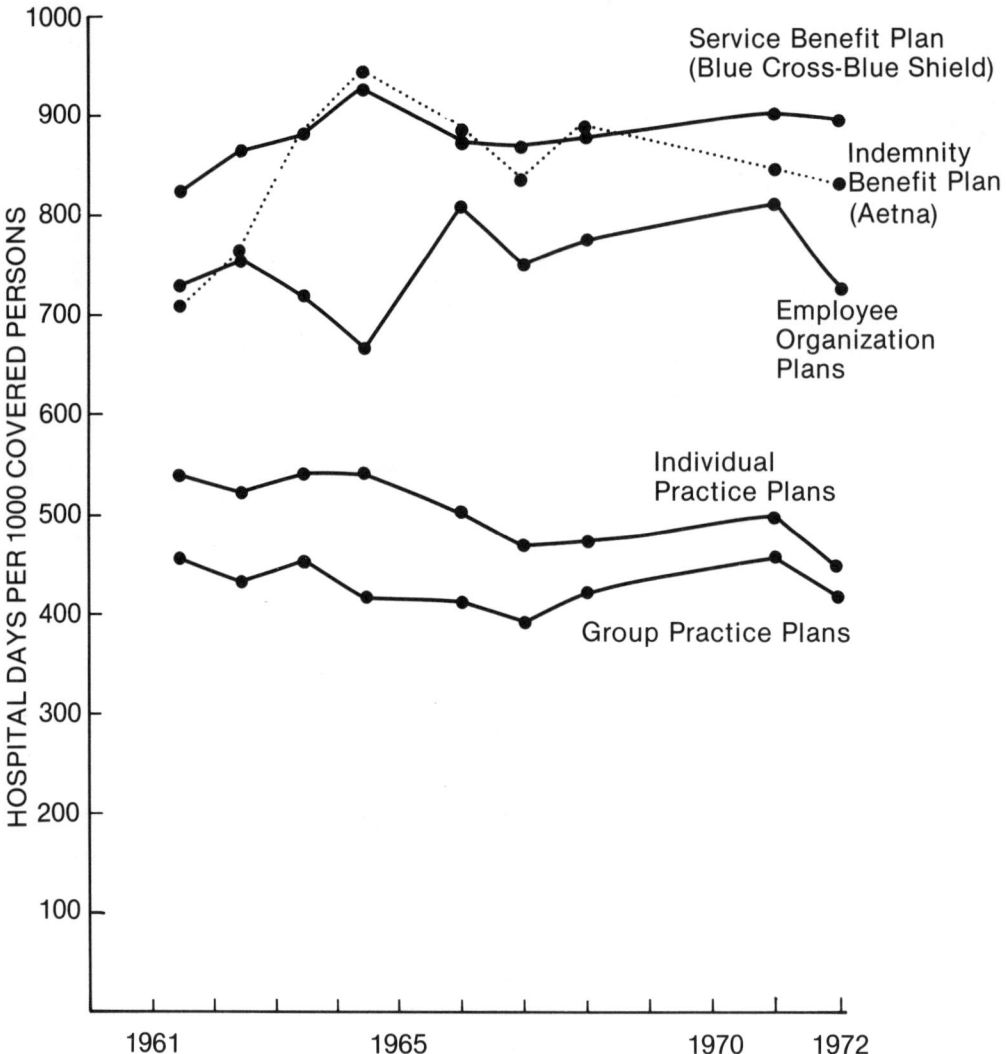

SOURCES: For 1961–1968: Perrott, George S., *The Federal Employees Health Benefit Program, Enrollment and Utilization of Health Services,* 1961–1968, Health Services and Mental Health Administration, DHEW, 1971, Table 6, p. 26; for 1969 and 1970: U.S. Civil Service Commission, *Fiscal Year Reports,* Bureau of Retirement, Insurance, and Occupational Health, Washington, D.C., report for year ended June 30, 1970, Table C-3, pp. 34–37, and report for year ended June 30, 1971, Table C-3, pp. 34–37; for 1971–1972: U.S. Civil Service Commission, *Annual Report of Financial and Statistical Data,* Bureau of Retirement, Insurance, and Occupational Health, Washington, D.C., for year ended June 30, 1972, Table D-4, pp. 34–35, for year ended June 30, 1973, Table D-4, pp. 34–35, and for year ended June 30, 1974, Table D-4, pp. 32–33.

Chart I-31

Admissions per 1000 Membership Years, Adjusted for Age and Sex, Federal Employees Health Benefits Program, by Type of Health Insurance Plan (U.S.A., 1970).[1]

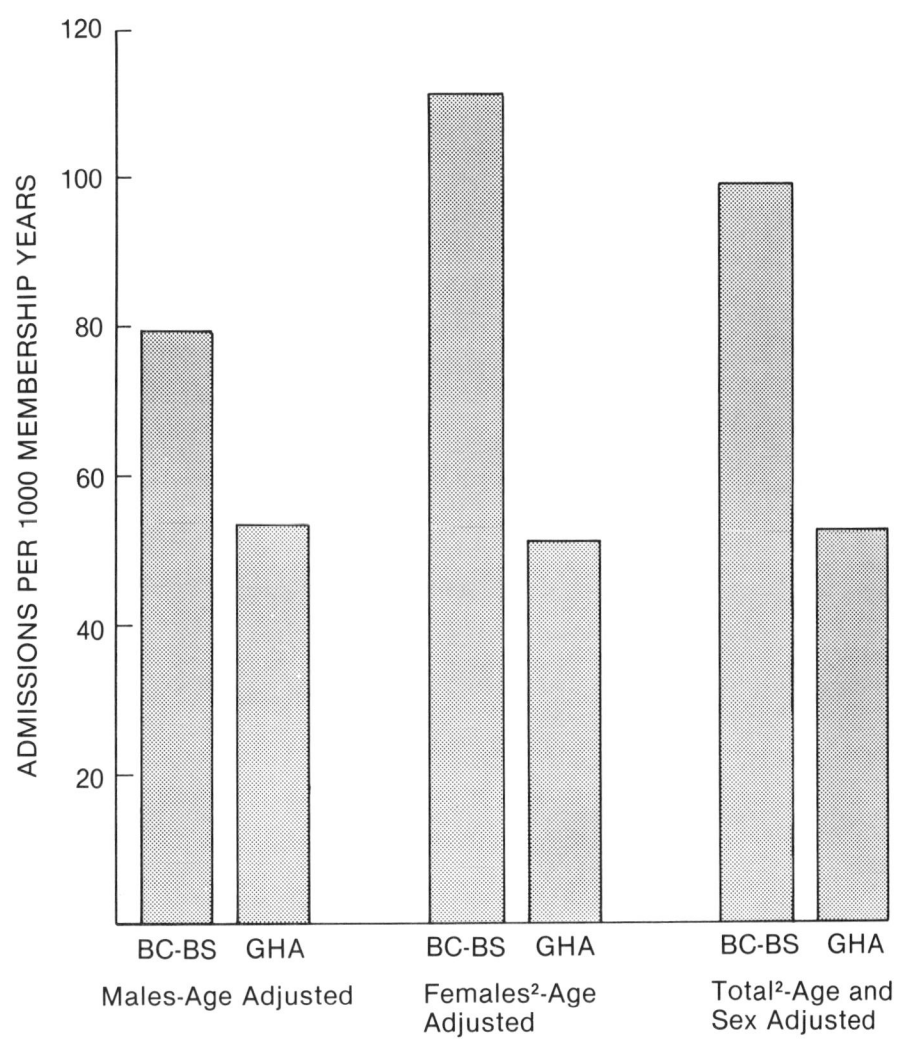

[1]The two comparison groups are Blue Cross-Blue Shield (BC-BS) subscribers, and members of Group Health Association (GHA), a group practice health maintenance organization.

[2]Obstetric admissions excluded.

SOURCE: Riedel, Donald C., et al., *Federal Employees Health Benefits Program, Utilization Study*, DHEW, Public Health Service, National Center for Health Services Research, Health Resources Administration, 1975, Table 8. p. 20.

Medical Care Insurance

Chart I-32

Selected Surgical Procedures per 1,000 Covered Persons, Federal Employees Health Benefits Program, by Whether Blue Shield or Group Practice Plan (U.S.A., January–December, 1968).

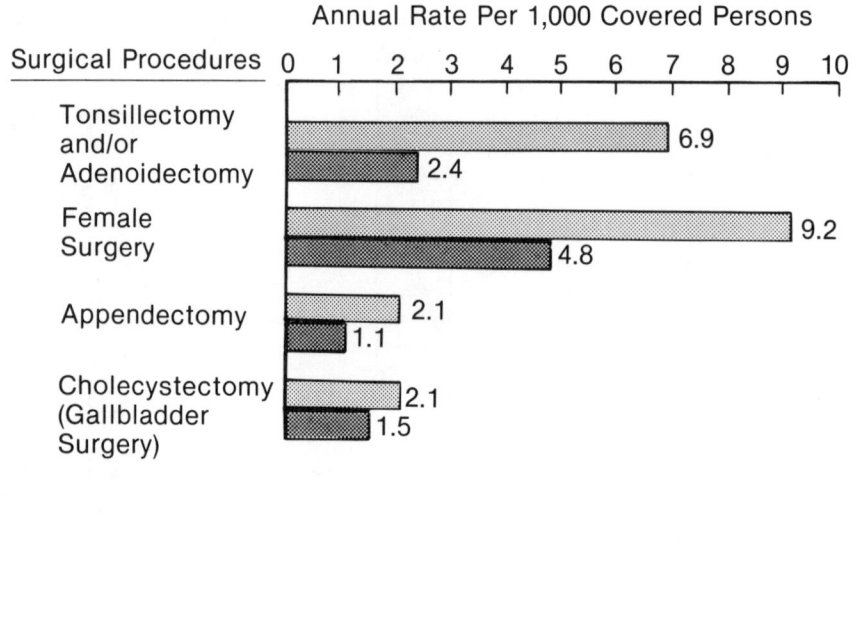

SOURCE: Perrott, George S., *The Federal Employees Health Benefits Program, Enrollment and Utilization of Health Services 1961–1968*, Health Services and Mental Health Administration, U.S. Department of Health, Education, and Welfare, 1971, Figure 7, p. 19.

Chart I-33

Relative Utilization Rates, Receipt of Preventive Services, Expenses and Satisfaction, by Type of Insurance Plan (Los Angeles County, California, 1967–1968).[1]

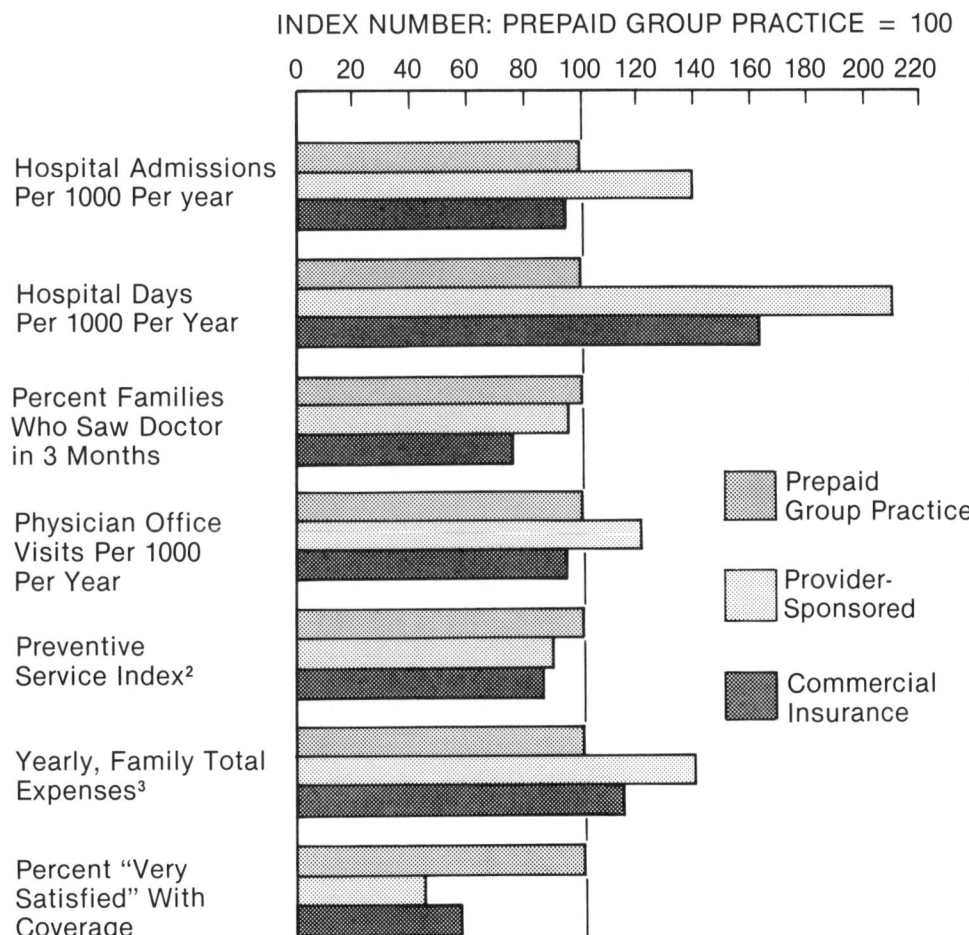

[1]Based on mail questionnaires, insurance records, and medical records, singly or in combination. About 3,000 families responded to questionnaire. Adjustments were made for 52% non-response by interviewing a sample of non-respondents.

[2]Preventive Service Index based on frequency of such services as "check-up" examinations of adults, vaginal cytology, routine rectal examinations, chest x-rays, serological tests and immunization as shown in a sample of medical records.

[3]Expenses exclude drugs and dental care.

SOURCE: Roemer, M.I., et al., *Health Insurance Outputs: Services, Expenditures and Attitudes under Three Types of Plan*, Bureau of Public Health Economics, Research Series No. 16, School of Public Health, University of Michigan, 1972.

Chart I-34

Percent of Primary Subscribers Who Report Specified Degrees of Satisfaction With Financial Coverage and Medical Care Received, by Type of Health Insurance Plan (Los Angeles County, California, 1967-1968).[1]

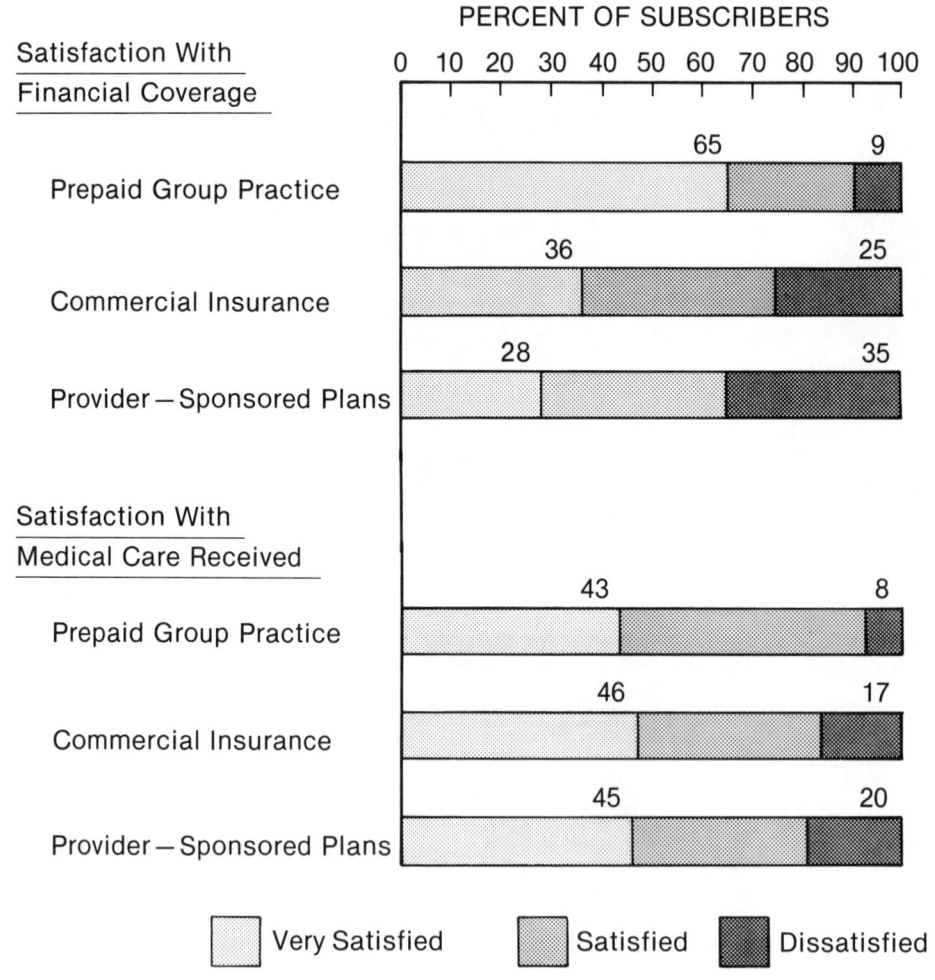

[1]Based on questionnaire responses mailed to about 6,000 families of whom 48 percent responded. Adjustments were made for non-response by interviewing a sample of non-respondents.

SOURCE: Roemer, M.I., et al., *Health Insurance Outputs: Services, Expenditures and Attitudes under Three Types of Plan*, Bureau of Public Health Economics, Research Series No. 16, School of Public Health, University of Michigan, 1972.

Chart I-35

Consumer Preference for Physicians to Work in Groups or Alone, by Age of Respondent (Detroit 1964-65, Cleveland 1968-70, and Cincinnati 1969).[1]

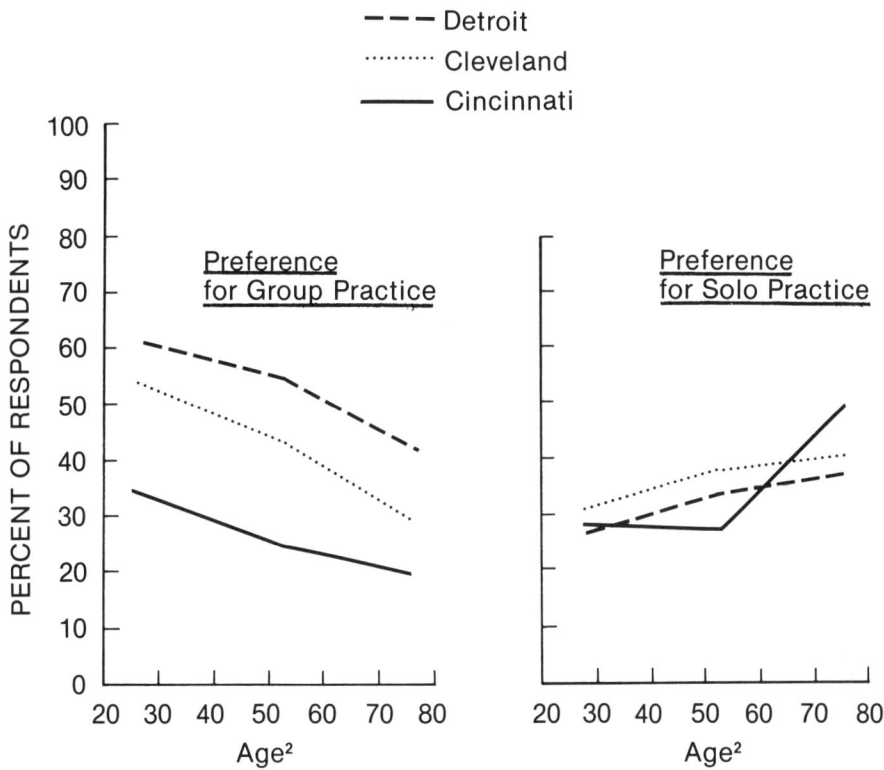

[1]The question asked was: Some people think it is important that family doctors and specialists work together in the same place as a group, while others think that family doctors can handle most illnesses by themselves and don't need to work in the same place with specialists. Which would you rather have: family doctors and specialists as a group or family doctors by themselves?

[2]The midpoint of the age group 65 and over is plotted at 75 years.

SOURCE: Metzner, Charles A., Rashid L. Bashshur, and Gary W. Shannon, "Differential Public Acceptance of Group Medical Practice," *Medical Care*, Vol. 10, July-August 1972, Table 4.

Chart I-36

Percent of Persons Approving of Multispecialty Group Practice[1], by Social Class ("Regionville,"[2] 1946–1950 and 1973).

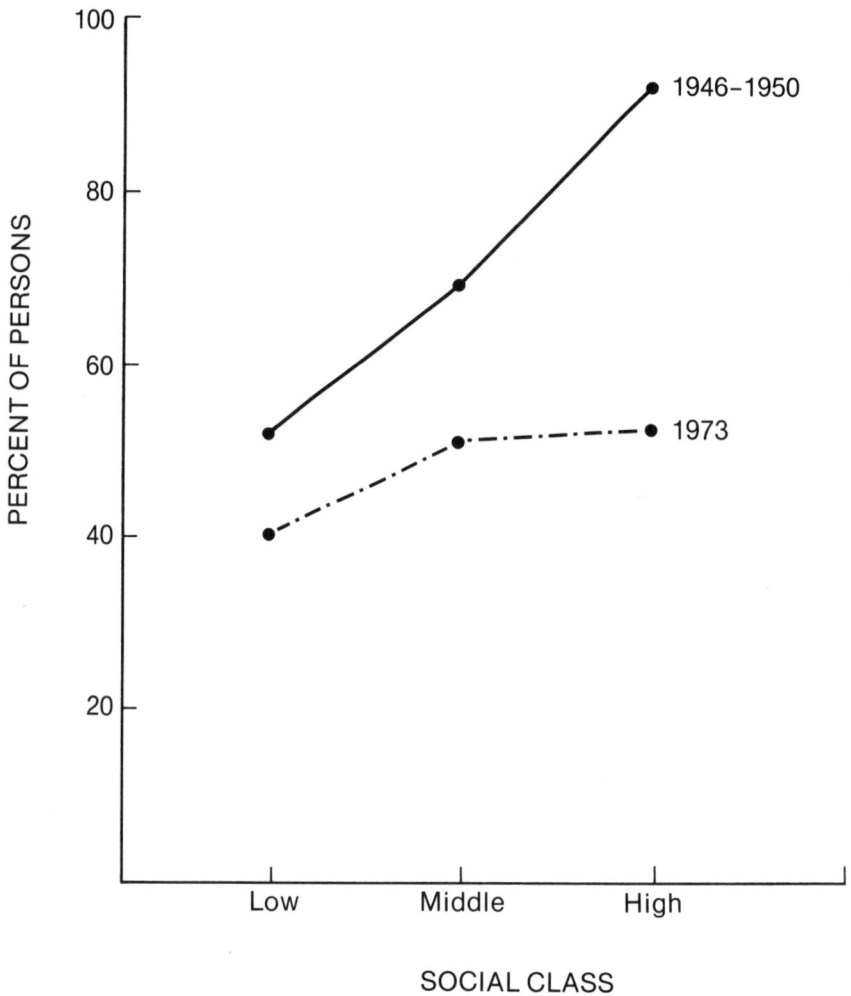

[1]This chart reflects responses to the question: "Would you prefer to go to a physician's office where a number of different doctors, each being a specialist in one branch of medicine, would work together in treating your illness, or would you prefer to go to a doctor who practices alone."

[2]A rural community in New York State.

SOURCE: Kunitz, S. J., A.A. Sorenson, and S.B. Cashman, "Changing Health Care Opinions in Regionville, 1946–1973," *Medical Care*, Vol. XIII, No. 7, July 1975, Table 11, p. 559.

Chart I-37

Cumulative Number of Losses to a Cohort of 1,000 Medicaid Enrollees Due to Voluntary Disenrollment, Loss of Eligibility, and Both Reasons Combined, East Baltimore Medical Plan, November 1971 through September 1973.

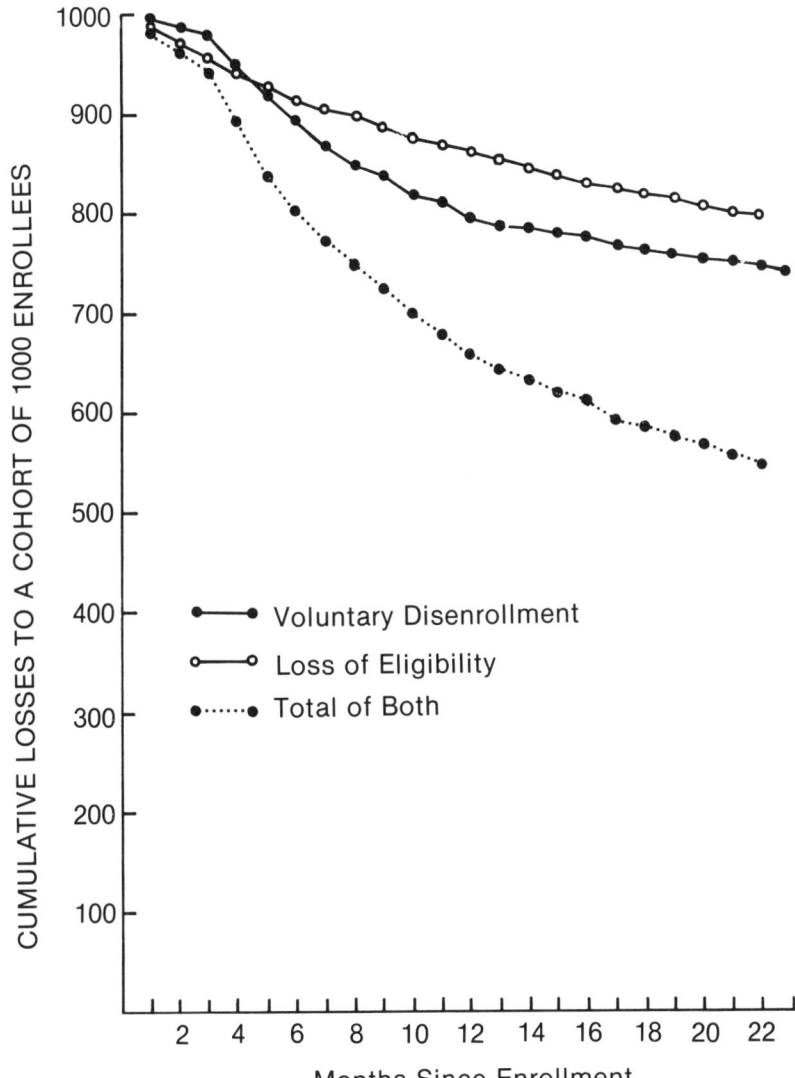

SOURCE: Wollstadt, L.J., S. Shapiro, and T. Bice, "Disenrollment From a Prepaid Group Practice: An Actuarial and Demographic Description," *Inquiry,* Vol. 15, June 1978, Table 2, page 145.

Chart I-38

Percent of Families Who Reported Having a Private Physician Prior to Selection of a Health Insurance Plan, by Type of Plan Selected (Rochester, New York, 1974).[1]

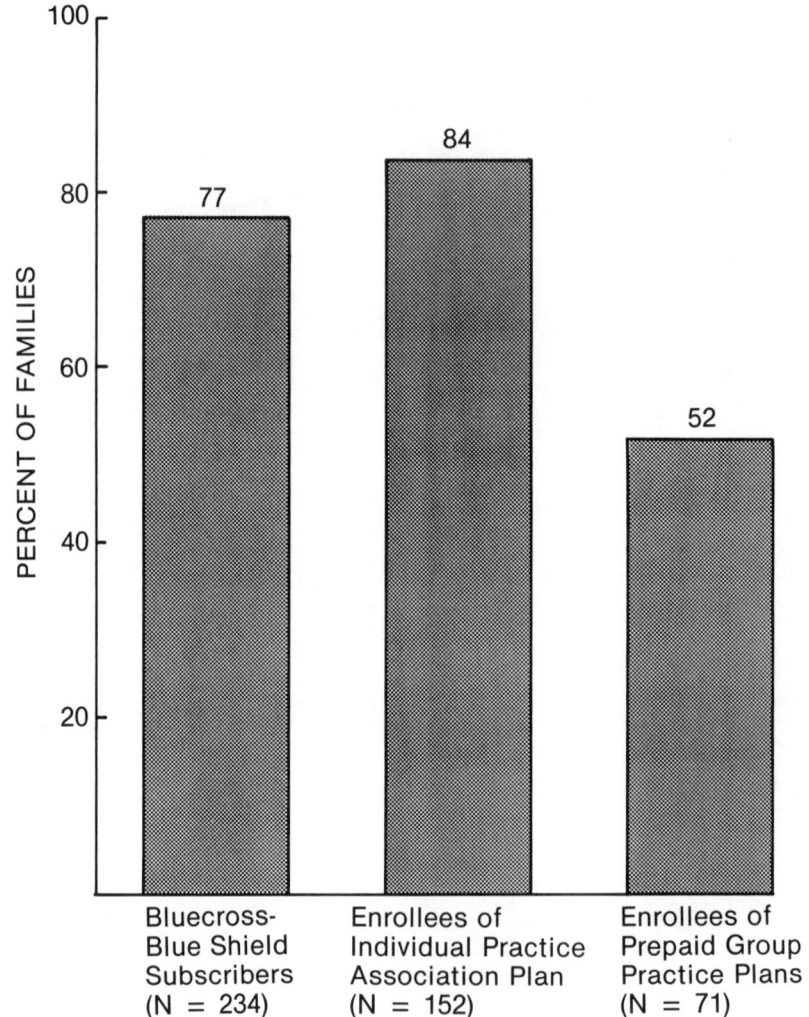

[1]Based on a study of industrial plant hourly employees who had a choice between three types of plans, with all preimiums full paid by the employer.

SOURCE: Berki, S.E., et al., "Enrollment Choice in a Multi-HMO Setting: The Role of Risk, Financial Vulnerability, and Access to Care," *Medical Care,* Vol. 15, No. 2, February 1977, Table 5, p. 109.

Medical Care Insurance

APPENDIX
Geographic Terms

SMSA Definition

The concept of a Standard Metropolitan Statistical Area (SMSA) was developed for use in statistical reporting and analysis. Except in the New England States, an SMSA is a county or a group of contiguous counties containing at least one city of 50,000 inhabitants or more or "twin cities" with a combined population of at least 50,000. In addition, contiguous counties are included in an SMSA if they are essentially metropolitan in character (based on criteria of labor force characterisitcs and population density) and are socially and economically integrated with the central city or cities.

Regions and Census Divisions of the United States

Regions	Northeast		North Central	
Divisions	New England	Middle Atlantic	East North Central	West North Central
States	Maine New Hampshire Vermont Massachusetts Rhode Island Connecticut	New York New Jersey Pennsylvania	Ohio Indiana Illinois Michigan Wisconsin	Minnesota Iowa Missouri North Dakota South Dakota Nebraska Kansas

Regions	South			Pacific	
Divisions	South Atlantic	East South Central	West South Central	Mountain	Pacific
States	Delaware Maryland District of Columbia Virginia West Virginia North Carolina South Carolina Georgia Florida	Kentucky Tennessee Alabama Mississippi	Arkansas Louisiana Oklahoma Texas	Montana Idaho Wyoming Colorado New Mexico Arizona Utah Nevada	Washington Oregon California Alaska Hawaii

Appendix

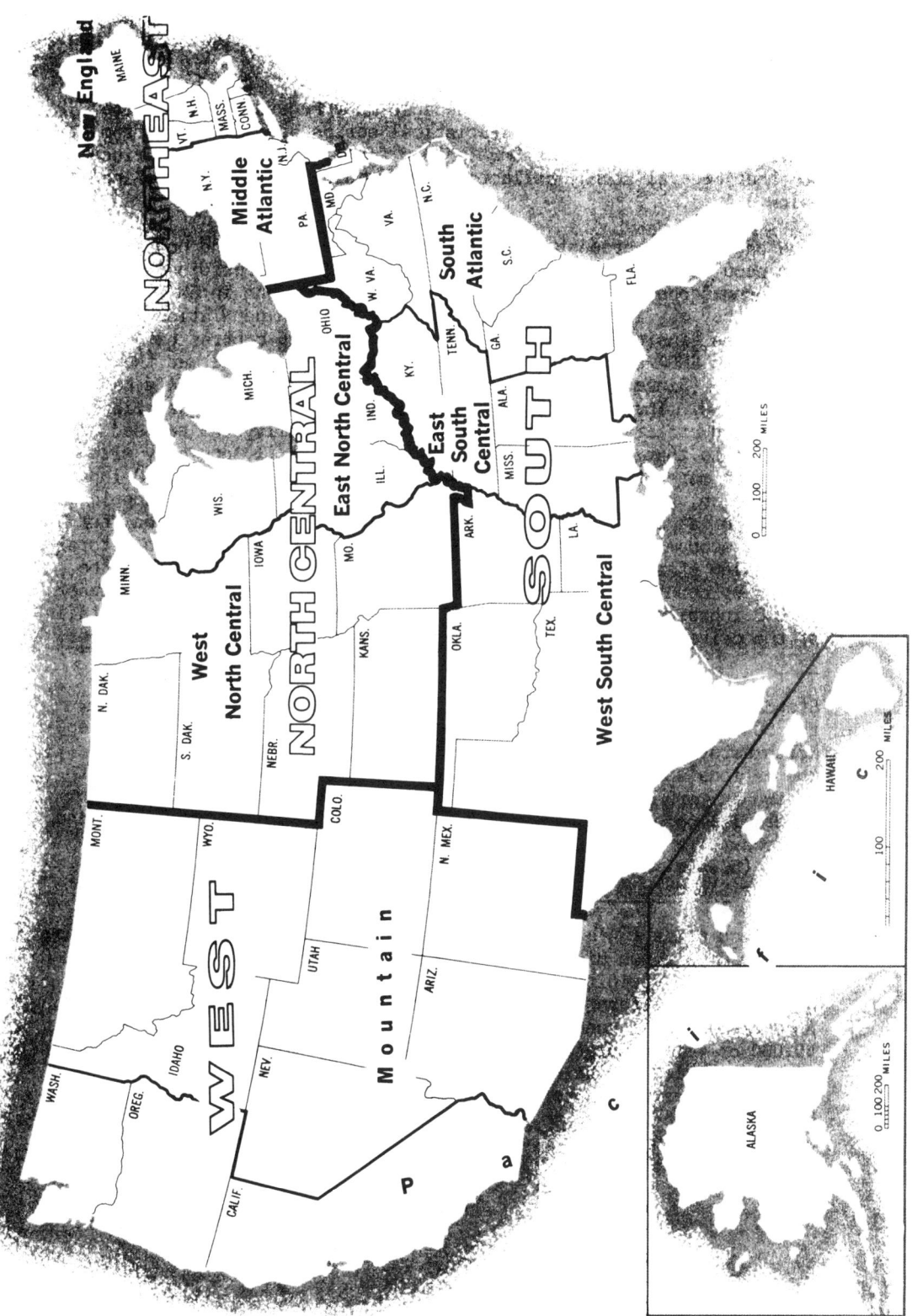

Appendix

Index

abortions, legalization, 67
activity restriction, 26, 27, 28, 29, 30, 149
   appendectomy, 275
   income, 31, 32, 48
   physician distribution, 150
acute conditions, 26, 27
   age, 27
admissions, see hospital utilization
age
   acute conditions, 27
   chronic conditions, 29, 30, 32
   dental visits, 76, 77
   disability days, 27, 30
   drugs, prescribed, 99
   emergency department care, 232
   hospital utilization, 82, 83, 213, 344, 345
   insurance coverage, 338, 370
   lifetime earnings, 107
   medical care expenditures, 130, 131
   nursing home care, 245
   physician visits, 38, 39, 40, 76, 77
   physician workweek, 173
aged
   dental visits, 76, 77
   drugs, prescribed, 99
   emergency department care, 232
   home care, 254
   hospital utilization, 82, 83, 209, 213, 214, 254, 325, 344, 345
   insurance coverage, 338, 370
   life expectancy, 16, 19
   medical care expenditures, 130, 131, 347, 348, 349, 350, 355
   medical care need, 254
   Medicare, see Medicare
   number, 3
   nursing facility utilization, 254
   physician visits, 38, 39, 40, 76, 77
   psychiatric services, 254
   x-ray exams, 303

ambulatory care, 227, 230, 295, 297, 298, 300, 301, 343, 346, 358, 382, 383
appointment keeping, 69, 70
appropriateness, see hospital utilization

British National Health Service, 51

Canadian Medicare, see Medicare, Canada
child health care, 268, 269, 276, 282, 295, 296, 297, 308, 319, 326, 355, 358
chiropractor services, 98
chronic conditions, 28
   age and income, 32
   age and sex, 29, 30
color
   dental visits, 78, 79
   dentists, 194
   disability, 17
   drugs, prescribed, 99
   emergency department care, 232
   health personnel, 162
   hospital utilization, 36, 84, 345
   income, 8, 9
   infant mortality, 22, 24
   insurance coverage, 372
   life expectancy, 15, 16, 17
   maternity care, 145
   outpatient visits, 36
   physicians, 152, 194
   physician visits, 36, 37, 78
   prenatal care, 56
   rheumatic fever, 326
compliance
   referrals, 69
   treatment recommendations, 50
costs and expenditures
   age, 130, 131, 347, 348
   aged, 349, 350, 355
   appendectomy, 275

cost and expenditures (continued)
  consumer dollar, 125, 126
  Consumer Price Index, 119, 120, 122
  day care, 253
  dental services, 115, 120, 126, 129, 131
  direct and third-party, 91, 117, 349
  drugs, 115, 120, 126, 129, 131, 132, 134, 135, 306, 347
  Economic Stabilization Program, 122
  emergency department, 230
  expenses met by insurance, 117, 349, 379, 397
  extended care facility, 347
  family, 127, 128, 129, 397
  federal outlays, portions of, 332
  Gross National Product, portion of, 108, 110, 111, 331
  health services and supplies, 115, 116
  home health care, 248
  homemaker service, 253
  hospital services, 91, 115, 116, 120, 121, 122, 123, 126, 129, 131, 225, 275, 347
  illness, 105, 106
  international comparisons, 110, 111
  lab tests, 302
  Medicaid, 116, 242, 339, 349, 353, 354, 355, 356, 357, 359
  medical care, 109, 111, 112, 113, 114, 116, 117, 118, 124, 125, 126, 127, 128, 129
  medical indigent, 355
  Medicare, 116, 123, 224, 242, 253, 339, 341, 342, 348, 349, 350, 351, 353, 393
  national, 108, 109, 110, 111, 112, 113, 114, 115, 116, 117, 118, 124, 125, 126, 127, 128, 134, 135, 331, 332, 333
  nursing home care, 115, 131, 242, 347
  out-of-pocket, 127, 128, 129, 130, 347, 349, 350, 379
  payments by state, 356
  per capita, 130, 131, 132, 253, 349
  personal health care, 117, 118, 124, 126, 127, 128, 129, 130, 131, 348, 349
  physician services, 71, 72, 75, 115, 120, 122, 126, 129, 131, 178, 347
  preventive services, 178
  private, 109, 112, 113, 114, 117, 125, 126, 127, 128, 347, 348, 349, 350, 379, 397
  program category, 109, 113
  public, 108, 109, 112, 113, 114, 116, 117, 331, 332, 333, 334, 335, 337, 339, 341, 348, 349, 353, 354, 355, 356, 357, 359
  public assistance recipients, 355

cost and expenditures (continued)
  social welfare, 331
  state and local, 109, 116, 355, 356
  surgery, 71, 272, 275
  trends, 105, 108, 112, 114, 115, 116, 117, 118, 120, 121, 122, 124, 126, 130, 225, 248, 331, 332, 333, 334, 337, 339, 347, 348, 349, 350, 379
  vendor payments, see tax-supported programs

daycare, 253
dental care costs, see costs and expenditures
dental visits
  age, 76, 77
  age and sex, 76
  aged, 76, 77
  color, 78, 79
  education, 79
  education, color and geographic area, 79
  geographic area, 79
  income, 78, 98
  income, residence and color, 78
  insurance status, 90
  multiple insurance, 90
  residence (urban or rural), 78
  sex, 76
  time since last visit, 77
dentists
  ancillary personnel, 180
  Black, 194
  distribution
    geographic area, 181
    practice type, 184
    state income, 182
  family, 49
  fees, 120
  income, 185
  productivity
    age, 186
    ancillary personnel use, 187
  ratio, 142, 181, 182
  supply, 142, 145, 180, 181, 182, 183, 184
  trends, 180, 184, 185
  type of practice, 183, 184, 185
disability, 26
  color, 17
  income, 32
  sex, 17
  See also activity restriction
disability days, 26

disability days (continued)
  age, 27, 30
  age and sex, 30
  appendectomy, 275
  income, 31, 48
  sex, 30
disability insurance, see insurance
discharges, see hospital utilization
drug costs
  age, 130, 131, 347, 348
  generic equivalents, 134, 135
  income, 129
  population characteristics, 132
  potential savings, 134, 135
  trends, 115, 120, 126, 347
drug manufacture
  new products, 133
  profitability, 134, 136
drug quality, 304, 305, 306
drugs, over-the-counter, 305
drugs, prescribed, 99, 134, 135, 297, 298, 304, 305

education level
  corrective lenses, 97
  dental visits, 79
  eye care, 97
  infant mortality, 25
  physician visits, 39
  prenatal care, 43, 44
emergency department, see hospitals and hospital utilization
employment, 4
expenditures, see costs and expenditures
extended care facilities, see Medicare
eye care, 97, 308, 309
federal employees, see insurance
federal expenditures, see public expenditures
foreign medical graduates, 157, 158

general practice, see physicians and quality
geographic area (region or state)
  urban or rural, see residence
  dental visits, 79
  dentists, 181, 182
  drugs, prescribed, 99
  group practice, 167, 399
  hospital beds, 199
  hospitals, 199
  hospital utilization, 85, 216, 217, 345
  length of stay, 85, 216

geographic area (continued)
  length of stay by diagnosis, 217
  medical vendor payments, 356
  nurses, 189
  nursing facilities, 239
  physicians, 143, 146, 149, 167
  surgery, 71
governmental expenditures, see public expenditures
group practice
  ambulatory care, 297, 300
  consumer preference, 399, 400
  form of organization, 169, 170
  geographic area, 167, 399
  hospital utilization, 96, 287, 391, 392, 394, 397
  multispecialty groups, 400
  outpatient departments, 297
  outpatient visits, 74
  physician income, 176
  physicians in, 158, 167, 168, 169, 171, 172, 176, 400
  physician stability, 172
  physician visits, 62, 73, 176, 391, 397, 400
  practice satisfaction, 171
  prepaid, see prepaid group practice
  quality, 171, 287, 289, 290, 291, 296, 297, 300
  size of groups, 168
  trends, 158, 166

health maintenance organizations, see prepaid health plans
health personnel
  see also individual personnel categories such as physicians and nurses
  Black, 194
  new and extended roles
    certification, 161
    child health associate, 161
    color and sex, 162
    licensure, 161
    Medex, 161, 162
    nurse-midwife, 161
    nurse practitioner, 161, 162
    pediatric nurse practitioner, 161
    physician assistant, 161, 162
    primary care, 162
    supply, 162
    training, 161
  supply, 141, 142, 145, 162, 193

health personnel (continued)
  trends, 141, 142, 193
home care services, 221, 226, 227, 247, 249, 250, 251, 254
home health agencies, see nursing facilities
homemaker service, 253
hospital care costs, see costs and expenditures
hospital care quality, see quality
hospital costs
  length of stay, 123
  Medicare, 123, 224, 393
  size of hospital, 123
  trends, 115, 116, 120, 121, 122
hospitals
  accreditation, 210, 211, 218, 264, 283
  audit, see quality
  average daily census, 198
  beds
    federal, 198, 200, 201, 202, 240
    geographic area, 199
    hospital type, 202, 204, 205
    international comparisons, 80
    major services, 94
    nonfederal, 198, 200, 201, 202, 206, 207, 240
    ratio, 80, 197, 199, 205
    trends, 197, 201, 205
  Blue Cross participation, 218
  coronary care, 302
  emergency department, 36, 52, 221, 228, 229, 230, 231, 232, 233, 234, 235, 236 299
  general, 204, 205
  long-term, 202, 203, 204, 205, 225, 226, 227
  maternity care, 94, 212, 261
  Medicare, see Medicare
  occupancy, 208
  optimal care by type, 283, 284
  osteopathic, 262
  outpatient departments, see outpatient departments
  ownership
    current, 198, 200, 202, 211, 240
    trends, 201, 203
  payroll expenses, 225
  personnel, 225
  proprietary, 198, 201, 203, 211, 260, 264, 282, 283, 284, 285
  PSRO areas, in, 324

hospitals (continued)
  psychiatric, 84, 202, 204, 205
  quality of care, see quality
  selected services, 219, 220, 221, 222
  size
    accreditation, 210, 211
    emergency department, 233
    hospital type, 205
    length of stay, 94, 209
    major services, 94, 212, 261
    maternity care, 212, 261
    nonfederal, 94, 205, 206, 207, 208, 210, 211
    quality, 290
    selected services, 220
    trends, 205
    utilization, 94, 208
  supply, 80, 197, 198, 199, 200, 201, 202, 204, 205, 206, 207, 210, 211, 218, 221, 240
  teaching, 218, 258, 263, 265, 276, 279, 282, 283, 284, 285, 290, 291, 296, 297, 299, 302, 313
  trends, 197, 201, 205, 218, 219, 220, 222, 225, 228, 236
  tuberculosis, 204, 205
  type of, 204, 205
  voluntary, 240, 264, 282, 283, 284
hospital utilization
  admissions, 80, 81, 84, 92, 93, 94, 95, 198, 203, 228, 250, 251, 281, 282, 283, 284, 286, 287, 319, 321, 322, 382, 392, 395, 397
  board-certified specialists, 285
  age, 82, 83, 87, 213, 254, 344
  age and color, 232
  age and sex, 82
  aged, 82, 83, 209, 213, 214, 232, 254, 325, 344, 345
  appropriateness, 91, 92, 226, 227, 232, 235, 281, 282, 286, 287, 316, 319, 320, 322
  bed size, 94, 208, 212
  births, 212
  Canadian Medicare, 52
  cardiac care, 222, 250, 251
  certification, 315, 318, 321, 322, 323, 324, 325
  color, 36, 84, 345
  days of care, 81, 82, 83, 86, 87, 89, 92, 94, 95, 96, 216, 222, 250, 251, 325, 344, 345, 381, 382, 389, 391, 394, 397

hospital utilization (continued)
  diagnosis, specific, 84, 93, 217, 222, 250, 251
  discharges, 83, 85, 213, 214, 215, 216, 317, 325, 344, 391
  emergency department, 36, 52, 228, 229, 230, 231, 232, 234, 235
  federal employees, 395
  geographic area, 85, 216, 217, 345
  high utilizers, 96
  income, 88, 345
  individual practice associations, 389
  insurance, group vs. nongroup, 382
  insurance status, 52, 86, 89, 90, 91, 230, 381, 391, 392, 394, 397
  insurance status and age, 87
  insurance status and income, 88
  insurance status and sex, 395
  international comparisons, 80, 86
  length of stay, 80, 81, 83, 85, 87, 89, 94, 208, 209, 213, 214, 215, 286, 287, 315, 316, 317, 318, 319, 320, 321, 322, 325, 344
  length of stay by diagnosis, 217
  length of stay by region, 85, 216, 217
  maternity care, 212
  Medicaid, 235, 316, 320, 344, 345, 390
  Medicare, 235, 317, 320, 325, 342, 344, 345
  multiple insurance, 90
  myocardial infarction, 222
  outpatient department, see outpatient visits
  patient opinions, 257
  prepaid group practice, 96, 287, 389, 391, 392, 394, 395, 397
  prepaid health plans, 389
  PSROs, 321, 322, 323, 324, 325
  psychiatric care, 254
  psychiatric intervention, 96
  psychiatric hospitals, 84
  public assistance, 235
  regulation, 316
  residence (urban or rural), 345
  sex, 82
  trends, 81, 228, 344, 345, 381, 394
  type of insurance, 86, 90, 230, 382, 391, 392, 397
  type of insurer, 235, 316, 390, 395
  type of service, 94, 222, 319
  uninsured, 390
  utilization review, 316
  workers' compensation, 235

income
  chiropractic care, 98
  chronic conditions, 32
  color, 8, 9
  dental visits, 78, 98
  dentist distribution, 182
  dentists, 185
  disability, 31, 32, 48
  hospital utilization, 88, 345
  infant mortality, 25
  insurance coverage, 372
  lifetime earnings, 105, 106, 107
  maternity care, 54
  medical care expenditures, 127, 128, 129
  medical school applicants and students, 154
  perception of need, 46
  pharmacist services, 55, 305
  physician distribution, 150
  physicians, 171, 175, 176, 177
  physician visits, 40, 41, 42, 48, 51, 53, 78, 98
  podiatric care, 98
  poverty level, 11
  prenatal care, 44, 46, 54
  preventive care, 42
  share of aggregate income, 10
  trends, 8, 9, 10, 11
individual practice associations, 388, 389
  see also prepaid health plans
infant mortality
  color, 22, 24
  education level, 25
  hebdomadal deaths, 310
  income, 25
  international comparisons, 21
  neonatal deaths, 22, 23
  risk category, 24
  social class, 23
injections, see quality
insurance, 336
  aged, 338, 349, 370
  benefit payments, 380
  Canadian Medicare, see Medicare, Canada
  color, 372
  disability insurance, 116, 336, 337, 365, 368, 377
  disenrollment, 401
  employee-benefit plans, 377
  expenses met, 117, 349, 379, 397
  federal employees, 368, 378, 395
  income, 372

insurance (continued)
  income loss from sickness, 367, 368
  loss ratio, 380
  Medicaid, see Medicaid
  Medicare, see Medicare
  membership duration, effect of, 401
  multiple insurance, 90
  number covered, 338, 369, 370, 371, 373, 374, 375, 376, 377
  OASDHI, 336, 337, 338, 365
  population characteristics, 372
  preventive index by plan, 397
  satisfaction by plan, 397, 398
  selected benefits, 369, 370, 373, 374, 375, 376, 377
  sick leave, 368
  termination, 401
  trends, 337, 338, 366, 368, 369, 370, 371, 373, 374, 377, 379
  type of insurer, 373, 374, 375, 378, 380, 397, 398
  typology, 365
  unemployment insurance, 336, 337
  wage and salary workers, 377
  workers' compensation, 336, 365, 366
    benefits, 366, 367
    trends, 116, 337, 366
insurance, use of benefits
  Canadian Medicare, 52, 53, 54, 55
  dental visits, 90
  emergency department, 52, 230, 235
  federal employees, 394, 395, 396
  hospital utilization, 86, 87, 88, 89, 90, 91, 316, 381, 382, 389, 390, 391, 392, 394, 395, 397
  individual practice associations, 389
  insurance status, 390
  Medicaid, see Medicaid
  Medicare, see Medicare
  membership duration, effect of, 384
  multiple insurance, 90
  other countries, 51, 52, 53, 54, 55
  outpatient visits, 52, 74, 382
  patient visits, 384
  pharmacist services, 55
  physician visits, 52, 53, 55, 62, 73, 90, 383, 390, 391, 397
  prenatal care, 56
  prepaid group practice, 56, 62, 73, 384, 389, 395
  prepaid health plans, 389
  preventive index by plan, 397
  preventive services, 390

insurance, use of benefits (continued)
  receipt of services, 56, 62, 73, 75, 383
  surgery, 71, 272, 383, 392, 396
  trends, 381
  type of insurer, 235, 316, 390, 395
  uninsured, 390
  utilization review, 316
  workers' compensation, 235
international comparisons
  hospital bed ratio, 80
  hospital utilization, 80, 86
  infant mortality, 21
  life expectancy, 18, 19
  medical care expenditures, 110, 111
  physician ratio, 139, 140
  risk of hysterectomy, 60
internships, see medical education

laboratory tests, see quality
labor force, see employment
length of stay, see hospital utilization
life expectancy
  color, 15, 16, 17
  international comparisons, 18, 19
  trends, 15
lifetime earnings, 105, 106, 107
long-term care, see hospitals, long-term and nursing facilities

maternity care
  cesarean section, 58
  color, 45
  hospital size, 94, 212, 261
  income, 54
  insurance status, 54
  quality, 212, 259, 260, 261, 262, 296
  referral patterns, 66
  type of physician, 45, 165, 260
  see also prenatal care
Medicaid, 336, 365
  ambulatory care, 230, 298, 346, 358
  child health care, 358
  eligibility categories, 355
  eligibility loss, 401
  emergency department care, 235
  expenditures, 116, 242, 339, 349, 353, 354, 355, 356, 357, 359
  hospital care, 316, 320, 390
  hospital utilization, 344, 345
  injections, approved, 298
  insurance coverage, 401
  length of stay, 316, 320, 344
  medical indigent, 355

Medicaid (continued)
  nursing home care, 242
  osteopathic care, 298
  outpatient visits, 346
  payments by state, 356, 357
  physician care, 298, 390
  place of visit, 346
  preventive services, 390
  quality, 298, 316, 320
  recipients, 354, 356, 401
  selected services, 353, 359
  source of care, 230, 358
  trends, 339
  utilization review, 316
  vendor payments, 353, 356
medical care need, 46, 47, 226
  perception of need, 46, 47, 70
medical education
  applicants, 153
  applicants, family income, 154
  Black enrollment, 152
  choice of specialty, 163
  enrollment, 151
  foreign graduates, 157, 158
  graduates, 151, 152, 155
  internships and residencies, 155, 157, 158, 218
  schools, 151
  students, family income, 154
  trends, 151
  women, 151
medical indigent, see Medicaid
Medicare, 336, 365
  ambulatory care, 230, 343, 346
  Canada, 52, 53, 54, 55
  day care, 253
  days of care, 325
  deductible and coinsurance, 351
  deductibles and premiums, 350
  discharges, 317, 325
  emergency department care, 235
  enrollment, 342
  expenditures, 116, 242, 248, 253, 339, 341, 342, 348, 349, 353, 393
  extended care facilities, 246, 342, 343
  extended care utilization, 342
  funding, source of, 340
  home health agencies, 246, 248, 252, 253
  homemaker service, 253
  hospital care, 320, 325
  hospital certification, 210, 218
  hospital charges, 123, 224

Medicare (continued)
  hospital costs, 123, 393
  hospital insurance, 340, 350
  hospital utilization, 317, 342, 344, 345
  length of stay, 320, 325, 344
  nursing facilities, 246, 342, 343
  nursing home care, 242
  outpatient visits, 343, 346
  physician perceptions, 352
  place of visit, 343, 346
  prepaid group practice, 393
  PSROs, 325
  quality, 317, 320, 325
  reimbursable charges, 351, 393
  selected services, 353, 393
  source of care, 230
  supplementary medical insurance, 340, 350
  trends, 248, 339, 340, 342, 344, 346, 347, 348, 350
  trust funds, 340
mobility, 7
morbidity
  economic loss, 105, 106
  migrant workers, 68
  presence of clinic, 68
  preventive program, 326
  physicians' wives, 60
mortality
  appendicitis, 267
  causes, 20, 263
  economic loss, 105, 106
  hebdomadal, effects of review, 310
  infant, see infant mortality
  international comparisons, 21
  maternal, 261, 262
  neonatal, 22, 23
  perinatal, 66, 259, 260
  postoperative, 266, 275
  postoperative ratio, 265
  rate, by hospital type, 260, 263
  stillbirths, 23
myocardial infarction, 222

neighborhood health centers, 172, 269
nurses
  distribution by geographic area, 189
  education, 190, 191, 218
  graduates, 191
  nurse-midwife, see health personnel
  nursing facilites, in, 243
  ratio, 142, 189
  supply, 142, 145, 188, 191, 192

nurses (continued)
  type of employment, 192
nursing care quality, 307
nursing facilities
  appropriateness, 226, 227, 244, 245
  beds, 237, 239, 240, 241
  costs and expenditures, 115, 131, 248, 253, 347
  geographic area, 239
  home health agencies, 226, 246, 247, 248, 249, 252, 253, 254
  Medicaid, see Medicaid
  Medicare, see Medicare
  nurses in, 243
  ownership, 240, 245
  patient characteristics, 242, 245
  personnel, 243
  ratio, 239
  size, 241, 245
  skilled nursing care, 244, 245
  source of payment, 242
  supply, 237, 238, 239, 240, 241
  trends, 237, 247, 248
  type of care, 238, 252
  type of facility, 245
  utilization, 242, 254, 342
nursing homes, see nursing facilities

OASDHI, see insurance
occupation, 45, 372
ophthalmologist services, 97
optometrist services
  education, 97
  quality, 309
osteopathic physicians, see physicians
outpatient departments, 219, 221, 227, 279, 296, 297
outpatient visits
  appointment keeping, 69, 70
  Canadian Medicare, 52
  color, 36
  insurance, group vs. nongroup, 382
  insurance status, 52
  Medicaid, 346
  Medicare, 343, 346
  prepaid group practice, 74
  quality, 279, 296, 297
  trends, 228

pharmaceutical services, see drugs and quality
pharmacist services, 55, 305

physicians
  antibiotic use, 304
  Black, 152, 194
  board-certified, 164, 285
  choice of specialty, 156, 163
  distribution
    activity restriction, 150
    activity restriction incidence, 149
    county size, 144
    geographic area, 143, 146, 149, 150, 167
    income of area, 146, 148, 149, 150
    ratio, 150
    residence (urban or rural), 144, 145
    socioeconomic status, 148
  drug prescribing, 297, 298, 304
  emergency department, 236
  employment stability, 172
  family, 49, 69
  fees, 71, 120, 122, 178
  foreign physicians, 157, 158
  general practice, 61, 66, 144, 147, 148, 156, 159, 160, 163, 168, 169, 173, 174, 177, 178, 183, 288, 292, 293, 294, 303
  group practice, see group practice
  income, 171, 175, 176, 177
  internships and residencies, see medical education
  lab test use, 302
  medical education, see medical education
  method of payment, 72, 179
  neighborhood health centers, 172
  obstetrician-gynecologists, 173
  osteopathic, 145, 262, 298
  practice satisfaction, 171
  productivity
    specialty, 174
    type of practice, 171, 176
  quality of care, see quality
  radiologists, 173
  ratio, 61, 62, 140, 142, 143, 144, 147, 148, 149, 150, 160
    international comparisons, 139, 140
  referral patterns, 66, 229
  specialists
    certification, 164
    fees, 178
    income, 177
    workweek by age, 173
  supply, 139, 140, 141, 142, 143, 144, 145, 147, 148, 149, 150, 151, 155, 158, 159, 160, 167, 183

physicians (continued)
  supply (continued)
    primary care, 143, 144, 147, 148, 159, 160, 168, 169, 183
    specialists, 59, 144, 147, 148, 159, 164, 169, 183
    trends, 151, 158, 164
  type of practice, 158, 167, 168, 169, 170, 171, 176, 183, 287, 289, 399, 400
  women, 151
  workweek by age, 173
  x-ray use, 303
physicians care costs, see costs and expenditures
physicians care quality, see quality
physician visits
  age, 38, 39, 40, 76, 77
  age and income, 40
  age and sex, 38, 76
  aged, 38, 39, 40, 76, 77
  Canadian Medicare, 52, 53, 54, 55
  color, 36, 37, 78
  consumer preference, 400
  education, 39
  general practice, 37, 61
  group practice, 62, 73, 176, 400
  income, 40, 41, 42, 48, 51, 78, 98
  income and insurance, 53
  income and sex, 51
  income, residence and color, 78
  insurance status, 52, 53, 54, 55, 62, 73, 90, 272, 383, 390, 391, 397
  maternal care, 58
  Medicaid, see Medicaid
  Medicare, see Medicare
  method of payment, 72, 272
  multiple insurance, 90
  other countries, 52, 53, 54, 55
  place of visit, 35, 36, 52, 174, 250, 346, 383
  PSRO, 321, 322, 323
  prepaid group practice, 62, 73, 391, 397
  residence, 39, 78
  rural, 65
  sex, 38, 51, 76
  surgery, see surgery
  symptom response ratio, 390
  time since last visit, 77
  travel distance, 65
  type of insurer, 390
  type of specialty, 37
  type of visit, 42
  uninsured, 390
podiatrist services, 98

poor
  pharmacist services, 305
  physician ratio, 147
  poverty level, 11
population characteristics
  See individual characteristic entries for correlation with other data
  age, 16, 19
  aged, 3
  color, 8, 9, 15, 16, 17
  employment, females, 4
  income, 8, 9, 10, 11
  life expectancy, 15, 16, 17, 18, 19
  lifetime earnings, 105, 106, 107
  mobility, 7
  poor, 11
  residence (urban or rural), 5, 6
  trends, 4, 5, 6, 11
prematurity, 260
prenatal care
  attitudes toward, 46
  color, 56
  education, 43, 44
  education and income, 44
  income, 44, 46, 54
  insurance status and color, 56
  unmet need, 46
  see also maternity care
prepaid group practice
  ambulatory care, 297, 300
  appropriate admissions, 287
  consumer preference, 400
  enrollment, 388
  federal employees, 395
  hospital utilization, 96, 287, 389, 391, 392, 394, 395, 397
  medicaid, 401
  Medicare reimbursement, 393
  membership duration, effect of, 384, 401
  number of, 388
  outpatient departments, 297
  outpatient visits, 74
  patient visits, 384
  physicians in, 171, 172, 400
  physician stability, 172
  physician visits, 62, 73, 391, 397, 400
  preventive services, 397
  prescribing patterns, 297
  quality, 171, 287, 290, 291, 297, 300
  satisfaction, 171, 397, 398
  service patterns, 56, 62, 73, 384, 389, 395

prepaid group practice (continued)
  surgery rates, 392, 396
  terminations, 401
prepaid health plans
  see also individual practice associations and prepaid group practice
  enrollment, 386, 387, 388
  hospital utilization, 389
  number of, 385, 386, 388
  qualified, federally, 386, 389
  size, 387
  trends, 385
  type of practice, 388, 389
preventive services, 42, 68, 178, 295, 383, 390, 397
Professional Standards Review Organizations, 321, 322, 323, 324, 325
proprietary hospitals, see hospitals
psychiatric hospitals, see hospitals and hospital utilization
psychiatric services
  aged, 254
  hospitals, in, 219
  social class, 50
  utilization, see hospital utilization
public assistance, see tax-supported programs
public programs, see tax-supported programs

quality
  admissions, 321, 322
  aged, 303
  alerter system, 310
  ambulatory care, 295, 297, 298, 300, 301
  anemia, 297
  antibiotic use, 304
  appendectomies, 267, 270, 272, 273, 274, 275, 276, 312
  audit, external, 278
  board-certified specialists, 285, 298
  cancer survival, 258
  case fatality rates, 263, 266, 275
  child health care, 268, 269, 276, 282, 295, 296, 297, 308, 319
  Children and Youth Program, 296
  cholecystectomy, 266
  criteria, adherence to, 295, 300, 301, 319
  diagnostic work-up, 300
  discharge ratio, 317
  discharges, 325
  drug prescribing, 304, 306

quality (continued)
  drugs
    over-the-counter, 305
    prescribed, 305
    prescribing, 297, 298
  emergency departments, 299
  eye care, 308, 309
  fractures, hip, 266
  gastrointestinal symptoms, 299
  general practice, 288, 292, 293, 294, 295, 303
  group practice, 171, 287, 289, 290, 291, 296
  gynecological disorders, 278, 297
  gynecological surgery, 311
  health accounting method, 314
  heart disease, 297, 302
  hebdomadal deaths, 310
  hospital care, 212, 257, 258, 260, 261, 262, 263, 264, 265, 266, 279, 280, 281, 282, 283, 284, 285, 286, 287, 290, 291, 296, 299, 310, 315, 316, 317, 318, 319, 320, 321, 322, 323, 324, 325, 327
  hospital certification, 315, 318
  hospital size, 212, 261
  hypertension, 295, 297
  hysterectomies, 271, 278
  incorrect surgical diagnosis, 273
  infant care, 282, 296
  injections, 298
  insurance status, 316
  internists, 295, 301
  interns and residents, 299, 302, 313
  lab tests results, 313
  lab test use, 302
  length of stay, 315, 316, 317, 318, 319, 320, 321, 322, 325
  management strategy, 276
  Maternal and Infant Care Program, 296
  maternity care, 212, 259, 260, 261, 262, 296
  Medicaid, 298, 316, 320
  medical audit, 304, 311
  Medicare, 317, 320, 325
  mortality, 259, 260, 263, 264, 265, 310
  myocardial infarction, 302
  neighborhood health centers, 296
  neurologists, 319
  nursing care, 307
  OEO, 296
  optometric care, 309
  osteopathic care, 262, 298
  otitis media, 295

quality (continued)
  outcome assessment, 300, 314
  outpatient departments, 279, 296, 297
  pain
    abdominal 276, 295
    chest, 295
  patient opinions, 257
  pediatricians, 276, 295, 319
  peer review, 298, 301, 321
  performance scores, 286, 287, 288, 289, 290, 291, 296, 297, 301, 302
  perinatal mortality, 259, 260
  pharmacy, 306
  pharmacist services, 305
  pharyngitis, 295, 297
  physicians care, 171, 257, 258, 260, 261, 262, 266, 267, 268, 269, 270, 271, 272, 273, 274, 275, 276, 277, 278, 279, 281, 282, 284, 285, 286, 287, 288, 289, 290, 291, 292, 293, 294, 295, 297, 298, 299, 300, 301, 302, 303, 304, 311, 312, 313, 314, 319, 321, 322, 323, 327, 390
  place of service, 285, 295, 297, 305
  postoperative deaths, 265, 266, 275
  poverty area, 305
  prepaid group practice, 171, 287, 290, 291, 297, 300
  preventive services, 295
  proprietary hospitals, 285
  PSRO, 321, 322, 323, 324, 325
  public assistance recipients, 303, 327
  respiratory infections, 300
  second-opinion programs, 277
  specialist care, 260, 276, 281, 282, 284, 285, 286, 288, 289, 291, 295, 298, 301, 303, 319
  surgery, 265, 266, 267, 268, 269, 270, 271, 272, 273, 274, 275, 276, 281, 285, 311, 312, 319
    elective, 277, 278
    unnecessary, 277, 278
  symptom response ratio, 390
  teaching hospitals, 258, 263, 265, 276, 279, 285, 296, 297, 299, 302, 313
  tissue committee, 312
  tonsillectomies, 268, 269
  tonsillitis, 297
  type of medical specialty, 281
  type of practice, 287, 289, 297
  urinary tract infection, 279, 295, 297, 300, 327
  utilization review, 315, 316, 318
  x-ray examinations, 303

race, see color
referral patterns, 66, 229
research expenditures, 109, 113, 334
residence (urban or rural)
  dental visits, 78
  hospital utilization, 345
  insurance coverage, 372
  physician visits, 39, 78
  place of, see population characteristics
  region or state, see geographic area
residencies, see medical education
rheumatic fever, 326
risk
  appendectomy, 275
  cholecystectomy, 266
  fracture, hip, 266

second opinion programs, see quality
sex
  chronic conditions, 29, 30
  dental visits, 76
  disability, 17
  disability days, 30
  drugs, prescribed, 99
  employment, females, 4
  health personnel, 162
  hospital utilization, 82, 395
  life expectancy, 15, 16, 17, 19
  lifetime earnings, 107
  medical students, 151
  physician visits, 38, 51, 76
sick leave, see insurance
social class
  family physician and dentist, 49
  group practice, attitudes toward, 400
  infant mortality, 23
  perception of need, 47
  psychiatric services, 50
social insurance programs, see tax-supported programs
specialty practice, see physicians
surgery
  appendectomy, 58, 59, 63, 267, 270, 272, 273, 274, 275, 276, 312, 396
  bed availability effect, 63
  board-certified specialists, 285
  cesarean section, 58
  cholecystectomy, 58, 63, 266
  colectomy, 63
  costs and expenditures, 71, 272, 275
  elective, 277, 278
  fractures, hip, 266
  geographic area, 71

surgery (continued)
  gynecological, 58, 60, 63, 278, 311
  hysterectomy, 58, 59, 60, 63, 271, 278
  incorrect diagnosis, 273
  insurance plan, 71, 272, 383, 392, 396
  leucotomy, 57
  mortality, 265, 266, 275
  office visits by color, 37
  other countries, 57, 59, 60, 63, 278
  prepaid group practice, 392, 396
  physician supply effect, 63
  quality, see quality
  second-opinion programs, see quality
  tonsillectomy, 58, 59, 63, 268, 269, 392, 396
  trends, 58, 268
  type of procedure, 57, 58, 59, 63, 266, 267, 268, 269, 270, 271, 272, 273, 274, 275, 276, 278, 311, 312, 392, 396
  unnecessary, 277, 278

tax-supported programs
  See also Medicaid and Medicare
  aged, 338, 348, 349, 350, 354, 355
  Aid to Families with Dependent Children, 336, 354, 355
  Aid to the Blind, 354, 355
  Aid to the Disabled, 354, 355
  armed forces, 116
  cash benefit payments, 337
  child care, 355
  Children and Youth Program, 296
  coverage, 336, 338, 354
  dependency, for, 336
  emergency department care, 235
  federal employees, see insurance
  general assistance, 336

tax-supported programs (continued)
  income maintenance programs, 336, 337
  Maternal and Infant Care Program, 296
  medical care benefit payments, 341
  national health expenditures, see costs and expenditures, national
  OASDHI, see insurance
  OEO, 172, 296
  Old Age Assistance, 303, 338, 355
  public assistance, 116, 235, 242, 272, 303, 327, 337, 348, 349, 354, 355
  public expenditures, 108, 109, 112, 113, 114, 116, 117, 331, 332, 333, 334, 335, 337, 339, 340, 341, 348, 349, 353, 354, 355, 356, 357, 359
  quality of care, 296, 303, 327
  research expenditures, 109, 113, 334
  retirement programs, 336, 337
  special population groups, 296
  state and local expenditures, 109, 116, 355, 356
  trends, 108, 112, 114, 116, 117, 331, 332, 333, 334, 337, 338, 339, 348, 350
  VA, 116, 335, 336, 337
  vendor payments, 116, 348, 353, 356
travel distance to provider, 64, 65, 66

unemployment insurance, see insurance
uninsured, 390

voluntary hospitals, see hospitals

well-baby care, 295
well-child care, 295
workers' compensation, see insurance